Principles and Techniques of
Practical Biochemistry

In this new, fifth edition of a highly popular text, undergraduate students are introduced to all the basic experimental techniques used routinely in practical biochemistry today. Most attention is given to techniques that students will encounter in their practical classes, with the principles and theories behind them explained in detail to aid understanding. As a further aid to students, example calculations and worked answers appear at the ends of most chapters. 'Key terms' to understand are also included to help students thoroughly review each topic.

No contemporary book on modern biochemical techniques would be complete without chapters on molecular biology, recombinant DNA technology, genetic analysis, protein purification and biomolecular interactions, and these topics have been extensively covered in this new edition.

The book is essential reading for all bioscience undergraduate students and preclinical medical students for whom practical biochemistry, molecular biology and immunology form part of the syllabus.

KEITH WILSON is Professor of Pharmacological Biochemistry and Director of Research Degrees, and JOHN WALKER is Professor and Head of the Department of Biosciences, both at the University of Hertfordshire.

Principles and Techniques of
Practical Biochemistry

Edited by Keith Wilson and John Walker

Fifth edition

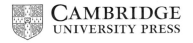

CAMBRIDGE
UNIVERSITY PRESS

PUBLISHED BY THE PRESS SYNDICATE OF THE UNIVERSITY OF CAMBRIDGE
The Pitt Building, Trumpington Street, Cambridge, United Kingdom

CAMBRIDGE UNIVERSITY PRESS
The Edinburgh Building, Cambridge CB2 2RU, UK
40 West 20th Street, New York, NY 10011-4211, USA
10 Stamford Road, Oakleigh, VIC 3166, Australia
Ruiz de Alarcón 13, 28014 Madrid, Spain
Dock House, The Waterfront, Cape Town 8001, South Africa

http://www. cambridge.org

First published by Edward Arnold 1975
as *A biologist's guide to principles and techniques of practical biochemistry*
Second edition 1981
Third edition 1986
Third edition first published by Cambridge University Press 1992
Reprinted 1993
Fourth edition published by Cambridge University Press 1994 as
Principles and techniques of practical biochemistry
Reprinted 1995, 1997
Fifth edition 2000
Reprinted 2001

Printed in the United Kingdom at the University Press, Cambridge

Typeset in Proforma 9.5/13pt, and Dax, in QuarkXPress™   [SE]

A catalogue record for this book is available from the British Library

Library of Congress Cataloguing in Publication data

Principles and techniques of practical biochemistry/edited by Keith Wilson and John M. Walker. – 5th
ed.
        p.   cm.
Includes bibliographical references and index.
ISBN 0 521 65104 2 (hardbound)
1. Biochemistry – Methodology.   I. Wilson, Keith, 1936–   .
    II. Walker, John M., 1948–   .
QP519.7.P75   1999
572–dc21   98–37214   CIP

ISBN   0 521 65104 2 hardback (fifth edition)
ISBN   0 521 65873 X paperback (fifth edition)
ISBN   0521 41769 4 (fourth edition)

Contents

Preface to the fifth edition

Teachers of genetics, cell biology, biochemistry and physiology are acutely aware of the rapid expansion of the knowledge base of their subjects that has taken place in the recent past. Each weekly batch of journals provides new discoveries for inclusion in an already crowded curriculum. Much of this expansion is the direct result of developments in molecular genetics, in particular of protocols for gene cloning and expression, which have resulted in routine procedures for the identification, cloning, sequencing and expression of genes for proteins ranging in function from metabolic enzymes and structural proteins to membrane receptors and regulatory proteins. The advent of such routine procedures has revolutionised our understanding of biological processes at the molecular level and has resulted in the coalescing of previously disparate disciplines. At the same time, this new knowledge of the molecular nature of biological processes has been exploited to medical and commercial advantages. Even the layperson has been made aware of application of molecular biology to areas as divergent as archaeology, plant and animal breeding, diagnostic tests for a wide range of inherited conditions, and new approaches to the diagnosis and treatment of chronic illnesses, particularly cancer. The decoding of the genome of many unicellular organisms and rapid progress on the Human Genome Project, which is now projected to be completed in the early years of the new millennium, promises even more spectacular applications in the future.

These advances in molecular biology have been paralleled, and in some cases made possible, by equally fundamental developments in immunology, cell culture, protein analysis and techniques such as chromatography, electrophoresis, mass spectrometry and various forms of spectroscopy. In planning this new edition of our book, our challenge has been to incorporate details of these developments whilst retaining our original aim, namely to concentrate on those techniques and principles which underlie practical exercises that undergraduates in all the biological sciences can expect to encounter in their practical classes and to cover in less detail the more sophisticated techniques that have made possible the advances they will learn about in their lectures and associated reading. In accordance with this aim, we have decided to cover techniques in molecular biology in greater detail than in earlier editions. There are now two chapters devoted to this area. Chapter 2 deals with the basic theoretical and practical details and Chapter 3 concentrates on their applications. Both chapters have been written by Dr Ralph Rapley, a new contributor to our book. Chapter 4, on immunological techniques, has also been completely rewritten by Susan and Robin Thorpe, from the National Institute for Biological Standards and Control, also new contributors to the book. A new chapter on protein purification has been introduced to emphasise its central importance in modern practical biology (Chapter 6). Whilst previous editions have devoted a chapter to enzyme techniques, no opportunity has previously been taken to emphasise similarities between enzyme–substrate (or inhibitor) binding and the binding of ligands to membrane receptors and membrane transporters. In view of the fundamental and physiologically important advances that have been made in our understanding of cell–cell interactions and the associated signal transduction and amplification processes, a new chapter has been introduced covering these important topics (Chapter 8).

The two chapters on spectroscopic and spectrometric techniques have been revised so that they are now presented in three chapters. Chapters 9 and 10 deal with those methods that are based on quantum principles and cover such important techniques as visible and ultraviolet spectroscopy, fluorimetry, luminescent spectroscopy, circular dichroism, turbidimetry, nephelometry and atomic absorption (Chapter 9), and infrared spectroscopy, electron spin resonance spectroscopy and nuclear magnetic resonance spectroscopy (including magnetic resonance imaging) (Chapter 10). Chapter 11 gives a detailed account of the various forms of mass spectrometry and includes a discussion of its use in protein structure determination, an application unthought of only a few years ago. Throughout the three chapters, opportunities have been taken to stress the complementary nature of spectroscopic and spectrometric data by considering the applications of the various techniques to the molecule phenacetin.

The chapters on centrifugation techniques (Chapter 5), electrophoresis (Chapter 12), chromatography (Chapter 13), radioisotope techniques (Chapter 14), and electrochemical techniques (Chapter 15) have all been updated. Throughout the book, emphasis has been placed on the quantitative nature of practical biochemistry. Nearly all chapters, therefore, now include a set of calculations, with answers, to enable students to test their understanding of the principles being covered. To further help students identify the key topics, each chapter also includes a section of 'key terms' to understand, together with another on suggestions for further reading. Inevitably, many of the chapters deal with common topics and every effort has been made to cross-reference to other chapters and minimise unnecessary duplication. However, a small amount of duplication between chapters has deliberately been retained, particularly in places where the slightly different approaches adopted by the authors were felt to add to the overall understanding and presentation. Many chapters make reference to common thermodynamic principles and equations. To strengthen, and thereby emphasise, the importance of thermodynamics to biochemical principles, a new section on the subject has been introduced in Chapter 1. This chapter now also includes worked numerical examples, some of a very fundamental, practical kind, which are truly basic to all practical work, but which many undergraduates initially have difficulty in handling. Examples include the difference between concentration and amount, calculation of pH and various thermodynamic values. We hope the innovation will prove helpful to our readers. In producing the new edition we have attempted to incorporate the many helpful suggestions made by readers of the fourth edition. We continue to welcome comments from all those who use the book as part of their studies and wish to express our gratitude to the many authors who have granted us permission to reproduce their copyright figures.

KEITH WILSON

JOHN WALKER

Contributors

Professor D. B. Gordon
Department of Biological Sciences
Metropolitan University of Manchester
Chester Street
All Saints
Manchester M15 6BH, UK

Dr A. Griffiths
Department of Biological Sciences
Oxford Brookes University
Headington
Oxford OX3 0BP, UK

Dr R. Rapley
Department of Biosciences
University of Hertfordshire
Hatfield Campus
College Lane
Hatfield
Herts AL10 9AB, UK

Dr P. K. Robinson
Department of Applied Biology
University of Central Lancashire
Preston
Lancs PR1 2HE, UK

Dr I. Simpkins
Department of Biosciences
University of Hertfordshire
Hatfield Campus
College Lane
Hatfield
Herts AL10 9AB, UK

Professor R. J. Slater
Department of Biosciences
University of Hertfordshire
Hatfield Campus
College Lane
Hatfield
Herts AL10 9AB, UK

Professor R. Thorpe
National Institute for Biological Standards and Control
Blanche Lane
South Mimms
Potters Bar
Herts EN6 3QG, UK

Dr S. Thorpe
National Institute for Biological Standards and Control
Blanche Lane
South Mimms
Potters Bar
Herts EN6 3QG, UK

Professor J. M. Walker
Department of Biosciences
University of Hertfordshire
Hatfield Campus
College Lane
Hatfield
Herts AL10 9AB, UK

Professor K. Wilson
Department of Biosciences
University of Hertfordshire
Hatfield Campus
College Lane
Hatfield
Herts AL10 9AB, UK

Abbreviations

The following abbreviations have been used throughout this book without definition:

AMP	adenosine 5′-monophosphate
ADP	adenosine 5′-diphosphate
ATP	adenosine 5′-triphosphate
bp	base-pairs
CHAPS	3-[(3-chloramidopropyl)dimethylamino]-1-propanesulphonic acid
c.p.m.	counts per minute
DDT	2,2-bis-(p-chlorophenyl)-1,1,1-trichlorethane
DNA	deoxyribonucleic acid
d.p.m.	disintegrations per minute
e^-	electron
EDTA	ethylenediaminetetra-acetate
EGTA	[ethylenebis (oxonitrilo)] tetra-acetic acid
e.m.f.	electromotive force
FAD	flavin adenine dinucleotide
FMN	flavin mononucleotide
HAT	hypoxanthine, aminopterin, thymidine medium
Hepes	4(2-hydroxyethyl)-1-piperazine-ethanesulphonic acid
kb	kilobase-pairs
log	logarithm to the base 10
M_r	relative molecular mass
min	minute
NAD^+	nicotinamide adenine dinucleotide (oxidised)
NADH	nicotinamide adenine dinucleotide (reduced)
$NADP^+$	nicotinamide adenine dinucleotide phosphate (oxidised)
$NADPH^+$	nicotinamide adenine dinucleotide phosphate (reduced)
Pipes	1,4-piperazinediethanesulphonic acid
P_i	inorganic phosphate
PP_i	inorganic pyrophosphate
p.p.m.	parts per million
RNA	ribonucleic acid
s.t.p.	standard temperature and pressure
Tris	2-amino-2-hydroxymethylpropane-1,3-diol

Chapter 1

General principles of biochemical investigations

1.1 THE NATURE OF BIOCHEMISTRY

Biochemistry is an interdisciplinary science that integrates systematically the principles of mathematics, physics and chemistry to attempt to explain the distinctive characteristics of life processes in terms of structure–function correlations. Advances in biochemistry have therefore largely exploited principles and techniques first applied in the physical sciences. Biochemistry is no longer simply an academic discipline but an applied science in which scientific discovery is expected to lead to material benefits. In recent years the fusion of biochemistry, cell biology and microbiology to form molecular biology has led to spectacular advances in the understanding and control of biological processes in medicine, agriculture, pharmaceutics and the food and drinks industry. This justifies to many the widely held belief that biotechnology will become the pre-eminent industry of the new millennium.

Biochemistry is quintessentially both analytical and quantitative in using model biological systems of different physiological complexities to explain cause-and-effect relationships in molecular terms. Analysis means literally 'getting to the bottom of things', i.e. taking to pieces. Analysis is useful only, however, when combined with synthesis, the piecing together, through interpretation and extrapolation of observations made on the disassembled parts, into the working whole. Analysis and synthesis therefore in combination define the boundaries between systems and surroundings, i.e. what components are part of the system and consequently affect the system directly in contrast to external factors that affect it only indirectly. Repeated investigations lead in many cases to the definition of a system.

In analytical biochemistry, for example, experimental models are subjected first to qualitative analysis, in which predominantly heterogeneous biological material is subjected to disruption techniques and the constituent parts separated, concentrated and identified. Qualitative analytical biochemistry is concerned with identifications mainly at the molecular level but sometimes at the electronic level. Quantitative analysis is concerned with measuring amounts and/or concentrations (amount per unit of volume) of constituents identified by qualitative analysis. The technique relies heavily on assay methods and instruments measuring the values of biochemical samples, representative of the whole population of biomolecules, within desirable limits of accuracy and precision of the population's true mean values. Quantitative estimations must therefore be supported by appropriate statistical analysis to establish whether or not numerical values are meaningful in terms of the objectives being set, whether data may have been obtained by chance or whether there is a valid pattern to the results. Accuracy (nearness to the true value) and precision (the variation in quantitative measurement around the norm) are both statistical terms.

Analysis, combined with microscopy (Section 1.7) and centrifugation (Chapter 5), not only has identified the cell as the basic unit of life but has led to an appreciation of biochemical compartmentalisation within subcellular systems of the cytoplasm and cell membranes. Biochemical compartmentalisation is least within prokaryotes, simple organisms lacking a true nucleus and possessing a single periplasmic membrane, and greatest in eukaryotes, which normally have not only a nucleus but also a nuclear membrane cytoplasmic extension, the endoplasmic reticulum, together with associated Golgi bodies and other membrane-bound organelles, ribosomes, mitochondria, peroxisomes, and plastids (in plants), all held together by an intricate web of microtubules and filaments.

Extensive study of membrane structure and function substantiated the classical Singer–Nicholson fluid mosaic model for membranes in which a hydrophobic lipid bilayer is loosely bound by mainly weak van der Waals' forces to both surface (extrinsic) and deep-seated (intrinsic) proteins. 'Proteins floating in a sea of lipid' is a well established, but still extremely apt, image for cell membranes. Intensive study has been made of the structure–function correlation between membrane proteins and transport, which has revealed the importance of α-helices (Section 6.2), which completely span the membrane, creating hydrophilic channels and thus allowing passage of a huge array of polar molecules (Section 8.4). Examples include lactose permease in *Escherichia coli*, glycophorin in erythrocyte membranes, bacteriorhodopsin in *Halobacterium halobium*, cytochrome oxidase in mitochondria, the H^+-ATPase of chloroplasts and mitochondria, the Na^+, K^+ pump of the nerve cells and Ca^{2+} channels in secretory epithelial tissue. Entry into a channel is, of course, selective, being controlled either directly by stereochemical binding at a receptor site (Section 8.3) or indirectly by gating mechanisms that open or close the channel by means of conformational change in the protein, which is induced occasionally by hormonal intervention (Section 8.4.1).

The self-assembly of non-polar lipids (glycolipids, sulpholipids and sterols) into lipid bilayers and spherical micelles was a key event in biochemical evolution, not only because it allowed membranes to organise biochemical processes into discrete subsystems but also because it facilitated the establishment of ion gradients. Such gradients were formed initially between the primaeval cell and its environment and later, after the establishment of the multicellular state, intercellularly. These ion gradients represent primary energy stores that can be exploited for performing biological work (transport, motion, biosynthesis, etc.). The uniqueness of living organisms lies in their ability to trap environmental energy and transform it through the process of anabolism into chemical bonds. These bonds typically comprise $C - C, C - N, C - O, N - H, O - H, O - P$. The energy conserved in these bonds is capable of being released to perform work. Compared to eukaryotes, the prokaryote kingdom displays a much greater capacity to exploit different environmental niches and to use alternative energy sources. Primitive organisms were probably subject to natural selection based on biochemical pathways for energy transduction and biosynthesis of macromolecules.

Prokaryotes established standardised mechanisms for energy generation via substrate level, oxidative and photosynthetic phosphorylation. These permitted natural selection within eukaryotes, after the arrival of endosymbiosis with prokaryotes, to operate physiologically on the basis of differentiation of cells into organs for performing specialised physiological functions. Each different cell type in a multicellular organism must reflect accompanying biochemical and physiological differences operating within these cells and invoke mutual cooperation of cells in physiological processes. As a consequence, a large part of developmental biochemistry is concerned with elucidating, at the molecular level, mechanisms of selective gene expression that lead to differentiation.

In genetic terms there are significant differences between species that prevent cross-fertilisation and gene mixing through DNA hybridisation (phylogenetic differences). Despite these differences there remain sufficient common chemical constituents and processes to allow for a mode of biochemical deduction based on extrapolation of results obtained in one species to be applied to another. Frequently, extrapolation is made to humans from, for example, microorganisms, animal tissue cultures or laboratory animals for monitoring the biochemical, physiological, pharmacological or toxicological responses to foreign exogenous compounds (xenobiotics) as a prelude to their commercial or medical use. This approach must be treated with caution however, since biological variation between cell types or species is possible and there may be gross physiological differences, particularly between unicellular and multicellular species. Any form of either chemical analysis or sample preparation for microscopy inevitably creates artefacts by destroying biological integrity, which means that *in vivo* extrapolation might be unjustified. Despite this criticism, however, the 'outside-in' analytical approach with 'bottom-up' extrapolation to the whole, has facilitated great insight into the unity and diversity of life forms and provided theoretical underpinning for other biological disciplines such as ecology, physiology, pharmacology, microbiology, botany, zoology and the environmental sciences which comprise biological systems.

Bioanalysis of the central information-processing molecules, DNA and RNA, in recent years, has led to an unequivocal and clearer appreciation of the connection between definable base sequences in the hereditary material, DNA, and how specific proteins are formed, thereby allowing for a more accurate explanation of how cells differentiate during development. Complementary advances in the artificial synthesis of DNA, exploiting the polymerase chain reaction (PCR) and methods for both multiplying and transferring DNA to unnatural recipients in genetic engineering (Section 3.7), have facilitated an 'inside-out' approach to solving problems in biochemistry that were hitherto much more difficult to pursue using the more traditional biochemical approaches.

1.2 **BIOENERGETICS**

1.2.1 **Laws of thermodynamics**

Bioenergetics is the study of energy and biomatter transformation in biosystems and is very closely related biochemically to metabolism, the sum of all chemical reactions in an organism. Bioenergetics is founded on thermodynamic laws, so-called because they were concerned historically with heat (enthalpy) exchanges in chemical and physical processes in closed systems. Closed systems allow energy, but not matter, to pass the system's boundary. The principal interrelated variables involved in closed systems are pressure, volume, temperature and con-centration changes that establish an equilibrium condition, at which point there is no exchange of energy with their surroundings. An example of a closed system and its surroundings is a chemical solution in a sealed phial transferred from 25 °C to a beaker of water at a higher temperature. A closed system removed from its equilibrium state is therefore capable of either taking up energy from or giving up energy to its surroundings.

Thermodynamics is concerned solely with measuring the difference in energy status across a boundary under non-equilibrium conditions and hence *not* with either the method of achieving this state or the rate at which the process occurs. Cells are, by contrast, open systems that exchange both energy and matter with their surroundings when temperature, volume and pressure remain constant.

Bioenergetics is concerned with the interconversion of kinetic, thermal, mechanical, electrical, electromagnetic (light) and osmotic energy in biosystems. Bioenergetics also incorporates the energy changes associated with biomolecules changing from one chemical form to another in metabolism. Degradative reactions, involving release of energy on breaking of bonds, constitutes catabolism, whereas energy conservation in bond formation constitutes anabolism. Anabolic reactions typically involve adding hydrogen atoms (reduction) and removing water molecules (dehydration) both to stabilise and to concentrate molecules, thus providing more energy on subsequent oxidation. Enzymic reduction *in vivo* is facilitated by reduced forms of coenzymes, principally NADPH. Oxidation not only invokes coenzymes such as NAD or the flavin prosthetic groups FMN or FAD in dehydrogenases but also the agency of proteins that combine either with oxygen, for example cytochrome oxidase , or with alternative electron acceptors as, for example, in the sulphate-reducing bacteria that grow anaerobically and produce large amounts of hydrogen sulphide (H_2S) from sulphate. Terminal electron acceptors that are alternatives to oxygen are found exclusively in prokaryotes.

The first and second laws of thermodynamics underpin bioenergetics. The first law states that 'Energy can be neither created nor destroyed but can be converted from one form to another', implying that the energy of the system plus its surroundings must remain constant. As a consequence, chemical reactions, in which bonds are broken and reformed, move to a position of equilibrium either by taking heat from the surroundings (as in endothermic reactions) or release heat to the surroundings (exothermic reactions). Endothermic reactions are recognised by a temperature decrease in the surroundings but show an increase in enthalpy (H) within the system, i.e. the change in enthalpy (ΔH) is positive. Exothermic reactions represent the converse, in which ΔH is negative when the external solution heats up. Enthalpy changes are expressed normally in J mol^{-1}. An enthalpy change ΔH always accompanies the establishment of an equlibrium involving either an exothermic or an endothermic reaction. At equilibrium, conditions are isothermal. Enthalpy changes are related to the equilibrium constant K_{eq} for a reaction, as given by the van't Hoff equation:

$$\frac{\mathrm{d}\ln K_{eq}}{\mathrm{d}T} = \frac{\Delta H}{RT^2} \tag{1.1}$$

which states that the rate of change of K_{eq} with temperature is logarithmic. Equation 1.1 may be integrated to give

$$\ln K_{eq} = -\frac{\Delta H}{RT} + c \tag{1.2}$$

where c is an integration constant, R is the molar or gas constant (8.314 J mol^{-1} K^{-1}) and T the absolute temperature (K). Consequently a plot of $\ln K_{eq}$ against $1/T$ for a reversible reaction would produce a straight line graph with a slope of $-\Delta H/RT$ allowing ΔH to be calculated. Some biochemists prefer to work in log$_{10}$ rather than natural logarithms. In such cases it must be remembered that $\ln x = 2.303 \log_{10} x$.

The second law of thermodynamics relates to the direction of energy flow by stating that 'All chemical and physical processes are pulled towards equilibrium by the forces of entropy (S) which represent a condition of chaotic, random molecular movement'. Entropy is consequently a function of temperature and in energy terms is represented as $T\Delta S$ expressed in J mol^{-1} K^{-1}. Entropy is greatest, for example, when a chemical reaction in a closed system is at equilibrium. Entropy is a part of enthalpy that cannot be used directly to perform useful work.

Biosystems are, however, orderly, organised states in which energy flow is directed towards the conversion of precursor molecules of greater entropy into biopolymers with decreased entropy. Furthermore, biosystems exist characteristically as non-equilibrium steady states. The living state does not contradict the second law of thermodynamics, since life is made possible by the exploitation of increases in entropy in the surroundings, i.e. ultimately the universe. As a consequence, entropy is, paradoxically, the driving force operating on living systems.

Josiah Gibbs (1839–1903) was responsible for introducing the notion of a measurable Gibbs free energy component of enthalpy, designated G, which could perform useful work and could also act as a reliable indicator of whether a reaction would proceed to equilibrium spontaneously or not from a given set of conditions, i.e. without the input of energy from the surroundings. Gibbs combined enthalpy, entropy and free energy in the equation

$$\Delta H = \Delta G + T\Delta S \tag{1.3}$$

which uses the first and second laws of thermodynamics but operates only under conditions of constant temperature, pressure and volume. This equation is frequently rearranged as

$$\Delta G = \Delta H - T\Delta S \tag{1.4}$$

Provided the free energy status of the products of a reaction is less than for the reactants, i.e. ΔG has a negative sign, the reaction is termed exergonic and will proceed spontaneously towards equilibrium, irrespective of whether the reaction is exothermic or endothermic. The converse process in which the free energy status of the products of a reaction are greater than the reactants, where ΔG has a positive value, is termed endergonic and will not proceed to equilibrium without the input of energy from the surroundings. A negative value for ΔG does not give an indication of the rate of the reaction, however, which is governed by kinetic factors relating mainly to the energy of activation being lowered significantly in enzyme-catalysed reactions (Section 7.3.6). Metabolism operates through the coupling of exergonic and endergonic reactions to achieve chemical synthesis at the expense of an increase in the entropy of the universe. All biochemical reactions are spontaneous therefore when viewed from this perspective.

Spontaneous reactions accompanying positive enthalpy changes are demonstrated, for example, when crystalline salts such as potassium chloride (KCl) are dissolved in water. The solution becomes cold by taking heat out of the solvent to break hydrogen bonds in the crystal lattice. In this case ΔS resulting from the increased mobility of the ions in water is greater than ΔH, making ΔG negative overall. A spontaneous reaction associated with a negative ΔH is observed, however, when anhydrous calcium sulphate dissolves: the temperature of the solution increases. Spontaneous reactions induced by a positive ΔS of the surroundings, in contrast, are seen in protein folding and in the organisation of polar lipids into micelles. The principal driving force in both of these cases is the hydrophobic action of non-polar groups (aromatic rings and alkyl groups of amino acids, and alkyl residues in fatty acids) forcing water molecules to organise as layers or shells on the outside surface. This happens because water molecules interact more strongly with each other, forming hydrogen bonds, with the non-polar groups. The initial interaction is not spontaneous in each case, however, because ΔH is slightly positive and entropy is decreased as the water molecules are forced to organise externally. Protein folding follows when hydrophobic groups exposed at the surface become more stabilised within the interior of the protein by non-covalent van der Waals' forces. Any hydrophilic amino groups drawn into the hydrophobic interior reduce their polarity by hydrogen bonding to form α-helices and β-pleated sheets, thus stabilising the protein structure. This infolding allows external water molecules to become more mobile and consequently the entropy of the solvent increases, making the overall process spontaneous. A similar increase in S of the surrounding water is achieved when phospholipids aggregate spontaneously first into monolayers and then into spherical micelles.

Gibbs free energy values in J mol^{-1} can be calculated in relation to four principal functions: chemical potential, electrical potential, hydrostatic potential and gravitational potential. Chemical potential and electrical potential are the most important in biochemical terms.

1.2.2 Standard energy status

The chemical potential of a solution is the product of its molar concentration (M) multiplied by its activity coefficient α. Activity coefficients for physiological solutions, which are usually in the mM or μM range, are sufficiently close to 1 that concentrations will substitute effectively for chemical activity. The standard energy status (or standard electrochemical potential) of μ^0, a unique property of the molecule resulting from the interaction of its chemical bonds, relates to the free energy of a solution containing 1 mol dm^{-3} at atmospheric pressure and at a given temperature, normally 25 °C, representing the standard state. Increases or decreases in the molar concentration changes the energy status to μ by a logarithmic factor according to the equation

$$\mu = \mu^0 + RT \ln [A] \tag{1.5}$$

where [A] is the concentration of solute A in mol dm^{-3}. When [A] equals 1 M in equation 1.5, $\mu = \mu^0$, since ln 1 = 0.

The difference in μ, $\Delta\mu$, if the concentration were to be changed from [A] to a lower concentration [A$_1$], would be

$$\underset{\text{new status}}{(\mu^0 + RT \ln [A_1])} - \underset{\text{old status}}{(\mu^0 + RT \ln [A])}$$

$$\Delta\mu = RT \ln \left(\frac{[A_1]}{[A]} \right) \tag{1.6}$$

assuming the molecule remained chemically unaltered. ΔG would have a negative sign in this case and free energy would be available potentially to perform work. Biological membranes play an important role in energy conservation by maintaining such solute gradients when selectively preventing solute transport. When membranes are permeable to the substance in question it would move spontaneously from the higher to the lower concentration, moving down the concentration gradient to dissipate the potential energy.

Chemical potential can be used to work out the thermodynamic feasibility of a chemical reaction, i.e. whether or not it will proceed spontaneously to equilibrium, when the concentration of the reactants and products are known, provided the equilibrium constant for the reaction is also known. This relationship may be derived from considering the hypothetical reaction A $\rightleftharpoons$ B, in which case

$$\mu[B] = \mu^0[B] + RT \ln [B]$$
$$\text{and } \mu[A] = \mu^0[A] + RT \ln [A]$$
$$\Delta\mu = (\mu^0[B] + RT \ln [B]) - (\mu^0[A] + RT \ln [A])$$

$$\Delta\mu = (\mu^0[B] - \mu^0[A]) + RT \ln \left(\frac{[B]}{[A]} \right) \tag{1.7}$$

where [B]/[A] represents the mass action ratio.

But if both B and A are at standard 1 M concentrations then

$$RT\ln\left(\frac{[B]}{[A]}\right) = 0$$

from which $\Delta\mu = \mu^0[B] - \mu^0[A] = \Delta G^0$, which defines the standard free energy change for a reaction. The standard free energy change, ΔG^0, constitutes the difference in free energy between the equilibrium state where $G = 0$ and that when reactants and products are maintained artificially under standard states at μ^0, i.e. at a uniform concentration of 1 mol dm^{-3} at atmospheric pressure (101 kPa), hydrogen ion concentration of 1 mol dm^{-3} (pH 0, Section 1.2.5) and at a given temperature, usually 25 °C (298 K).

For any other molar concentrations of B and A

$$\Delta\mu = \Delta G = \Delta G^0 + RT\ln\left(\frac{[B]}{[A]}\right) \tag{1.8}$$

Under equilibrium conditions

$$\Delta G = 0 \text{ and } K_{eq} = \frac{[B]}{[A]}$$

therefore $\Delta G^0 = -RT\ln\left(\frac{[B]}{[A]}\right) = -RT\ln K_{eq}$ \hfill (1.9)

1.2.3 Standard free energy change

ΔG^0 has very little relevance in biological systems because the value of cellular pH is normally around neutrality (6.0 to 7.5). As a consequence $\Delta G^{0\prime}$ is used as the standard free energy change at pH 7.0, when the equation that applies is

$$\Delta G^{0\prime} = -RT\ln K_{eq} \tag{1.10}$$

The units for the equilibrium constant in equation 1.10 will change according to whether a single product is formed from a single reactant (no units) to M (where two products are produced from a single reactant) to M^{-1} (where two products give rise to a single product). This does not affect the units of measurement for $\Delta G^{0\prime}$, which remain J mol^{-1}. For this reason units for K_{eq} are frequently omitted.

For non-standard, non-equilibrium mass action ratios, the relevant free energy equation is therefore

$$\Delta G' = \Delta G^{0\prime} + 2.303 RT\log\left(\frac{[\text{products in mol dm}^{-3}]}{[\text{reactants in mol dm}^{-3}]}\right) \tag{1.11}$$

The phosphorylation of fructose 6-phosphate (F6P) by ATP to fructose 1,6-bisphosphate (FBP) by phosphofructokinase-1 (PFK-1) may be used to illustrate the significance of this equation.

The equilibrium constant $K_{eq} = \left(\dfrac{[FBP]}{[ATP][F6P]} \right)$

$$= 3.08 \times 10^2 \, M^{-1}$$

If FBP, ATP and F6P were to be maintained at pH 7.0 away from equilibrium at standard 1 M concentrations, the Gibbs free energy at t(K) is given by the equation

$$\Delta G' = \Delta G^{0\prime} + 2.303RT\log\left(\dfrac{[FBP]}{[ATP][F6P]} \right)$$

but, since

$$\left(\dfrac{[FBP]}{[ATP][F6P]} \right) = 1$$

because reactants and products are at unit concentration, $\Delta G' = \Delta G^{0\prime}$.

At equilibrium $\Delta G' = 0$ and $\Delta G^{0\prime} = -2.303RT \log K_{eq}$ (equation 1.10). Hence in the example for PFK-1 above, at 25 °C, pH 7, ΔG^0 can be calculated as follows:

$$\Delta G^{0\prime} = -2.303 \times 81314 \, J \, mol^{-1} \, K^{-1} \times 298 \, K \times \log(3.08 \times 10^2)$$
$$= -14\,199.3 \, J \, mol^{-1}$$

Putting the mass action ratio at exactly 1 would make approximately 14.2 kJ of free energy available to perform work if the reaction were allowed to move to the equilibrium position. Whenever $K_{eq} > 1$, therefore, an equimolar solution of products and reactants would proceed spontaneously to equilibrium. The converse applies for reactions where $K_{eq} < 1$, in which case energy would need to be provided from the surroundings to attain the equilibrium condition.

For coupled reactions involving a common intermediate

i.e. K_{eq1} K_{eq2}
   $A \rightleftharpoons B \rightleftharpoons C,$

where B is the common intermediate, the overall K_{eq} for the conversion of A to C is the product $K_{eq1} \times K_{eq2}$. In coupled reactions that include a reaction proceeding in the backward direction, a reciprocal value for K_{eq} is used to calculate the overall K_{eq}. Examples of calculations of $\Delta G^{0\prime}$ involving coupled reactions are shown below.

Example 1

The pentose phosphate pathway (PPP) is the metabolic sequence for the synthesis of pentose sugars. Ribose 5-phosphate and xylulose 5-phosphate are typical pentose sugars found in the PPP. What is the standard free energy for the formation of ribose 5-phosphate from xylulose 5-phosphate at 37 °C, given

$$\text{ribulose 5-phosphate} \xrightleftharpoons{\quad K_{eq} = 2.30 \quad} \text{ribose 5-phosphate}$$

$$\text{ribulose 5-phosphate} \xrightleftharpoons{\quad K_{eq} = 0.67 \quad} \text{xylulose 5-phosphate}$$

Answer	The overall K_{eq}	$= [(1/0.67) \times 2.30] = 3.433$
	Hence $\Delta G^{0\prime}$	$= -2.303 \times 8.314\,J\,mol^{-1}\,K^{-1} \times 310\,K \times \log 3.433$
		$= -3179.55\,J\,mol^{-1}$

Hence the difference in free energy between products and reactants poised at 1 M concentrations would be 3179.55 J less than when they are at equilibrium conditions. This represents a form of potential energy that is theoretically available to perform work such as coupling to endergonic reactions.

Example 2 An important stage in the breakdown of sugars via the Embden–Meyerhof (glycolytic) pathway occurs by the coupling of glyceraldehyde 3-phosphate dehydrogenase with phosphoglycerate kinase to form ATP in a substrate level phosphorylation. If the coupled reactions occurred together in solution at pH 7 and 38 °C, what would be the standard free energy change for the formation of ATP from glyceraldehyde 3-phosphate and P_i?.

$$K_{eq} = 0.875 \times 10^{-1}$$

glyceraldehyde 3-phosphate + inorganic phosphate $\rightleftharpoons$ 1,3-bisphosphoglycerate

NAD   NADH + H$^+$

1,3-bisphosphoglycerate + ADP $\xrightarrow{K_{eq} = 1.746 \times 10^3}$ 3-phosphoglycerate + ATP

Answer	The overall $K_{eq} = 0.0875 \times 1746 = 152.78$
	$\Delta G^{0\prime} = -2.303 \times 8.314\,J\,mol^{-1}\,K^{-1} \times 311\,K \times \log 152.78$
	$\quad = -13.005\,kJ\,mol^{-1}$

The $\Delta G^{0\prime}$ generated from the phosphoglycerate kinase reaction alone is equal to $-18.5\,kJ\,mol^{-1}$ under the conditions specified. This is considerably less than the $\Delta G^{0\prime}$ for ATP synthesis from ADP and P_i under the same conditions, which amounts to approximately $-30.5\,kJ\,mol^{-1}$. Substrate-level phosphorylation is achieved *in vivo* in the phosphoglycerate kinase reaction by exploiting mass action ratios.

Example 3 In the case of PFK-1 cited earlier, if the concentrations of FBP, ATP and F6P were, respectively, 80 μM, 8 mM and 1.5 mM, what would be the actual free energy change?

Answer

$$\Delta G' = \Delta G^{0\prime} + 2.303\,RT\log\left(\frac{[FBP]}{[F6P][ATP]}\right)$$

$$= -14199.3\,J\,mol^{-1} + 2.303 \times 8.314\,J\,mol^{-1}\,K^{-1} \times 298\,K$$

$$\times \log\left(\frac{80 \times 10^{-6}}{1.5 \times 10^{-3} \times 8 \times 10^{-3}}\right)$$

$$=-14199.3\,\text{J}\,\text{mol}^{-1}+4701.1\text{J}\,\text{mol}^{-1}$$
$$=-9498.2\,\text{J}\,\text{mol}^{-1}$$

Physiological concentrations of FBP are maintained in a steady state, well removed from near-equilibrium conditions, making this reaction metabolically irreversible. The constraint on PFK *in vivo* is achieved by allosteric regulation (Section 7.3.4).

Example 4 $\Delta G^{\circ\prime}$ for ATP synthesis under standard conditions at 25 °C = 30 540 J mol^{-1}. The concentrations of ATP, ADP and P$_i$ in cells is normally such that considerably more energy than 30 540 J mol^{-1} is necessary to synthesise 1 mole of ATP from ADP and P$_i$. If the steady state concentrations of ATP, ADP and P$_i$ in isolated chloroplasts under full illumination at pH 7.0 and 25 °C were, respectively, 8 mM, 0.5 mM and 5 mM, what would be ΔG_p (the phosphorylation potential), the free requirement for the synthesis of 1 mole of ATP under these conditions?

Answer
$$\Delta G_p = \Delta G^{0\prime} + 2.303\,RT\log\left(\frac{[\text{ATP}]}{[\text{ADP}][\text{P}_i]}\right)$$

$$=-30\,540\,\text{J}\,\text{mol}^{-1}+2.303\times8.314\,\text{J}\,\text{mol}^{-1}\,\text{K}^{-1}\times298\,\text{K}$$

$$\times\log\left(\frac{8\times10^{-3}}{0.5\times10^{-3}\times5\times10^{-3}}\right)$$

$$=-30\,540\,\text{J}\,\text{mol}^{-1}+19\,999\,\text{J}\,\text{mol}^{-1}$$
$$=50.54\,\text{kJ}\,\text{mol}^{-1}$$

Frequently, *in vivo* ΔG_p is of the order of 50 kJ mol^{-1}.

Many reactions that represent a thermodynamic barrier as judged by positive $\Delta G^{0\prime}$ values can be made spontaneous by manipulating the mass action ratio. An illustration occurs in the synthesis of glyceraldehyde 3-phosphate (G3P) from 3-phosphoglycerate (3PGA) via 1,3-bisphosphoglycerate (1,3-BPGA) in the photosynthetic carbon reduction cycle (Calvin–Benson cycle). The first stage involves phosphoglycerate kinase:

$$3\text{PGA} + \text{ATP} \rightleftharpoons 1,3\text{-BPGA} + \text{ADP}$$
$$\Delta G^{0\prime} = 18.5\,\text{kJ}\,\text{mol}^{-1}$$

This reaction is endergonic under standard conditions and consequently ATP is not being used to drive the reaction. However,

$$\text{since } \Delta G^{\prime} = \Delta G^{0\prime} + 2.303\,RT\log\left(\frac{[\text{ADP}][1,3\,\text{BPGA}]}{[3\text{PGA}][\text{ATP}]}\right)$$

the thermodynamic barrier is reduced *in vivo* and the reaction made exergonic for a number of reasons. First, 3PGA levels are high following ribulose bisphosphate carboxylase (Rubisco) activity; secondly, ATP levels are high as a result of photo-phosphorylation; thirdly, 1,3-BPGA is low through coupling of phosphoglycerate kinase to glyceraldehyde-3-phosphate dehydrogenase. This enzyme represents the second stage of the process:

1,3-BPGA + NADPH $\rightleftharpoons$ G3P + NADP
$\Delta G^{0\prime} = -6.3 \text{ kJ mol}^{-1}$

Despite the low concentrations of 1,3-BPGA, the reaction is made more exergonic under physiological conditions by the generation of large amounts of NADPH from NADP as a result of the light reactions of photosynthesis. Glyceraldehyde-3-phosphate dehydrogenase also has a very high affinity for both 1,3-BPA and NADPH (K_m 1,3-BPA = 1 μM, K_m NADPH = 4 μM). (Details on the importance of K_m for enzyme-catalysed reactions are given in Section 7.3.2.)

1.2.4 Reduction–oxidation (redox)

Many biological molecules are known to exist in either a reduced (red) or oxidised (ox) form as a result of either gaining or losing electrons to molecules with similar properties. Such substances are known as redox couples or half-cells. (Further details on theoretical and practical aspects of redox substances are given in Section 15.3). When two half-cells are mixed, electron transfer takes place in a redox chemical reaction such that the oxidising half-cell becomes reduced and the reducing half-cell oxidised, thus establishing an equilibrium condition when electron transfer ceases. Free energy changes accompanying such redox reactions are typified hypothetically as

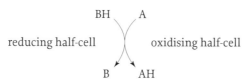

in which A/AH and B/BH represent two substances in their oxidised and reduced forms, respectively.

The free energy expressed in electrical terms for a 1 M standard solution containing a monovalent cation (C^+) is the product nFE, where nF coulombs is the charge on one mole of the substance. In the case of a monovalent ion $n = 1$. The Faraday constant, F, is the product of the charge on a single electron (1.602×10^{-19} C) and Avogadro's number (6.022×10^{23}) (the number of molecules in one mole; see Section 1.4.4). Thus $F = 9.648 \times 10^4$ C. The term E relates to the electric potential to which the charge is subjected. An individual half-cell can be set up such that its oxidised and reduced forms are both at 1 M concentration (50% oxidised), i.e. under the same standard state as for chemical potential described earlier. When two half-cells are arranged to form a cell, such that each half-cell is in its standard state, a potential difference is set up between them. This ΔE is dependent upon the different affinities that each half-cell has for electrons, as measured by their individual electrode potentials. Electrode potentials are measured for any given half-cell against the hydrogen half-cell in a standard state, in which a 1 M solution of HCl (at pH 0) is equilibrated with H_2 gas (Section 15.2). The standard electrode potential for a given half-cell is known as the redox potential and is designated as E^0 (pH 0) or $E^{0'}$ (pH 7.0). The E^0 for the hydrogen half-cell is 0.0 V at pH 0; at pH 7.0 it is -0.3200V (Section 15.3). Redox potentials are consequently ordered as either being more negative or more positive than the hydrogen half-cell. In moving towards an equilibrium position, any substance with a more negative standard redox potential than the hydrogen half-cell will spontanously reduce it, causing H_2 gas to be liberated at the hydrogen half-cell. Conversely any substance having a standard redox potential more positive than the hydrogen half-cell will spontaneously oxidise it in moving towards equilibrium, but H_2 gas will not be produced. If equilibrium were obtained, a single redox potential would be achieved and electron flow would cease. Table 15.1 (p. 743) lists some standard redox potentials ($E^{0'}$ values) of biological importance.

For two half-cells maintained under standard states, the potential energy available represents the standard free energy change $\Delta G^{0'}$, and is equal to $nF\Delta E^{0'}$, where $\Delta E^{0'}$ is the difference in the standard redox potentials between the two half-cells. Subtracting the equilibrium state where there is no free energy available from the standard state produces a negative term in the expression

$$\Delta G^{0'} = -nF\Delta E^{0'} \tag{1.12}$$

If $\Delta E^{0'}$ is negative, i.e. $E^{0'}$ for the oxidising half-cell is less than $E^{0'}$ for the reducing half-cell $\Delta G^{0'}$ would be positive and equimolar concentrations of reactants and products would require an input of energy from the surroundings.

In general terms, the redox potential of a given half-cell will change according to the proportion of its oxidised and reduced forms as given by the Nernst equation:

$$\text{i.e. } E' = E^{0'} + 2.303\frac{RT}{nF}\log\left(\frac{[\text{ox}]}{[\text{red}]}\right) \tag{1.13}$$

where $E^{0'}$ is the half-oxidised (midpoint redox potential) and nF is the charge per mole. Physiological values for redox potential relate therefore to the logarithmic ratio of [ox]/[red] which means that they are independent of concentration as long as dilute solutions are used. Equation 1.13 also shows that, at 50% oxidation for a given half-cell, $E' = E^{0'}$. The Nernst equation may be used to facilitate exergonic reactions, for example when the redox potential is lowered in chloroplasts when large amounts of light-generated NADPH are used for the glyceraldehyde-3-phosphate dehydrogenase reaction described earlier.

In cases where products and reactants are away from their half-oxidised condition, the mass action ratio has to be taken into account to calculate the new value for $\Delta E'$. Hence for the hypothetical reaction

BH   A

B   AH

$$E'_{A/AH} = E^{0'}_{A/AH} + 2.303 \frac{RT}{nF} \log\left(\frac{[A]}{[AH]}\right)$$

$$E'_{B/BH} = E^{0'}_{B/BH} + 2.303 \frac{RT}{nF} \log\left(\frac{[B]}{[BH]}\right)$$

$$\Delta E'_{(ox-red)} = E'_{A/AH} - E'_{B/BH} - (E^{0'}_{A/AH} - E^{0'}_{B/BH}) + 2.303 \frac{RT}{nF} \log\left(\frac{[A]}{[AH]}\right) - \log\left(\frac{[B]}{[BH]}\right)$$

$$\Delta E'_{(ox-red)} = \Delta E^{0'} - 2.303 \frac{RT}{nF} \log\left(\frac{[AH][B]}{[A][BH]}\right) \tag{1.14}$$

allowing the value of $\Delta G'$ to be calculated from $\Delta G' = - nF\Delta E'$.

Some examples of the application of redox potential for calculating $\Delta G^{0'}$ are shown below:

Example 5   What is the equilibrium constant for the oxidation of acetaldehyde (ethanal) to acetate (ethanoate) by ferredoxin at pH 7.0 and 30 °C?

acetaldehyde $\rightleftharpoons$ acetate $+ 2H^+ + 2e$ $(E^{0'} = -0.60 \text{ V})$
ferredoxin $(Fe^{2+}) \rightleftharpoons$ ferredoxin $(Fe^{3+}) + e$ $(E^{0'} = -0.432 \text{ V})$

Answer   The redox reaction is represented by

acetaldehyde   2 ferredoxin (Fe^{3+})

reducing half-cell   oxidising half-cell

acetate   2 ferredoxin (Fe^{2+})

$$\Delta G^{0'} = - nF\Delta E^{0'} = -2.303 \, RT \log K_{eq}$$

$$\log K_{eq} = \frac{nF \, \Delta E^{0'}}{2.303 \, RT}$$

$$= \frac{\{2 \times 96\,860 \text{ J V}^{-1} \text{mol}^{-1} \times [(-0.432 \text{ V}) - (-0.60 \text{ V})]\}}{(2.303 \times 8.314 \text{ J mol}^{-1} \text{K}^{-1} \times 303 \text{ K})}$$

$$= \frac{(2 \times 96\,860 \text{ J V}^{-1} \text{mol}^{-1} \times 0.168 \text{ V})}{(2.303 \times 8.314 \text{ J mol}^{-1} \text{K}^{-1} \times 303 \text{ K})}$$

$$= \frac{32544.96}{5801.58}$$

$$\log K_{eq} = 5.6097$$

$$K_{eq} = 4.07 \times 10^5$$

Example 6

In mitochondria, energy resulting from electron transport is made available for proton pumping by the oxidation of protons arising from dehydrogenase activity in the tricarboxylic acid (or Krebs) cycle to water. How many moles of ATP could theoretically be produced under standard conditions of pH 7.0, and 25 °C from the proton gradient established, given $\Delta G^{0\prime}$ for ATP synthesis from ADP = 30 540 J mol^{-1}?

$$\text{NADH} \rightarrow \text{NAD}^+ + \text{H} + 2e \qquad (E^{0\prime} = -0.320 \text{ V})$$

$$\text{H}_2\text{O} \rightarrow \tfrac{1}{2}\text{O}_2 + 2\text{H}^+ + 2e \qquad (E^{0\prime} = +0.816 \text{ V})$$

Answer

$$\Delta G^{0\prime} = -nF\Delta E^{0\prime} = -2 \times 96\,860\,\text{J V}^{-1}\text{mol}^{-1} \times [(0.816 \text{ V}) - (-0.320 \text{ V})]$$
$$= -2 \times 96\,860\,\text{J V}^{-1}\text{mol}^{-1} \times (1.136 \text{ V})$$
$$= -220.066 \text{ kJ mol}^{-1}$$

$$\text{Number of moles of ATP} = \frac{-220.066 \text{ kJ mol}^{-1}}{-30.540 \text{ kJ mol}^{-1}}$$
$$= 7.21 \text{ moles}$$

This is considerably greater than the experimentally observed value of 2.5, highlighting inefficiencies in the coupling process.

Example 7

In photosynthetic electron transport, light quanta are transformed into ATP by the light reactions of photosynthesis involving the excitation of chlorophyll molecules. The effective wavelength range for higher plant photosynthesis is approximately 400 nm to 710 nm for O_2 evolution resulting from the photolysis of H_2O, i.e. oxygenic photosynthesis. Show by means of calculations that one photon of 710 nm light could provide enough energy to reduce NADP following oxidation of water, assuming $E^{0\prime}$ values for the H_2O/O_2 and NADPH/NADP half-cells to be, respectively, +0.816 V and −0.342 V ($\Delta E^{0\prime} = +1.14$ V).

Answer

The energy per quantum is given by the equation

$$E = \frac{hc}{\lambda} \qquad (1.15)$$

where c is the velocity of light (2.998 × 10^8 ms^{-1}), h is the Planck constant = 6.626 × 10^{-34} J s, and λ is the wavelength. The energy per quantum (E) is expressed in J photon^{-1}.

Hence, when $\lambda = 710$ nm,

$$E = \frac{6.626 \times 10^{-34}\,\text{J s} \times 2.998 \times 10^8 \text{ ms}^{-1}}{710 \times 10^{-9}\,\text{m}}$$

$$= 2.798 \times 10^{-19}\,\text{J photon}^{-1}$$

Since this unit is very small, it is more convenient to express energy as J einstein^{-1}, where 1 einstein is equivalent to one mole of photons, which is Avogadro's number of photons.

The energy per einstein of 710 nm light $= 2.789 \times 10^{-19} \times 6.023 \times 10^{23}$ photons mol^{-1}

$$= 168.52 \times 10^3 \, \text{J mol}^{-1}$$
$$= 168.52 \, \text{kJ mol}^{-1}$$

This amount of energy may be converted into V by dividing it by the Faraday constant, $9.6485 \times 10^4 \, \text{J V}^{-1} \, \text{mol}^{-1}$.

Hence $168.52 \, \text{kJ mol}^{-1} = \dfrac{168.52 \times 10^3 \, \text{J}}{9.6485 \times 10^4 \, \text{J V}^{-1}}$

$$= 1.75 \, \text{V}$$

Note that this value of 1.75 V can also be obtained by considering the displacement of a single electron by a single photon when

$$\frac{2.789 \times 10^{-19} \, \text{J photon}^{-1}}{1.602 \times 10^{-19} \, \text{J V}^{-1}} = 1.75 \, \text{V}$$

where $1.602 \times 10^{-19} \, \text{J V}^{-1}$ is the charge on a single electron $=$ Faraday constant (F)/Avogadro's number.

This means, in principle, that one photon of 710 nm wavelength light could provide enough energy to reduce NADP after oxidation of water. In practice, however, two photons are involved cooperatively in transferring a single electron from water to NADP. The reasons for this include the facts that redox carriers more positive than H_2O/O_2 (in particular an oxidised form of chlorophyll at the manganese reaction centre of photosystem II) and more negative than NADPH/NADP are involved (notably the non-haem protein ferredoxin), redox carriers are not in their standard states, energy transfer losses are incurred, and ATP, ADP and P$_i$ mass action ratios require a ΔG_p value of around 50 kJ mol^{-1} under physiological conditions. *In vitro* chloroplast preparations have shown that 710 nm represents a cut-off point for oxygenic photosynthesis, although 710 nm will continue to reduce ferredoxin in a cyclic flow involving a chlorophyll reaction centre (Section 15.3).

1.2.5 Electrochemical potential

Chemical and electrical potential for an electrolyte (A) may be combined as the electrochemical potential by the equation

$$\mu = \mu^0 + RT \ln [A] + nF\Delta E \tag{1.16}$$

As a consequence, charged ions in solution are able to exert an electromotive force on other ions by virtue of their electrochemical potential. This equation is exploited in cells by the differential permeability of membranes that establish equilibrium conditions of electrochemical potential by creating different electrical potentials in adjacent compartments whilst holding solutions at different concentrations. This property is vital in, for example, maintaining osmotic balance between cells to facilitate water absorption. The difference in electrical potential across a membrane associated with such asymmetric solute concentrations represents a potential energy source and is defined in volts (V) as the Nernst potential.

The Nernst potential may be derived by considering the electrochemical potentials of a cation $[C^+]$ distributed in two compartments inside (i) and outside (o), separated by a membrane freely permeable to $[C^+]$ but not to any counterion $[A^-]$. If the concentration of $[C^+]$ at equilibrium is represented by $[C^+]_i$ and $[C^+]_o$ respectively, then the difference in molar energies in the two compartments is given by

$$\Delta\mu = \mu_i - \mu_0$$

$$= (RT \ln [C^+]_i + nFE_i) - (RT \ln [C^+]_o + nFE_o)$$

$$= (RT \ln [C^+]_i - RT \ln [C^+]_o) + (nFE_i - nFE_o)$$

$$= RT \ln \left(\frac{[C^+]_i}{[C^+]_o} \right) + nF (E_i - E_o)$$

$$= RT \ln \left(\frac{[C^+]_i}{[C^+]_o} \right) + nF (E_M) \tag{1.17}$$

where $E_M = (E_i - E_o)$ is the membrane potential.

But at equilibrium $\Delta\mu = 0$ when $E_M = E_N$, the Nernst potential. Hence the equilibrium Nernst potential equation may be written as

$$E_N = \frac{RT}{nF} \ln \left(\frac{[C^+]_o}{[C^+]_i} \right) \tag{1.18}$$

This is the electromotive force in volts associated with maintaining a particular ion gradient across a membrane. RT/nF is a constant for a univalent ion equal to 0.0295 V at 25 °C.

A term may be found for $\ln ([C^+]_i/[C^+]_o)$ by inverting the previous equation to

$$-E_N = \frac{RT}{nF} \ln \left(\frac{[C^+]_i}{[C^+]_o} \right)$$

when $\ln \left(\dfrac{[C^+]_i}{[C^+]_o} \right) = -E_N \dfrac{nF}{RT}$

Equation 1.17 may therefore be rewritten as

$$\Delta\mu = -E_N nF + nFE_M$$
$$= nF (E_M - E_N) \tag{1.19}$$

This equation represents the energy stored in a membrane ion gradient maintained under non-equilibrium conditions. Considerable amounts of energy may be used *in vivo* to set up such conditions.

The Nernst equation has considerable physiological application where potential differences are established between cells that are subject to change under exitable conditions. For example, the resting potential of the squid giant axon, a favourite model system, may be calculated from the Nernst equation at 16 °C to be approximately −75 mV when the concentrations of [K$^+$] outside is 20 mM and inside is 400 mM. Experimental values are typically nearer −60 mV at this temperature, however, after the concentrations and differential permeability of other ions such as Na$^+$, Cl$^-$ and endogenous amino acid anions are taken into account. Frog muscle is another example of tissue that produces a resting potential across the membrane of approximately −90 mV when the outside concentrations of Na$^+$, K$^+$, and Cl$^-$ are respectively 120 mM, 2.5 mM and 120 mM and when the internal concentrations of the same ions are, respectively, 10 mM, 140 mM and 4 mM.

When this principle is applied to the distribution of H$^+$ across biological membranes, for example the inner mitochondrial membrane, another useful term may be derived, which Mitchell and Moyle, in 1968, called the proton motive force (p.m.f.). In this case H$^+$ accumulates in the intermembrane space as electrons are conveyed from reduced hydrogen carriers NADH or FADH towards oxygen (Section 15.3). If the suffixes i and o are taken to represent the matrix side (where the Kreb's cycle is located) and the intermembrane space respectively, then

$$\Delta\mu^{[H^+]} = \mu^{[H^+]}_i - \mu^{[H^+]}_o$$

Substituting in equation 1.17, in which n = 1, gives

$$\Delta\mu^{[H^+]} = RT\ln\left(\frac{[H^+]_i}{[H^+]_o}\right) + F(E_i - E_o)$$

$$= -RT\ln\left(\frac{[H^+]_o}{[H^+]_i}\right) + F(E_i - E_o)$$

$$= -2.303\,RT\log\left(\frac{[H^+]_o}{[H^+]_i}\right) + F(E_i - E_o)$$

But pH $= -\log$ H$^+$ (Section 1.4.5).

Therefore, $\Delta\mu^{[H^+]} = 2.303\,RT\Delta pH_{o-i} + F(E_i - E_o)$

where ΔpH_{o-i} is the difference in pH across the membrane.

This is usually expressed the other way around as

$$\Delta\mu^{[H^+]} = FE_{M_{i-o}} + 2.303\,RT\Delta pH_{o-i} \tag{1.20}$$

$\Delta\mu^{[H^+]}$ is converted into volts by dividing by F to give

$$\text{p.m.f.} = E_{M_{i-o}} + 2.303\,\frac{RT}{F}\Delta pH_{o-i}$$

i.e. $\text{p.m.f.} = E_{M_{i-o}} + z\Delta pH_{o-i}$ $\tag{1.21}$

where z is a constant for a given temperature.

An electrochemical gradient of any ion represents a potential energy store, since energy release would follow translocation of the ions down an electrochemical gradient through a channel in the membrane. In oxidative and photosynthetic phosphorylation, electrochemical gradients are established through H^+ accumulation against a concentration gradient in the periplasmic space of bacteria, the intermembrane space of mitochondria and the interthylakoid (lumen) of chloroplasts. This accumulation exploits the equation $\Delta G' = -nF\Delta E'$. The proton gradient then allows protons to traverse the membrane through a proton channel represented by the protein complex ATP synthase. *In vivo* this enzyme is also capable of ATPase activity that actively pumps protons in the opposite direction. The coupling of energy-releasing electron flow to the establishment of electrochemical gradients was accommodated in Peter Mitchell's chemiosmotic theory. It involved oxidation of hydrogen carriers by electron carriers, releasing protons into the intermembrane space, with electron flow continuing until it reached the terminal electron acceptors. Evidence in favour of the chemiosmotic theory has derived mainly from mitochondrial and chloroplast preparations using O_2 electrodes, pH electrodes and sophisticated spectrophotometric techniques (Section 15.1.2).

1.2.6 **Group transfer molecules**

In metabolism, exergonic and endergonic reactions are frequently coupled through the agency of a class of intermediates known as group transfer molecules. These comprise nucleoside di- and triphosphates (e.g. adenosine triphosphate and diphosphate), acylphosphates (e.g. acetyl phosphate, 1,3-bisphosphoglyceric acid), enol phosphates (e.g. phosphoenolpyruvate) and acyl-CoA derivatives (e.g. acetyl-CoA and succinyl-CoA). Synthesis of such group transfer molecules is dependent on the ambient conditions of concentration and the reduction–oxidation states of participating molecules, allowing for energy release to be captured in chemical bonds. Table 1.1 shows the major classes of group transfer molecule that act as the energy currency in metabolism. These molecules are especially energy rich because they have a specific set of chemical bonds that are readily capable of being changed as a result of hydrolysis to molecules of lower energy status (greater entropy) with the concomitant release of energy. Factors contributing to free energy changes include lowering of negative charge repulsion, stabilisation of products through isomerisation and electron sharing by resonance. *In vivo* hydrolysis of group transfer molecules does not normally occur, but instead energy is conserved in the biosynthesis of new chemical bonds.

The structures of ATP and 1,3-bisphosphoglycerate are shown in Fig. 1.1, which illustrates the principles involved. The enzymic transfer of a phosphate group from a group transfer molecule to ADP is known as substrate-level phosphorylation (SLP). Substrate level phosphorylation is ubiquitous in living organisms but is especially important in anaerobes. ATP and ADP are the most important group transfer molecules because they are very stable in water and are frequently covalently bonded to the active site of many enzymes, usually as the magnesium salt, whenever phosphorylation/dephosphorylation is involved. This includes the phosphorylation of proteins by protein kinases (Section 8.4.3).

Table 1.1 Common group transfer molecules

Type	General formula	Examples	$\Delta G^{o\prime}$ for hydrolysis at 25 °C (kJ mol^{-1})
Phosphate derivatives			
Pyrophosphates	$$\begin{array}{ccc} O & & O \\ \parallel & & \parallel \\ R-O-P-O \sim P-OH \\ \mid & & \mid \\ OH & & OH \end{array}$$	PP$_i$	− 33.4
		ATP ADP GTP GDP etc.	− 30.5
Acylphosphates	$$\begin{array}{cc} O & O \\ \parallel & \parallel \\ R-C-O \sim P-OH \\ & \mid \\ & OH \end{array}$$	1,3-BPGA	− 43.9
Enolphosphates	$$\begin{array}{cc} CH_2 & O \\ \parallel & \parallel \\ R-C-O \sim P-OH \\ & \mid \\ & OH \end{array}$$	PEP	− 61.9
Amidine phosphates	$$\begin{array}{cc} NH_2 & O \\ \parallel & \parallel \\ R-C-NH-O \sim P-OH \\ & \mid \\ & OH \end{array}$$	Creatine phosphate	− 43.0
Thioesters	$$\begin{array}{c} O \\ \parallel \\ RS \sim C-R' \end{array}$$	CH$_3$CO $\sim$ SCoA Acetyl CoA	− 31.4

1,3-BPGA, 1,3-bisphosphoglyceric acid; PEP, phosphoenolpyruvate.

ATP and ADP may also bind, as allosteric effectors, to proteins to induce conformational change, for example phosphofructokinase (PFK-1, Section 7.3.4). ATP is commonly regarded as the cell's 'energy currency' because it is readily produced from other phosphorylated group transfer molecules. Neither ATP or ADP can be stored at high concentration in cells as they are normally turned over rapidly and their concentration within cells is regulated closely within narrow limits. Approximate average concentrations of ATP, ADP and P$_i$ in the cytoplasm would be 10 mM, 1 mM and 10 mM, respectively. Following exercise, for example, ATP levels are reduced in skeletal muscle, with a simultaneous rise in ADP. Conversely, ATP levels are increased when there is a demand for energy for precursor biosynthesis. The pyridine nucleotides NAD(P)/NAD(P)H are another major group of water-soluble coenzyme molecules that are continuously turned over in metabolism through their involvement in oxidation–reduction reactions, which comprise a substantial part of metabolism. Very generally, NADPH is used for biosynthetic reactions whereas NAD is used for degradative sequences. Typical cytoplasmic levels of NAD and NADH would be, respectively, 0.50 mM and 0.05 mM. Group transfer molecules and reduced pyridine nucleotides generated in catabolism are turned over continuously in metabolism.

The nutritional classification of organisms is based on both the external source of electrons for reduction purposes and the energy source. Organisms that rely on inorganic electron donors are said to be lithotrophic whereas those that rely on organic sources are said to be organotrophic. To each of these classes may be added the prefix 'photo' if energy is provided by light within the visible and far-red region of the spectrum, or 'organo' if energy is provided by the oxidation of either organic or inorganic compounds.

1.3 METHODS FOR INVESTIGATING METABOLISM

1.3.1 General principles

Certain generalities may be applied to the way in which metabolic pathways are elucidated and, once they are known, to determine whether or not a particular organelle, cell, organ or organism is exploiting a specific pathway. These approaches are mainly, although not exclusively, applied to *in vitro* preparations (Section 1.6) and thus may also be used, along with microscopy (Section 1.7), to evaluate the integrity of organelles, etc. Preliminary evidence for identifying whether or not a particular pathway is operating may be inferred from yield (biomass production) studies on microorganisms growing on a particular substrate, or by measurements of gaseous exchange processes. This approach, which relies on prior knowledge of stoichiometry and of the pathways for dissimilation, is considered in more detail in the specialist literature listed in Section 1.10. Experiments may be performed in which, for example, all intermediates and enzymes involved in a pathway are first identified and quantified by chromatographic, spectroscopic or other means. When tissue extracts are supplemented with these intermediates, the rate of processes in the pathway would be expected to accelerate in a predictable manner due to faster turnover. Changes in metabolic rate may also be achieved by altering environmental conditions, for example glucose breakdown via the Embden–Meyerhof pathway (EMP) in facultative anaerobes such as the yeast *Saccharomyces cerevisiae* is accelerated by switching from aerobic to anaerobic conditions. Such metabolic perturbations closely relate to changes in kinetic activities of key regulatory enzymes as they respond to the binding of different positive or negative effector ligands which induce allosteric changes in the enzymes (Section 7.3.4). The identification and characterisation of so-called rate-limiting enzymes, for example PFK-1, has been important in studies on the regulation of metabolic pathways. In general terms, there must be a positive correlation between the rate of overall physiological process and the kinetic and regulatory properties of key enzymes. The specific activity of key enzymes involved in a metabolic pathway, for example, would be expected to be high.

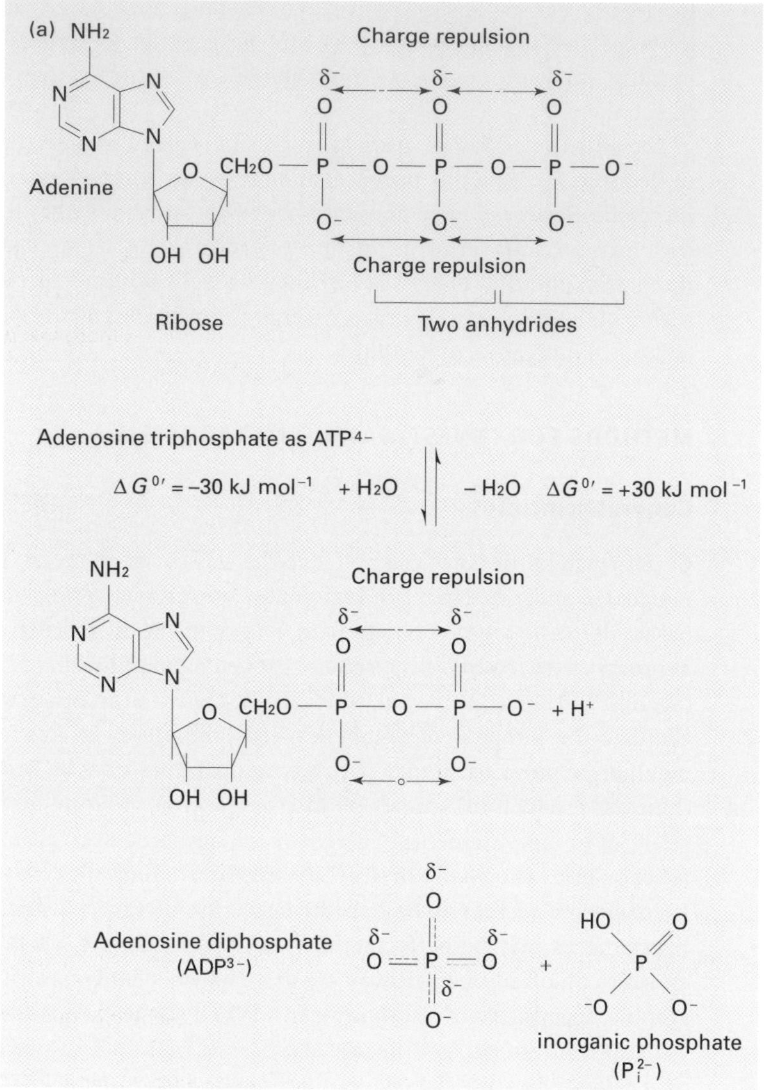

Fig. 1.1. (a) Acid anhydride structure of ATP and the free energy changes on hydrolysis and condensation. *In vivo* ATP and ADP are complexed as their magnesium salts MgATP^{2-} and Mg ADP^{2-}; this reduces the negative charge on these molecules and assists in binding to either active or allosteric sites of enzymes.

1.3.2 **Enzyme inhibitors**

Addition of enzyme inhibitors (Section 7.3.8) will cause intermediates to accumulate before the blockage point, thereby aiding identification of intermediates and confirming a known pathway in a novel experimental model. For example, iodoacetic acid is a powerful non-competitive inhibitor of glyceraldehyde 3-phosphate dehydrogenase in the EMP by forming covalent C $-$ S bonds with cysteine resi-

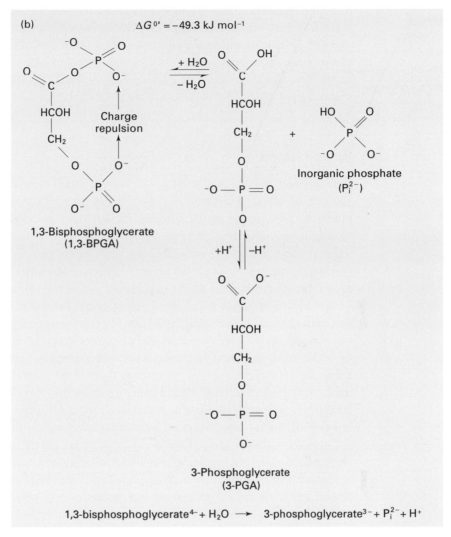

Fig. 1.1. (b) Acid anhydride structure of 1,3-bisphosphoglycerate and free energy changes on hydrolysis and condensation.

dues at the active site of the enzyme whereas monofluoroacetic acid (MFA) is a powerful inhibitor of citrate synthetase in the Krebs cycle, causing pyruvate to accumulate at the end of the glycolytic sequence. Inhibitors are particularly useful for working out the order of redox carriers in electron transport chains (Section 15.3), since carriers are left in a reduced state before the blockage point and show characteristic changes in absorption spectrum. For example, in the mitochondrial electron transport chain rotenone blocks some of the iron sulphur polypeptides of the NADH complex (complex I), whereas antimycin A blocks cytochrome b in the cytochrome bc_1 complex (complex III) and tetramethyl-p-phenylenediamine (TMPD) inhibits mobile cytochrome c. Photosynthetic inhibitor examples include dichloromethylurea (DCMU), which blocks the path of electron flow from pheophytin to plastoquinone in photosystem II and methyl-viologen (paraquat) which is a competitive inhibitor of NADP$^+$ reductase and diverts electrons away from NADP$^+$ to reduce O_2 instead. Highly destructive $O_2^{\pm}$ and $O_2^{2\pm}$ free radicals are generated in chloroplast membranes after paraquat treatment, thereby destroying them. As a consequence paraquat is a very effective herbicide.

1.3.3 Isotopic tracers

Isotopic tracers are very powerful tools for identifying the metabolic fate of precursors and for following metabolic turnover. Heavy isotopes are tracked using techniques of mass spectrometry whereas radioisotopes are exploited using the techniques described in Section 14.6. The great advantage of radiolabelling is in its sensitivity and specificity. In radiolabelling studies either universally labelled (U) or specifically labelled atoms are incorporated into molecules applied to the experimental model, at a specific activity (μC_i μmol^{-1}, Chapter 14) conducive for easy qualitative and/or quantitative analysis. Suitable specific activities may have to be determined by trial and error if the scientific literature gives no clear guide. Labelled test compounds are available commercially under most circumstances. Normal metabolism follows assuming there is no isotopic discrimination. The experimental models are sometimes given preliminary doses of the unlabelled compound of interest to stimulate metabolism and hence uptake of the label. Often different elements in compounds may be labelled (dual labelling) and this aids in discriminating biosynthetic origins in pathways, as, for example, in amino acid metabolism.

Time course studies and pulse chase techniques are the two main approaches employed in metabolic studies in which radiolabelled compounds are identified and recovered. In a time course study, labelled compounds are applied to the experimental system for increasing but normally very short time intervals, usually involving seconds of exposure. As the period of exposure to the radioactive tracer is progressively increased, a greater number of compounds become labelled. Metabolism is then stopped by adding a strong protein precipitant (frequently boiling ethanol) to denature the enzymes before the labelled intermediates are identified and possibly quantified after suitable chromatographic separation against known standards. In a pulse chase experiment, a few seconds of exposure of the system to a radiolabelled compound establishes a pool of labelled compounds which is diluted by the metabolism of a second pulse of the identical, but unlabelled, compound. In pulse chase experiments, compounds that become labelled earliest will be the first to lose the label and show decreases in specific activity on dilution with the unlabelled pulse. Autoradiography (Section 14.2.3) involves the identification of radiolabelled compounds shown as dark patches on photographic film laid in the dark over a completed chromatograph containing radioactive compounds. It is sometimes used for qualitative analysis by comparing the migration characteristics of the sample on the autoradiograph with those of unlabelled standards on a normal chromatograph. The dark patches on the film, in this case, are caused by radioactive emissions that cause chemical changes in the photographic emulsion.

Quantification of label is achieved either after elution of the compounds or by direct scanning of the chromatograph resolving the radiolabelled mixtures, using techniques described in Section 13.11.5. Chemical or enzymic cleavage of molecules allows individual atoms in a radiolabelled compound to be assessed quantitatively for radiolabel, which frequently allows the label to be followed from one compound to the next, thereby aiding the elucidation of metabolic sequences and culminating in a complete pathway. The order of radiolabelling can be worked out by meticulously visually comparing autoradiographs and quantifying radioactivity in compounds identified by chromatography. The method is particularly effective when combined with enzyme assay and inhibitor studies.

Numerous examples of the application of radiolabelling may be found in standard biochemistry texts such as those indicated in Section 1.10. The classical model is probably the Calvin–Benson photosynthetic carbon reduction cycle (PCRC) in which 3PGA was identified as the first stable product of carboxylation in a process involving a reversal of both the oxidative pentose phosphate pathway (PPP) and the EMP. The crucial discovery was the presence of ^{14}C from $H^{14}CO_3^-$ in the C-1 carboxylate group of 3PGA following carboxylation of ribulose 1,5-bisphosphate by the enzyme ribulose bisphosphate carboxylase oxygenase (Rubisco). ^{14}C later appeared in the C-3 and C-4 atoms of fructose- 1,6-bisphosphate, following aldolase activity, thereby confirming gluconeogenesis as the principal pathway of carbohydrate synthesis in this system. Pulse chase experiments involving $H^{14}CO_3^-$ and HCO_3^- showed that label was lost first from 3PGA and last from ribulose 1,5-bisphosphate, thereby supporting other experimental evidence indicating a direct cyclical relationship between these key molecules in the path of carbon in photosynthesis.

Another example is that the combined operation of the EMP followed by the Krebs cycle, in the complete oxidation of carbohydrates to CO_2 and water, can readily be demonstrated in a model system such as the action of baker's yeast *Saccharomyces cerevisiae* by using separate time course studies involving glucose, specifically labelled with [^{14}C]glucose, in either the C-1, C-2, C-3, C-4, C-5 or C-6 positions and quantitatively measuring $^{14}CO_2$ produced for each specifically labelled glucose molecule in a manometric study (Section 1.3.4). In this case, the order the label appears is as follows: first, $^{14}CO_2$ from C-3 and C-4 (from pyruvate dehydogenase activity) which are identical; second C-2 and C-5 (also identical), which appear only after the second turn of the Krebs cycle (from isocitrate dehydrogenase and α-oxoglutarate dehydrogenase respectively); third, from C-1 and C-6 (also identical), which appear after the third event of the Krebs cycle (from isocitrate dehydrogenase and α-oxoglutarate dehydrogenase). Consequently the C-6/C-1 ratio for CO_2 is close to 1 for the combined operation of these pathways. This compares with a normally much lower C-6/C-1 ratio for CO_2 for the PPP for glucose oxidation, which occurs in tissues such as the lactating mammary gland, owing to the specific release of CO_2 from the C-1 carbon atom of glucose following 6-phosphogluconate decarboxylase activity. The C-6/C-1 ratio for CO_2 in the PPP approximates to 1.0 in longer-term incubations with either [14]C-1 glucose or [14]C-6 glucose owing to recycling of pentose sugars back to glucose, i.e. label will move from the C-6 position to the C-1 position as recycling proceeds, thereby releasing a gradually increasing proportion from the C-6 carbon. Details of the EMP, Krebs cycle and PPP may be found in specialist metabolism texts cited in Section 1.10.

1.3.4 Manometric techniques

Manometry may be used to measure either uptake or evolution of both CO_2 and O_2, whereas O_2 and CO_2 electrodes simply monitor changes in O_2 and CO_2 levels respectively, albeit with greater sensitivity. Manometry also has the distinctive feature of allowing the simultaneous determination of O_2 and CO_2 exchange and has the advantage that the magnitude of the exchange is independent of the partial pressure of the gas at the beginning of the experiment. Studies are carried out in a small flask attached to some form of manometer that measures changes in the amount of gas in the flask. In all types of manometer, the flasks, immersed in a water bath with a temperature control of ± 0.5 deg.C, are shaken mechanically at rates of 100 to 120 oscillations per minute to ensure that respiratory gas exchange is not limited by diffusion of gas into the liquid phase. The total volume of liquid in the flask should generally not exceed 4 cm³ because of gas diffusion limitations. The two principal types of manometer are the Warburg constant volume manometer (Fig. 1.2) and the Gilson constant pressure manometer.

Respiratory quotients (RQ), defined as the relationship between the volume of CO_2 produced and the volume of O_2 consumed during respiration, i.e.

$$RQ = \frac{CO_2 \text{ evolved}}{O_2 \text{ absorbed}} \tag{1.22}$$

may give an indication of the nature of the endogenous substrate being metabolised. The complete oxidation of a simple carbohydrate gives an RQ of 1, whereas a fat gives a value of approximately 0.7 and a protein 0.8. Deviations from these values are sometimes obtained because some CO_2 may be reincorporated into cellular material, lowering the volume of CO_2 evolved. The rate at which an organism or tissue consumes O_2 or evolves CO_2 is expressed by a metabolic quotient Q_x, where X is the gas being measured. Thus Q_{O_2} is defined as the volume of O_2 taken up per milligram dry weight of biological material per hour. In some cases it may be expressed in terms of milligrams of nitrogen (generally determined by the Kjeldahl method (Section 6.3.2)) or milligram of protein or DNA. In such cases it is expressed as follows:

$$Q_{O_2}(N) = mm^3\, O_2\, (mg \text{ tissue N})^{-1}\, h^{-1}$$

Metabolic quotients may also be determined in atmospheres of different or varying gas composition, for example pure N_2, in which case an additional suffix is added to the quotient, thus

$$Q_{CO_2}^{N_2}(N) = mm^3\, CO_2\, (mg \text{ tissue N})^{-1}\, h^{-1} \text{ in an atmosphere of } N_2 \text{ gas}$$

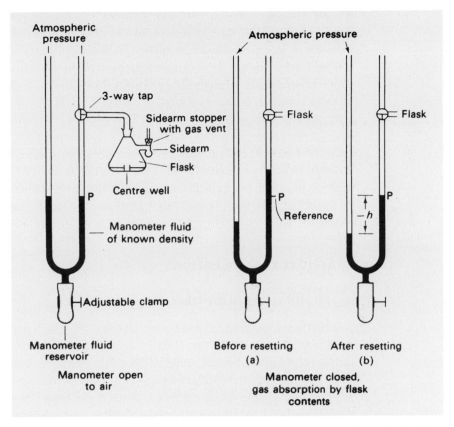

Fig. 1.2. Diagram of a constant volume Warburg manometer. CO_2 gas is being absorbed in the experimental flask and the resulting decrease in pressure forces the fluid level in the right-hand limb to rise and that in the left-hand limb to fall. At regular time intervals the meniscus of the fluid in the left-hand limb is returned to the reference point P by withdrawing fluid into the reservoir using the adjustable clamp, thereby measuring the resultant decrease in pressure $-h$ mm.

The change h is related to the quantity X of gas evolved at s.t.p. by the equation:

$$X = h\left(\frac{V_g\dfrac{273}{T} + V_l\alpha}{P_0}\right)$$

where V_g is the volume of the gas space in the flask, including that of the capillary from the flask to the reference mark P (mm^3); V_l is the volume of liquid in the flask (mm^3); α is the solubility of the gas in the liquid in the flask; T is the temperature of the water bath in K; P_0 is the standard pressure expressed in millimetres of manometric fluid. Since, for a given experimental flask being used to study a particular reaction under defined conditions, all values within the brackets in the equation are constant, $X = kh$, where k is the flask constant. Flask constants for particular manometers are usually supplied by manufacturers or can be obtained by a suitable form of calibration.

If there is a possibility of confusion, the quotients may be cited as positive or negative, indicating the production or removal respectively, of metabolite. Manometric techniques have been applied in studies on tissue slices and homogenates, with attendant problems of homogeneity of gas supply and artefacts, in mitochondrial studies for the study of respiratory control, and in the effect of inhibitors on mitochondrial respiration (although the technique is less sensitive than the O_2 electrode (Section 15.6)). When manometry is used for photosynthetic studies it is necessary to carry out a control determination in darkness and to keep the partial pressure of one gas constant during the experiment. This may be achieved by maintaining a constant partial pressure of CO_2 by using carbonate–bicarbonate buffers or by removing all the O_2 by chemical means. This has limited value, however, since it is known that the rate of CO_2 exchange is dependent on the O_2 content of the atmosphere.

1.4 PRACTICAL CONSIDERATIONS

1.4.1 Health and safety in the laboratory

Scientific work is conducted under a legal framework, which governs not only the health and safety of workers but also the conducting and recording of experiments for protection of intellectual property (IP) rights. Industrial laboratories work to good laboratory practice (GLP) conditions, which specify the organisational process and conditions under which studies are planned, performed, monitored, recorded and repeated. GLP seeks to ensure, as far as possible, the quality and integrity of data for non-clinical laboratory studies. GLP regulations were first published by the USA's Food and Drug Administration (FDA) in 1976. At that time the FDA identified significant problems in the manner in which non-clinical studies were being performed in the USA. Deficiencies were found during inspections of major pharmaceutical firms, private testing facilities and government laboratories. The result of these experiences heralded the birth of GLP. Essential elements of GLP include personnel, management, the responsibilities of study directors, quality assurance, laboratory operations, equipment testing, standard operating procedures (SOPs), reporting and storing in archives, together with other aspects of regulatory compliance. Although academic institutions such as universities operate mainly outside GLP regulations, the model is followed as closely as is practicable. Further details of GLP may be found in the suggestions for further reading (Section 1.10).

Most biochemical work is performed in purpose-built laboratory suites whose ergonomic design is critically important for efficient work and management. Biochemical laboratories are most effectively designed with large centrally sited areas for housing either heavy general equipment (e.g. high speed centrifuges) or stores, wash-up and supportive administrative facilities. Specialised laboratories for weighing, spectrophotometry or various forms of chromatography may also be found in larger departments. Many laboratories are now designed on a flexible modular basis for possible change of purpose. All laboratories are potentially dangerous places to work and therefore eating, drinking, smoking and physical horseplay of any kind are forbidden.

Health and safety for all laboratory workers, has become a key issue in recent years, with government legislation enforcing strict codes of practice. In the UK, for example, detailed COSHH forms (Control of Substances Hazardous to Health) must be completed either by individuals for personal use or by managers in charge of laboratory workers, detailing precisely the experimental procedures and levels of exposure to potentially hazardous chemicals. Toxicity data for potentially hazardous substances are available through a variety of databases. Section 1.10 gives some examples. Many toxicity data are incomplete, however, so great care should be taken in cases of uncertainty. Hazard warning labels are frequently provided by suppliers of laboratory equipment and chemicals. The extent of personal protection necessary will vary according to the nature of the experiment. Safety spectacles and lightweight disposable gloves should be worn at all times, along with buttoned-up laboratory coats. High-necked buttoned gowns must be worn for microbiological work. Heavy-duty leather gloves should be worn either for ultra-low temperature work or for handling highly corrosive liquids. The main physical danger in laboratories comes from fire and smoke, from explosion of volatile solvents and gases, from vacuum implosion of glass vessels, from sources of ionising radiation, from lasers and ultraviolet light and from ultrasonic vibration.

Potential biological hazards also arise from work with laboratory animals, either through allergies or by transmission of certain diseases to humans, from body fluids (especially hepatitis B virus from infected serum), from working either with pathogenic animals or cell tissue cultures and from all microorganisms, including those which may have been genetically engineered. Work with either tissue cultures or microorganisms should, therefore, take place inside safety cabinets in which a sterile air flow moves vertically away from the operator. Manipulative skills in aseptic technique are absolutely essential for all experiments using such models.

Despite even the most stringent attention to good safety practice, accidents do happen and it is very important to have available qualified first-aiders to deal with emergencies. Key telephone numbers for emergency servies should be clearly and conveniently posted. The disposal of unused chemicals, radioactive isotopes and infected material should be subject to clear procedural guidelines and detailed records kept of such disposals. Corrosive chemicals such as acids and alkalis must be neutralised before being washed away down the sink. All organic solvents must be stored in metal drums, with chlorinated solvents stored separately, before chemical incineration at high temperature. Radioactive waste, in particular, is subject to stringent disposal regulations that are legally enforceable. All spent or contaminated tissue or cell cultures or microbial cultures must be sterilised by autoclaving before disposal.

1.4.2 Professional skills

Academic and professional qualifications are particularly important in the employability of biochemists and continuing professional development (c.p.d.) training for employees is becoming the norm for practising biochemists. In the context of the world of work, good personal transferable skills (PTS) are equally as important as technical knowledge and skills for ensuring the efficient working of biochemical laboratories. PTS are needed at all levels, from leaders of research units or heads of quality control sections to students on supervised work experience. PTS skills include listening, learning, speaking, writing, self-management and coping, thinking and group work, together with project management and information retrieval methods. Individual or group project work is probably the first major simulation of the 'world of work' that many undergraduates experience in integrating theory, practical, work, self-management and communication skills. Researchers, in particular, need to become familiar with the range of specialist library facilities and services. Good information retrieval skills are absolutely essential for workers to become aware of new developments impinging on fields of interest. Training should focus on modern methods of retrieval (abstracts/indices, CD-Roms, networking, on-line databases), on types of literature (methods, reviews, patents, statistics, accounts, current awareness, conferences, theses). The overall objective is to develop a critical approach to acquiring relevant information from the plethora available and to develop an awareness of the advantages and limitations of different types of information tools.

Basic manual dexterity and good recording skills are essential for workers to be safe and useful in a laboratory environment. Training involving repeated trials under qualified supervision should be provided before independent work is undertaken and competence demonstrated, for example, in lifting and transporting apparatus, use of gas cylinders, vacuum and compressed air pumps, use of rotary evaporators for concentrating solutions, freeze dryers, small and medium centrifuges, the use of mechanical and electronic balances, pH meters, burettes, pipettes micropipettes and microsyringes, etc.

1.4.3 Units of measurement

The international nature of science demands standardisation of nomenclature and units of measurement to simplify communication. Mathematical formulae and the labelling of elements in biochemicals frequently use letters from the Greek alphabet (Table 1.2), which should be memorised, since they are so common in a biochemist's vocabulary. Many examples taken from Table 1.2 appear, for example, in the various chapters of this book.

The French Système International d'Unités (the SI system) is the accepted convention for units of measurement. Table 1.3 gives some important SI units and Table 1.4 lists physical constants expressed in SI terms. Table 1.5 shows common prefixes to ease expressions for the extremes found in biological systems.

Volumes of liquids used in practical biochemistry are frequently very small. Despite recommendations that they be abandoned in exact scientific work, litres (l), millilitres (ml), microlitres (μl) and nanolitres (nl) not only remain in common usage but are accepted terms for most scientific journals probably because they are easier both to pronounce and to write down than their SI equivalent. Table 1.6 gives some non-SI units of volume and their SI equivalents.

Table 1.2   The Greek alphabet

A	B	Γ	Δ
α	β	γ	δ
alpha	beta	gamma	delta
E	Z	H	Θ
ε	ζ	η	θ
epsilon	zeta	eta	theta
I	K	Λ	M
ι	κ	λ	μ
iota	kappa	lambda	mu
N	Ξ	O	Π
ν	ξ	ο	π
nu	xi	omicron	pi
P	Σ	T	Y
ρ	σ	τ	υ
rho	sigma	tau	upsilon
Φ	X	Ψ	Ω
φ	χ	ψ	ω
phi	chi	psi	omega

Non-SI terms are also to be found in older published work. As a consequence it is important to have some appreciation of the interconversion of units for interpretation. Table 1.7 shows some common units and their SI equivalents. More detailed tables may be found in reference texts cited in Section 1.10.

1.4.4 Preparing and dispensing solutions

Chemicals may be subdivided, in simplified terms, into three classes:

Strong electrolytes	Weak electrolytes	Non-polar hydrophobic
Highly polar substances which ionise completely in an aqueous solvent, e.g. NaCL	Only partially ionise in aqueous solution, e.g. ethanoic (acetic) acid	Substances that dissolve only in organic solvents such as chloroform, e.g. hydrocarbons

Ions will be either positively charged cations or negatively charged anions. Water is very weakly ionised in the forms of the hydroxonium ion (H_3O^+) and hydroxyl ion (OH^-) (see Section 1.4.5). Electrolytes share the common property of conductivity, i.e. the ability to conduct an electric current. Weak electrolytes will partition into a mixture of aqueous and organic solvents according to their relative partition coefficients (Section 8.8). Certain electrolytes, for example the so-called 'neutral' amino acids such as glycine, exist as mixed charge ions (zwitterions) carrying no net charge because they have one charged amino group and one charged carboxylate group when the pH is around 7.0 (Section 6.1). Some small heterocyclic compounds,

Table 1.3 Commonly used SI units, physical quantities and units

Physical quantity	Name of SI unit	Symbol
Length	metre	m
Area	square metre	m^2
Volume	cubic metre	m^3
Time	second	s
Velocity	metres per second	$m\,s^{-1}$
Acceleration	metres per square second	$m\,s^{-2}$
Mass	kilogram	kg
Amount of substance	mole	mol
Concentration	moles per cubic metre	$mol\,m^{-3}$
Density	kilograms per cubic metre	$kg\,m^{-3}$
Temperature	kelvin	K
Pressure	pascal	Pa
Electric charge	coulomb	C
Electric current	ampere	A
Electric potential difference	volt	V
Electric resistance	ohm	Ω
Electric field strength	volts per metre	$V\,m^{-1}$
Electric capacitance	farad	F
Wavelength	metre	m
Luminous intensity	candela	cd
Force	newton	N
Energy	joule	J
Power	watt	W
Frequency	hertz	Hz
Magnetic flux density	tesla	T
Magnetic field strength	amperes per metre	$A\,m^{-1}$
Dipole moment	coulomb metre	C m
	bequerel	Bq
	curie	ci

Table 1.4 Values for some physical constants in SI units

Avogadro's number (molecules per mole, N)	6.0225×10^{23}
Boltzmann constant (k)	$1.38 \times 10^{-23}\,J\,K^{-1}$
Dalton (atomic mass unit, Da)	1.661×10^{24}
Elementary charge (of proton) (e)	$1.602 \times 10^{-19}\,C$
Faraday constant (F)	$9.648 \times 10^{4}\,C\,mol^{-1}$
Molar or universal gas constant (R)	$8.314\,J\,mol^{-1}\,K^{-1}$
Molar volume of an ideal gas at standard temperature and pressure (s.t.p.)	$22.41\,dm^3\,mol^{-1}$
Planck constant (h)	$6.626 \times 10^{-34}\,J\,s$
Velocity of light in a vacuum (c)	$2.998 \times 10^{8}\,m\,s^{-1}$

Table 1.5 Common unit prefixes associated with quantitative terms

Multiple	Prefix	Symbol
10^{18}	exa	E
10^{15}	peta	P
10^{12}	tera	T
10^{9}	giga	G
10^{6}	mega	M
10^{3}	kilo	k
10^{2}	hecto	h
10^{1}	deca	da
10^{-1}	deci	d
10^{-2}	centi	c
10^{-3}	milli	m
10^{-6}	micro	μ
10^{-9}	nano	n
10^{-12}	pico	p
10^{-15}	femto	f
10^{-18}	atto	α

Table 1.6 Interconversion of non-SI and SI units of volume

1 litre (l)	10^{3} ml	= 1 dm^{3}	= 10^{-3} m^{3}
1 millilitre (ml)	1 ml	= 1 cm^{3}	= 10^{-6} m^{3}
1 microlitre (μl)	10^{-3} ml	= 1 mm^{3}	= 10^{-9} m^{3}
1 nanolitre (nl)	10^{-6} ml	= 1 nm^{3}	= 10^{-12} m^{3}

Table 1.7 Conversion factors for changing common units to their SI equivalents

Unit	Symbol	SI equivalent
ångström	A	10^{-10} m
inch	in.	0.0254 m
ounce	oz	28.3 g
pound	lb	0.4536 kg
Centigrade degree	°C	$(t\,°C + 273)$ K
		$[(5/9)(°F - 32)]°$
millimetres of mercury	mmHg (torr)	133.322 Pa
atmosphere	atm	101 325 Pa
bar	bar	10^{5} Pa
pounds force per square inch	lbf in.$^{-2}$	6894.76 Pa
calorie	cal	4.186 J
erg	erg	10^{-7} J
electron volt	eV	1.602×10^{-19} J
ln x (natural logarithm of x)	ln x	2.303 $\log_{10} x$ (logarithm to the base 10)
curie	Ci	3.7×10^{10} Bq

having a ring structure to which hydroxyl groups are attached, are also soluble in water, for example soluble sugars such as glucose or sucrose. Section 1.10 cites texts that give an in-depth coverage of solution properties and the importance of water as the biological milieu.

Concentrations are expressed most commonly in terms of weight by volume (w/v) in which a given amount of solid is dissolved in a solvent to a fixed total volume, including the solute. Various units of concentration are therefore possible, for example $mg\,cm^{-3}$, $g\,dm^{-3}$, etc. If the concentration is very low it is common for either parts per million (p.p.m.) or parts per billion (p.p.b.) to be used, the assumption being made that the density of water approximates to $1\,g\,cm^{-3}$. Gas mixture concentrations are expressed as p.p.m. or p.p.b. on a volume/total volume basis.

Molarity (M) is another very common expression of concentration. It expresses the number of moles of a substance that are present in a given volume of solution. A mole of a substance in grams (the gram mole) is numerically equal to its molecular mass. Thus, for sodium chloride, which has a molecular mass of 58.5 daltons (from atomic weights: Na = 23 daltons, Cl = 35.5 daltons) one mole is 58.5 g. A 1 M solution of a substance contains one mole of the substance in 1 litre of solution. In the case of sodium chloride, a 1 M solution therefore contains 58.5 g in 1 litre of solution. The concept of molarity can be applied to pure water (H_2O) to calculate its molarity. Since water has a molecular mass of 18 daltons, from the definition of molarity above, the molarity of water is equal to 1000/18 or 55.6 M, since 1 litre of water weighs 1000 g. Less frequently solutions are expressed as weight/weight (w/w), in which case a fixed mass of solvent is added to dissolve the solute.

Solutions of equal molarity contain an identical number of molecules, defined by Avogadro's number, and as a consequence have some identical physiological properties such as osmotic pressure (water potential), depression of freezing point of water, and elevation of the boiling point of water. Equally importantly, one mole of any substance in the gas phase occupies $22.4\,dm^3$ at standard temperature (273 K) and pressure ($1.05 \times 10^5\,Pa$).

It is important to note that although atomic mass and molecular mass are both expressed in daltons, biochemists very commonly prefer to use the term relative molecular mass (M_r), which is defined as the ratio of the molecular mass of a molecule relative to one-twelfth of the mass of ^{12}C isotope. M_r therefore has no units. This topic of relative molecular mass is discussed further in Question 5 in Section 5.13, and in Chapter 11, p. 555.

Biological substances are found most frequently at very low concentrations and the volumes taken for analysis are very small; as a consequence the units mM, μM and nM are often more pertinent in biochemistry than M. Table 1.8 is included as an *aide-mémoire* for interconversion of units for the preparation of solutions.

Simple dilutions of concentrated solutions may be made either using the dilution formula $M_1V_1 = M_2V_2$ where M_1 and M_2 represent the initial and final molarities and V_1 and V_2 represent the initial and final volumes, where three of the variables are known. In many cases, however, first principles are best applied from manipulating terms shown in Table 1.8.

Some examples of preparing solutions of different concentrations follow.

| Table 1.8 | Interconversion of mol, mmol and μmol in different volumes to give different concentrations | |

M	mM	μM
1 mol dm^{-3}	1 mmol dm^{-3}	1 μmol dm^{-3}
1 mmol cm^{-3}	1 μmol cm^{-3}	1 nmol cm^{-3}
1 μmol mm^{-3}	1 nmol mm^{-3}	1 pmol mm^{-3}

Example 8

An incubation medium to prepare ribosomes from wheatgerm contains 90 mM potassium chloride, 2 mM calcium chloride, 1 mM magnesium acetate, 6 mM potassium bicarbonate. How is 100 cm³ of this solution prepared given that the molecular masses of these compounds are: KCl 74.55 daltons, $CaCl_2.6H_2O$ 219.08 daltons, $Mg(CH_3COO)_2.4H_2O$ 214.46 daltons, $KHCO_3$ 100.1 daltons?

Answer

Remember that a 1 mM solution contains 1 mmol dm^{-3} or 1 μmol cm^{-3} or 0.1 mmol per 100 cm³ (see Table 1.8 for these important conversions) and that a millimole of a substance, in milligrams, is numerically equal to one-tenth of the molecular mass.

The required amounts are therefore:

$$\text{potassium chloride} = 90 \times 7.455 \text{ mg} = 670.95 \text{ mg}$$

$$\text{calcium chloride} = 2 \times 21.908 \text{ mg} = 43.82 \text{ mg}$$

$$\text{magnesium acetate} = 1 \times 21.45 \text{ mg} = 21.45 \text{ mg}$$

$$\text{potassium bicarbonate} = 6 \times 10.01 \text{ mg} = 60.06 \text{ mg}$$

These quantities are dissolved in a minimal volume of water and the solution made up to 100 cm³ in a measuring cylinder. Volumetric flasks introduce unnecessary accuracy for this type of experiment.

Example 9

A 0.1 mM solution of *p*-nitrophenol (PNP) requires dilutions to give a maximum amount of 2 μmol in 5 cm⁻³ of a borate buffer and three intermediate amounts to prepare a calibration curve to verify the Beer–Lambert law (Section 9.4.1). How is a table prepared for this experiment, showing volumes of reagents used, amounts of PNP added and concentrations of PNP, expressed in μM?

Answer

0.1 mM PNP solution contains 0.1 μmol cm^{-3}.
2 cm³ of 0.1 mM PNP would therefore contain 0.2 μmol.
The reagent blank would not contain any PNP.

$$0.2 \text{ μmol PNP per 5 cm}^3 \text{ is equivalent to } \frac{0.2}{5} \text{ μmol cm}^{-3} = 0.04 \text{ μmol cm}^{-3}$$

$$= 0.04 \text{ mM} = 40 \text{ μM}$$

A typical table would therefore be represented as:

0.1 mM PNP (cm³)	Borate buffer (cm³)	μmol PNP	mM PNP
0	5.0	0	0
0.5	4.5	0.05	10
1.0	4.0	0.10	20
1.5	3.5	0.15	30
2.0	3.0	0.20	40

The solutions would be prepared in at least duplicate for the experiment.

Example 10

When carrying out *in vitro* protein synthesis the following mixture is to be prepared:

Phosphate buffer	30 μl
1.0 M KCl	19 μl
0.3 M dithiothreitol	3 μl
0.01 GTP	1 μl
Distilled water	10 μl
Amino acid mixture	10 μl
mRNA (10 μg)	20 μl
Ribosome solution	125 μl

Sufficient magnesium acetate solution (M_r 214.46) has to be added to give a final volume of 260 μl and a Mg^{2+} concentration of 6 mM. How much and what concentration of magnesium acetate solution should be added? How many micrograms of magnesium acetate is being added? How many milligrams of magnesium acetate is needed to make up 1 cm³ of a stock solution of the required molarity?

Answer

The combined volume of the mixture without the magnesium is 238 μl, which means that 22 μl of magnesium acetate solution must contain sufficient Mg^{2+} to give a final concentration of 6 mM. The concentration of magnesium acetate solution (x mM) may be found by applying the dilution formula $M_1V_1 = M_2V_2$.

Hence x mM × 22 μl = 6 mM × 260 μl

$$x = 70.91 \text{ mM}$$

22 μl of a 70.91 mM solution contains $22 \times 70.91 \times 10^{-6} \times 214.46$ μg magnesium acetate = 0.3346 μg. A 1 cm³ stock solution of magnesium acetate would contain $1 \times 70.91 \times 214.46$ μg = 15.21 mg.

Delivering volumes of solutions with the accuracy and precision pertinent to a particular experimental model is a core skill. In this context, 'accuracy' refers to the difference between the desired volume and the volume actually delivered, and 'precision' to the reproducibility of delivery. Various types of pipette are available for different purposes. For example, transfer or bulb pipettes deliver a fixed volume and are more accurate than graduated pipettes. For safety reasons, automatic fillers must always be used with pipettes. Small volumes, in the 1 to 1000 μl range, are conveniently delivered using an adjustable volume micropipette fitted with disposable plastic tips. Microsyringes, on the other hand, deliver volumes as low as 1 μl and have graduated divisions of 0.01 μl. The Hamilton microsyringe is the most common type of graduated ultra low volume pipette, with an accuracy of approximately 1%. Repetitive volumes of solution may often be delivered, without loss of accuracy or precision, from a burette or microburette. Automated devices for volume delivery are now common in laboratories.

1.4.5 pH and buffer solutions

The intracellular environment of cells is essentially aqueous. Water has many important chemical and physical properties, not least of which is its very slight tendency to ionise as hydroxonium ions (H_3O^+) and hydroxyl ions (OH^-). When an H_2O molecule binds a proton to form H_3O^+ it is acting as a base, whereas when it forms OH^- it is acting as an acid.

The equilibrium constant for H_2O ionisation is

$$K_{eq} = \frac{[H^+][OH^-]}{[H_2O]} = 1.8 \times 10^{-16}\,M$$

where concentrations are expressed in molarity.

H_2O has been shown to be 55 M in Section 1.4.4 and therefore

$$[1.8 \times 10^{-16}][55] = [H^+][OH^-]$$
$$1 \times 10^{-14}\,M^2 = [H^+][OH^-]$$

$1 \times 10^{-14}\,M^2$ is known as the ion product of water (K_W) which is constant.

Electrolytes that react with water to increase the proportion of OH^- are bases, whereas acids increase the proportion of H^+. Pure water is electrically neutral, i.e. $[H^+] = [OH^-] = 10^{-7}\,M$. A convenient term for expressing concentrations of H^+ is as its negative logarithm (pH), i.e. $pH = -\log[H^+]$. By the same token pOH is $-\log[OH^-]$ and therefore $pH + pOH = 14$. For example a $10^{-3}\,M$ solution of an acid completely dissociated in water would have a pH of 3 and a ten-fold difference in the concentration of H^+ would mean a difference of 1 in pH.

Organisms and cells can generally withstand large variations in the pH of their external environment. In contrast, cellular processes are sensitive to pH changes and take place in a medium the pH of which is carefully regulated. There may, however, be localised intracellular pH variations, for example at membrane surfaces. The majority of intracellullar processes occur at a pH maintained near neutrality. This neutral pH is generally the one at which the various metabolic processes occur at their maximum rate. The hydrolases of lysosomes, however, have their maximum activity at a pH in the region of 5, a pH that prevails following the death of the cell. The gastric juice of mammals is quite exceptional in having a pH of approximately 1. The enzyme pepsin, which initiates the digestion of dietary proteins in the stomach, has its maximum activity at pH 1.

The control of a virtually constant pH in biological systems is achieved by the action of efficient buffering systems, the chemical nature of which is such that they can resist pH changes due to the metabolic production of acids such as lactic acid and bases such as ammonium. The major buffering systems found in cellular fluids involve phosphate, bicarbonate, amino acids and proteins.

The sensitivity of biological processes to pH may be due to one of several reasons. The process may be catalysed by H^+ or may involve an H^+ as a reactant or product. Alternatively, a pH change may alter the distribution of a compound or ion across a membrane, possibly by altering the permeability of the membrane. Membranes, like many other biological structures and molecules, possess ionisable groups the precise state of ionisation of which influences their molecular conformation and thus their biological activity. This is particularly true of proteins and thus of enzymes. Some proteins rely on a slight change in the pH of their environment to complete their biological function. In the case of haemoglobin, whose primary function is to transport oxygen from the lungs to the tissues, a slight decrease in the pH of the tissues, due to carbon dioxide and hydrogen ion production as a result of the active respiration of the tissue, helps to facilitate the unloading of the oxygen when and where it is required. The unloading of oxygen is accompanied by the uptake of protons by the haemoglobin, thus simultaneously helping to buffer the system. *In vitro* studies of metabolic processes require the use of buffers. Deliberate changes in pH, however, may help in the analytical study of certain groups of molecules, for example amino acids, proteins and nucleic acids, by such techniques as electrophoresis and ion-exchange chromatography.

A buffer solution resists change in hydrogen ion concentration on the addition of acid or alkali. This resistance is called the buffer action. The magnitude of the buffer action is called the buffer capacity (β), and is measured by the amount of strong base required to alter the pH by one unit:

$$\beta = \frac{db}{d(pH)} \tag{1.23}$$

where d(pH) is the increase in pH resulting from the addition db of base.

In practice, buffer solutions usually consist of a mixture of a weak acid or base and its salt, for example acetic acid and sodium acetate (in the Brönsted and Lowry nomenclature, a mixture of a weak acid and its conjugate base). In a solution of a weak acid (RCOOH) and its salt (RCOO$^-$), added H^+ are neutralised by the anions of the salt, which act, therefore, as a weak base, and, conversely, added OH$^-$ are removed by neutralisation of the acid. It is clear from this that the buffer capacity of a particular acid and its conjugate based will be a maximum when their concentrations are equal, i.e. when pH = pK_a of the acid. Buffer capacity also depends upon the total concentrations of acid and salt as well on their relative proportions

– the greater the total concentration, the greater the buffer capacity. The usual concentration of acid and salt in buffer solutions is of the order of 0.05–0.20 M and generally the mixtures posses acceptable buffer capacity within the range $pH = pK_a \pm 1$. The criteria for buffers suitable for use in biological research may be summarised as follows. They should

   (i) possess adequate buffer capacity in the required pH range;
  (ii) be available in a high degree of purity;
 (iii) be very water soluble and impermeable to biological membranes;
 (iv) be enzymically and hydrolytically stable;
  (v) possess a pH that is minimally influenced by their concentration, the temperature and the ionic composition or salt effect of the medium;
 (vi) not be toxic;
(vii) only form complexes with cations that are soluble;
(viii) not absorb light in the visible or ultraviolet regions.

Needless to say, not all buffers that are commonly used meet all these criteria. Phosphates tend to precipitate polyvalent cations and are often metabolites or inhibitors in many systems and Tris is often toxic or may have inhibitory effects. However, a number of zwitterionic buffers of the Hepes and Pipes type fulfil the requirements and are often used in tissue culture media containing sodium bicarbonate or phosphate solutions as nutrients. They suffer from the disadvantage that they interfere with Lowry protein determinations.

Physiologically, proteins comprise an important group of buffers. By virtue of their large numbers of weak acidic and basic groups in the amino acid side-chains, proteins have a very high buffer capacity. For example, haemoglobin is the main compound responsible for the buffering capacity of blood.

Some commonly used buffers are listed in Table 1.9. To obtain buffer solutions covering an extended pH range, but derived from the same ions, mixtures of different systems may be used. The McIlvaine buffers cover the pH range 2.2 to 8.0 and are prepared from citric acid and disodium hydrogen phosphate.

The state of ionisation of a weak electrolyte is dependent upon the prevailing pH and the numerical value of its ionisation constant. For weak acids, which ionise according to the equation

$RCOOH = RCOO^- + H^+$
acid   conjugate
            base

the ionisation constant K_a is given by the expression:

$$K_a = \frac{[RCOO^-][H^+]}{[RCOOH]} \tag{1.24}$$

In the case of weak bases such as amines, which ionise according to the equation:

$RNH_2 + H_2O = RNH_3^+ + OH^-$
base   conjugate
              acid

Table 1.9 pK_a values of some acids and bases that are commonly used as buffer solutions

Acid or base	pK_a (at 25 °C)
Acetic acid	4.75
Barbituric acid	3.98
Carbonic acid	6.10, 10.22
Citric acid	3.10, 4.76, 5.40
Glycylglycine	3.06, 8.13
Hepes[a]	7.50
Phosphoric acid	1.96, 6.70, 12.30
Phthalic acid	2.90, 5.51
Pipes[a]	6.80
Succinic acid	4.18, 5.56
Tartaric acid	2.96, 4.16
Tris[a]	8.14

[a] See List of abbreviations at the front of this volume.

the ionisation constant may be expressed in terms of a K_b value:

$$K_b = \frac{[RNH_3^+][OH^-]}{[RNH_2][H_2O]} \tag{1.25}$$

or more commonly in terms of the K_a value of the conjugate acid:

$$K_a = \frac{[RNH_2][H^+]}{[RNH_3^+]} \tag{1.26}$$

In such cases, the product of K_a and K_b for a weak base is equal to K_W, the ion product of water.

In practice, since K_a values are numerically very small, it is customary to use pK_a values, where p$K_a = -\log_{10}K_a$. It follows that, for weak bases, pK_a + pK_b = 14. The precise way in which the state of ionisation of a weak electrolyte varies with pH is given by the Henderson–Hasselbalch equation. For a weak acid, this takes the form

$$pH = pK_a + \log\left(\frac{[\text{conjugate base}]}{[\text{acid}]}\right)$$

$$\text{or } pH = pK_a + \log\left(\frac{[\text{ionised form}]}{[\text{unionised form}]}\right) \tag{1.27}$$

In the case of a weak base, expressing the equation in terms of the ionisation of the conjugate acid we obtain

$$pH = pK_a + \log\left(\frac{[\text{base}]}{[\text{conjugate acid}]}\right)$$

$$\text{or } pH = pK_a + \log\left(\frac{[\text{unionised form}]}{[\text{ionised form}]}\right) \tag{1.28}$$

It can be appreciated from these equations that weak acids will be predominantly unionised at low pH values and ionised at high pH values. The exact opposite is the case for weak bases; at low pH values the conjugate acid will predominate and at high pH values the unionised free base will exist. This sensitivity to pH of the state of ionisation of weak electrolytes is important both physiologically, as for example in the absorption by passive difussion from the gastrointestinal tract of weak electrolytes and their excretion by the kidney, and in investigations *in vitro* employing such techniques as electrophoresis and ion-exchange chromatography. A few calculations on pH and buffers are set out below to illustrate the principles involved.

Example 11 Calculate the pH obtained by dissolving 1.025 g of anhydrous sodium acetate (M_r 82) in 100 cm^3 of 0.25 M acetic acid, given that the pK_a of acetic acid is 4.75.

Answer The concentration of acetate is 10.25 g dm^{-3} = 0.125 M, which when applied in the Henderson–Hasselbalch equation gives

$$pH = pK_a + \log\left(\frac{[\text{acetate}]}{[\text{acetic acid}]}\right)$$

$$= 4.75 + \log\left(\frac{0.125}{0.250}\right)$$

$$= 4.75 - 0.30$$

$$= 4.45$$

In this example the concentration of acetic acid is taken to be 0.250 M because its ionisation as a weak electrolyte is insignificant.

Example 12 How many grams of solid NaH_2PO_4 and Na_2HPO_4 are needed to prepare 1 dm^3 of 0.1 M phosphate buffer, pH 7.1, given pK_{a2} = 6.8 and the atomic weights Na = 23, P = 31 and O = 16.

Answer The calculation is concerned only with

$$H_2PO_4^- \rightleftharpoons HPO_4^{2-} + H^+$$

for which pK_{a2} = 6.8.

Hence, $7.1 = 6.8 + \log\left(\dfrac{[HPO_4^{2-}]}{[H_2PO_4^-]}\right)$

$$0.3 = \log\left(\frac{[HPO_4^{2-}]}{[H_2PO_4^-]}\right)$$

$$2.0 = \left(\frac{[HPO_4^{2-}]}{[H_2PO_4^-]}\right)$$

Since the total concentration of HPO_4^{2-} plus $H_2PO_4^-$ is 0.1 M, $[HPO_4^{2-}]$ is 0.067 moles and $[H_2PO_4^-]$ is 0.033 moles, respectively; i.e. $[HPO_4^{2-}]$ is (0.067×142) g = 9.46g and $[H_2PO_4^-]$ is (0.033×120) g = 4.00 g.

1.4.6 **Physiological solutions**

Physiological solutions may be classified broadly according to their use for short-term incubations, supporting long-term growth of microbes, plant or animal tissue cultures, or for nutritional studies involving whole animals and plants. The chemical and physical properties of physiological solutions are designed to minimise artefacts and their chemical composition is sometimes based on reformulating mixtures identified by prior biochemical analysis of natural fluids. Occasionally a medium is formulated empirically. Chemically defined solutions are preferable but not always possible because of the very stringent growth requirements of many tissue cultures. Crucial factors are maintaining the medium isotonic with the tissue (i.e. possessing the same water potential) and buffering to a physiological pH.

1.5 *IN VIVO* MODELS

In vivo techniques apply to multicellular organisms and use either whole animals or parts of animals in which isolated organs are perfused with nutrients or whole plants or parts of plants suspended in a physiological solution.

1.5.1 **Animal studies**

The use of animals for biochemical experiments *in vivo* is extensive, since alternative model techniques such as cell culture are often considered physiologically too simplistic to meet the needs of the investigation. Animals are used for fundamental research, for medical and clinical research, for veterinary and agricultural research, in the manufacture of vaccines, antibodies and hormones, for testing the potency of drugs or other biological products where chemical determination is not feasible, and also for toxicological testing. Much animal work is directed towards the study of the metabolism of xenobiotics (drugs, food additives) and extrapolation of results to humans as a prerequisite to clinical trials. Mice, rats and guinea-pigs are most commonly used because of their lower cost and east of handling, but rabbits, cats, dogs and primates are also used. The animals are bred specifically for experimental purposes and in the UK their husbandry is subject to scrutiny by the Home Office Inspectorate, who issues vivisection licences for work involving live vertebrates. Biological strain, age, sex, nutritional state, circadian rhythms and stress state of the animals all have to be closely regulated to minimise variability in results. Experiments are normally performed, therefore, on small groups of animals, as physiologically similar as possible, and the collated results analysed statistically. When metabolic responses to xenobiotics are being monitored, the results obtained must be compared with a control group that has received a placebo (a completely inert substance such as lactose). In humans or laboratory animals the fate of an administered compound, the xenobiotic, can be traced by monitoring the concentrations of the compound and/or its metabolites in blood, urine, faeces, bile, expired air, sweat or saliva. Excretion patterns of small laboratory animals are best studied by placing the animal in a metabolic cage for the duration of the experiment. Such cages allow urine and faeces to be collected separately and expired carbon dioxide to be trapped. If ^{14}C-labelled compounds are used, the cage is supplied with CO_2-free air and the expired $^{14}CO_2$ absorbed in sodium hydroxide solution. The assay of $^{14}CO_2$ expired allows an estimate of the extent of complete degradation of the compound to be made. Since many excretion products in urine and faeces are conjugated (i.e. linked to polar molecules such as glucuronic acid, sulphate and glycine), it is essential that samples are hydrolysed, enzymically or chemically, before the free metabolites are extracted and identified by established analytical techniques such as gas–liquid chromatography (GLC) and high-performance liquid chromatography (HPLC).

The technique of whole-body autoradiography (Section 14.2.3) has proved very useful as a method of visualising the distribution of radioactive materials administered to small animals. Experimental information on distribution, relative accumulation in tissues, rates of excretion and ability to cross biological membranes is obtainable by this technique. At a suitable time interval after injection with a radioactively labelled compound, the animal is killed by anaesthetisation and cooled rapidly in an acetone–solid CO_2 mixture at $-78\,°C$ or in liquid N_2 (less than $-195\,°C$). The frozen animal is embedded in an aqueous solution of resin (gum acacia) at low temperature. After the resin has set, the animal's body may either be sliced by machine to a suitable level with a blade attached to an electric drill, or serial sections made using a microtome which has a special tungsten carbide blade. The prepared animal surface is placed in close contact with X-ray film at a low temperature for one to two weeks after which time the film is developed (see Fig. 14.12).

The fate of a compound in a living laboratory animal may also be studied through the vascular perfusion of an attached organ such as the liver or kidney. This procedure involves infusing the compound through a fine hollow needle inserted into the artery carrying blood to the organ and performing subsequent analysis on the blood being transported from that organ by the corresponding vein.

Ethical issues surrounding whole animal experimentation are leading to increased effort being directed towards finding suitable alternatives as well as reducing the number of animals used for essential experimentation. The main approach being increasingly adopted is to change to *in vitro* methods where appropriate. A guide to alternative animal experimentation is listed in Section 1.10.

1.5.2 Plant studies

Higher plants have traditionally been used to further basic understanding of the biochemistry of fundamental processes such as pathways for photosynthesis, respiration, photorespiration, nitrogen assimilation, etc., which are aspects of primary metabolism relating to ATP and pyridine nucleotide turnover. Increasingly, however, plants are now being used for 'applied' research in fields such as plant breeding, plant pathology, food research, environmental pollution, xenobiotic testing and in the search for so-called secondary products. These secondary products are part of biochemical pathways not concerned primarily with energy production and conservation but which have been shown occasionally to have considerable economic importance as pharmaceuticals, pigments, perfumes and natural agrochemicals. Much of the future of plant biochemistry is now clearly associated with using molecular biological techniques to clone genes involved in secondary product synthesis for expression in microbial hosts (Section 3.3). Progress with this has been held back by the relative paucity of knowledge of secondary metabolism and its regulation in plants.

Methods for studying the metabolism of whole plants depends on the objectives of the experiment. Whole plants may be grown either outside in field plots or in more controlled environments inside glasshouses or environmental cabinets, where factors such as temperature, light, relative humidity (RH) and gaseous environment can be controlled within specified limits. Any test compound may be added to either relatively ill-defined compost or to sand/rockwool mixtures when plants are grown hydroponically in chemically defined nutrient solutions. The mineral composition of a nutrient solution supporting the hydroponic growth of plants is qualitatively similar to that used for microorganisms except that it usually contains additional essential microelements such as Mn^{2+}, B^{2+}, Zn^{2+}, Cu^{2+} and Mo^{2+}. Test compounds may be injected into roots, included in the rhizosphere or applied to foliage by painting or spraying. Dilute organic solvents and mild detergents promote uptake through the waxy cuticle. Gaseous uptake proceeds through open stomata under conducive RH conditions. The subsequent distribution of the compound proceeds either locally by plasmodesmata or over longer distance through the vascular system. Radiolabelling techniques may be conveniently used for metabolic investigations. A major difficulty in studying plant metabolism in general is that plant organs do not contain enzymes in such high concentrations as animal organs because the metabolic rate of plants is usually lower.

1.6 *IN VITRO* MODELS

In vitro methods involve the incubation of biologically derived material in artificial physical and chemical environments. The term *in vitro* is equally applicable to enzyme preparations, to isolated organelles, to intact microorganisms and to excised parts of animals and plants. Conditions may be chosen to promote a limited degree of growth, differentiation and development, as for instance in cell, tissue and organ culture. The specific advantage of cell and tissue culture methods is that they reduce the physiological and biochemical constraints imposed by contiguous cells. The methodology has found widespread application in the biosciences. In its most fundamental sense, cell culture facilitates the investigation of the developmental potential (totipotency) of cells, i.e. the capacity, within the limits of its genetic constitution, of one cell to form any other type of cell, given an appropriate artificial chemical and physical environment. A general criticism of experimentation *in vitro* is that it is the study of artefacts and extrapolation to the situation *in vivo* may be unjustified.

1.6.1 **Homogenates**

The simplest type of *in vitro* model for multicellular organisms is a homogenate. Homogenisation simply disrupts the tissue and releases intracellular compounds to form a brei. Such crude mixtures may be useful directly in enzyme assays or for studies where uptake of a metabolite or a xenobiotic into intact tissue may be difficult, but frequently homogenisation is used as a preliminary step for partial purification of cellular organelles to investigate metabolic compartmentalisation.

The choice of tissue, the physical and chemical properties of physiological solutions used and the choice of cell disruption method employed in practice is very important for successful homogenisation. Methods for disrupting cells and tissues are considered in Section 6.3.3. The biological material should be rich in specific organelles and be very active in the particular metabolic pathways of interest. Fresh liver or cauliflower curd, for example, are excellent model animal and plant tissues for crude mitochondrial preparations, whereas hepatocytes are good sources of liposomes, and thymus tissue is excellent for nuclear isolations. The specific activity of key enzymes can be used to assess the quality of the preparation. The first route to finding a suitable medium in which to suspend tissue for homogenisation is to consult the literature. If this fails, trial experiments using a range of media have to be carried out. In addition to a buffered, balanced salt solution, media usually contain a carbon source. Sucrose is used commonly to provide sufficient osmotic potential to prevent organelles swelling and bursting but it interferes with certain enzyme assays and is sometimes replaced with either mannitol or sorbitol, which is usually metabolised very slowly by plant and animal tissues. Many different recipes are used to try to preserve organelle and metabolic integrity, sometimes by preventing enzyme inactivation. As well as maintaining isoosmotic conditions and an appropriate pH, critical levels of certain inorganic ions may also be important. For example Mg^{2+} help to maintain both nuclear and ribosome integrity. On the other hand, chelating agents such as EDTA or EGTA may be added to remove divalent cations such as Mg^{2+} or Ca^{2+} when it is important to inactivate membrane proteases. Inhibitors such as di-isopropylphosphofluoridate (for serine residues) or *N*-ethylmaleimide (for sulphydryl groups) may be included in extraction media to inhibit protease activity. Alternatively, artificial protease substrates such as bovine serum albumin (BSA) may also be added to ameliorate protease activity.

Many enzymes need to be maintained with their sulphydryl groups in a reduced state, which means adding reducing agents to the extraction medium such as 2-mercaptoethanol, dithiothreitol, reduced glutathione or cysteine, at concentrations around 30 mM. Polyvinylpyrrolidone either in water-soluble form or as the cross-linked polymer Polyclar may be added to a medium to remove phenolics by filtration. An organic-based aqueous medium is sometimes preferred to salt solutions in tissue extractions. For example, citrate has been used in the isolation of nuclei because of its ability to inactivate neutral deoxyribonucleases, and glycerol, ethyleneglycol and ethyleneglycol polymers have been used for preparation of plastids. A non-aqueous medium may also be used in the isolation of organelles. The suspending fluid is usually a blend of a light and heavy organic solvent such as ether–chloroform or benzene–carbon tetrachloride. The density of the medium can be varied so that the required organelles either float or sediment from the remainder of the homogenate in the subsequent centrifugation states (Section 5.9). Non-aqueous fractionation procedures have been used, for example in the preparation of chloroplasts and also of haemosiderin granules from spleen. The technique does have some disadvantages in that morphological alterations may occur in some tissues and most enzymes are inactivated by organic solvents.

1.6.2 Organ and tissue slice techniques

In perfusion of isolated organs such as liver, kidney or heart, the organ is first removed from a recently killed animal and maintained at constant temperature in suitable apparatus. The metabolic fate of the perfused compound in the organ may then be determined as for *in vivo* perfusion. The perfusion fluid may be passed through the organ either by gravity feed or by using a small pump. If the perfusion fluid is recirculated, pumps must be used. The flow of fluid through the organ is usually achieved with peristaltic pumps, which ensure a pulsatile flow that closely resembles the type of flow produced by the heart.

Superfusion is a simpler technique in which the incubation fluid simply trickles over the surface of the organs which are suspended in a bath. When mechanical responses of isolated tissue are being investigated, clamped organs are attached to a force transducer that 'reads' tissue movement. Electrophysiological techniques may also be used for organs such as brains or muscle, in which case microelectrodes attached to tissue detect voltage changes across membranes that are detected on an oscilloscope or similar recording device.

Slice techniques utilise tissue slices thin enough to enable oxygen to reach the innermost layers of the slice and also allow adequate removal of waste products by diffusion. Slices 0.5 to 5 mm thick generally meet the above requirements whilst allowing the proportion of disrupted cells to intact cells to remain small. The organ under study should be removed immediately after the animal is killed in order to minimise any postmortem changes. Cutting of the slices is done by using razor blades, or, for more uniform preparations, using a microtome. The tissue slices are transferred to a vessel containing a suitable suspending medium. The metabolism of the slices may then be studied and the effects of added compounds on the metabolic processes determined. Slices need 95% oxygen to be used in the gas phase in order to achieve aeration of the innermost cells of the slices. An obvious disadvantage of this technique, however, is that by trying to ensure adequate diffusion of oxygen to the innermost cells of the slices, toxic concentrations of oxygen may be in contact with the outer layers of cells. Figure 1.3 illustrates the use of rat liver slices in a dynamic agar culture system for the study of rat hepatic drug metabolism.

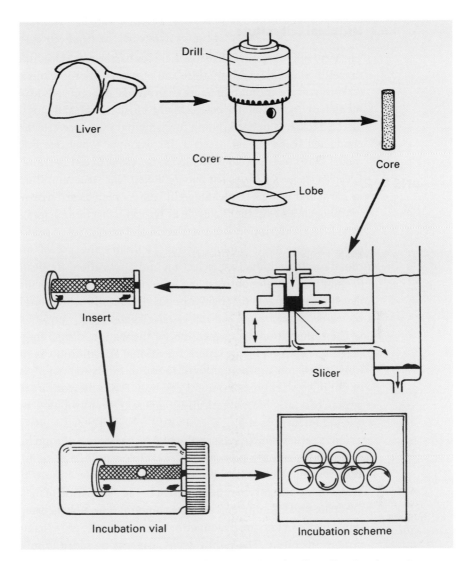

Fig. 1.3. Schematic representation of the preparation of rat liver slices in a dynamic organ culture system. *Slice preparation*: the slices are produced by pulling an immobilised core across a motor-driven oscillating blade. The thickness of the slices produced is controlled by a combination of the distance between an adjustable plate at the bottom of the holder and the weight applied to the piston on top of the tissue core. Freshly sectioned slices, produced at a rate of one every 3 to 4 s are swept away to a collecting chamber by a stream of buffer. (Reproduced, with permission, from Barr, J., Weir, A. J., Brendel, K. and Sipes, I. G. (1991) *Xenobiotica*, **3**, 331–9.)

1.6.3 **Microbial cell culture**

The term microorganism usually includes bacteria, fungi, actinomycetes, yeasts, unicellular and filamentous algae and protozoa. Microorganisms grown in pure (axenic) culture are simpler to use than animal or plant cells in culture for experimental or industrial purposes. Many biochemical and physiological studies directed towards understanding fundamental life processes have therefore been conducted using model bacteria, for example *Escherichia coli, Bacillus subtilis*, model yeasts (e.g. *Saccharomyces cerevisiae, Candida albicans*) and model algae (e.g. *Chlorella vulgaris, Chlamydomonas dysosmos*). The structural simplicity of bacteria in particular is a great advantage in studies such as self-assembly processes, in morphogenesis (e.g. the life cycle of lysogenic bacteriophages), in DNA replication, RNA transcription and translation and in control of gene expression, especially because their haploid nature facilitates the use of mutants. Types of mutation, their induction, selection and application are dealt with briefly in Section 1.6.6. Studies on yeast and bacterial genetics in particular have led to the development of genetic engineering techniques in which foreign DNA may be increased, characterised and expressed (Chapter 2).

The composition of the medium for incubation of microorganisms *in vitro* is determined largely by the latter's nutritional classification as either chemolithotroph, chemoorganotroph, photolithotroph or photoorganotroph, and whether or not it is a wild-type or mutant cell line. Typically, a minimal medium for the growth of a fully biosynthetically competent (prototrophic) chemoorganotroph would contain salts of Na^+, K^+, Ca^{2+}, Mg^{2+}, NH_4^+ or NO_3^-, Cl^-, HPO_4^{2-}, and SO_4^{2-} and a simple carbon source such as glucose. A chemoorganotroph mutated, such that synthesis of alanine is prevented, for example, would be an alanine auxotroph and as such would have to be supplied with alanine in the culture medium. Different auxotrophic mutants may be exploited in the elucidation of metabolic pathways. Complex organic supplements may sometimes be added either when the nutritional requirements are ill defined or to accelerate the growth rate of chemoorganotrophs in culture. The gelling agent agar may be added to solidify the medium and facilitate the surface growth of microorganisms. Preformulated medium is available in powdered form from commercial suppliers. More extensive consideration of factors affecting the design of media for industrial application may be found in the further reading in Section 1.10.

Microbial growth can be in either closed or open systems. In closed systems a finite amount of medium is supplied and growth continues until either one factor in the medium becomes limiting or a toxic by-product of growth accumulates. In open systems of so-called continuous culture, outflow from the system of both cells and medium is balanced by the addition of an equivalent volume of fresh medium.

Closed systems, which use a single volume of growth medium are called batch cultures. The disadvantage of batch cultures is that they usually give rise to unbalanced growth in which a relatively heterogeneous population is present at any given point in the life cycle. If fresh medium is added periodically, thereby increasing the total culture volume and stimulating further growth, they are called fed-batch cultures. The objective of fed-batch culture is to control important nutrients within a narrow concentration range. Open, continuous culture systems enable nutrients, biomass and waste products to be controlled by varying the dilution rate (the rate at which culture is removed and replaced). Open systems are referred to as either chemostats, where growth is controlled at sub-maximum levels by the rate of dilution of the medium containing a single limiting nutrient, or biostats, where the cell population is maintained within narrow predetermined limits by monitoring some physiological property of the culture (e.g. the concentration of outlet gas or cell population), which then acts as a signal for dilution and wash out of excess cells. Fresh medium is introduced from reservoirs to the vessel by triggering the opening of solenoid valves. The specific advantage of continuous cultures over batch cultures is that they facilitate growth under steady-state conditions in which there is tight coupling between cell division and biosynthesis. All facets of metabolism are therefore proceeding at a steady state preset by the dilution rate employed (i.e. the supply of the limiting nutrient). It follows that if the rates of cell division and biosynthesis are constant and equal, the mean composition of the cells in culture does not vary with time when growth is said to be balanced. Balanced growth is extremely useful in many biochemical studies and contrasts with either batch or fed-batch culture, where cellular composition and physiological state varies throughout the growth cycle.

Microbial cultures have widespread industrial uses for large-scale production of alcohols, amino acids, coenzymes, growth regulators, organic acids, polysaccharides, solvents, sterols, surfactants, vitamins and much more. Microbial degradation of waste products, particularly those from the agricultural and food industries, is another important industrial application of microbial cells in culture, especially in the degradation of toxic wastes, for example pesticides, or in the bioconversion of wastes to useful end-products. Biomass production as single-cell protein (SCP) following growth of microorganisms on different substrates is a further important use. Microorganisms also have value in replacing animals in preliminary toxicological testing of xenobiotics.

The application of recombinant DNA techniques, described in Chapter 3, has led to an ever-expanding list of improved native microbial product following gene manipulation and heterologous (foreign) proteins. A good example of the combination of gene cloning, *in vitro* mutagenesis and amino acid analogue resistance is the commercial production of phenylalanine in *E. coli*. Examples of recombinant proteins derived from microbial sources licensed for therapeutic use include factor VIII for haemophilia, insulin for diabetes, interferons α and β for anti-cancer chemotherapy and erthyropoietin for anaemia. Further details of the isolation, preservation and improvement of industrially important microorganisms may be found in the specialist reading cited in Section 1.10.

1.6.4 **Plant cell and tissue culture**

This term refers to the long-term *in vitro* incubation of parts of mosses, liverworts and vascular plants (ferns, gymnosperms and angiosperms) in or on a suitable medium under defined environmental conditions. The technique started as a model system for investigating the potential of plant cells incubated *in vitro* to show totipotency. *In vitro* models, based on culture techniques, are now very widely used to investigate problems across practically the whole of the plant sciences. Much of the success of using molecular biological techniques for plant improvement, for example, relies on the control of organogenesis and embryogenesis *in vitro* and the establishment of plantlets *ex vitro*.

A wide range of different types of medium is available, much of which comes from commercial suppliers in powder form, for the proliferation of plant cells and tissue *in vitro*. Tissue culture medium has to be either autoclaved or filter sterilised before use. Common examples of media include, Murashige and Skoog, Gamborg B5, Nitsche, Shenck and Hildebrandt, and McCown's Woody Plant Medium (WPM). In addition to a balanced mixture of macro- and microelements, which contribute to the correct water potential of medium, most of the osmotically active solute is provided as soluble carbon sources (typically 1% to 5%, w/v), because plant tissue *in vitro* is, almost always, never fully photosynthetic, even if it contains some photosynthetic pigments. Nitrogen is most commonly supplied in inorganic form, either as NO_3^- or NH_4^+, which may be supplemented with organic sources such as urea, glutamine or casein hydrolysate. Vitamin inclusions for coenzyme production are normally from the B group. Most non-tumour cultures require auxin-like regulators that promote cell expansion, such as naturally occurring indol-3-yl acetic acid (IAA) or synthetic compounds such as naphthalene acetic acid (NAA) or 2,4-dichlorophenoxyacetic acid (2,4-D). Cytokinins included to stimulate cell division may be the naturally occurring zeatin or synthetic analogues such as 6-furfurylaminopurine (kinetin). Gibberellins are rarely essential for growth *in vitro*. The induction and maintenance of growth depends additionally on an appropriate balance of growth regulators as well as on their absolute concentrations. The majority of media currently used are chemically defined but some may include complexes such as coconut milk or yeast extract. Organic buffers are not normally included and antibiotics are used only when essential to clean up highly contaminated explants. Medium may contain activated charcoal (0 % to 3 %, w/v) or polyvinylpyrrolidone (PVP) at concentrations up to 250 mg dm^{-3} and antioxidants such as citrate, ascorbate, thiourea or dithiothreitol (DTT) to prevent browning due to phenol release, oxidation and polymerisation. Non-ionic surfactants such as the poloxyethylene–polypropylene copolymer Pluronic F68 are sometimes included in medium to increase plasma membrane permeability. Oxygen-saturated perfluorochemicals (PFCs), for example perfluorodecalin (Flutec PP5), may also stimulate growth by improving the oxygen supply to cells. Microporous nylon meshes or cellulose nitrate filters have also been reported to improve cell aeration and improve growth *in vitro*. Growth-retarding chemicals such as Paclobutrazol may be added to medium to ameliorate anatomical and physiological abnormalities associated with tissue incubation for long periods, under high RH. Such vitrification is reduced when the medium is solidified with agar to approximately 1% (w/v) final concentration. As a naturally occurring coloid, agar is of variable chemical composition and quality.

The brand of agar may have a marked influence on the ease of organogenesis. Since agar is comparatively expensive, synthetic gelling agents such as Gelrite are now gaining popularity. Physical support of tissue cultures in liquid media may involve paper rafts or rods or nylon mesh filters.

Making up culture medium containing different concentrations of carbon sources and plant growth regulators is simple when planned in advance. The following example is intended to illustrate the procedure:

Example 13 Basal Murashige and Skoog (MS) medium is available commercially in powder form, in which all ingredients are supplied other than the carbon source, plant growth regulators and agar. Assuming that this powder is required at 4.2 g dm^{-3}, how would the planning process proceed for making 250 cm^3 of medium containing either 2.0 % (w/v) sucrose or 5% (w/v) sucrose with 2,4-dichlorophenoxy-acetic acid (2,4-D) at either 0.1 mg dm^{-3} or 1.0 mg dm^{-3} at each sucrose concentration and with kinetin added at either 0.25 mg dm^{-3} or 2.50 mg dm^{-3} at each 2,4-D concentration?

Answer The first step is to draw out a table of the different combinations of media to work out the volumes containing each of the constituents, bearing in mind that volumes of stock solutions of the growth regulators will need to be prepared by initially dissolving the solids in absolute ethanol because they are non-polar and hence poorly soluble in water. After being dissolved, the growth regulators may be made up to the correct volume for the stock solution in either deionised or distilled water.

	2.0% sucrose		5% sucrose	
2,4-D (mg dm^{-3})	0.1	1.0	0.1	1.0
Kinetin (mg dm^{-3})	0.25 2.50	0.25 2.50	0.25 2.50	025 2.50

pH to 5.8.

Agar 1% in each case.

Stock solutions are prepared 10 times more concentrated than the final concentration.

Measuring cylinders are sufficiently accurate for the volume measurements.

Total volume of medium required = 8 × 250 cm^3 = 2 dm^3.

Volume containing 2% (w/v) sucrose and 5% sucrose = 1 dm^3.

Volume containing 2,4-D at either 0.1 mg dm^{-3} or 1.0 mg dm^{-3} = 500 cm^3.

Volume containing kinetin at 0.25 mg dm^{-3} or 2.5 mg dm^{-3} = 250 cm^3.

MS salts required = 2 × 4.2 g = 8.4 g.

Dissolve the salts in a convenient volume of distilled or deionised water and make up to a volume that is suitable for splitting into two portions to incorporate the two different sucrose concentrations: 500 cm^3 would be a suitable volume in this case.

Divide into two 250 cm³ samples using a 500 cm³ measuring cylinder and transfer each solution to a 500 cm³ conical or round-bottomed flask. Label flasks as 2% sucrose and 5% sucrose, respectively.

Add 20 g of sucrose and 50 g of sucrose to the appropriate flask, swirling to dissolve.

Make up the contents of each flask to 500 cm³ with deionised water and divide each into two 250 cm³ samples, labelling the flasks with the appropriate sucrose and 2,4-D concentrations.

Add either 5.0 cm³ or 50 cm³ or 2,4-D stock solution to the appropriate flask and make up the contents of each flask to 400 cm³.

Divide each 400 cm³ volume into two 200 cm³ samples and label with the appropriate sucrose, 2,4-D and kinetin concentrations.

Add either 2.5 cm³ or 25 cm³ of kinetin stock solution to the correct flask and adjust the pH of the contents of each flask to 5.8 using 0.1 M HCl (and 0.1 M NaOH if overshoots occur).

Make up the volume in each flask to 250 cm³, add 1.0 g of agar to each flask to 250 cm³ and then add 1.0 g of agar powder to each flask. The additional contribution that the agar makes to the total volume of medium is insignificant. If the medium is to be poured into sterile vessels after autoclaving, the agar will dissolve during autoclaving. If the medium is to be inoculated with cells or tissue directly, however, each flask of medium must be heated separately above 70 °C to dissolve the agar, before distribution into smaller samples for autoclaving prior to subsequent inoculation.

The volumes used above are, of course, *for illustrative purposes only* and can be adjusted according to personal choice, the main error to avoid is making early volumes too large such that later additions of stock solutions overshoot the final volume. If the plan is drawn out before starting, this error can be spotted and hence no damage is done. It is most important when preparing media to strike out the stage immediately completed because interruptions can lead to a muddle and the whole process has to be begun again. Unexpected growth results can often be traced back to faulty medium preparation.

Setting up a plant cell or tissue or culture begins with the excision and surface sterilisation of explants which may be chosen from any part of the plants, depending on the objective of the study. Leaves are frequently preferred for protoplast isolation (cells without walls), anthers for production of haploids, shoot meristems for proliferating shoot cultures and root tips for root cultures. The explant may be either sterile or infected systemically, for example with a virus. Explants may be excised either in the field or from glasshouse-grown plants or seedlings incubated under aseptic conditions. Surface sterilisation most frequently employs several minutes exposure to a 1% to 10% (w/v) sodium hypochlorite solution (proprietary domestic bleaches will do) in which chlorine gas acts as biocide. After the set time (of the order of 5 min) excess hypochlorite must be removed immediately by copious washing in sterile distilled water.

Explants   are most likely to survive *in vitro* when the tissue chosen is physiologically active (i.e. not dormant). Many types of explant contain meristematic tissue capable of cell division. Undifferentiated callus is formed soon after excision and comprises cells with a small amount of cytoplasm but large vacuoles. Such tissue may, however, develop localised growth centres, called meristemoids, from which caulogenesis (shoot induction) rhizogenesis (root initiation) or both may ensue. The ability of callus to undergo such organogenesis is genetically controlled but may be encouraged *in vitro* by manipulating the cytokinin to auxin ratio in the medium. A high cytokinin to auxin ratio usually favours shoot proliferation, whereas a low cytokinin to auxin ratio usually promotes rooting. In practical terms, whole plantlets can be produced *in vitro* from organogenic callus by first encouraging shoot proliferation on a cytokinin-rich medium and then transferring leafy shoots to auxin-rich medium for root induction. Roots may also be developed *in vivo*, provided plants are protected from desiccation. The biochemical explanation of this phenonomen, which has been known for nearly 50 years, is still incomplete. Organogensis from callus is not generally recommended for plantlet multiplication *in vitro* (micropropagation) because there is considerable evidence that it results in genetically aberrant plants being recovered. A greater degree of chromosomal stability can be achieved by using shoot meristems as initial explants for reasons that are, as yet, ill defined. Meristem cultures are consequently a convenient starting material for micropropagation. Meristem culture can also be used sometimes to cure plants infected wth viruses, following the use of high temperature treatments (thermotherapy) and/or chemicals (chemotherapy).

Callus   is often used as the starting material for suspension culture, in which a mixture of both single cells and cell aggregates are incubated in a liquid medium that has to be artificially aerated to prevent cells from becoming waterlogged. The ease of suspension formation is largely genetically controlled but friability can be improved empirically in certain cases by reducing calcium levels in the medium, altering the gas mix, changing the plant growth regulator régime, or adding antioxidants or combinations of such variables.

Plant cell suspensions   may be grown as batch, fed-batch or continuous culture on a small, medium or large scale. For example, single individual cells may be grown in incubated microscope slide chambers, where knowing the clonal origin of the plants is a prerequisite for the study. The wide-necked Erlenmeyer flask, shaken on horizontal platform orbital shakers, is a favourite container for small-scale batch cultures. Fermenters from 1 to 50 000 dm^3 capacity have been designed in which cells are mainly gassed by sparging with air and rather than by swirling with metal impeller blades because of the low shear strength of plant cell walls.

Cell suspensions provide excellent model systems for studies on cell division, cell expansion, cell differentiation and intermediary metabolism, because of the ease of adding test compounds and of harvesting cells and medium for analysis.

The physiological properties of plant suspensions render them more difficult to exploit than microbial cells, however, because they are much larger (greater than 10^5 μm^3), they contain more than 90% (v/v) water, the cell-doubling time is slow (1–2 days usually) and they do not normally excrete metabolites into the medium but compartmentalise them within vacuoles. Secondary product synthesis in plant suspensions is also mainly growth linked. These features coupled with the higher cost of plant culture medium, long fermentation time (usually of the order of weeks), higher downstream processing costs and ploidy instability on prolonged subculture, significantly detracts from their usefulness as a source of economically important drugs, food additives, perfumes, biocides, etc.

Despite these difficulties, research is being conducted using cell fermenters for plant secondary product synthesis because such compounds are either not possible or economically impractical to synthesise chemically. Since many desirable compounds are derived from plants found only in environmentally sensitive areas, there is added pressure on chemical manufacturers to turn to alternative sources of supply. Genetic engineering of complex plant secondary-product genes into microorganisms is difficult because many genes might be involved that may be subject to *in vivo* regulation. Cell lines yielding higher levels of secondary product *in vitro* have been shown for some species following the plating of low density cell suspensions onto Petri dishes (Bergmann plating) and then screening for elevated secondary product synthesis using radioimmunoassay (RIA) or enzyme-linked immunosorbent array (ELISA) techniques (Section 4.7). Plant cell suspensions are also useful in experiments in which mutants are selected by growing colonies in the presence of the selecting agent. Ideally, suspensions comprising only single haploid cells should be used for mutant selection. Single-cell suspensions may be obtained by sequential filtration through a graded series of filters down to 50 μm^2. Single-cell clones selected for superior yields are usually transferred to a production medium, possibly involving mild stress, which suppresses cell division whilst promoting some degree of differentiation.

Higher yields of secondary metabolites in plant cell cultures may follow cell immobilisation on calcium alginate beads or a variety of inert supports, although the method has so far rather limited industrial application in higher plant systems. Similarly biotransformation using either free or immobilised cells, in which low value precursor is converted into higher value-added product, has also been shown to be feasible using plant cell culture systems but so far has had limited application on a large scale.

If single-cell clones are intended for whole plant regeneration, the regenerated cells must transmit the selected trait via seed production. Certain species, for example carrot or oil palm, form somatic embryos in suspension as expressions of totipotency, from which artificial 'seeds' may be produced by coating these propagules with protective resins. This offers potential for direct liquid drilling of artificial seeds into soil.

Single-cell suspensions may also be derived from pectinase digestion of leaves or other starting material. Such pectinases are supplied under various trade names such as Macerozyme R10, Pectolyase Y23 and Rhozyme HP150, and are used normally as solutions in the concentration range 0.03% to 0.2% (w/v). Pectinases are normally used, however, in conjunction with cellulases to prepare protoplasts. Cellulases are supplied under trade names such as Cellulase, Cellulysin and Driselase, and are used normally within the 1% to 2% (w/v) concentration range.

Medium for preparing protoplasts has to be buffered appropriately and of sufficient water potential to prevent protoplasts bursting. Mannitol or sorbitol up to 15% (w/v) is often used for this. Protoplasts are best prepared from thin strips of leaf by static overnight digestion in small Petri dishes in the dark at 25 °C. Protoplasts released into the incubation medium are then purified, following filtration to clear all debris, by low speed density gradient centrifugation (Section 5.7). Protoplasts concentrated at interfaces are removed by drawing them off with Pasteur pipettes. Strict attention to maintaining aseptic conditions is necessary if protoplasts are to be used for plating experiments, hence antibiotics are often incorporated into culture medium.

Protoplasts may be incubated successfully in a variety of ways, but, prior to incubation, protoplasts must be washed and counted to find an effective inoculum density for growth. Cell counting may be performed in a haemocytometer or in a particle counter, for example the Coulter counter. Protoplast viability must also be assessed using either fluorescein diacetate (FDA) and ultraviolet microscopy or Evans Blue stain using visible light microscopy. FDA staining works on the principle that the dye, which is non-fluorescent, readily crosses membranes to be converted into fluorescein by endogenous esterases. Evans Blue, on the other hand, is excluded by living membranes. Protoplasts may be plated in agar (a 1.2% (w/v) medium) or on liquid medium on agar medium, in 4.5% (w/v) agarose medium or in a hanging drop on the lid or base of a Petri dish. The inoculum density is usually about 10^4 cells cm^{-3}. Protoplast cultures are normally static. The temperature range is usually 25 to 30 °C, and low density continuous illumination may be provided of the order of 50 μmol m^{-2} s^{-1}. Protoplasts will not start to divide until new walls have formed, which takes about 24 h. Growth of colonies will ensue over a two-week interval and, to enhance growth rate, the colonies are transferred to fresh medium that is at a lower osmotic pressure. If plantlets are required, regenerative media have to be used, incorporating an appropriate balance of growth regulators. Protoplasts have very widespread application in plant sciences, including infection by viruses, uptake of organelles and cell wall regeneration. Their greatest use, however, has been in genetic transformation and somatic hybridisation. Protoplast fusion is especially valuable in plant breeding experiments because it may be used to overcome sexual incompatibility mechanisms between genera that prevent the formation of viable zygotes.

Successful hybridisation depends on developing effective techniques for protoplast fusion, for selection of fusion hybrids, for regeneration of plantlets and for analysis of regenerated plants. Fusion methods are either chemical or physical (electrofusion). Chemical methods either use incubation solutions incorporating high concentrations, about 30% (w/v), of polyethyleneglycol (PEG) of M_r 6000 or high pH, calcium solutions (pH 10.4 in 1.1% (w/v) CaCl$_2$, 6H$_2$O in 10% (w/v) mannitol). Fusion is generally achieved in less than 30 min. PEG is the preferred

Table 1.10 Some applications of plant cell and tissue culture

System	Process investigated
Protoplasts	
Nicotiana tabacum	Cell wall regeneration; clonal propagation of mutant plants; interspecific hybrids; uptake of *Rhizobium*; homologous and heterologous gene expression
Solanum tuberosum	Somaclonal variation in cultivar Russet Burbank; genetic transformation using Ti plasmid; transformation by cocultivation of protoplasts with isolated *Agrobacterium tumefaciens* cells; direct protoplast transformation
Arabidopsis thaliana	Intergeneric hybridisation, model for molecular biological investigations
Glycine max	Isolation of viable bacteroids from root nodule protoplasts, molecular model for investigating nitrogen fixation
Cell suspensions	
Acer pseudoplatanus	Control of cell division and expansion in single cells, batch and continuous cultures, with monitoring of associated biochemical changes
Daucus carota	Somatic embryogenesis in higher plants
Nicotiana tabacum	Industrial fermentation of biomass for tobacco industry; ubiquinone production; selection, regeneration and sexual transmission in regenerants resistant to the herbicide picloram
Digitalis purpurea	Biotransformation of digitoxin to digoxin
Catharanthus roseus	Ajmalacine and serpentine production
Lithospermum erythrorhizon	Commercial shikonin
Callus	
Phaseolus vulgaris	Physiology and biochemistry of differentiation
Vicea faba	Cytogenetic studies indicating chromosome instability
Elaeis guinensis	Cloning of oil palm plantlets and crop improvement
Solanum tuberosum	Somaclonal variation
Nicotiana tabacum	Shoot regeneration following exposure to electric currents
Anther and microspores	
Brassica napus	Embryogenesis from cultured microspores
Vitis vinifera	Transformation and regeneration of grapevine
Nodal stem segments	
Baciopa monniera	Micropropagation of a medicinal plant
Embryos	
Papaver somniferum	Plant breeding; direct pollination of excised ovules to overcome prezygotic barriers to fertility
Hordeum vulgare	Production of mutants resistant to lysine analogues

Table 1.10 (*Cont.*)	
System	Process investigated
Meristem	
Solanum tuberosum	Elimination of potato virus X by thermotherapy followed by plantlet regeneration
Chrysanthemum morifolium	Breeding of radiation-induced mutants
Leaf discs	
Brassica napus	Transformation using *A. tumerfaciens* of glyphosphate resistance genes
Lycopersicum esculentum	Transformation using *A. tumefaciens* of antisense genes to inhibit fruit ripening

method when two types of mesophyll protoplast are fused, since they tend to burst at high pH. Fusion medium must be removed before transfer of protoplast to incubation medium.

Electrofusion   is an alternative method for protoplast fusion that involves two steps. In the first, protoplasts are placed in a medium of low conductivity between two electrodes (platinum wires arranged in parallel on a microscope slide). A high frequency alternating field (0.5 to 1.5 MHz) is applied between the electrodes, which causes the protoplasts to align in a process known as di-electrophoresis. In the second step, one or more short (10–200 μs) direct current pulses (of 1–3 kV cm^{-1}) are applied, which causes pores to form in the membranes of protoplasts and allows fusion to take place where there is close membrane contact. This technique allows a higher degree of control over the fusion process than chemical methods do and consequently is becoming more widely used.

Fusion is a random process and the result of a fusion treatment can be a mixture of unfused homokaryon parental protoplasts, fused homokaryons and fused heterokaryons. Following fusion, heterokaryons containing nuclei of both species in a common (mixed) cytoplasm regenerate a new wall. Nuclear fusion, if achieved, will result in a somatic hybrid cell which must be totipotent if hybrid whole plants are to be produced. Various techniques have been devised for identification and recovery of somatic hybrids, which are frequently based on complementation of biochemical mutants (Section 1.6.6). Morphologically distinct or fluorescently labelled protoplasts can also be identified under an inverted microscope and removed with micromanipulation. Fluorescence-activated cell sorting (FACS, Section 4.8.5) methods may also be used for separating different protoplast populations.

Protoplasts were used for early genetic transformation experiments because of the relative ease of infection with *Agrobacterium tumefaciens*. In this case, sterile protoplasts were suspended at 25 °C in a buffered plasmid preparation (concentration 10 μg poly-L-ornithine cm^{-3}. After incubation, which is best conducted under vacuum, washed protoplasts are plated, at a suitable inoculum density, onto an appropriate selection medium. The selection medium can take a variety of forms but is most frequently based on the introduction of a linked resistance gene into the cloning vector, for example kanomycin or hygeromycin. The use of *A. tumefaciens* was initially limited to those species that are naturally infected by Gram-negative bacteria, which, until recently, meant that cereals were excluded from this technology. Supervirulent strains of *A. tumefaciens* have been discovered recently that can achieve transformation of monocotyledonous tissue cultures.

Protoplasts may also be transformed using direct DNA injection, by electroporation, by liposome invasion, by particle bombardment (biolistics) or by using silicon carbide fibres that punch holes in the membrane. Electroporation involves incubating protoplasts with cloned DNA in specially designed cuvettes. A direct current of short duration is applied that causes pore formation, allowing the DNA to penetrate more easily. Biolistics is now gaining in popularity for transformation studies because it can be carried out directly on explants much more easily than with *A. tumefaciens* or other cloning agents. Currently there are many examples of successful introduction and expression of foreign DNA in host plants, examples include freezing resistance, virus resistance and fungal resistance as indicated in the suggested reading in Section 1.10.

Haploid plant tissue and cell cultures are also important in the context of providing a source of mutants for comparative biochemical studies (Section 1.6.6) for protoplast fusion experiments and for improvement of agronomic traits principally by micropropagation of resistance mutants, for example salinity, herbicides and desiccation. Such haploid material is derived by diverting an immature gametophyte (pollen grain) away from its normal developmental pathway. Haploid tissue can be produced *in vitro* by either anther culture or microspore (pollen) culture. In anther culture, immature anthers are removed from donor plants, grown under very precise environmental conditions to ensure that the stage of pollen development is best for recovery of haploids. This generally corresponds either to the period immediately following meiosis or to the first pollen grain mitosis, according to the species. Aseptically removed anthers from different genera have separate but exacting nutritional requirements. Isolated microspores are much more difficult to grow *in vitro* because their nutritional requirements are so exacting. If regeneration of haploid plantlets can be achieved, homozygous diploids may be induced by treating the roots with dilute solutions of the alkyloid colchicine.

The range of applications of plant tissue and cell culture is very extensive. Table 1.10 gives a few examples. More extensive coverage is given in the suggestions for further reading (Section 1.10).

1.6.5 **Animal cell culture**

The distinction between simple techniques of incubation *in vitro*, such as perfusion and cell and tissue culture, is to some extent arbitrary, since conditions chosen for cell culture may not permit cell division. However, the maintenance of viable cells for periods in excess of 24 h generally leads to them being referred to as cells in culture. Advances in animal cell and tissue culture applications have been profound in recent years because of the versatility of the techniques and the ready availability of media, cells and culture vessels from specialist suppliers. The major drawback to the technique is that it may be expensive to operate and requires specialist training. Table 1.11 lists some strengths and weaknesses of the methodology.

Many physiological salt solutions have been developed for short-term work with animal tissues, for example Tyrode's, Young's, Locke's, Meng's and Da Jalon's, many being derived from Ringer's solution, which was one of the first to be formulated. One of the most common is Krebs–Ringer bicarbonate, the bicarbonate solution having been designed, originally, to approximate to the ionic composition of mammalian serum. Typically such salt solutions contain different combinations of the major salts NaCl, KCl, $MgSO_4$, $CaCl_2$, $NaHCO_3$ and KH_2PO_4, in various concentrations.

The control of gaseous exchange and pH are critically important for long-term maintenance of cells in culture. Medium buffered with 30 mM bicarbonate has to be maintained in air containing 5% CO_2 to keep the pH between 7.3 and 7.5. Phenol red dye, which adopts an orange red colour at this pH, is usually included as a check on correct pH value. Medium containing zwitterionic buffers such as Hepes does not require this treatment. Calcium ion levels are critical for the growth of anchorage-dependent cells but have to be omitted for suspension cultures. Other inclusions are typically vitamins, carbon sources, amino acids and proteins. Examples of defined medium include Delbecco's Modified Eagle's Medium (DMEM), Ames Medium and McCoy's 5A medium. The use of serum-free medium (SFM) is particularly important when effects of hormones and growth factors on cell differentiation are being investigated. A range of SFM types is available commercially and they contain known amounts of some of the purified serum components. Such media are very expensive.

Protein inclusions in chemically undefined medium usually comprise either plasma or serum. Serum contains important growth factors such as insulin-like growth factor (IGF), epidermal growth factor (EGF) or platelet-derived growth factor (PDGF), which are essential for long-term growth of more highly differentiated excised tissues. Antibiotics active against a range of contaminating microorganisms may be incorporated, filter sterilised, at concentrations from 2.5 to 100 $\mu g\,cm^{-3}$ and are claimed to be effective for 5 to days at 37 °C. Most medium is supplied in liquid form and has a limited shelflife under refrigeration. Some types of medium are available commercially in powdered form, which extends storage life especially when the medium is kept cold. Medium should always be batch tested for its ability to maintain growth of either specified cell lines or primary cultures before using it for a specific experiment. Further details on the choice of medium for the growth of animal cells *in vitro* may be found in the reading list in Section 1.10.

Excised tissue is usually heterogeneous and cell types are typically categorised according to their mesenchyme or haemopoietic embryonic origin. Examples of

| Table 1.11 | Strengths and weaknesses of animal cell and tissue culture |

Strengths

Range of cell types in culture is now very large including genetically defined clones.

Ready availability of media, cells and culture vessels from commercial suppliers.

Methods for isolation of primary cells and storage of cell lines is now well documented.

Viability and physiology of tissue is easily monitored.

Increased control of environmental variables, e.g. temperature, pH, medium constituents.

Ease of application of test compound with improved tissue specificity and easier recovery of metabolites.

Large-scale replication of experiments may be performed readily in small space and short time.

Scale of experimentation in model system is from single cell to organ.

Scale-up offers scope for biotechnology.

Reduction of animals killed for experimentation/bioproducts processing, e.g. in cytotoxicity testing and antibody production.

High batch-to-batch consistency when compared with sources for isolation of serum proteins.

Weaknesses

Method may be considered to be too specialised and laborious for routine use.

Resources needed are expensive, e.g. fetal calf serum.

Lack of *in vivo* specificity.

cells in culture include macrophages, T and B lymphocytes and polymorpho-nuclear leukocytes. Pioneering studies established that varying degrees of growth of tissues was possible *in vitro* in sterile medium containing salts, carbohydrates, vitamins and amino acids, and serum supplements. Animal cells may be subdivided broadly into those that remain viable only when attached to a solid substrate (e.g. primary cultures or diploid fibroblast cells) and those that will proliferate as suspensions (e.g. human tumour cells, HeLa cells and hybridomas). Newly isolated or primary cell cultures of non-tumour cells typically show anchorage dependence by growing *in vitro* only when attached to a surface, which may be either other cells (as *in vivo*) or plastic, gelatin or collagen, but rarely glass. Primary cell lines spread over the surface as monolayers but will not overlayer owing to contact inhibition of adjacent cell membranes. Such cultures are said to show confluence, which severely limits cell density in culture. This problem can be overcome by using cell support systems (microbeads or hollow fibres), which are considered below.

In general terms, highly differentiated excised tissue is more difficult to establish *in vitro* as primary cell lines either because the cells tend to dedifferentiate immediately or because they will not subculture in medium devoid of growth factors or steroid hormone supplements typically found in serum, e.g. IGF, EGF, PDGF or oestrogen.

Continuous subculture is possible only in transformed cell lines which have become either naturally aneuploid or chemically mutated (e.g. with 3,4-benz-pyrene or nitrosomethyl urea) or infected with a virus (e.g. simian virus 40 (SV40) or Rous sarcoma virus). Transformed cells, for example baby hamster kidney (BHK) cells, typically show reduced contact inhibition, an ability to grow in suspension, changes in shape and loss of differentiation (neoplasia), and a requirement for much less stringently defined culture medium. Interestingly, some transforming viruses may introduce viral oncogenes coding for proteins that substitute for growth factors normally supplied in serum. Transformed cell lines frequently induce tumour formation when injected into suitable hosts. The close similarity between transformed and tumour cells is often exploited experimentally, transformed cells being used instead of tumour cells because of the former's tendency to be cytologically more homogeneous.

Cells may be grown in either batch or continuous culture. Either way, control of gaseous exchange and pH are critically important. If the vessels are sealed, then medium must be gassed with either 5% or 10% CO_2 at inoculation. Vented flasks have to be kept within CO_2 incubators, which automatically control temperature and CO_2 concentration and maintain a high humidity. The growth characteristics of cells have had profound effects on the design of culture vessels. Small-scale static culture of cells up to, say, 1 cm³ is conveniently established either in microtitre plate wells or in specialised tissue culture plates with wells of varying cubic capacity that may be precoated with gelatin. Scintillation vials may also be employed. Plastic Petri dishes and flat-sided bottles of glass or plastic may be used for slightly larger cultures, up to 50 cm³. Batches of roller bottles, which rotate at 1 r.p.m. or less on proprietary or homemade machines, provide increased surface area for up to 1 dm³ of growth medium, especially when the inner surface is corrugated. However, cells then have to be removed by trypsin treatment. Specialised, and expensive, cell factories or capillary perfusion beds are also available, which employ either glass bead columns or hollow fibres to support cells in which medium, previously equilibrated with 5% CO_2 in air, is circulated.

Suspension culture of cells such as lymphocytes or hybridomas is possible, especially in small-scale fermenters of up to 10 dm³ capacity in which cells are gently stirred magnetically. Alternatively, small-scale airlift fermenters may be employed. Free cell suspension culture has very limited application, however, and has been surpassed in biotechnological application by the development of microcarriers, which allow for large-scale suspension culture of anchorage-dependent cells.

Microcarriers consist of a cross-linked polymer such as dextran, polyacrylamide, polystyrene or plastic, usually containing either fixed positive or fixed negative charges which facilitate attachment. Trade name examples of positively charge microcarriers are Cytodex and Superbeads; Rapid Cell G and Biosolon are examples of negatively charged microcarriers. Non-charged, gelatin-coated beads are also commercially available, for example Gele-beads. A major problem associated with the isolation of free cells and cell aggregates from organs is that of releasing the cells from their supporting matrix without affecting the integrity of

Table 1.12 Some applications of animal cell and tissue culture

Baby hamster kidney (BHK) cells	Large-scale production of foot and mouth vaccines
WI 38 (*ex* human embryo lung tissue)	Production of rubella vaccine
Simian kidney epithelial cells	Production of polio vaccines
Murine lymphoblastoid cells	Production of histocompatibility (H-2^K) and differentiation specific (Thy-1) antigens
Myeloma cell lines	Production of monoclonal antibodies
T helper cells	Production of lymphokines
Leukocytes	Production of α-interferon
Diploid fibroblasts	Production of β-interferon
B or T lymphocytes	γ-Interferon
Porcine kidney cells	Production of urokinase

the cell membrane. The earliest approaches to this problem employed mechanical techniques such as forcing the tissue through cheesecloth or silk, or shaking the tissue with glass beads in an appropriate buffer. These procedures inevitably caused considerable cell damage and resulted in a low cell yield, which posed the practical question of determining whether or not the isolated cells were representative of those originally present in the tissue. The use of a biochemical, rather than a mechanical, approach has largely overcome these problems. In the case of hepatocyte isolation, the use of collagenase and hyaluronidase in a calcium-free medium to digest the matrix has enabled cells with a viability in excess of 95% to be isolated on a routine basis. The liver may be removed, thinly sliced and then incubated with the enzymes, or it can be cannulated *in situ*, perfused with an oxygenated, calcium-free medium containing the enzymes, and then removed and broken up with a blunt spatula. The latter technique requires greater practical expertise but appears to give a greater and more reproducible cell yield and viability. In all cases, viability is generally assessed by the ability of the cells to exclude the dye trypan blue, but other procedures based upon respiration or protein synthesis are probably better.

The proliferation of animal cells in culture has many applications including their use as model systems for biochemical, physiological and pharmacological studies and the production of growth factors, blood factors, monoclonal antibodies, interferons, enzymes, vaccines and hormones. A brief outline of some of the specific uses of particular animal cell and tissue cultures is given in Table 1.12.

1.6.6 **Mutants**

Much of biochemistry is concerned with defining the structural and metabolic consequences of mutations, i.e. altering the base sequences of DNA. Indeed, much of our knowledge of the principles of linkage, genetic mapping and the control of transcription and translation in cells is based largely on the exploitation of mutant organisms. The special value of mutations, if expressed, is that they form the basis of a comparative study with the normal (wild-type) cells.

In chemical terms, there are several classes of mutation, which may either occur naturally or be induced when cells are treated with physical or chemical mutagens, for example X-rays, ultraviolet radiation, hydroxylamine, alkylating agents such as ethylmethane sulphonate or acridine dyes such as proflavin. The use of restriction endonucleases and genetic recombination *in vitro* (Section 3.6.2) facilitates directed mutagenesis, the intentional alteration of a gene at a specific location for a specific purpose. A point mutation is said to occur when a single base in DNA is changed, and a double mutation when there are two such changes. Deletions and deletion substitutions refer either to removal of a base or to exchange base-pairing in parts of a gene.

Microorganisms have traditionally been used for studies in biochemical genetics because they are predominantly haploid, have short generation times, can be grown in/on defined media (making mutant isolation easier), and can be propagated as large biomasses of biochemically uniform cell populations in industrial-scale fermenters. The genetic transfer systems of microorganisms are also simpler than those of eukaryotes and are now relatively well defined both in terms of genetic mapping and in complementation tests.

Largely as a result of microbial studies, mutations may be further classified according to the conditions under which the mutation is expressed. So-called non-conditional mutants display the mutant phenotype under all (natural) conditions. Examples of non-conditional mutants include auxotrophy, where mutation results in an enzyme deficiency or inactivity which may be rectified by supplements of the products of those defective enzymes, provided they can be transported into the cell. Prototrophs are non-conditional mutants in which auxotrophs gain a biosynthetic function leading to autonomy from a nutritional supplement. Regaining a wild-type phenotype in this way is called reversion and is usually associated with point mutations. A resistance mutation confers increased resistance to an anti-metabolite or environmental stress. Anti-microbial (drug) resistance in bacteria, yeast or plasmids is an example of resistance mutation often of single-gene origin.

A conditional mutant is one that does not always display the mutant phenotype. Suppressor-sensitive mutations (*sus*) do not display the mutant characteristic in the presence of the gene product from a wild-type suppressor gene. Hence the mutation expression is being suppressed. For example, a bacteriophage carrying a *sus* mutation will produce progeny when it infects a host cell expressing the su^+ gene (the so-called permissive condition) but will not do so when the host cell lacks the suppressor gene (su^-), under so-called non-permissive conditions. Another good example of a conditional mutant is a temperature-sensitive mutant in which a physiologically active protein is rapidly inactivated above or below a critical temperature. The particular value of conditional mutants for biochemical studies is that they are conditionally or potentially lethal and enable investigations to be made on enzymes that cannot be corrected by nutritional supplements. For example, mutants of DNA and RNA polymerases or aminoacyl tRNA synthases cannot be corrected by simple nutritional supplements to the medium as these enzymes are involved in the metabolism of complex macromolecules.

The application of mutants in genetic, biochemical or physiological studies presupposes that such mutants can be selected from a mixed population. *In vitro* techniques are widely exploited for such selection procedures. Selection of biochemical auxotrophs is usually based on incorporating effective concentrations of antibiotics (e.g. penicillin or streptomycin) into minimal media of bacterial suspensions to kill dividing, wild-type cells. Auxotrophs present will be incapable of growth but remain viable and may be recovered after centrifugation and washing to remove excess penicillin. Surviving cells can then be incubated on a supplemented medium. The nature of the supplement to minimal medium will biochemically characterise the auxotroph. Replica plating from complete medium to minimal medium using a sterile velvet pad is another potential means of detecting auxotrophic colonies on subsequent transfer to complete medium.

A convenient way of isolating prokaryotic auxotrophs is by initial exposure of the microorganism to an effective concentration of 5-bromodeoxyuridine (BUdR). Prototrophs then take up the thymidine analogue and are killed when the BUdR is degraded by exposure to light. Auxotrophs that fail to take up the analogue survive but will grow only on a medium enriched with nutrients. Specific auxotrophs can be picked up by progressively simplifying the number of nutrient supplements.

In eukaryotes there is still no reliable replica plating technique. Selection for auxotrophism is currently based either on the laborious total isolation, used originally for *Neurospora*, in which supplements are added on a trial-and-error basis, or on using alternative scavenging pathways. In the latter case, enzyme detection means that when anti-metabolite analogues are added to minimal medium to kill wild-type dividing cells, auxotrophs do not incorporate the compounds and survive when alternative pathways for synthesis are available. For this to occur, either chromosomal aberration of the allele must have created a stage of functional hemizygosity or the gene in question lies on the X chromosome. Examples of this principle are the isolation of thymidine kinase (TK) mutants, which survive because cells fail to incorporate 5-BUdR but can synthesise dTMP from an alternative folic acid pathway and HRPT (hypoxanthine phosphoribosyl transferase) mutants that fail to incorporate 8-thioguanine into inositol monophosphate (IMP) but survive because IMP is also synthesised from the secondary scavenging folic acid pathway. In this pathway, selective amplification of the gene for the key enzyme dehydrofolate reductase can be achieved by selecting for resistance to aminopterin and amethopterin (methotrexate), which are analogues of folic acid. TK⁻ and HRPT⁻ strains are of critical importance in the HAT selection technique for the production of monoclonal antibodies (Section 4.2.3).

Eukaryotic cell lines are also critically important as starting material for the selection of somatic cell hybrids resulting from protoplast fusion experiments. A good example of this approach is the selection of a somatic hybrid from leaf protoplasts of *Nicotinia glauca* and *Nicotinia langsdorfii*. A sexual cross of these species produces a teratoma that overproduces auxins and cytokinins, both of which are necessary to support growth of cell lines of *N. glauca* and *N. langsdorfii*. Only the fusion hybrid colonies will grow in medium devoid of auxin and cytokinin. Scion grafts of the somatic hybrid onto either *N. glauca* or *N. langsdorfii* as stock causes a teratoma to develop.

1.6.7 **Cryopreservation**

Repeated subculture of cell lines may result in genetic aberration and hence loss of biosynthetic capacity or morphogenetic potential. Various strategies are possible to alleviate these difficulties, including methods either for slowing down growth in stock cultures or for freeze-drying for certain microbial cultures. Cryopreservation in liquid nitrogen is the preferred method for most eukaryotes and is based on the principle that the only reactions that occur at -196 °C, the boiling point for liquid nitrogen, are ionisations due to background irradiation, which are very rare. Biochemical reactions cease at about -130 °C. Various experimental protocols have been devised, often empirically, for different tissue types. Successful cryopreservation requires that viability is maintained after the sample has been held for indefinite periods in liquid nitrogen. The rate of freezing is very important, since too-rapid freezing causes large crystals of ice to form intracellularly. Such crystals, on thawing, lyse cell membranes. Slow freezing rates favour the deposition of extracellular ice at subzero temperatures, provided the internal concentration of solutes is sufficiently high to make the internal water potential lower than that externally. This process may be assisted by adding a penetrating cryoprotectant such as glycerol to the medium supporting the specimen. When ice has formed extracellularly, water is withdrawn from the cells because the vapour pressure density of ice is lower than that of the predominantly aqueous cytoplasm. Water moves out until the vapour pressure densities are equilibrated. During this process, the protoplast shrinks and plant and microbial cells may become plasmolysed temporarily. Alternatively, non-penetrative cryoprotective agents such as PEG and PVP may be used to ensure that cell dehydration proceeds smoothly during slow freezing. If the dehydration is too rapid, denaturation of proteins may occur because of localised high salt (solution effects), which may cause protein precipitation. At a critical temperature corresponding to the eutectic point (i.e. the freezing point for the equilibrium mixture of solid and liquid) for the cytoplasm, the cell contents freeze, without ice crystals forming.

Slow cooling rates are best achieved with samples held in ampoules within commercial units that cool at rates of 0.1 to 10 deg.C min^{-1}. Such units consist of containers enclosing a low melting point liquid alcohol, cooled by a refrigeration coil. Stepwise cooling, which may be equally effective, involves holding the specimen for prescribed periods at a given temperature in improvised units. When the temperature reaches either -50 °C to -70 °C for the improvised units, or -100 °C for controlled freezing, the ampoules are transferred directly to liquid nitrogen.

Thawing of samples is best achieved rapidly by removing them to a water bath held at 30 °C to 40 °C for a few minutes, whilst applying gentle agitation. Washing to remove the cryoprotectant should not be necessary, as cryprotectants should be non-toxic. Damage to tissue during an experimental protocol may be estimated by employing light or electron microscopic techniques (Section 1.7). Viability may be assessed either by monitoring respiration, by cytological staining (e.g. exclusion of Evans Blue stain from viable cells) or by regrowth in appropriate media.

1.6.8 Culture collections

The increasing importance of culture techniques for experimental purposes relies heavily on reference collections of plant, animal and microbial cell lines being readily available, so as to enable coincidental comparative studies to be made in different laboratories. Special characteristics of particular cell lines may include biochemical markers, karyotype analyses, nutritional mutants, drug resistance or sensitivity, tumour production, cellular inclusions (e.g. microbial contaminants, phage or other episomes) or secretory products (e.g. hormones or immunoglobulins). An example of a culture collection is the National Collection of Type Cultures, Central Public Health Laboratory, Colindale Avenue, London.

1.7 MICROSCOPY

1.7.1 General principles

Biochemical analysis is frequently accompanied by light and electron microscopic examination of tissue, cell or organelle preparations to evaluate the integrity of samples and to correlate structure with function. Microscopy serves two independent functions of enlargement (magnification) and improved resolution (the rendering of two objects as separate entities). Light microscopes employ optical lenses to sequentially focus the image of objects, whereas electron microscopes use electromagnetic lenses. Light and electron microscopes work either in a transmission or scanning mode depending on whether the light or electron beam either pass through the specimen and are diffracted or whether they are deflected by the specimen surface. Polarised light microscopes detect optically active substances in cells, for example particles of silica or asbestos in lung tissue or starch granules in amyloplasts. Light microscopes in phase contrast mode are often used to improve image contrast of unstained material, for example to test cell or organelle preparations for lysis. Changes in phase of emergent light may be caused either by diffraction by the specimen, or even by differences in thickness of the specimen. At their point of focus, the converging light rays show interference, resulting in either increases or decreases in the amplitude of the resultant wave (constructive or destructive interference, respectively), which the eye detects as differences in brightness.

Microscopes using visible light will magnify approximately 1500 times and have a resolution limit of about 0.2 μm whereas a transmission electron microscope is capable of magnifying approximately 200 000 times and has a resolution limit for biological specimens of about 1 nm. The excellent resolving power of transmission electron microscopy (TEM) is largely a function of the very short wavelength of electrons accelerated under the influence of an applied electric field. (An accelerating voltage of 100 kV produces a wavelength of 4×10^{-3}nm). Scanning electron microscopes (SEM) use a fine beam of electrons to scan back and forth across the metal-coated specimen surface. The secondary electrons that are generated from this surface are collected by a scintillation crystal, which converts each electron impact into a flash of light. Each light flash inside the crystal is amplified by a photomultiplier and used to build up an image on a fluorescent screen. The principal application of SEM is the study of surfaces such as those of cells. The resolution limit of a scanning electron microscope is about 6 nm. Figure 1.4 illustrates the application of TEM and SEM in biological investigations.

1.7.2 Preparation of specimens

TEM requires thin sample specimens, i.e. squashes, smears, hanging drops or very thin sections. Preservation and integrity of cellular components requires initial tissue fixation, which may be achieved either by rapid freezing or by chemical treatment to stabilise and cross-link protein and lipid components of membranes. Fixation with formaldehyde (principally used in light microscopy) and glutaraldehyde (alone or in combination with formaldehyde for electron microscopy) is the result of the formation of methylene bridges with side-chain amino groups of proteins, whilst osmium tetroxide, a common fixative in electron microscopy, cross-links mainly with unsaturated fatty acid side-chains (Fig. 1.5). Fixed tissue is then subjected to sequential processes of staining and sectioning.

Samples for ion probe analysis (Section 1.7.3) are prepared either by chemical fixation or, more successfully, by ultrarapid freezing methods, such as immersion in liquid propane or nitrogen slush, which serve to immobilise ions. Where frozen tissue is used, sections must be extremely thin and may require the use of an ultra-cryomicrotome. Histological stains are used to produce contrast, which aids resolution. Many stains used in light microscopy rely on anionic and cationic reactions with intracellular ampholytes, and their efficiency is profoundly influenced by pH. Cytoplasmic components are mostly cationic in the slightly acid pH range, implying preferential binding to anionic (acidic) stains such as eosin. Chromatin and DNA at pH 6.0 are anionic and thus bind to cationic stains such as methylene blue. Contrast in material for TEM is improved by incorporating heavy-metal salts into the specimens to induce a greater extent of electron absorption. This can be achieved by exploiting the binding of uranium to nucleic acids and proteins and of lead to lipids.

Fixed tissue, when not frozen, needs supporting before sections are cut for microscopic study. Embedding media such as waxes and epoxyresins (Araldite or Epon) are immiscible with both water and alcohol, which necessitates the initial dehydration and equilibrium of fixed tissues by passing them through solutions containing increasing concentrations of ethanol, followed by transfer to xylene or propylene oxide, before infiltration with an appropriate embedding medium in its liquid phase. Sections 10 μm thick cut from tissue frozen at $-20\,°C$ in a refrigerated microtome called a cryostat are good for rapid examination by light microscopy

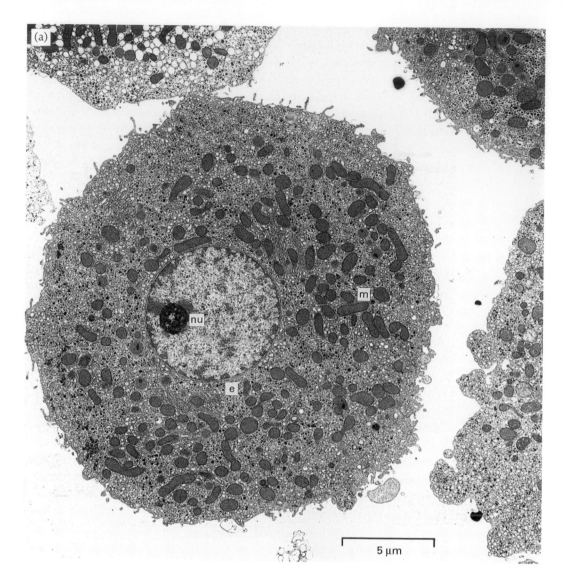

Fig. 1.4. (a) Transmission electron micrograph of a transverse section of isolated rat hepatocyte, demonstrating intact cytoplasmic and nuclear membranes with well-defined microvilli around the nuclear membrane. Cell organelles are intact together with the nucleus (Nu), mitochondria (m), smooth and rough endoplasmic reticulum (e). Cells were fixed in phosphate-buffered (0.067 M, pH 7.4) 2% (w/v) glutaraldehyde. Selected specimens were postfixed in 1% (w/v) osmium tetroxide in 0.12 M phosphate buffer (pH 7.4) and processed into epoxy resin. Ultrathin sections (60 to 90 nm) were stained with uranylacetate and lead acetate. Photomicrographs were exposed during the examination of specimens on photographic film, which was then processed.

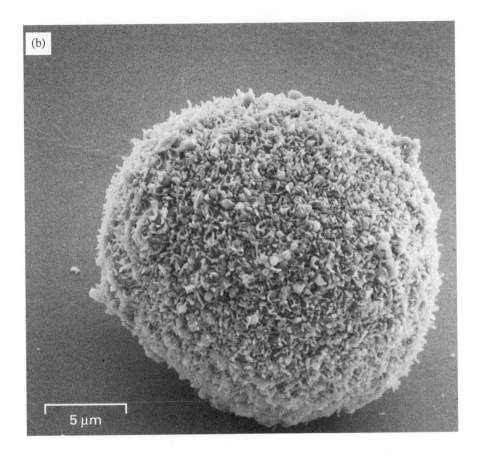

(b)

5 μm

Fig. 1.4. (*cont.*) (b) Scanning electron micrograph of isolated rat hepatocyte. Hepatocytes are spherical, with prominent microvilli covering the surface. Cells were attached to glass coverslips coated with poly L-lysine for 2 h before being fixed in phosphate-buffered (0.067 M, pH 7.4) 2% glutaraldehyde for 4 h at room temperature. Critical-point drying followed serial dehydration in alcohol, and cells were sputter-coated with gold–palladium. (Photomicrograph kindly provided by Glaxo Wellcome Research, Stevenage.)

but suffer damage if thawed. Wax sections, 5 μm thick, are floated on warm water, placed on glass slides, dried and subsequently dewaxed and stained for light microscope examination. Ultrathin sections for TEM (less than 100 nm) are cut with ultramicrotomes using diamond as the cutting edge from an area of block face trimmed to about 0.1 mm^2. Section ribbons are floated onto water and mounted on fine copper grids for staining and examination. Cell organelles are examined in the electron microscope in isolated, intact form rather than in thin sections.

In negative staining, a heavy metal stain, often phosphotungstic acid, is allowed to dry in a puddle around the surfaces of isolated cell particles supported on a thick carbon or plastic film. The stain molecules are deposited into surface crevices in the specimen during drying and produce a ghost image in which the specimen appears light against a dark background, often outlining details very clearly. The contrast

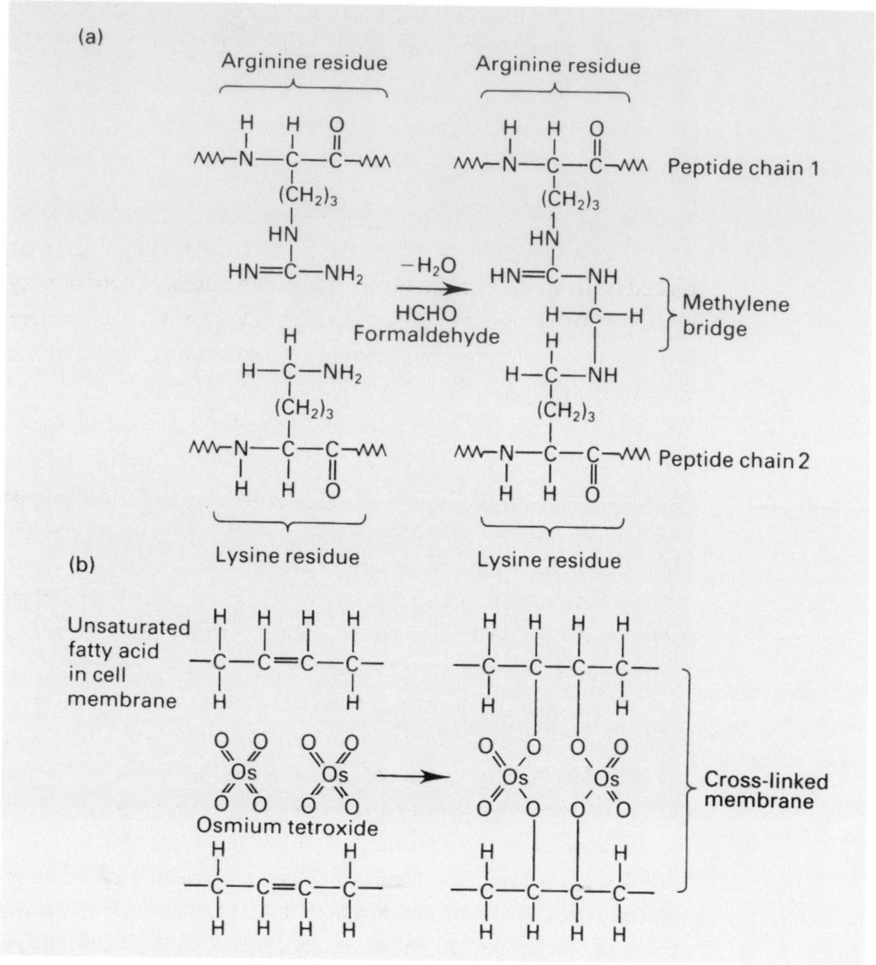

Fig. 1.5. Cross-linking by some chemical fixatives: (a) formaldehyde, (b) osmium tetroxide.

and surface details of isolated specimens are also frequently increased by the technique of shadowing. A thin layer of a heavy metal such as platinum is deposited on the surface of the specimen from one side. The effect in the electron microscope is as if a strong light is directed toward the specimen from one side, placing surface depression in deep shadow. Antibodies prepared against specific cellular proteins, which have absorbed colloidal gold are frequently used for staining in TEM because the gold is electron dense. Several antigens can be localised simultaneously if different antibodies are labelled with gold particles of different sizes.

Freeze-fracture techniques in which frozen samples are cleaved with a knife along fracture planes in membranes, utilise this shadowing technique to produce replicas of broken cellular material that show the membrane surface structure on, and within, cell organelles. Microscopic images using light microscopy and electron microscopy are best recorded using photomicrography, which requires the operator to have considerable experience of microscopes, film and processing to reproduce high quality images that are accurate and repeatable. Further details of photomicrographic methods may be found in the suggestions for further reading (Section 1.10).

1.7.3 Ion probe analysis

Electron microscopes may be equipped to perform X-ray spectrochemical analysis. When a specimen is irradiated by an electron beam, an electron may be displaced from an inner to an outer orbital. The vacated orbital may be infilled by an electron from a higher energy orbital with the emission of an X-ray photon characteristic of the difference in energy levels of the two orbitals. The binding energy of the electrons in an orbital is related to the charge on the nucleus; hence each element produces its own characteristic emission spectrum. Emitted photons are usually detected by energy-dispersive analysis, using lithium drifted solid-state detectors. Each photon emitted reacts with silicon atoms to produce an electrical pulse proportional to the energy of the photon. An electronic pulse height analyser and microcomputer are used to process the spectral data, which are normally displayed on a video monitor. X-ray spectrochemical analysis permits the measurement of ion distributions *in situ* in SEM and TEM by combining the high spatial resolution of electron microscopy with the ability to determine subcellular elemental composition. Areas as small as 100 nm^2 can be analysed under optimal conditions and detection of any element with an atomic number greater than 10 is possible. Measurement is made in terms of total concentration of the element rather than free ion activity and in this sense the method is comparable to flame photometry (Section 9.9) though with a higher sensitivity.

Another highly sensitive method for the analysis of elements in biological materials uses a high energy proton beam to excite characteristic X-rays. This technique is known as proton induced X-ray emission (PIXE) and has spatial resolution of 1 μm, with normally an analytical sensitivity of 10 p.p.m., although under optimal conditions a sensitivity of one part in 10^7 can be achieved for many elements. The principle of the technique closely resembles that of X-ray spectrochemical analysis, although in PIXE X-rays are produced by collisions between protons rather than between electrons and the target atoms. The technology associated with electron focusing cannot be applied directly to the PIXE method as the lenses are too weak to cope with high energy protons. Consequently, strong focusing magnetic quadruple lenses have been developed. An advantage of PIXE is that high energy protons penetrate much further than electrons, being less easily deflected by atomic collisions. Thus, the resolution of the proton beam is maintained through thicker specimens.

1.7.4 Cytochemistry

Cytochemical techniques may be used to identify specific chemical components, especially enzymes, in cells by direct microscopic observations of tissue sections *in situ*. The technique is based on the colorimetric detection of the components or of their metabolic products. The products of most enzymic reactions are soluble

Table 1.13 Some examples of the cytochemical assay of enzymes by light microscopy (LM) and electron microscopy (EM)

Enzyme	Cellular function	Localisation methods
Acyl transferases	Catalyse transfer of acyl group through CoA	Localisation depends on production of free sulphydryl group and can involve: (i) production of electron-dense ferrocyanide precipitate, or (ii) incubation in the presence of cadmium/lanthanum ions to form insoluble mercaptides
Cytochrome oxidase	Terminal cytochrome in electron transfer chain involved in the transfer of electrons from flavoproteins to O_2	'Nadi' reaction. Naphthol plus aromatic diamine mixed in the presence of cytochrome c gives coloured indophenol. Modification for EM involves the formation of an indoaniline product that yields a coordination polymer
DNase and RNase	Release nucleotides from DNA and RNA	Precipitation with lead, plus an extra initial step, e.g. hydrolysis of nucleotide by phosphatase
Esterases	Hydrolyse a range of carboxylic acid esters	For EM, thioacetic acid is used as substrate. If incubation medium includes lead nitrate, an electron-dense lead sulphide is produced. Alternatively, for LM and EM, azo dye methods can be used
Sulphatases	Catalyse the hydrolytic cleavage of sulphate esters	For LM, naphthol sulphates substituted as substrates and liberated naphthols coupled to diazonium salts give an insoluble dye product (Azo dye method). For EM, heavy-metal trapping agents used, e.g. lead and barium

and must be made insoluble before visualisation can be achieved. The formation of insoluble electron-dense precipitates suitable for electron microscopic studies involves such so-called capture mechanisms. Table 1.13 gives some specific examples of enzyme cytochemical techniques. Cytochemical techniques have been very useful in locating the enzymes associated with, for example, oxidative phosphorylation, β-oxidation, and fatty acid synthesis.

Immunocytochemical microscopy exploits the capacity of cell constituents to act as antigens and to bind specifically to antibodies produced against them. For example, purified monoclonal antibodies (usually from mouse) will bind to a labelled antigen. The presence of the mouse antibody may then be detected using a second labelled anti-mouse antibody, raised in another species. Alternatively an immunoglobulin antibody, isolated and purified chromatographically from the blood of an inoculated animal (say a rabbit) may be used to produce a second antibody in another animal (usually a goat). Methods for visualisation of the label commonly include fluorescence, enzymic reactions, and gold with silver enhancement. A fluorescent dye, such as fluorescein or rhodamine isocyanate is attached to the goat anti-rabbit antibody which may be observed to detect conjugation between rabbit antibodies and the host antigens as a characteristic fluorescence under an ultra violet light microscope fitted with a suitable filter. This indirect method has the advantage that goat anti-rabbit antibody may be used with different rabbit antibodies. The method is also quick and can reveal more than one antigen on the same section, but has the disadvantage that little structural detail is revealed. Sometimes direct labelling of the primary antibody is sufficient. More in-depth coverage of immunological aspects of cytology is given in Section 4.8.5.

Fluorescent analogue cytochemistry permits a study of the spatial organisation of cellular components in living cells by covalently labelling functional molecules or organelles with fluorescent probes and reincorporating these fluorescent analogues into cells, for example the molecular organisation of the cytoskeletal protein actin, labelled with s-iodoacetamidofluorescein, injected into cells by hypoosmotic shock treatment may be followed using fluorescence microscopy. Simultaneous differential analysis of cellular components may be achieved by conjugating fluoroscein and rhodamine isocyanate to antibodies showing differing specificity to antigens. In recent years, confocal micrscopy has been developed for high resolution three-dimensional viewing of fluorescent labels in biological samples. The technique has been adapted to a scanning mode by the use of lasers for fluorescence activation. Details of the theory and application of confocal microscopy is given in Section 1.10. Fluorescent analogues and fluorescent antibodies may both be used in cell-sorting methods (Section 4.8.5). Enzymic antibody labels may also be exploited if conjugated with suitable cross-linking reagents. For example, horseradish peroxidase may be bound by a bifunctional disulphide agent such as N-succinimidyl-3-(2-pyridyldithio)propionate (SDPD), which forms disulphide bonds with lysine residues. Antigen–antibody reactions are detected by applying suitable chromogenic reagents. Gold particles attaching to specific cell antigen may be visualised by silver precipitation in light microscopy but require electron microscopy for quantification of target antigens.

1.7.5 Micrometry, image analysis and video microscopy

These techniques permit measurements of length, area, depth, shape, surface density and other topographical features that may then be correlated with biochemical parameters. Micrometry, in simple terms, may be carried out using the eyepiece of a compound microscope fitted with an eyepiece graticule (calibrated against a stage micrometer) to measure, for example, the degree of opening of stomata in epidermal strips to a range of different incubation conditions. So called quantitative light microscopy may be used to define three-dimensional images in two-dimensional form as in morphometry or, alternatively, similar methods may take a two-dimensional image and use it to derive a three-dimensional structure as in stereology. These methods usually include a range of eyepiece graticules with simple set ruling, short lines or wavy lines that permit scoring of the number of

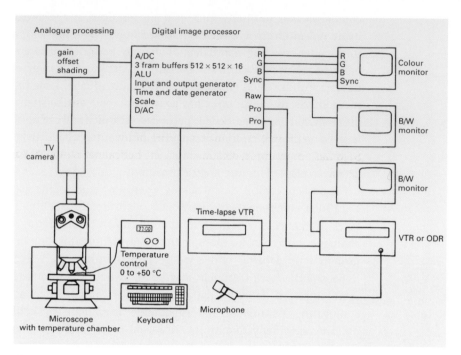

Fig. 1.6. A possible schematic layout for video microscopy. At least one black-and-white (B/W) monitor is required. The colour monitor and time-lapse recorder are optional. Pro, processed images: Sync, synchroniser; Raw, raw image; VTR, video taperecorder; ODR, optical disc recorder. (Reproduced, with permission, from Weiss, D. G. and Galfe, G. (1992) in *Image Analysis in Biology*, ed. D.-P. Häder, CRC Press, Boca Raton, FL.)

either points or intersections of reference objects of interest when the slide is moved randomly with a mechanical stage. Bias is avoided in electron microscopy by taking random micrographs. An especially important measurement based on these principles is the surface area to volume ratio, which is particularly important in physiological investigations.

The advent of microcomputers has greatly extended numerical data manipulation for microscopic investigations. For example, digitiser pads allow operators to electronically trace with a pen the outline either of images directly projected onto the pad or of photographs attached to the pad. The movements of the pen are then passed electronically to a digital computer programmed for morphometry. Image analysers use television cameras to project the image onto a photocathode tube to produce a digitised picture of, say, 512×512 elements (pixels). Usually, each pixel can take the form of 256 shades of grey from 0 (black) to 255 (white). Digitised images are then stored in the computer memory or on disc for later processing and analysis.

Video microscopy can improve microscopic images in three ways: video enhancement (VEM), which increases low contrast images electronically; video intensification (VIM), which amplifies low light images, for example from bioluminescence or fluorescence; and digital image processing. The basic equipment needed for video microscopy is shown in Fig. 1.6.

Video microscopy has great advantages for biochemical investigations because it allows not only for image enhancement and improved resolution of low contrast images of living material, but also for quantitative measurement of specific molecules to be followed over a specific time period. For example, the use of video microscopy has revealed structures that include micelles actively transcribing rDNA genes and microtubule gliding involving ATPase activity.

Scanning tunnelling microscopy (STM) is another technique for viewing the three-dimensional molecular structure of hydrated specimens. Image-processed STM has, for example, demonstrated the helical nature of DNA at approximately 2.5 nm thick.

1.8 KEY TERMS

anabolism
analysis
analytical separations
analytical standards
anion
artefact
auxotroph
auxotrophy
Avogadro's number
axenic culture
batch cultures
buffer action
buffer capacity
Bergmann plating
bioenergetics
biolistics
biomass
biostats
Brönsted and Lowry
callus
catabolism
cation
caulogenesis
chemical fixation
chemical potential
chemolithotroph
chemo-organotroph
chemostat
chemotherapy
closed systems
compartmentalisation
conditional mutant
conductivity
confluence
confocal microscopy
conjugate acid
conjugated molecules
continuous cultures
Control of Substances Hazardous to
    Health
coupled reactions
cryopreservation
cryoprotectant

cryostat
deletions
deletion-substitutions
di-electrophoresis
differentiation
digital image processing
directed mutagesis
Einstein
electrical potential
electrochemical potential
electrofusion
electroporation
embedding media
endergonic reaction
endothermic reaction
enlargement
enthalpy
entropy
equilibrium conditions
equilibrium constant
eukaryote
exergonic reaction
exothermic reaction
Faraday constant
fed-batch cultures
first law of thermodynamics
fluorescence-activated cell sorting
fluoroscent analogue cytochemistry
freeze-fracture
ghost image
Gibbs free energy
good laboratory practice
gram mole
group transfer molecule
half-cell
Henderson–Hasselbalch equation
heterokaryon
homokaryon
hydrophilic
homogenate
homogenisation
hydroponics
immunocytochemical microscopy

ion gradient
lithotrophic
manometry
mass action ratio
membrane potential
meristematic tissue
meristemoids
metabolism
metabolic quotient
microcarriers
micrometry
micropropagation
minimal medium
molar
molar or gas constant
molarity
mole
molecular mass
morphometry
mutant
negative staining
Nernst potential
non-conditional mutant
open systems
organotrophic
oxidative phosphorylation
perfusion
personal transferrable skills
pH
phase contrast
phosphorylation potential
photolithotroph
photo-organotroph
photosynthetic phosphorylation
phylogenetic
pK_a
placebo
point mutation
polar molecules
polarised light microscopes
prokaryote
proton gradient
proton-induced X-ray emission

proton motive force	secondary products	thermodynamic barrier
protoplast fusion	single-cell protein	thermotherapy
prototrophic	slice techniques	tissue fixation
prototrophs	somatic embryos	totipotency
pulse chase	somatic hybridisation	transmission electron miscroscopy
qualitative analysis	specific labelling	ultramicrotome
quantitive analysis	spontaneous reactions	universal labelling
quantitative light microscopy	standard energy status	vascular perfusion
redox couples	standard free energy change	video enhancement
redox potential	standard state	video intensification
relative molecular mass	steady-states	weak acid
resistance mutation	stereology	weak base
resolution	substrate-level phosphorylation	weak electrolyte
respiratory quotient	suppressor-sensitive mutations	whole-body autoradiography
rhizogenesis	superfusion	wild-type
scanning electron microscopy	synthesis	xenobiotic
scanning tunnelling microscopy	Système International d'Unités	X-ray spectrochemical analysis
second law of thermodynamics	temperature-sensitive mutant	zwitterion

1.9 CALCULATIONS

Question 1

An enzyme reaction has been carried out in a volume of 10 cm^3 and calcium chloride ($CaCl_2.6H_2O$) has to be added to stop the reaction to give a final concentration of 10 mM calcium chloride. How many milligrams of $CaCl_2.6H_2O$ needs to be added, given the M_r of $CaCl_2.6H_2O$ = 219.08?

Answer
10 mM = 10 mmol cm^{-3}
μmoles required = $10 \times 10 = 100$ μmol = $100 \times 219.08 \times 10^{-3}$ mg
= 21.91 mg

Question 2

Trypsin in powdered form has to be added to 10 cm^3 of a 1 mg cm^{-3} of bovine serum albumin (BSA) in buffer (pH 8) to give an enzyme to substrate ratio of 1:500 (w/w). How much solid BSA is added?

Answer
$$\frac{\text{Weight trypsin}}{\text{Weight BSA}} = \frac{500}{1}$$

But weight of BSA = 10 mg. Therefore weight of trypsin = 10/500 mg = 0.02 mg.

Question 3

A solution contains 2 μmol glucose cm^{-3} and 0.5 mmol fructose cm^{-3}. What would be the final molar concentration with respect to (i) glucose and (ii) fructose if 10 cm^3 of the solution was made up to a final volume of 30 cm^3 with distilled water? (iii) What additional weight of fructose would you need to add to this 30 cm^3 solution to make it 0.2 M with respect to fructose given that M_r for fructose is 180?

Answer
(i) Concentration of glucose = $\dfrac{10 \times 2}{30}$ μmol cm^{-3} = 0.667 μmol cm^{-3} = 6.67×10^{-4} M

(ii) Concentration of fructose $= \dfrac{10 \times 0.5}{30}$ mmol cm^{-3} = 0.167 mmol cm^{-3} = 0.167 M

(iii) Additional weight of fructose $= 30$ cm$^3 \times (0.200$ M $- 0.167$ M$)$
$$= 30 \times 0.033 \times 180 \text{ mg}$$
$$= 178 \text{ mg}$$

Question 4

(a) Calculate the theoretical RQ for the complete oxidation of (i) pyruvic acid and (ii) glycerol.

(b) During the metabolism of acetic acid by the yeast *Saccharomyces cerevisiae*, 10 μmoles of acetic acid was found to give an oxygen uptake of 220 μl over a period of 1 h. Endogenous metabolism over the same period gave oxygen uptake of 42 μl. What is the percentage acetic acid incorporated into cellular material over this time period, assuming 100% uptake.

Answer

(a) Since the chemical formula for pyruvic acid is $CH_3COCOOH$, the stoichiometry for oxidation is

$$C_3H_4O_3 + 5[O] \Longrightarrow 3CO_2 + 2H_2O$$

$$RQ = \frac{3CO_2}{2.5O_2} = 1.20$$

Since the chemical formula for glycerol is

$$CH_2OH$$
$$CHOH$$
$$CH_2OH$$

the stoichiometry for oxidation is

$$C_3H_8O_3 + 7[O] \Longrightarrow 3CO_2 + 4H_2O$$

$$RQ = \frac{3CO_2}{3.5O_2} = 0.86$$

(b) Since the chemical formula for acetic acid is CH_3COOH, the stoichiometry for the oxidation is

$$C_2H_4O_2 + 4[O] \Longrightarrow 2CO_2 + 2H_2O$$

Oxygen uptake due to acetate metabolism $= (220 - 42)$ μl $= 178$ μl. Thus, 10 μmoles of acetic acid approximates to 10×22.4 μl, assuming s.t.p. conditions.

Hence percentage respired $= \dfrac{178}{224} \times 100\%$

$$= 79.46\%$$

which leaves the percentage incorporated as 20.54%.

Question 5

The enzyme phosphoglucomutase catalyses the interconversion of glucose 1-phosphate to glucose 6-phosphate. At 30 °C and pH 7.0, the equilibrium mixture contains 2.99×10^{-5} M of the 1-phosphate and 5.68×10^{-4} M of the 6-phosphate. Calculate the standard free energy change for the reaction, given $R = 8.314$ J mol^{-1} K^{-1}.

| Answer | $\Delta G^{0\prime} = -RT\ln K_{eq}$ |

$$K_{eq} = \frac{5.68 \times 10^{-4}\,M}{2.99 \times 10^{-5}\,M}$$

$$= 19.0$$

$$\Delta G^{0\prime} = 8.314\,J\,mol^{-1}\,K^{-1} \times 303\,K \times \ln 19.0$$

$$= 7417.5\,J\,mol^{-1}$$

1.10 SUGGESTIONS FOR FURTHER READING

ANDERSON, D. and CONNING, D. M. (1993). *Experimental Toxicology: The Basic Issues*, 2nd edn. The Royal Society of Chemistry, London. (A detailed consideration of model systems for toxicological testing.)

ATKINS, P. W. and JONES, L. L. (1997). *Chemistry, Molecules, Matter and Change*, 3rd edn. W. H. Freeman & Co., New York. (A good undergraduate foundation on general chemistry, including a CD-ROM.)

BEVAN, M. W., HARRISON, B. D. and LEAVER, C. J. (ed.) (1994). *The Production and Uses of Genetically Transformed Plants*. The Royal Society/Chapman & Hall, London. (Specific examples of practical applications of plant molecular biology.)

BEYNON, R. J. (1993). *Postgraduate Study in the Biological Sciences: A Researchers Companion*. Portland Press Ltd, London. (Suitable for undergraduates, covering advice on practical experimental skills, scientific writing, oral presentations and the use of computers.)

GAMBORG, O.L. and PHILLIPS, G. C. (1996). *Plant Cell, Tissue and Organ Culture, Fundamental Methods*. Springer-Verlag, Berlin, Heidelberg, New York. (A comprehensive treatise on plant tissue culture applications.)

FURR, A. K. (ed.) (1995). *CRC Handbook of Laboratory Safety*, 4th edn. CRC Press, Boca Raton, FL. (A complete guide to laboratory safety.)

GARNER, W. Y., BARGE, M. S. and USSUARY, J. P. (eds.) (1992). *Good Laboratory Practice Standards: Applications for Field and Laboratory Studies*, ACS Professional Handbook. American Chemical Society, Washington, DC. (A good GLP handbook.)

GEORGE, E. F. (1996). *Plant Propagation by Tissue Culture*, vols. 1 and 2, 3rd edn. Exegetics Ltd, Edington, Wilts. (Detailed coverage of medium used for plant cell and tissue applications.)

HARRIS, D. A. (1995). *Bioenergetics at a Glance*. Blackwell Science, Oxford. (A modular guide incorporating structural and molecular biology studies into mechanistic explanations of energy transformations in biosystems.)

HARRIS, D. C. (1995). *Quantitive Chemical Analysis*, 4th edn. W. H. Freeman & Co. New York. (A thoroughly comprehensive treatment of chemical analysis.)

JOSEPH, P. D. (1997). *Molecular Toxicology*. Oxford University Press Inc., New York. (Molecular biology applications in toxicology and comprehensive coverage of xenobiotic metabolism.)

LOWE, K. C., DAVEY, M. R. and POWER, J. B. (1996). Plant tissue culture: past, present and future. *Plant Tissue Culture & Biotechnology*, **2**, 175–86. (A short review of recent advances in plant tissue culture methods.)

LEHNINGER, A. L., NELSON, D. L. and COX, M. M. (1993). *Principles of Biochemistry*, 2nd edn. Worth Publishers, New York. (A thoroughbred textbook on biochemistry for undergraduates; excellent for calculations.)

MORGAN, S. J. and DARLING, D. C. (1994). *Animal Cell Culture: Introduction to Biotechniques*. Bios Scientific, Oxford. (A comprehensive consideration of animal cell culture methods.)

PAWLEY, J. B. (ed.) (1995). *Handbook of Biological Confocal Microscopy*, 2nd edn. Plenum Press, New York. (A reference text on all aspects of confocal microscopy.)

SALWAY, J. G. (1994). *Metabolism at a Glance*, Blackwell Science, Oxford. (A concise overview of metabolism with excellent metabolic charts.)

SAMUELS, M. L. (1991). *Statistics for the Life Sciences*. Dellen Publishing Co./Collier Macmillan Inc., San Francisco. (A basic introduction to statistical validation of experiments and experimental design.)

STANBURY, P. F., WHITAKER, A. and HALL, S. J. (1998). *Principles of Fermentation Technology*, 2nd edn. Elsevier Science Publishers, BV, Amsterdam. (An easy-to-read text that covers most aspects of microbial fermentations.)

SMITH, C. and WOOD, E. J. (eds.) (1991). *Energy in Biological Systems – Molecular and Cell Biochemistry*. Chapman & Hall, London. (A readily understandable text linking bioenergetics and metabolism.)

TUFFERY, A. A. (1995). *Laboratory Animals: An Introduction for Experimenters*, 2nd edn. John Wiley & Sons, Chichester. (A manual for qualified licence holders.)

Chapter 2

Molecular biology and basic techniques

2.1 INTRODUCTION

One of the key macromolecular elements essential for the maintenance, integrity and functioning of all cells is proteins. Proteins are an essential yet diverse group of biomolecules encompassing enzymes, antibodies, transport and structural proteins, to name but a few. The synthesis of proteins is itself catalysed by enzymes and proteins; however, this process is ultimately directed by the genetic material deoxyribonucleic acid or DNA. DNA encodes all the information needed to specify the structure of every protein the cell can produce. The realisation that DNA lies behind all the cell's activities led to the development of molecular biology. Rather than a discrete area of biosciences, molecular biology is now accepted as a very important means of understanding and describing complex biological processes. The development of the methods and techniques to study processes at the molecular level has led to new and powerful ways of isolating, analysing, manipulating and exploiting nucleic acids. It has also given rise to the development of new and exciting areas of the biological sciences such as biotechnology, genome mapping, molecular medicine and gene therapy.

In considering the potential utility of molecular biological techniques it is important to understand some of the fundamental attributes of the structures of nucleic acids and gain an appreciation of how this dictates the function *in vivo* and *in vitro*. Indeed many techniques used in molecular biology mimic in some way the natural functions of nucleic acids, such as replication and transcription. This chapter is therefore intended to provide an overview of the general features of nucleic acid structure and function and describe some of the basic methods used in its isolation and analysis.

2.2 COMPONENTS AND PRIMARY STRUCTURE OF NUCLEIC ACIDS

DNA and RNA are macromolecular structures composed of regular repeating polymers formed from nucleotides. These are the basic building blocks of nucleic acids and are derived from nucleosides, which are composed of two elements: a five-membered pentose carbon sugar (2-deoxyribose in DNA and ribose in RNA), and a nitrogenous base. The carbon atoms of the sugar are designated 'prime' (1', 2', 3', etc.) to distinguish them from the carbons of nitrogenous bases

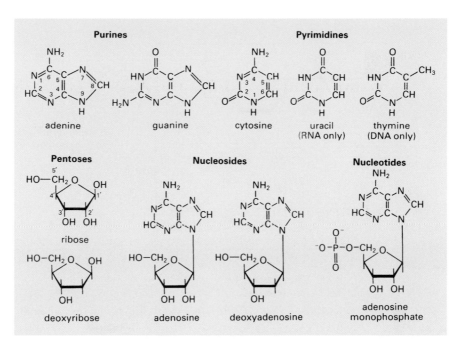

Fig. 2.1. Structures of bases, nucleosides and nucleotides.

of which there are two types, purines and pyrimidines. A nucleotide, or nucleoside phosphate, is formed by the attachment of a phosphate to the 5′ position of a nucleoside by an ester linkage (Fig. 2.1). Such nucleotides can be joined together by the formation of a second ester bond by reaction between the phosphate of one nucleotide and the 3′-hydroxyl of another, thus generating a 5′ → 3′ phosphodiester bond between adjacent sugars; this process can be repeated indefinitely to give long polynucleotide molecules (Fig. 2.2). DNA has two such polynucleotide strands, however, since each strand has both a free 5′-hydroxyl group at one end, and a free 3′-hydroxyl at the other end, each strand has a polarity or directionality. The polarity of the two strands of the molecule are in opposite directions, and thus DNA is described as an anti-parallel structure (Fig. 2.3).

The purine bases (composed of fused five- and six-membered rings), adenine (A) and guanine (G), are found in both RNA and DNA, as is the pyrimidine (a single six-membered ring) cytosine (C). The other pyrimidines are each restricted to one type of nucleic acid: uracil (U) occurs exclusively in RNA, whilst thymine (T) is limited to DNA. Thus it is possible to distinguish between RNA and DNA on the basis of the presence of ribose and uracil in RNA, and deoxyribose and thymine in DNA. However, it is the sequence of bases along a molecule that distinguishes one DNA (or RNA) from another. It is conventional to write a nucleic acid sequence starting at the 5′-end of the molecule, using single capital letters to represent each of the bases, for example CGGATCT. Note that there is usually no point in including the sugar or phosphate groups, since these are identical throughout the length

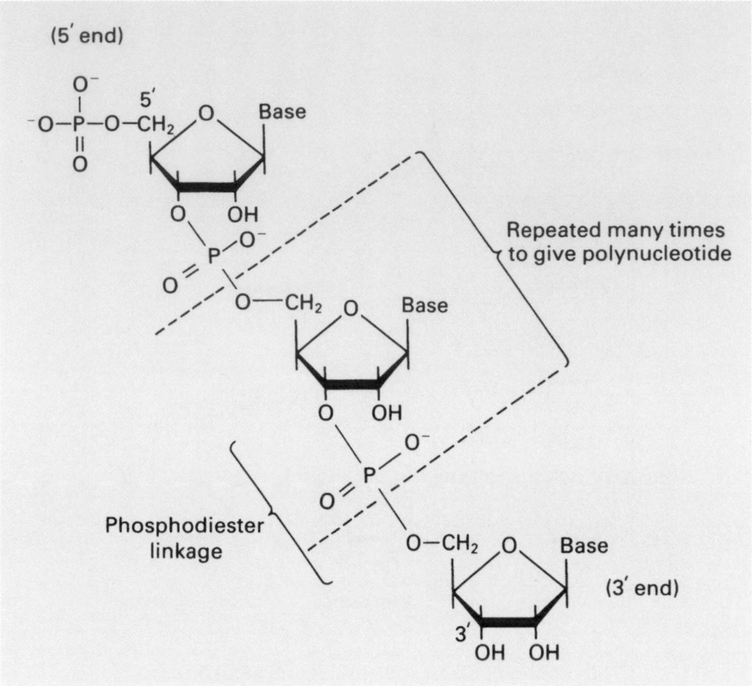

Fig. 2.2. Polynucleotide structure.

of the molecule. Terminal phosphate groups can, when necessary, be indicated by use of a 'p'; thus 5'-pCGGATCT-3' indicates the presence of a phosphate on the 5' end of the molecule.

2.2.1 **Secondary structure of nucleic acids**

The two polynucleotide chains in DNA are usually found in the shape of a right-handed double helix, in which the bases of the two strands lie in the centre of the molecule, with the sugar-phosphate backbones on the outside. A crucial feature of this double-stranded structure is that it depends on the sequence of bases in one strand being complementary to that in the other. A purine base attached to a sugar residue on one strand is always hydrogen bonded to a pyrimidine base attached to a sugar residue on the other strand. Moreover, adenine (A) always pairs with thymine (T) or uracil (U) in RNA, via two hydrogen bonds, and guanine (G) always pairs with cytosine (C) by three hydrogen bonds (Fig. 2.4). When these conditions are met a stable double-helical structure results in which the backbones of the two strands are, on average, a constant distance apart. Thus, if the sequence of one strand is known, that of the other strand can be deduced. The strands are designated as plus (+) and minus (−) and an RNA molecule complementary to the minus (−) strand is synthesised during transcription (Section 2.6.3). The base sequence may cause significant local variations in the shape of the DNA molecule

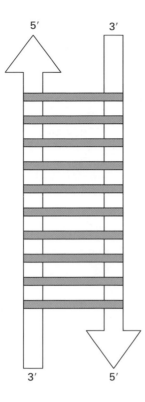

Fig. 2.3. The antiparallel nature of DNA. One strand of DNA in a double helix runs 5′ → 3′, whilst the other strand runs in the opposite 3′ → 5′. The strands are held together by hydrogen bonds between the bases.

and these variations are vital for specific interactions between the DNA and various proteins to take place. Although the three-dimensional structure of DNA may vary, it generally adopts a double-helical structure termed the B form or B-DNA *in vivo*. There are also other forms of right handed DNA, such as A and C, that are formed when DNA fibres are subjected to different relative humidities (Table 2.1).

The major distinguishing feature of B-DNA is that it has approximately 10 bases for one turn of the double helix; furthermore a distinctive major and minor groove may be identified (Fig. 2.5). In certain circumstances, where repeated DNA sequences or motifs are found, the DNA may adopt a left-handed helical structure termed Z-DNA. This form of DNA was first synthesised in the laboratory and is thought not to exist *in vivo*. The various forms of DNA serve to show that it is not a static molecule but dynamic and constantly in flux; it may be coiled, bent or distorted at certain times. Although RNA almost always exists as a single strand, it often contains sequences within the same strand which are self-complementary, and which can therefore base-pair if brought together by suitable folding of the molecule. A notable example is transfer RNA (tRNA), which folds up to give a clover leaf secondary structure (Fig. 2.6).

Table 2.1	The various forms of DNA			
DNA form	% humidity	Helix direction	Base/turn helix	Helix diameter (A)
B	92%	RH	10	19
A	75%	RH	11	23
C	66%	RH	9.3	19
Z	(Pu-Py)$_n$	LH	12	18

RH, right-handed helix; LH, left-handed helix; Pu, Purine; Py, Pyrimidine.
Different forms of DNA may be obtained by subjecting DNA fibres to different relative humidities. The B form is the most common form of DNA whilst the A and C forms have been derived under laboratory conditions. The Z form may be produced with a DNA sequence made up from alternating purine and pyrimidine nucleotides.

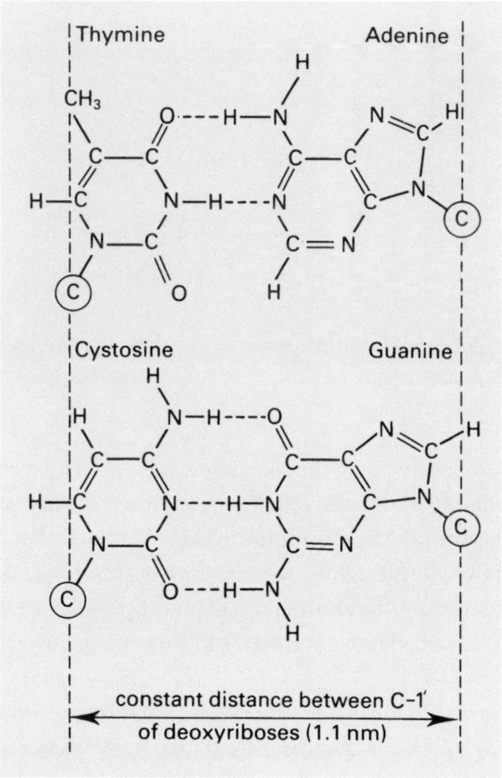

Fig. 2.4. Base-pairing in DNA. C in a circle represents carbon at the 1′ position of deoxyribose.

2.2.2 Separation of double-stranded DNA

The two anti-parallel strands of DNA are held together only by the weak forces of hydrogen bonding between complementary bases, and partly by hydrophobic interactions between adjacent, stacked base-pairs, termed base-stacking. Little energy is needed to separate a few base-pairs, and so, at any instant, a few short

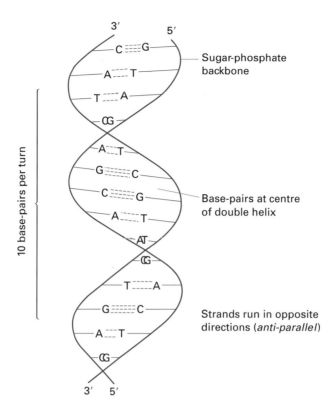

Fig. 2.5. The DNA double helix.

stretches of DNA will be opened up to the single-stranded conformation. However, such stretches immediately pair up again at room temperature, so the molecule as a whole remains predominantly double stranded.

If, however, a DNA solution is heated to approximately 90 °C or above there will be enough kinetic energy to denature the DNA completely, causing it to separate into single strands. This denaturation can be followed spectrophotometrically by monitoring the absorbance of light at 260 nm. The stacked bases of double-stranded DNA are less able to absorb light than the less constrained bases of single-stranded molecules, and so the absorbance of DNA at 260 nm increases as the DNA becomes denatured, a phenomenon known as the hyperchromic effect.

A plot of the absorbance at 260 nm against the temperature of a DNA solution indicates that little denaturation occurs below approximately 70 °C, but further increases in temperature result in a marked increase in the extent of denaturation. Eventually a temperature is reached at which the sample is totally denatured, or melted. The temperature at which 50% of the DNA is melted is termed the melting temperature or T_m, and this depends on the nature of the DNA (Fig. 2.7). If several different samples of DNA are melted, it is found that the T_m is highest for those DNAs that contain the highest proportion of cytosine and guanine, and T_m can actually be used to estimate the percentage C + G in a DNA

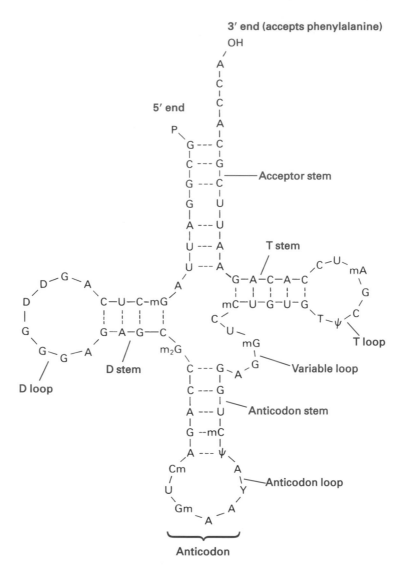

Fig. 2.6. Secondary structure of yeast tRNA^{Phe}. A single strand of 76 ribonucleotides forms four double-stranded 'stem' regions by base-pairing between complementary sequences. The anticodon will base-pair with UUU or UUC (both are codons for phenylalanine), and phenylalanine is attached to the 3'-end by a specific aminoacyl tRNA synthetase. Several 'unusual' bases are present: D, dihydrouridine; T, ribothymidine; ψ, pseudouridine; Y, very highly modified, unlike any 'normal' base. mX indicates methylation of base X (m$_2$X shows dimethylation); Xm indicates methylation of ribose on the 2' position.

sample. This relationship between T_m and C + G content arises because cytosine and guanine form three hydrogen bonds when base-paired, whereas thymine and adenine form only two. Because of the differential numbers of hydrogen bonds between A·T and C·G pairs, those sequences with a predominance of C·G pairs

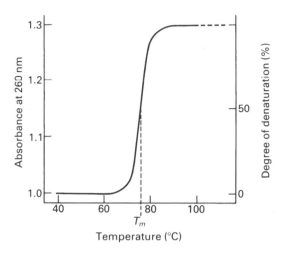

Fig. 2.7. Melting curve of DNA.

will require greater energy to separate or denature them. The conditions required to separate a particular nucleotide sequence are also dependent on environmental conditions such as salt concentration.

If melted DNA is cooled it is possible for the separated strands to reassociate, a process known as renaturation. However, a stable double-stranded molecule will be formed only if the complementary strands collide in such a way that their bases are paired precisely, and this is an unlikely event if the DNA is very long and complex (i.e. if it contains a large number of different genes). Measurements of the rate of renaturation can give information about the complexity of a DNA preparation (Section 2.3).

Strands of RNA and DNA will associate with each other, if their sequences are complementary, to give double-stranded, hybrid molecules. Similarly, a strand of radioactively labelled RNA or DNA, when added to a denatured DNA preparation, will act as a probe for DNA molecules to which it is complementary (Section 2.7). This hybridisation of complementary strands of nucleic acids is very useful for isolating a specific fragment of DNA from a complex mixture (Section 2.10). It is also possible for small single-stranded fragments of DNA (up to 40 bases in length) termed oligonucleotides to hybridise to a denatured sample of DNA. This type of hybridisation is termed annealing and again is dependent on the base sequence of the oligonucleotide and the salt concentration of the sample.

2.3 GENES AND GENOME COMPLEXITY

Each region of DNA that codes for a single RNA or protein is called a gene, and the entire set of genes in a cell, organelle or virus forms its genome. Cells and organelles may contain more than one copy of their genome. Genomic DNA from

Table 2.2 **Repetitive satellite sequences found in DNA, and their characteristics**

Types of repetitive DNA	Repeat unit size (bp)	Characteristics/motifs
Satellite DNA	5–200	Large repeat unit range (Mb) usually found at centromeres
Minisatellite DNA		
Telomere sequence	6	Found at the ends of chromosomes. Repeat unit may span up to 20 kb G-rich sequence
Hypervariable sequence	10–60	Repeat unit may span up to 20 kb
Microsatellite DNA	1–4	Mononucleotide repeat of adenine dinucleotide repeats common (CA). Usually known as VNTR (variable number tandem repeat)

bp, base-pairs; kb, kilobase-pairs.

nearly all prokaryotic and eukaryotic organisms is also complexed with protein and termed chromosomal DNA. Each gene is located at a particular position along the chromosome, termed the locus, whilst the particular form of the gene is termed the allele. In mammalian DNA, each gene is present in two allelic forms which may be identical (homozygous) or which may vary (heterozygous). The occurrence of different alleles at the same site in the genome is termed polymorphism. In general, the more complex an organism the larger its genome, although this is not always the case, since many higher organisms have non-coding sequences some of which are repeated numerous times and termed repetitive DNA. In mammalian DNA repetitive sequences may be divided into low copy number and high copy number DNA. The latter is composed of some repeat sequences that are dispersed throughout the genome and some that are clustered together. The repeat-cluster DNA may be defined as so-called classical satellite DNA, minisatellite or microsatellite DNA, the latter being composed mainly of dinucleotide repeats (Table 2.2). These sequences are polymorphic and vary between individuals; they also form the basis of genetic fingerprinting (Section 3.8.6).

Higher organisms may be identified by using the size and shape of their genetic material at a particular point in the cell division cycle, termed metaphase. At this point DNA condenses to form a number of very distinct chromosome structures. Various morphological characteristics of chromosomes may be identified at this stage, including the centromere and the telomere. The array of chromosomes from a given organism may also be stained with dyes and subsequently identified by light microscopy. The complete array of chromosomes in an organism is termed the karyotype. In certain genetic disorders aberrations in the size, shape and number of chromosomes may occur and thus the karyotype may be used as an indicator of the disorder (Section 3.8.2). Perhaps the best-known example of this is the correlation of Down's syndrome, where three copies of chromosome 21 (trisomy 21) exist rather than two as in the normal state.

2.3.1 **Renaturation kinetics and genome complexity**

When preparations of double-stranded DNA are denatured and allowed to renature, measurement of the rate of renaturation can give valuable information about the complexity of the DNA, i.e. how much information it contains (measured in base-pairs). The complexity of a molecule may be much less than its total length if some sequences are repetitive, but complexity will equal total length if all sequences are unique, appearing only once in the genome. In practice, the DNA is first cut randomly into fragments about 1 kb in length (Section 2.9), and is then completely denatured by heating above its T_m (Section 2.2.2). Renaturation at a temperature about 10 deg.C below the T_m is monitored either by decrease in absorbance at 260 nm (the hypochromic effect), or by passing samples at intervals through a column of hydroxylapatite (Section 13.5.2), which will adsorb only double-stranded DNA, and measuring how much of the sample is bound. The degree of renaturation after a given time will depend on C_o, the concentration (in nucleotides per unit volume) of double-stranded DNA prior to denaturation, and t, the duration of the renaturation in seconds.

For a given C_o, it should be evident that a preparation of phage λ DNA (genome size 49 kb) will contain many more copies of the same sequence per unit volume than a preparation of human DNA (haploid genome size 3×10^6 kb), and will therefore renature far more rapidly, since there will be more molecules complementary to each other per unit volume in the case of λ DNA, and therefore more chance of two complementary strands colliding with each other. In order to compare the rates of renaturation of different DNA samples it is usual to measure C_o and the time taken for renaturation to proceed half way to completion, $t_{\frac{1}{2}}$, and to multiply these values together to give a $C_o t_{\frac{1}{2}}$ value. The larger the $C_o t_{\frac{1}{2}}$, the greater the complexity of the DNA; hence λ DNA has a far lower $C_o t_{\frac{1}{2}}$ than does human DNA.

In fact, the human genome does not renature in a uniform fashion. If the extent of renaturation is plotted against log $C_o t$ (this is known as a Cot curve), it is seen that part of the DNA renatures quite rapidly, whilst the remainder is very slow to renature (Fig. 2.8). This indicates that some sequences have a higher concentration than others; in other words, part of the genome consists of repetitive sequences. These repetitive sequences can be separated from the single-copy DNA by passing the renaturing sample through a hydroxylapatite column early in the renaturation process, at a time which gives a low value of $C_o t$. At this stage only the rapidly renaturing sequences will be double stranded, and they will therefore be the only ones able to bind to the column.

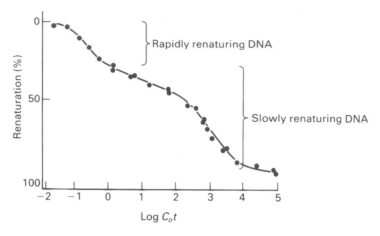

Fig. 2.8. Cot curve of human DNA. DNA was allowed to renature at 60 °C after being completely dissociated by heat. Samples were taken at intervals and passed through a hydroxylapatite column to determine the percentage of double-stranded DNA present. This percentage was plotted against log $C_o t$ (original concentration of DNA × time of sampling).

2.4 THE NATURE OF THE GENETIC CODE

DNA encodes the primary sequence of a protein by utilising sets of three nucleotides, termed a codon or triplet, to encode a particular amino acid. The four bases (A, C, G and T) present in DNA allow up to 64 triplet combinations; however, since there are only 20 naturally occurring amino acids, more than one codon may encode an amino acid. This phenomenon is termed the degeneracy of the genetic code. With the exception of a limited number of differences found in mitochondrial DNA and one or two other species, the genetic code appears to be universal. In addition to coding for amino acids, particular triplet sequences also indicate the beginning (Start) and the end (Stop) of a particular gene. Only one start codon exists (ATG), which also codes for the amino acid methionine, whereas three dedicated stop codons are available (TAT, TAG and TGA) (Fig. 2.9).

2.5 CELLULAR LOCATION OF NUCLEIC ACIDS

In general, DNA in eukaryotic cells is confined to the nucleus or organelles such as mitochondria or chloroplasts that contain their own genome. The predominant RNA species are, however, normally located within the cytoplasm. The genetic information of cells and most viruses is stored in the form of DNA. This information is used to direct the synthesis of RNA molecules, which fall into three classes. Figure 2.10 indicates the locations of nucleic acids in prokaryotic and eukaryotic cells.

(i) *Messenger RNA* (mRNA) contains sequences of ribonucleotides that code for the amino acid sequences of proteins. A single mRNA codes for a single

First Position (5'-end)	Second Position				Third Position (3'-end)
	T	**C**	**A**	**G**	
T	Phe	Ser	Tyr	Cys	T
	Phe	Ser	Tyr	Cys	C
	Leu	Ser	**Stop**	**Stop**	A
	Leu	Ser	**Stop**	Trp	G
C	Leu	Pro	His	Arg	T
	Leu	Pro	His	Arg	C
	Leu	Pro	Gln	Arg	A
	Leu	Pro	Gln	Arg	G
A	Ile	Thr	Asn	Ser	T
	Ile	Thr	Asn	Ser	C
	Ile	Thr	Lys	Arg	A
	Met	Thr	Lys	Arg	G
G	Val	Ala	Asp	Gly	T
	Val	Ala	Asp	Gly	C
	Val	Ala	Glu	Gly	A
	Val	Ala	Glu	Gly	G

Fig. 2.9. The genetic code. Note that the codons in blue represent the start codon (ATG) and the three stop codons.

    polypeptide chain in eukaryotes but may code for several polypeptides in prokaryotes.

(ii) *Ribosomal RNA* (rRNA) forms part of the structure of ribosomes, which are the sites of protein synthesis. Each ribosome contains only three or four different rRNA molecules, complexed with a total of between 55 and 75 proteins.

(iii) *Transfer RNA* (tRNA) molecules carry amino acids to the ribosomes, and interact with the mRNA in such a way that their amino acids are joined together in the order specified by the mRNA. There is at least one type of tRNA for each amino acid.

In eukaryotic cells alone a further group of RNA molecules termed small nuclear RNA (snRNA) is present; they function within the nucleus and promote the maturation of mRNA molecules. All RNA molecules are associated with their respective binding proteins and are essential for their cellular functions. Nucleic acids from prokaryotic cells are less well compartmentalised, although they serve similar functions.

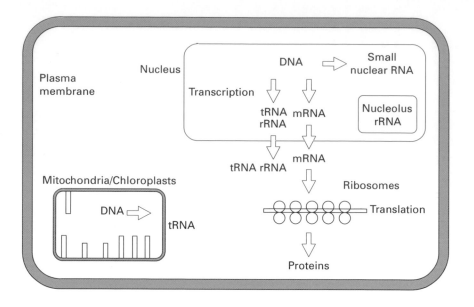

Fig. 2.10. Location of DNA and RNA molecules in eukaryotic cells and the flow of genetic information.

2.5.1 **The packaging of DNA**

The DNA in prokaryotic cells resides in the cytoplasm, although it is associated with nucleoid proteins, where it is tightly coiled and supercoiled by topoisomerase enzymes to enable it physically to fit into the cell. In contrast, eukaryotic cells have many levels of packaging of the DNA within the nucleus, involving a variety of DNA-binding proteins.

First-order packaging involves the winding of the DNA around a core complex of four small proteins, repeated twice, termed histones (H2A, H2B, H3 and H4). These are rich in the basic amino acids lysine and arginine and form a barrel-shaped core octomer structure. Approximately 180 bp of DNA is wound twice around the structure, which is termed a nucleosome. A further histone protein, H1, is found to associate with the outer surface of the nucleosome. The compacting effect of the nucleosome reduces the length of the DNA by a factor of 6.

Nucleosomes also associate to form a second order of packaging termed the 30 nm chromatin fibre, thus further reducing the length of the DNA by a factor of 7 (Fig. 2.11). These structures may be further folded and looped through the interaction with other non-histone proteins and ultimately form chromosome structures.

DNA is found closely associated with the nuclear lamina matrix, which forms a protein scaffold within the nucleus. The DNA is attached at certain positions within the scaffold, usually coinciding with origins of replication. Many other DNA binding proteins are also present, such as high mobility group proteins (HMG), which assist in promoting certain DNA conformations during processes such as replication or active gene expression.

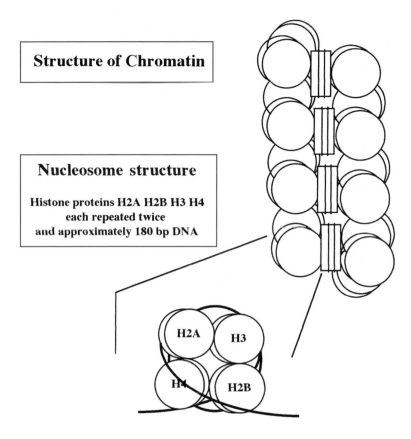

Fig. 2.11. Structure and composition of the nucleosome and chromatin.

2.6 THE CELLULAR FUNCTIONS OF DNA

2.6.1 DNA replication

The double-stranded nature of DNA provides a means of replication during cell division, since the separation of two DNA strands allows complementary strands to be synthesised upon them. Many enzymes and accessory proteins are required for *in vivo* replication, which in prokaryotes begins at a region of the DNA termed the origin of replication.

DNA has to be unwound before any of the proteins and enzymes needed for replication can act, and this involves separating the double-helical DNA into single strands. This process is carried out by the enzyme DNA helicase. Furthermore, in order to prevent the single strands from reannealing, small proteins termed single-stranded DNA-binding proteins (SSBPs) attach to the single DNA strands (Fig. 2.12)

On each exposed single strand a short, complementary RNA chain termed a primer is first produced, using the DNA as a template. The primer is synthesised by

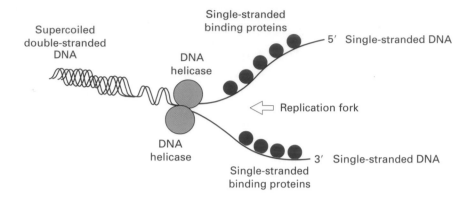

Fig. 2.12. Initial events at the replication fork involving DNA unwinding.

an RNA polymerase enzyme known as a primase, which uses ribonucleoside triphosphates and itself requires no primer to function. Then DNA polymerase III
(DNA pol III) also uses the original DNA as a template for the synthesis of a DNA
strand, using the RNA primer as a starting point. The primer is vital since it leaves
an exposed 3'-hydroxyl group. This is necessary, since DNA polymerase III can add
new nucleotides only to the 3' end and not the 5' end of a nucleic acid. Synthesis of
the DNA strand therefore occurs only in a $5' \rightarrow 3'$ direction from the RNA primer.
This DNA strand is usually termed the leading strand and provides the means for
continuous DNA synthesis.

Since the two strands of double-helical DNA are antiparallel, only one can be
synthesised in a continuous fashion. Synthesis of the other strand must take place
in a more complex way. The precise mechanism was worked out by Reiji Okazaki
in the 1960s. Here the strand, usually termed the lagging strand, is produced in relatively short stretches of 1–2 kb termed Okazaki fragments. This is still in a $5' \rightarrow 3'$
direction, using many RNA primers for each individual stretch. Thus, discontinuous synthesis of DNA takes place and allows DNA polymerase III to work in the
$5' \rightarrow 3'$ direction. The RNA primers are then removed by DNA polymerase I, which
has a $5' \rightarrow 3'$ exonuclease, and the gaps are filled by the same enzyme acting as a
polymerase. The separate fragments are joined together by DNA ligase to give a
newly formed strand of DNA on the lagging strand (Fig. 2.13).

The replication of eukaryotic DNA is less well characterised, involves multiple
origins of replication and is certainly more complex than that of prokaryotes. In
both cases, however, the process involves $5' \rightarrow 3'$ synthesis of new DNA strands.
The net result of the replication is that the original DNA is replaced by two molecules, each containing one 'old' and one 'new' strand; the process is therefore
known as semi-conservative replication. The ideas behind DNA synthesis, replication and the enzymes involved in them have been adopted in many molecular biological techniques and form the basis of many manipulations in genetic
engineering.

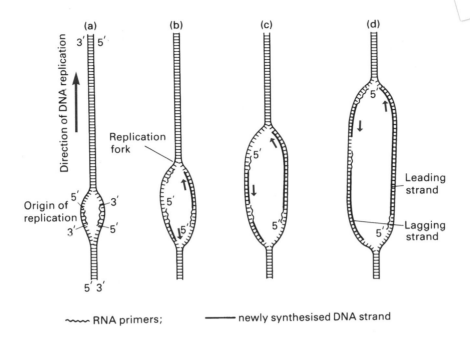

Fig. 2.13. DNA replication. (a) Double-stranded DNA separates at the origin of replication. RNA polymerase synthesises short DNA primer strands complementary to both DNA strands. (b) DNA polymerase III synthesises new DNA strands in a 5′ to 3′ direction, complementary to the exposed, old DNA strands, and continuing from the 3′-end of each RNA primer. Consequently DNA synthesis is in the same direction as DNA replication for one strand (the leading strand) and in the opposite direction for the other (the lagging strand). RNA primer synthesis occurs repeatedly to allow the synthesis of fragments of the lagging strand. (c) As the replication fork moves away from the origin of replication, polymerase III continues the synthesis of the leading strand, and synthesises DNA between RNA primers of the lagging strand. (d) DNA polymerase I removes RNA primers from the lagging strand and fills the resulting gaps with DNA. DNA ligase then joins the resulting fragments, producing a continuous DNA strand.

2.6.2 DNA protection and repair systems

Cellular growth and division require the correct and coordinated replication of DNA. Mechanisms that proofread replicated DNA sequences and maintain integrity of those sequences are, however, complex and are only beginning to be elucidated for prokaryotic systems. Bacterial protection is afforded by the use of a restriction modification system based on differential methylation of host DNA, so as to distinguish it from foreign DNA such as viruses. The most common is type II and consists of a host DNA methylase and restriction endonuclease that recognises short (4–6 bp) palindromic sequences and cleaves foreign unmethylated DNA at a particular target sequence. The enzymes involved in this process have been of enormous benefit for the manipulation and analysis of DNA, as indicated in Section 2.9.

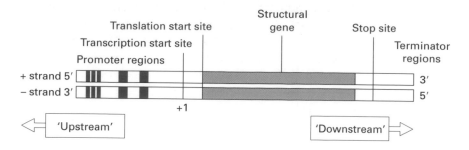

Fig. 2.14. Structure and nomenclature of a typical gene.

Repair systems allow the recognition of altered, mispaired or missing bases in double-stranded DNA and invokes an excision repair process. The systems characterised for bacteria are based on the length of repairable DNA during either replication (dam system) or in general repair (urr system). In some cases damage to DNA activates a protein termed RecA to produce an SOS response that includes the activation of many enzymes and proteins; however, this has yet to be fully characterised. The recombination–repair systems in eukaryotic cells may share some common features with prokaryotes, although the precise mechanism has yet to be established. Defects in DNA repair may result in the stable incorporation of errors into genomic sequences and these may underscore several genetic-based diseases.

2.6.3 Transcription of DNA

Expression of genes is carried out initially by the process of transcription, whereby a complementary RNA strand is synthesised by an enzyme termed RNA polymerase from a DNA template encoding the gene. Most prokaryotic genes are made up of three regions. At the centre is the sequence that will be copied in the form of RNA, this is called the structural gene. To the 5′ side (upstream) of the strand that will be copied (the plus (+) strand) lies a region called the promoter, and downstream from the transcription unit is the terminator region. Transcription begins when DNA-dependent RNA polymerase binds to the promoter region and moves along the DNA to the transcription unit. At the start of the transcription unit the polymerase begins to synthesise an RNA molecule complementary to the minus (−) strand of the DNA, moving along this strand in a 3′ to 5′ direction, and synthesising RNA in a 5′ → 3′ direction, using ribonucleoside triphosphates. The RNA will therefore have the same sequence as the plus strand of DNA, apart from the substitution of uracil for thymine. On reaching the stop site in the terminator region, transcription is stopped, and the RNA molecule is released. The numbering of bases in genes is a useful way of identifying key elements. Point or base + 1 is the residue located at the transcription start site, positive numbers denote 3′ regions, whilst negative numbers denote 5′ regions (Fig. 2.14).

In eukaryotes, three different RNA polymerases exist, designated I, II and III. Messenger RNA is synthesised by RNA polymerase II, whilst RNA polymerase I and III catalyse the synthesis of rRNA (I), tRNA and snRNA (III). Many non-expressed genes tend to have residues that are methylated, usually the C of a G-C dinucleotide and, in general, active genes tend to be hypomethylated. This is especially prevalent at the 5′-flanking regions and is a useful means of discovering and identifying new genes.

2.6.4 Promoter and terminator sequences in DNA

Promoters are usually to the 5′-end or upstream of the structural gene and have been best characterised in prokaryotes such as *Escherichia coli*. They comprise two highly conserved sequence elements: the TATA box (consensus sequence 'TATAAT') which is centred approximately 10 bp upstream from the transcription initiation site (−10 in the gene numbering system), and a further sequence which is centred about −25 bp upstream from the TATA box. This element is thought to be important in the initial recognition and binding of RNA polymerase to the DNA, while the −10 sequence is involved in the formation of a transcription initiation complex (Fig. 2.15a).

The promoter elements serve as recognition sites for DNA-binding proteins that control gene expression and these proteins are termed transcription factors or *trans*-acting factors. These proteins have a DNA-binding domain for interaction with promoters and an activation domain to allow interaction with other transcription factors. A well-studied example of a transcription factor is TFIID, which binds to the −35 promoter sequence in eukaryotic cells. Gene regulation occurs in most cases at the level of transcription, and primarily by the rate of transcription initiation, although control may also be by modulation of mRNA stability, or at other levels such as translation. Terminator sequences are less well characterised, but are thought to involve nucleotide sequences near the end of mRNA with the capacity to form a hairpin loop, followed by a run of U residues, which may constitute a termination signal for RNA polymerase.

In the case of eukaryotic genes numerous short sequences spanning several hundred bases may be important for transcription, compared to normally fewer than 100 bp for prokaryotic promoters. Particularly critical is the TATA box sequence, located approximately −35 bp upstream from the transcription initiation point in the majority of genes (Fig. 2.15b). This is analogous to the −10 sequence in prokaryotes. A number of other transcription factors also bind sequentially to form an initiation complex that includes RNA polymerase, subsequent to this, transcription is initiated. In addition to the TATA box, a CAT box (consensus GGCCAATCT) is often located at about −80 bp, which is an important determinant of promoter efficiency. Many upstream promoter elements (UPEs) have been described that are either general in their action or tissue (or gene) specific. Elements that contain the sequence GGGCG may be present at multiple sites and in either orientation and are often associated with housekeeping genes such as those encoding enzymes involved in general metabolism. Some promoter

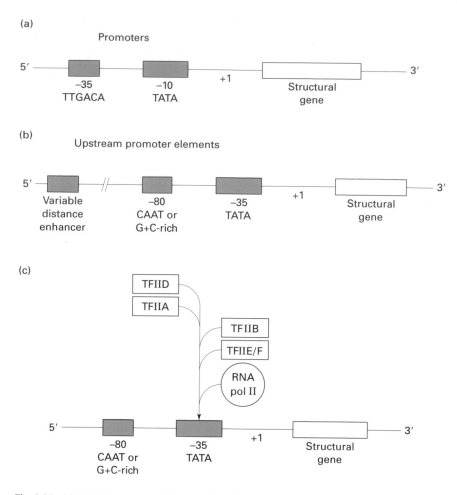

Fig. 2.15. (a) Typical promoter elements found in a prokaryotic cell (e.g. *E. coli*). (b) Typical promoter elements found in eukaryotic cells. (c) Generalised scheme of binding of transcription factors to the promoter regions of eukaryotic cells. Following the binding of the transcription factors IID, IIA IIB, IIE and IIF a preinitiation complex is formed. RNA polymerase II then binds to this complex and begins transcription from the start point +1.

sequence elements, such as the TATA box, are common to most genes, while others may be specific to particular genes or classes of genes.

Of particular interest is a class of promoter first investigated in simian virus 40 (SV40) and termed an enhancer. These sequences are distinguished from other promoter sequences by their unique ability to function over several kilobases either upstream or downstream from a particular gene in an orientation-independent manner. Even at such great distances from the transcription start point they may increase transcription by several hundred-fold. The precise interactions between transcription factors, RNA polymerase or other DNA-binding proteins and the DNA sequences they bind to may be identified and characterised by the technique of DNA footprinting (Section 3.8.3). For transcription in eukaryotic cells to proceed, a number of transcription factors need to interact with the promoters and with each other. This cascade mechanism is indicated in Fig. 2.15c and is termed a preinitiation complex. Once this has been formed around the −35 TATA sequence RNA polymerase II is able to transcribe the structural gene and form a complementary RNA copy (Section 2.6.6).

2.6.5 Transcription in prokaryotes

Prokaryotic gene organisation differs from that found in prokaryotes in a number of ways. Prokarotic genes are generally found as continuous coding sequences that are not interrupted. Moreover they are frequently found clustered into operons, which contain genes that relate to a particular function such as the metabolism of a substrate or synthesis of a product. This is particularly evident in the best-known operon identified in *E. coli*, termed the lactose operon, where three genes (*lacZ*, *lacY* and *lacA*) share the same promoter and are therefore switched on and off at the same time. In this model, the absence of lactose results in a repressor protein binding to an operator region upstream from the *Z*, *Y* and *A* genes and prevents RNA polymerase from transcribing them (Fig. 2.16a). However the presence of lactose requires the genes to be transcribed to allow its metabolism. Lactose binds to the repressor protein and causes a conformational change in its structure. This prevents it binding to the operator and allows RNA polymerase to bind and transcribe the three genes (Fig. 2.16b). Transcription and translation in prokaryotes is also closely linked or coupled whereas in eukaryotic cells the two processes are distinct and take place in different cell compartments.

2.6.6 Post-transcriptional processing

Transcription of a eukaryotic gene results in the production of a heterogeneous nuclear RNA transcript (hnRNA) that faithfully represents the entire structural gene (Fig. 2.17). Three processing events then take place. The first step involves the addition of a methylated guanosine residue (m^7Gppp) termed a cap to the 5′-end of the hnRNA. This may be a signalling structure or aid in the translation of the molecule (Fig. 2.18). In addition, 150 to 300 adenosine residues termed a poly(A) tail are attached at the 3′ end of the hnRNA by the enzyme poly(A) polymerase. The polyA tail allows the specific isolation of eukaryotic mRNA from total RNA by affinity chromatography (Section 2.8.2); its presence is thought to confer stability on the transcript.

Unlike prokaryotic transcripts, those from eukaryotes have their coding sequence (expressed regions or exons) interrupted by non-coding sequence (intervening regions or introns). Intron–exon boundaries are generally determined by the sequence GU . . . AG and need to be removed or spliced before the mature mRNA is formed (Fig. 2.18). The process of intron splicing is mediated by snRNAs, which exist in the nucleus as ribonuclear protein particles. These are often found in a large nuclear structure complex termed the spliceosome, where splicing takes

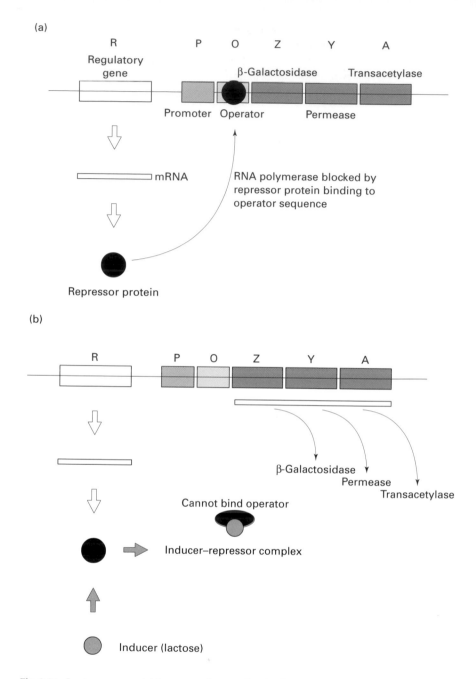

Fig. 2.16. Lactose operon (a) in a state of repression (no lactose present) and (b) following induction by lactose.

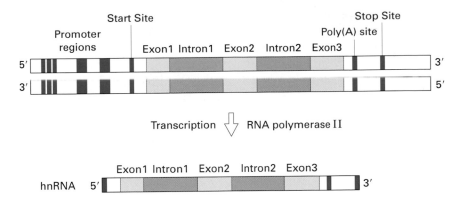

Fig. 2.17. Transcription of a typical eukaryotic gene to form heterogeneous nuclear RNA.

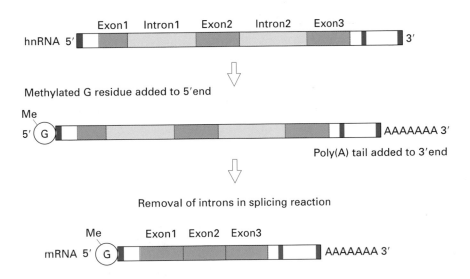

Fig. 2.18. Post-transcriptional modifications of heterogeneous nuclear RNA.

place. Introns are usually removed in a sequential manner from the 5' to the 3'-end and their number varies between different genes. Some eukaryotic genes, such as histone genes, contain no introns whereas the gene for dystrophin, the defective protein in muscular dystrophy, contains over 250 introns. In some cases, however, the same hnRNA transcript may be processed in different ways to produce different mRNAs coding for different proteins in a process known as alternative splicing. Thus a sequence that constitutes an exon for one RNA species may be part of an excised intron in another. The particular type or amount of mRNA synthesised from a cell or cell type may be analysed by a variety of molecular biological techniques (Section 3.8.1).

2.6.7 **Translation of mRNA**

Messenger RNA molecules are read and translated into protein by complex RNA–protein particles termed ribosomes. The ribosomes are termed 70 S or 80 S, depending on their sedimentation coefficient (Section 5.8). Prokaryotic cells have 70 S ribosomes whilst those of the eukaryotic cytoplasm are 80 S. Ribosomes are composed of two subunits that are held apart by ribosomal binding proteins until translation proceeds. There are sites on the ribosome for the binding of one mRNA and two tRNA molecules and the translation process is in three stages.

(i) *Initiation:* involving the assembly of the ribosome subunits and the binding of the mRNA.

(ii) *Elongation:* where specific amino acids are used to form polypeptides, this being directed by the codon sequence in the mRNA.

(iii) *Termination:* which involves the disassembly of the components of translation following the production of a polypeptide.

Transfer RNA molecules are also essential for translation. Each of these are covalently linked to a specific amino acid, forming an aminoacyl tRNA, and each has an exposed triplet of bases that is complementary to the codon for that amino acid. This exposed triplet is known as the anticodon, and allows the tRNA to act as an 'adaptor' molecule, bringing together a codon and its corresponding amino acid. The process of linking an amino acid to its specific tRNA is termed charging and is carried out by the enzyme aminoacyl tRNA synthetase.

In prokaryotic cells the ribosome binds to the 5′ end of the mRNA at a sequence known as the ribosome-binding site or sometimes termed the Shine–Dalgarno sequence, after the discoverers of the sequence. In eukaryotes the situation is similar, although less well understood, but is thought to involve a so-called Kozak sequence. The ribosome appears to scan the mRNA for this sequence before translation. Following translation initiation, the ribosome moves towards the 3′ end of the mRNA, allowing an aminoacyl tRNA molecule to base-pair with each successive codon, thereby carrying in amino acids in the correct order for protein synthesis. There are two sites for tRNA molecules in the ribosome (the A site and the P site) and when these sites are occupied, directed by the sequence of codons in the mRNA, the ribosome allows the formation of a peptide bond between the amino acids. The process is also under the control of the enzyme peptidyl transferase. When a ribosome encounters a termination codon (UAA, UGA or UAG) a release factor binds to the complex and translation stops, the polypeptide and its corresponding mRNA are released and the ribosome divides into its two subunits (Fig. 2.19). A myriad of accessory initiation and elongation protein factors are involved in this process. In eukaryotic cells the polypeptide may then be subjected to post-translational modifications such as glycosylation and by virtue of specific amino acid signal sequences may be directed to specific cellular compartments or exported from the cell.

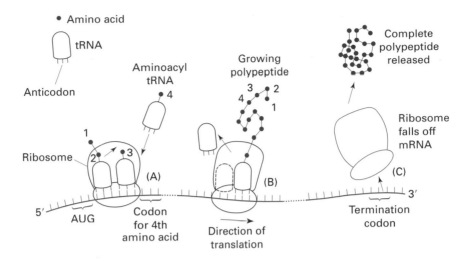

Fig. 2.19. Translation. Ribosome A has moved only a short way from the 5'-end of the mRNA, and has built up a dipeptide (on one tRNA) that is about to be transferred onto the third amino acid (still attached to tRNA). Ribosome B has moved much further along the mRNA and has built up an oligopeptide that has just been transferred onto the most recent aminoacyl tRNA. The resulting free tRNA leaves the ribosome and will receive another amino acid. The ribosome moves towards the 3' end of the mRNA by a distance of three nucleotides, so that the next codon can be aligned with its corresponding aminoacyl tRNA on the ribosome. Ribosome C has reached a termination codon, has released the completed polypeptide, and has fallen off the mRNA.

Since the mRNA base sequence is read in triplets, an error of one or two nucleotides in the positioning of the ribosome will result in the synthesis of an incorrect polypeptide. Thus it is essential for the correct reading frame to be used during translation. This is ensured in prokaryotes by base-pairing between the Shine–Dalgarno sequence and a complementary sequence of one of the ribosome's rRNAs, thus establishing the correct starting point for movement of the ribosome along the mRNA. However, if a mutation such as a deletion/insertion takes place within the coding sequence it will also cause a shift of the reading frame and result in an aberrant polypeptide. Genetic mutations and polymorphisms are considered in more detail in Section 3.8.5.

2.7 THE MANIPULATION OF NUCLEIC ACIDS: BASIC TOOLS AND TECHNIQUES

2.7.1 Enzymes used in molecular biology

The discovery and characterisation of a number of key enzymes have enabled the development of various techniques for the analysis and manipulation of DNA. In particular the enzymes termed type II restriction endonucleases have been found to play a key role in all aspects of molecular biology. These enzymes recognise

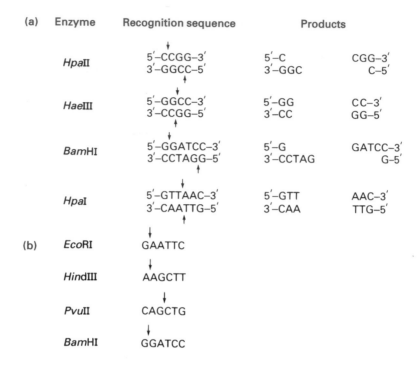

Fig. 2.20. Recognition sequences of some restriction enzymes showing (a) full descriptions and (b) conventional representations. Arrows indicate positions of cleavage. Note that all the information in (a) can be derived from knowledge of a single strand of the DNA, whereas in (b) only one strand is shown, drawn $5' \rightarrow 3'$; this is the conventional way of representing restriction sites.

certain DNA sequences, usually 4–6 bp in length, and cleave them in a defined manner. The sequences recognised are palindromic or of an inverted repeat nature; that is, they read the same in both directions on each strand. When cleaved they leave a flush-ended or staggered (also termed a cohesive-ended) fragment depending on the particular enzyme used (Fig. 2.20). An important property of staggered ends is that those produced from different molecules by the same enzyme are complementary (or 'sticky') and so will anneal to each other. The annealed strands are held together only by hydrogen bonding between complementary bases on opposite strands. Covalent joining of ends on each of the two strands may be brought about by the enzyme DNA ligase (Section 3.2.2). This is widely exploited in molecular biology to enable the construction of recombinant DNA, i.e. the joining of DNA fragments from different sources. Approximately 500 restriction enzymes have been characterised and recognise over 100 different target sequences. A number of these, termed isoschizomers, recognise different target sequences but produce the same staggered ends or overhangs. A number of other enzymes have proved to be of value in the manipulation of DNA, as summarised in Table 2.3, and are indicated at appropriate points within the text.

Table 2.3   Types and examples of typical enzymes used in the manipulation of nucleic acids

Enzyme	Specific example	Use in nucleic acid manipulation
DNA polymerases	DNA pol I	DNA-dependent DNA polymerase 5'→3'/3'→5' exonuclease activity
	Klenow	DNA pol I lacks 5'→3' exonuclease activity
	T4 DNA pol	Lacks 5'→3' exonuclease activity
	Taq DNA pol	Thermostable DNA polymerase used in PCR
	Tth DNA pol	Thermostable DNA polymerase with RT activity
	T7 DNA pol	Used in DNA sequencing
RNA polymerases	T7 RNA pol	DNA-dependent RNA polymerase
	T3 RNA pol	DNA-dependent RNA polymerase
	Qβ replicase	RNA-dependent RNA polymerase, used in RNA-amplification
Nucleases	DNase I	Non-specific endonuclease that cleaves DNA
	Exonuclease III	DNA-dependent 3'→5' stepwise removal of nucleotides
	RNase A	RNases used in mapping studies
	RNase H	Used in second strand cDNA synthesis
	S1 nuclease	Single-strand-specific nuclease
Reverse transcriptase	AMV-RT	RNA-dependent DNA polymerase, used in cDNA synthesis
Transferases	Terminal transferase (TdT)	Adds homopolymer tails to the 3' end of DNA
Ligases	T4 DNA ligase	Links 5'-phosphate and 3'-hydroxyl ends via phosphodiester bond
Kinases	T4 polynucleotide kinase (PNK)	Transfers terminal phosphate groups from ATP to 5'-OH groups
Phosphatases	Alkaline phosphatase	Removes 5'-phosphates from DNA and RNA
Transferases	Terminal transferase	Adds homopolymer tails to the 3' end of DNA
Methylases	*Eco*RI methylase	Methylates specific residues and protects from cleavage by restriction enzymes

PCR, polymerase chain reaction; RT, reverse transcriptase; cDNA, complementary DNA; AMV, avian myeloblastosis virus.

2.8 ISOLATION AND SEPARATION OF NUCLEIC ACIDS

2.8.1 Isolation of DNA

The use of DNA for analysis or manipulation usually requires that it is isolated and purified to a certain extent. DNA is recovered from cells by the gentlest possible method of cell rupture to prevent the DNA from fragmenting by mechanical shearing. This is usually in the presence of EDTA which chelate the Mg^{2+} needed for enzymes that degrade DNA, termed deoxyribonucleases (DNases). Ideally, cell walls, if present, should be digested enzymically (e.g. lysozyme treatment of bacteria), and the cell membrane should be solubilised using detergent. If physical disruption is necessary, it should be kept to a minimum, and should involve cutting or squashing of cells, rather than the use of shear forces. Cell disruption (and most subsequent steps) should be performed at 4 °C, using glassware and solutions that have been autoclaved to destroy DNase activity.

After release of nucleic acids from the cells, RNA can be removed by treatment with ribonuclease (RNase) that has been heat treated to inactivate any DNase contaminants. RNase is relatively stable to heat as a result of its disulphide bonds, which ensure rapid renaturation of the molecule on cooling. The other major contaminant, protein, is removed by shaking the solution gently with water-saturated phenol, or with a phenol/chloroform mixture, either of which will denature proteins but not nucleic acids. Centrifugation of the emulsion formed by this mixing produces a lower, organic phase, separated from the upper, aqueous phase by an interface of denatured protein. The aqueous solution is recovered and deproteinised repeatedly, until no more material is seen at the interface. Finally, the deproteinised DNA preparation is mixed with two volumes of absolute ethanol, and the DNA allowed to precipitate out of solution in a freezer. After centrifugation, the DNA pellet is redissolved in a buffer containing EDTA to inactivate any DNases present. This solution can be stored at 4 °C for at least a month. DNA solutions can be stored frozen, although repeated freezing and thawing tends to damage long DNA molecules by shearing. The procedure described above is suitable for total cellular DNA. If the DNA from a specific organelle or viral particle is needed, it is best to isolate the organelle or virus before extracting its DNA, since the recovery of a particular type of DNA from a mixture is usually rather difficult. Where a high degree of purity is required, DNA may be subjected to density gradient ultracentrifugation through caesium chloride, which is particularly useful for the preparation of plasmid DNA. A flowchart of DNA extraction is indicated in Fig. 2.21. It is possible to check the integrity of the DNA by agarose gel electrophoresis and determine the concentration of the DNA by using the fact that 1 absorbance unit equates to 50 μg DNA cm^{-3} and so

$$50 \times A_{260} = \text{concentration of DNA sample } (\mu g \, cm^{-3})$$

Contaminants may also be identified by scanning ultraviolet spectrophotometry from 200 nm to 300 nm. A ratio of absorbance at 260 nm to that at 280 nm of approximately 1.8 indicates that the sample is free from protein contamination, which absorbs strongly at 280 nm (Chapter 6).

2.8.2 Isolation of RNA

The methods used for RNA isolation are very similar to those described above for DNA; however, RNA molecules are relatively short, and therefore less easily damaged by shearing, so cell disruption can be rather more vigorous. RNA is very vulnerable to digestion by RNases, which are present endogenously in various concentrations in certain cell types and exogenously on human fingers. Gloves should therefore be worn, and a strong detergent should be included in the isolation medium to immediately denature any RNases. Subsequent deproteinisation should be particularly rigorous, since RNA is often tightly associated with proteins. DNase

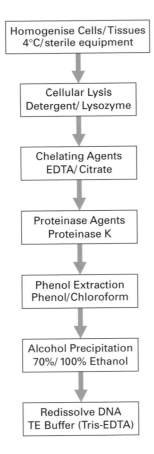

Fig. 2.21. General steps involved in extracting DNA from cells or tissues.

treatment can be used to remove DNA, and RNA can be precipitated by ethanol. One reagent in particular that is commonly used in RNA extraction is guanadinium thiocyanate, which is both a strong inhibitor of RNase and a protein denaturant. A flowchart of RNA extraction is indicated in Fig. 2.22. It is possible to check the integrity of an RNA extract by agarose gel electrophoresis. The most abundant RNA species are the rRNA molecules 23 S and 16 S in prokaryotes and 18 S and 28 S in eukaryotes. These appear as discrete bands on the agarose gel and indicate that the other RNA components are likely to be intact. This is usually carried out under denaturing conditions to prevent secondary structure formation in the RNA. The concentration of the RNA may be estimated by using ultraviolet spectrophotometry. At 260 nm 1 absorbance unit equates to 40 μg cm^{-3} of RNA and therefore:

$$40 \times A_{260} = \text{concentration of RNA sample } (\mu\text{g cm}^{-3})$$

Contaminants may also be identified in the same way as that for DNA by scanning ultraviolet spectrophotometry; however, in the case of RNA a 260 nm : 280 nm ratio of approximately 2 would be expected for a sample containing no protein (Section 2.8.1).

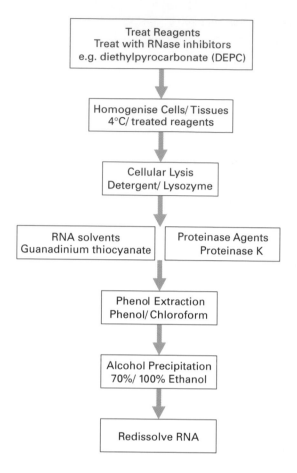

Fig. 2.22. General steps involved in extracting RNA from cells or tissues.

In many cases it is desirable to isolate eukaryotic mRNA, which constitutes only 2% to 5% of cellular RNA, from a mixture of total RNA molecules. This may be carried out by affinity chromatography (Section 13.9) on oligo(dT)–cellulose columns. At high salt concentrations, the mRNA containing poly(A) tails binds to the complementary oligo(dT) molecules of the affinity column, and so mRNA will be retained; all other RNA molecules can be washed through the column by further high salt solution. Finally, the bound mRNA can be eluted using a low concentration of salt (Fig. 2.23). Nucleic acid species may also be subfractionated by more physical means such as electrophoretic or chromatographic separations based on differences in nucleic acid fragment sizes or physicochemical characteristics.

2.8.3 Electrophoresis of nucleic acids

Electrophoresis in agarose or polyacrylamide gels is the usual way to separate DNA molecules according to size. The technique can be used analytically or

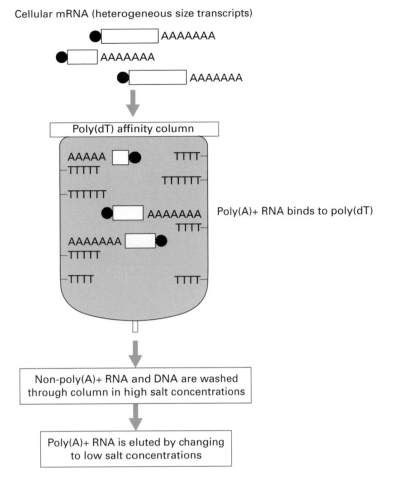

Fig. 2.23. Affinity chromatography of poly(A)+ RNA.

preparatively, and can be qualitative or quantitative. Large fragments of DNA such as chromosomes may also be separated by a modification of electrophoresis termed pulsed-field gel electrophoresis (PFGE). This is discussed in more detail in Section 12.4.3. The easiest and most widely applicable method is electrophoresis in horizontal agarose gels, followed by staining with ethidium bromide. This dye binds to DNA by insertion between stacked base-pairs (intercalation), and it exhibits a strong orange/red fluorescence when illuminated with ultraviolet light (Fig. 2.24). Very often electrophoresis is used to check the purity and intactness of a DNA preparation or to assess the extent of an enzymic reaction during, for example, the steps involved in the cloning of DNA. For such checks 'mini-gels' are particularly convenient, since they need little preparation, use small samples and give results quickly. Agarose gels can be used to separate molecules larger than about 100 bp. For higher resolution or for the effective separation of shorter DNA molecules, polyacrylamide gels are the preferred method.

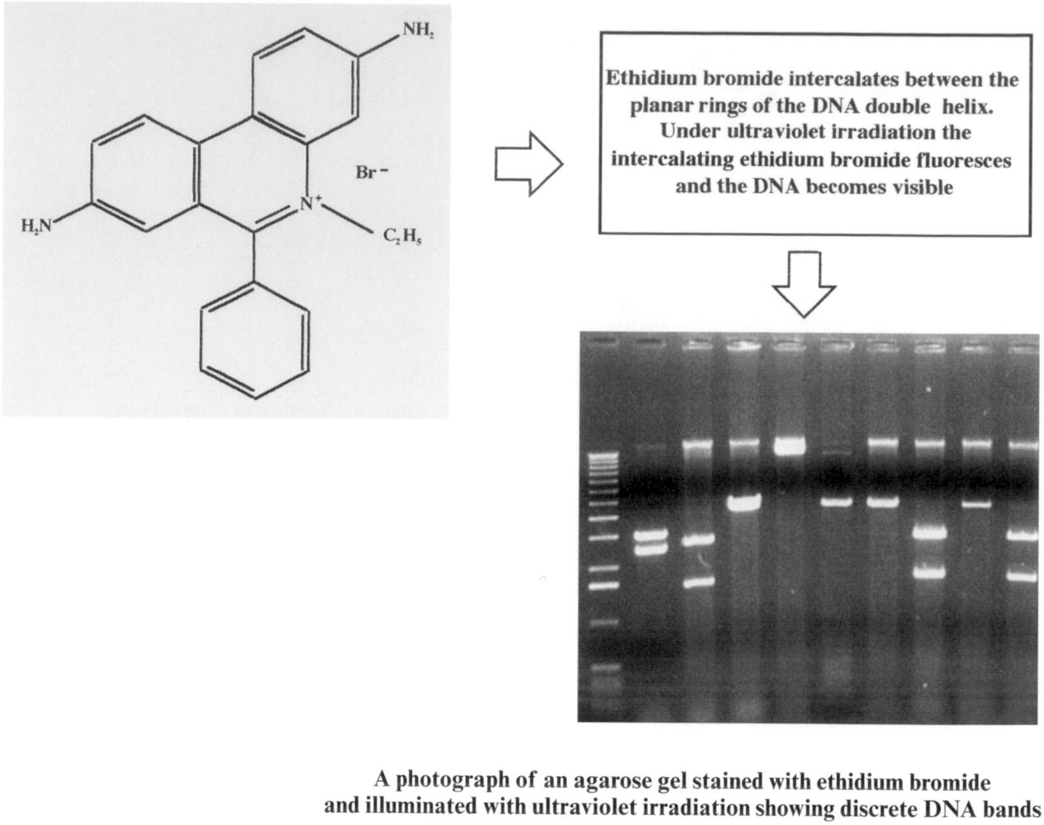

Ethidium bromide intercalates between the planar rings of the DNA double helix. Under ultraviolet irradiation the intercalating ethidium bromide fluoresces and the DNA becomes visible

A photograph of an agarose gel stained with ethidium bromide and illuminated with ultraviolet irradiation showing discrete DNA bands

Fig. 2.24. The use of ethidium bromide to detect DNA.

When electrophoresis is used preparatively, the piece of gel containing the desired DNA fragment is physically removed with a scalpel. The DNA may be recovered from the gel fragment in various ways. This may include crushing with a glass rod in a small volume of buffer, using agarase to digest the agrose, thus leaving the DNA, or by the process of electroelution. In this last method, the piece of gel is sealed in a length of dialysis tubing containing buffer and is then placed between two electrodes in a tank containing more buffer. Passage of an electrical current between the electrodes causes DNA to migrate out of the gel piece, but it remains trapped within the dialysis tubing, and can therefore be recovered easily.

2.9 RESTRICTION MAPPING OF DNA FRAGMENTS

Restriction mapping involves the size analysis of restriction fragments produced by several restriction enzymes individually and in combination (Section 2.7.1). The principle of this mapping is illustrated in Fig. 2.25, in which the restriction sites of two enzymes, A and B, are being mapped. Cleavage with A gives fragments 2 and 7 kb from a 9 kb molecule, hence we can position the single A site 2 kb from

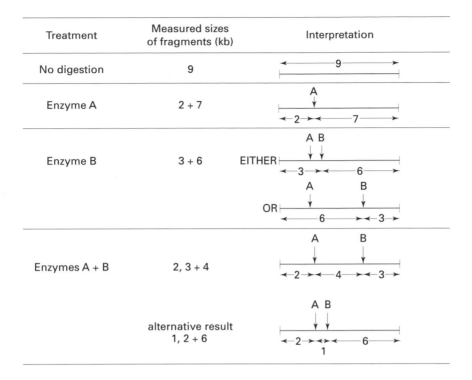

Fig. 2.25. Restriction mapping of DNA. Note that each experimental result and its interpretation should be considered in sequence, thus building up an increasingly unambiguous map.

one end. Similarly, B gives fragments of 3 and 6 kb, so it has a single site 3 kb from one end; but it is not possible at this stage to say whether it is near to A's site or at the opposite end of the DNA. This can be resolved by a double digestion. If the resultant fragments are 2, 3 and 4 kb, then A and B cut at opposite ends of the molecule; if they are 1, 2 and 6 kb, the sites are near each other. Not surprisingly, the mapping of real molecules is rarely as simple as this, and computer analysis of the restriction fragment lengths is usually needed to construct a map.

2.10 NUCLEIC ACID BLOTTING METHODS

Electrophoresis of DNA restriction fragments allows separation based on size to be carried out; however, it provides no indication of the presence of a specific, desired fragment among the complex sample. This can be achieved by transferring the DNA from the intact gel onto a piece of nitrocellulose or nylon membrane placed in contact with it. This provides a more permanent record of the sample, since DNA begins to diffuse out of a gel that is left for a few hours. First, the gel is soaked in alkali to render the DNA single stranded. It is then transferred to the membrane so that the DNA becomes bound to it in exactly the same pattern as that

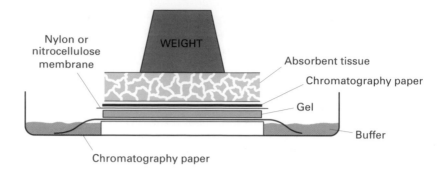

Fig. 2.26. Southern blot apparatus.

originally on the gel. This transfer, named a Southern blot after its inventor, Ed Southern, can be performed electrophoretically, or by drawing large volumes of buffer through both gel and membrane, thus transferring DNA from one to the other by capillary action (Fig. 2.26). The point of this operation is that the membrane can now be treated with a labelled DNA molecule, for example a gene probe (Section 2.11). This single-stranded DNA probe will hybridise under the right conditions to complementary fragments immobilised onto the membrane. The conditions of hybridisation, including the temperature and salt concentration, are critical for this process to take place effectively. This is usually referred to as the stringency of the hybridisation and it is particular for each individual gene probe and for each sample of DNA. A series of washing steps with buffer is then carried out to remove any unbound probe and the membrane is developed, after which the precise location of the probe and its target may be visualised. It is also possible to analyse DNA from different species or organisms by blotting the DNA and then using a gene probe representing a protein or enzyme from one of the organisms. In this way it is possible to search for related genes in different species. This technique is generally termed zoo blotting.

The same basic process of nucleic acid blotting can be used to transfer RNA from gels onto similar membranes. This allows the identification of specific mRNA sequences of a defined length by hybridisation to a labelled gene probe and is known as northern blotting. Not only is it possible with this technique to detect specific mRNA molecules but it may also be used to quantify the relative amounts of the specific mRNA. It is usual to separate the mRNA transcripts by gel electrophoresis under denaturing conditions since this improves resolution and allows a more accurate estimation of the sizes of the transcripts (Section 2.8.2). The format of the blotting may be altered from transfer from a gel to direct application to slots on a specific blotting apparatus containing the nylon membrane. This is termed slot or dot blotting and provides a convenient means of measuring the abundance of specific mRNA transcripts without the need for gel electrophoresis. It does not, however, provide information regarding the size of the fragments.

Polypeptide:		Phe	Met	Pro	Trp	His	
Corresponding nucleotide sequences:	5′	T TTC	ATC	T CCC A G	TGG	T CAC	3′

Fig. 2.27. Oligonucleotide probes. Note that only methionine and tryptophan have unique codons. It is impossible to predict which of the indicated codons for phenylalanine, proline and histidine will be present in the gene to be probed, so all possible combinations must be synthesised (16 in the example shown).

2.11 GENE PROBE DERIVATION

The availability of a gene probe is essential in many molecular biological techniques, yet in many cases it is one of the most difficult steps. The information needed to produce a gene probe may come from many sources but with the development and sophistication of genetic databases, gaining this knowledge is usually one of the first stages. There are a number of genetic databases throughout the world and it is possible to search these over the Internet and identify particular sequences relating to a specific gene or protein (Section 2.15). In some cases it is possible to use related proteins from the same gene family to gain information on the most useful DNA sequence. Proteins or DNA sequences that are similar but from different species may also provide a starting point with which to produce a so-called heterologous gene probe. Although in some cases probes are already produced and cloned, it is possible, armed with a DNA sequence from a database, to chemically synthesise a single-stranded oligonucleotide probe. This is usually undertaken by computer-controlled gene synthesisers that link dNTPs together on the basis of a desired sequence. It is essential to carry out certain checks before probe production to determine whether the probe is unique, and is neither able to self-anneal nor is self-complementary, both of which may compromise its use.

Where scant DNA information is available to prepare a gene probe it is possible in some cases to use the knowledge gained from analysis of the corresponding protein. Thus it is possible to isolate and purify proteins and sequence part of the N-terminal end of the protein (Section 6.4). From our knowledge of the genetic code, it is possible to predict the various DNA sequences that could code for the protein, and then synthesise appropriate oligonucleotide sequences chemically. Due to the degeneracy of the genetic code, most amino acids are coded for by more than one codon, therefore there will be more than one possible nucleotide sequence that could code for a given polypeptide (Fig. 2.27). The longer the polypeptide, the greater the number of possible oligonucleotides that must be synthesised. Fortunately, there is no need to synthesise a sequence longer than about 20 bases, since this should hybridise efficiently with any complementary sequences and should be specific for one gene. Ideally, a section of the protein should be chosen that contains as many tryptophan and methionine residues as possible, since these have unique codons and there will therefore be fewer possible base sequences that could code for that part of the protein. The synthetic oligonucleotides can then be used as probes in a number of molecular biological methods.

2.12 LABELLING DNA GENE PROBE MOLECULES

An essential feature of a gene probe is that it can be visualised by some means. Therefore a gene probe that hybridises to a complementary sequence may be used to identify the desired sequence from a complex mixture. There are two main ways of labelling gene probes. Traditionally this has been carried out using radioactive labels, but gaining in popularity are non-radioactive labels. Perhaps the most used radioactive label is phosphorus-32 (^{32}P), although for certain techniques sulphur-35 (^{35}S) and tritium (^{3}H) are used. These may be detected by the process of autoradiography, where the labelled probe molecule, bound to sample DNA, located for example on a nylon membrane, is placed in contact with an X-ray sensitive film. Following exposure, the film is developed and fixed just as a black-and-white negative and reveals the precise location of the labelled probe and therefore the DNA to which it has hybridised.

Non-radioactive labels are increasingly being used to label DNA gene probes. Until recently radioactive labels were more sensitive than their non-radioactive counterparts. However, recent developments have led to similar sensitivities in the latter, which, when combined with their improved safety, have led to their greater acceptance.

The labelling systems are termed either direct or indirect. Direct labelling allows an enzyme reporter such as alkaline phosphatase to be coupled directly to the DNA. Although this may alter the characteristics of the DNA gene probe, it offers the advantage of rapid analysis, since no intermediate steps are needed. However, indirect labelling is at present more popular. This relies on the incorporation of a nucleotide that has a label attached. At present three of the main labels in use are biotin, fluorescein and digoxygenin. These molecules are covalently linked to nucleotides using a carbon spacer arm of 7, 14 or 21 atoms. Specific binding proteins may then be used as a bridge between the nucleotide and a reporter protein such as an enzyme. For example, biotin incorporated into a DNA fragment is recognised with a very high affinity by the protein streptavidin. This may be either coupled or conjugated to a reporter enzyme molecule such as alkaline phosphatase. This is able to convert a colourless substrate p-nitrophenol phosphate (PNPP) into a yellow-coloured compound p-nitrophenol (PNP) and also offers a means of signal amplification. Alternatively, labels such as digoxygenin incorporated into DNA sequences may be detected by monoclonal antibodies, again conjugated to reporter molecules including alkaline phosphatase. Thus, rather than the detection system relying on autoradiography, which is necessary for radiolabels, a series of reactions resulting in a colour, a light or a chemiluminescence reaction takes place (Section 9.8). This has important, practical implications, since autoradiography may take 1 to 3 days, whereas colour and chemiluminescent reactions take minutes.

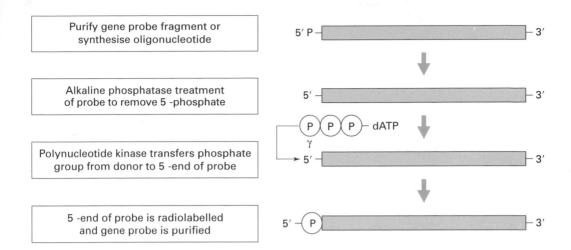

Fig. 2.28. End-labelling of a gene probe at the 5′-end with alkaline phosphatase and polynucleotide kinase.

2.12.1 **End-labelling of DNA molecules**

The simplest form of labelling DNA is by 5′- or 3′-end-labelling. 5′-End-labelling involves a phosphate transfer or exchange reaction where the 5′-phosphate of the DNA to be used as the probe is removed and in its place a labelled phosphate, usually ^{32}P, is added. This is carried out by using two enzymes: the first, alkaline phosphatase, removes the existing phosphate group from the DNA; then polynucleotide kinase, is added and catalyses the transfer of a phosphate group (^{32}P-labelled) to the 5′ end of the DNA. The newly labelled probe is then purified, usually by chromatography through a Sephadex column to remove any unincorporated radiolabel (Fig. 2.28).

Using the other end of the DNA molecule, the 3′-end, is slightly less complex. Here a new, labelled dNTP ($\alpha^{32}-$P]ATP or biotin-labelled dNTP) is added to the 3′ end of the DNA by the enzyme terminal transferase. Although this is a simpler reaction, a potential problem exists because a new nucleotide is added to the existing sequence and so the complete sequence of the DNA is altered, which may affect its hybridisation to its target sequence. End-labelling methods also suffer from the fact that only one label is added to the DNA so such methods are of a lower activity in comparison to others that incorporate label along the whole length of the DNA (Fig. 2.29).

2.12.2 **Random primer labelling**

The DNA to be labelled is first denatured and then placed under renaturing conditions in the presence of a mixture of many different random sequences of hexamers or hexanucleotides. These hexamers will, by chance, bind to the DNA sample wherever they encounter a complementary sequence and so the DNA will rapidly

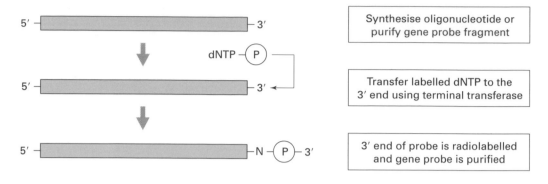

Fig. 2.29. End-labelling of a gene probe at the 3′ end using terminal transferase. Note that the addition of a labelled dNTP at the 3′-end alters the sequence of the gene probe.

acquire an approximately random sprinkling of hexanucleotides annealed to it. Each of the hexamers can act as a primer for the synthesis of a fresh strand of DNA catalysed by DNA polymerase, since it has an exposed 3′-hydroxyl group. The Klenow fragment of DNA polymerase is used for random primer labelling because it lacks a 5′ → 3′ exonuclease activity. This is prepared by cleavage of DNA polymerase with subtilisin, giving a large enzyme fragment which has no 5′ → 3′ exonuclease activity, but which still acts as a 5′ → 3′ polymerase. Thus, when the Klenow enzyme is mixed with the annealed DNA sample in the presence of dNTPs, including at least one which is labelled, many short stretches of labelled DNA will be generated (Fig. 2.30). In a similar way to random primer labelling the polymerase chain reaction may also be used to incorporate radioactive or non-radioactive labels (Section 2.13.5).

2.12.3 Nick translation

A traditional method of labelling DNA is by the process of nick translation. Low concentrations of DNase I are used to make occasional single-strand nicks in the double-stranded DNA that is to be used as the gene probe. DNA polymerase then fills in the nicks, using an appropriate deoxyribonucleoside triphosphate (dNTP), at the same time making a new nick to the 3′ side of the previous one (Fig. 2.31). In this way the nick is translated along the DNA. If labelled dNTPs are added to the reaction mixture, they will be used to fill in the nicks, and so the DNA can be labelled to a very high specific activity.

2.13 THE POLYMERASE CHAIN REACTION

There have been a number of key developments in molecular biological techniques; however, the one that has had the most impact in recent years is the polymerase chain reaction or PCR. One of the reasons for the adoption of the PCR is the elegant simplicity of the reaction and relative ease of the practical manipulation

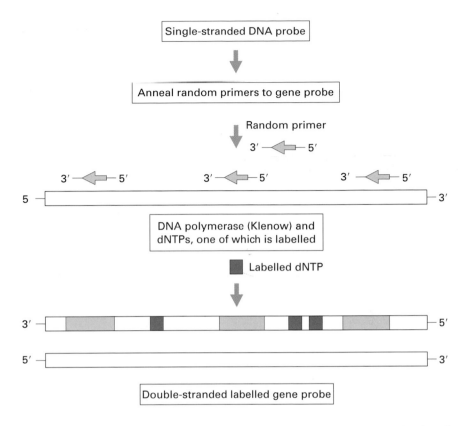

Fig. 2.30. Random primer gene probe labelling. Random primers are incorporated and used as a start point for Klenow DNA polymerase to synthesise a complementary strand of DNA whilst incorporating a labelled dNTP at complementary sites.

steps. Frequently this is one of the first techniques used when DNA is analysed; it has opened up the analysis of cellular and molecular processes to those outside the field of molecular biology.

The PCR is used to amplify a precise fragment of DNA from a complex mixture of starting material usually termed the template DNA and in many cases requires little DNA purification. It does require some knowledge of the DNA sequence information which flanks the fragment of DNA to be amplified (target DNA). From this information two oligonucleotide primers may be chemically synthesised, each complementary to a stretch of DNA to the 3′-side of the target DNA, one oligonucleotide for each of the two DNA strands (Fig. 2.32). It may be thought of as a technique analogous to the DNA replication process that takes place in cells, since the outcome is the same, the generation of new complementary DNA stretches based upon existing ones. It is also a technique that has replaced, in many cases, traditional DNA cloning methods, since it fulfils the same function, the production of large amounts of DNA from limited starting material. This is achieved, however, in a fraction of the time needed to clone a DNA fragment (Chapter 3).

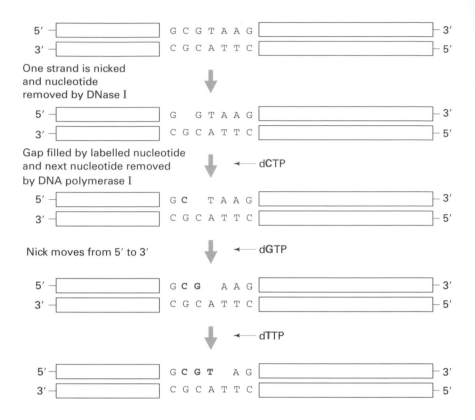

Fig. 2.31. Nick translation. The removal of nucleotides and their subsequent replacement with labelled nucleotides by DNA polymerase I increase the label in the gene probe as nick translation proceeds.

Although not without its drawbacks, the PCR is a remarkable development that is changing the approach of many scientists to the analysis of nucleic acids and continues to have a profound impact on core biosciences and biotechnology.

2.13.1 Stages in the PCR

The PCR consists of three defined sets of times and temperatures, termed steps: (i) denaturation, (ii) annealing and (iii) extension. Each of these steps is repeated 30–40 times or cycles (Fig. 2.33). In the first cycle the double-stranded template DNA is first denatured by heating the reaction to above 90 °C. Within the complex DNA the region to be specifically amplified (target) is made accessible. The temperature is then cooled to between 40 and 60 °C. The precise temperature is critical and each PCR system has to be defined and optimised. Reactions that are not optimised may give rise to other DNA products in addition to the specific target or may not produce any amplified products. The second, annealing, step allows the hybridisation of the two oligonucleotide primers, present in excess, to bind to their complementary sites, which flank the target DNA. The annealed oligonucleotides act as

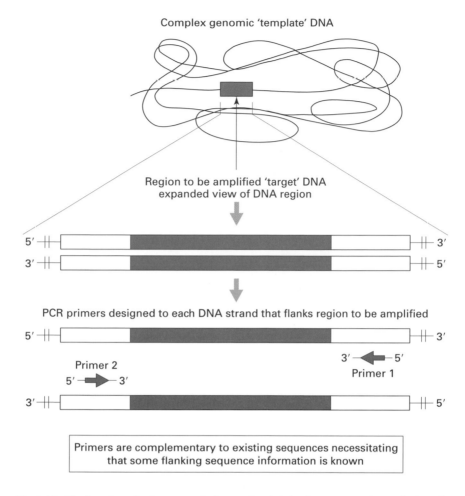

Fig. 2.32. The location of polymerase chain reaction (PCR) primers. PCR primers designed for sequences adjacent to the region to be amplified allowing a region of DNA (e.g. a gene) to be amplified from a complex starting material of genomic template DNA.

primers for DNA synthesis, since they provide a free 3′-hydroxyl group for DNA polymerase. The third step, DNA synthesis or extension, is carried out by a thermo-stable DNA polymerase, most commonly *Taq* DNA polymerase.

DNA synthesis proceeds from both of the primers until the new strands have been extended along and beyond the target DNA to be amplified. It is important to note that, since the new strands extend beyond the target DNA they will contain a region near their 3′ ends that is complementary to the other primer. Thus, if another round of DNA synthesis is allowed to take place, not only will the original strands be used as templates but also the new strands. Most interestingly, the products obtained from the new strands will have a precise length, delimited exactly by the two regions complementary to the primers. As the system is taken through successive cycles of denaturation, annealing and extension all the new strands

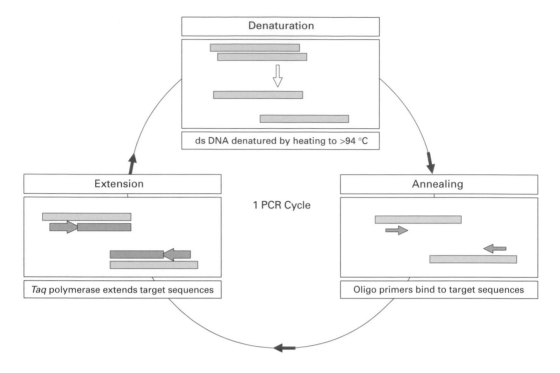

Fig. 2.33. A simplified scheme of one PCR cycle that involves denaturation, annealing and extension. ds, double-stranded.

will act as templates and so there will be an exponential increase in the amount of DNA produced. The net effect is to selectively amplify the target DNA flanked by the primers (Fig. 2.34).

One problem with the early PCR reactions was that the temperature needed to denature the DNA also denatured the DNA polymerase. However, the availability of a thermostable DNA polymerase enzyme isolated from the thermophilic bacterium *Thermus aquaticus* found in hot springs provided the means to automate the reaction. *Taq* DNA polymerase has a temperature optimum of 72 °C and survives prolonged exposure to temperatures as high as 96 °C and so is still active after each of the denaturation steps. The widespread utility of the technique is also due to the ability to automate the reaction and as such many thermal cyclers have been produced in which it is possible to programme-in the temperatures and times for a particular PCR reaction.

2.13.2 **Primer design in the PCR**

The key to the PCR lies in the design of the two oligonucleotide primers. These not only have to be complementary to sequences flanking the target DNA but must not be self-complementary or bind to each other to form dimers, since both reactions prevent DNA amplification. They also have to be matched in their

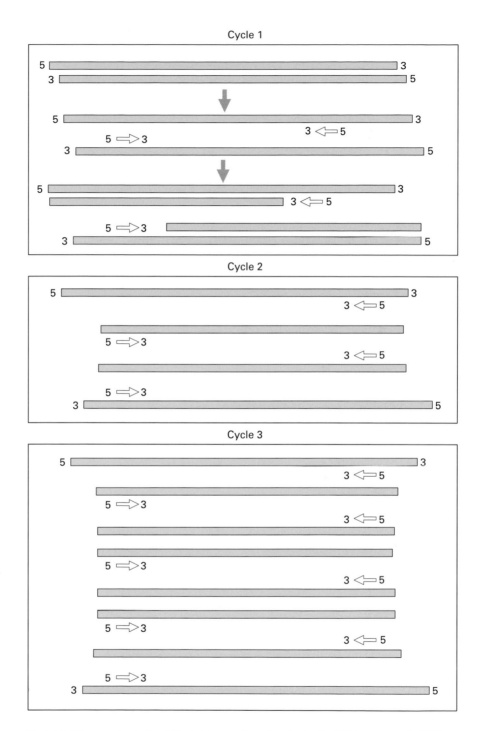

Fig. 2.34. Three cycles in the PCR. As the number of cycles in the PCR increases, the DNA strands that are synthesised and become available as templates are delimited by the ends of the primers. Thus specific amplification of the desired target sequence flanked by the primers is achieved. Primers are denoted as 5′ → 3′.

G + C content and have similar annealing temperatures. The increasing use of information from the Internet and the sequences held in gene databases (Section 2.15) are useful starting points when designing primers and reaction conditions for the PCR and a number of software developments have allowed the process of primer design to be straightforward. It is also possible to design primers with additional sequences at their 5′ ends, such as restriction endonuclease target sites or promoter sequences, however, modifications like these require that the annealing conditions be altered to compensate for the areas of non-homology in the primers. A number of PCR methods have been developed where either one of the primers or both are random. This gives rise to arbitrary priming in genomic templates but interestingly may also give rise to discrete banding patterns when analysed by gel electrophoresis. In many cases this technique may be used reproducibly to identify a particular organism or species. This is sometimes referred to as rapid amplification of polymorphic DNA (RAPDs) and has been used successfully in the detection and differentiation of a number of pathogenic strains of bacteria.

2.13.3 **PCR amplification templates**

The PCR may be used to amplify DNA from a variety of sources or templates. It is also a highly sensitive technique and potentially requires only one or two molecules for successful amplification. Unlike many manipulation methods used in current molecular biology the PCR technique is sensitive enough to require very little template preparation. Extraction from many prokaryotic and eukaryotic cells may involve a simple boiling step. Indeed the components of many extraction techniques such as sodium dodecyl sulphate (SDS) and proteinase K may adversely affect the PCR. The PCR may also be used to amplify RNA, a process termed reverse transcriptase–PCR (RT–PCR). Initially, a reverse transcription reaction that converts RNA to cDNA is first carried out (Section 3.2.5). This reaction normally involves the use of the enzyme reverse transcriptase, although some thermostable DNA polymerases used in the PCR such as that from *Thermus thermophilus (Tth)*, have a reverse transcriptase activity under certain buffer conditions. This allows mRNA transcription products to be effectively analysed. It may also be used to differentiate latent viruses (detected by standard PCR) or active viruses, which replicate and thus produce transcription products and are therefore detectable by RT–PCR (Fig. 2.35). In addition the PCR may be extended to determine relative amounts of a transcription product.

2.13.4 **Sensitivity of the PCR**

The enormous sensitivity of the PCR system is also one of its main drawbacks, since the very large degree of amplification makes the system vulnerable to contamination. Even a trace of foreign DNA, such as that contained in dust particles, may be amplified to significant levels and may give misleading results. Hence cleanliness is paramount when carrying out PCR and dedicated equipment and

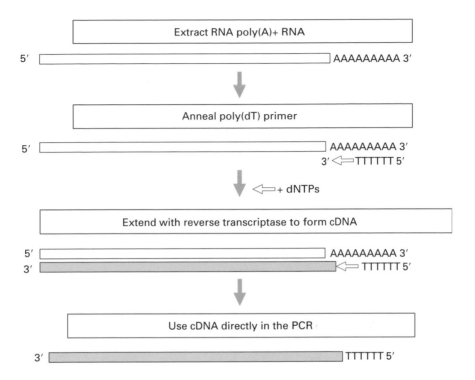

Fig. 2.35. Reverse transcriptase–PCR (RT–PCR). In RT–PCR, mRNA is converted to complementary DNA (cDNA) using the enzyme reverse transcriptase. The cDNA is then used directly in the PCR.

in some cases laboratories are used. It is possible that amplified products may also contaminate the PCR, although this may be overcome by ultraviolet irradiation to damage already amplified products so that they cannot be used as templates. A further interesting solution is to incorporate uracil into the PCR and then treat the products with the enzyme uracil *N*-glycosylase (UNG) which degrades any PCR products with incorporated uracil, rendering them useless as templates. Many traditional methods in molecular biology have now been superseded by the PCR and the applications for the technique appear to be unlimited. Some of the main techniques derived from the PCR are introduced in Chapter 3, while some of the main areas in which the PCR has been put to use are summarised in Table 2.4. The success of the PCR process has given impetus to the development of other amplification techniques based on either thermal or non-thermal (isothermal) cycling methods. The most popular alternative to the PCR is termed the ligase chain reaction or LCR. This operates in a fashion similar to the PCR but a thermostable DNA ligase joins sets of primers together that are complementary to the target DNA. Following this, a similar exponential amplification reaction takes place, producing amounts of DNA that are similar to those derived from the PCR. A number of alternative amplification techniques are listed in Table 2.5.

Table 2.4   Selected applications of the PCR. A number of the techniques are described in the text of Chapters 2 and 3

Field or area of study	Application	Specific examples or uses
General molecular biology	DNA amplification	Screening gene libraries
Gene probe production	Production/labelling	Use with blots/hybridisations
RNA analysis	RT–PCR	Active latent viral infections
Forensic science	Scenes of crime	Analysis of DNA from blood
Infection/disease monitoring	Microbial detection	Strain typing/analysis RAPDs
Sequence analysis	DNA sequencing	Rapid sequencing possible
Genome mapping studies	Referencing points in genome	Sequence-tagged sites (STS)
Gene discovery	mRNA analysis	Expressed sequence tags (EST)
Genetic mutation analysis	Detection of known mutations	Screening for cystic fibrosis
Quantification analysis	Quantitative PCR	5′ nuclease (TaqMan assay)
Genetic mutation analysis	Detection of unknown mutations	Gel-based PCR methods (DGGE)
Protein engineering	Production of novel proteins	PCR mutagenesis
Molecular archaeology	Retrospective studies	Dinosaur DNA analysis
Single-cell analysis	Sexing or cell mutation sites	Sex determination of unborn
In situ analysis	Studies on frozen sections	Localisation of DNA/RNA

RT, reverse transcriptase; RAPDs, rapid amplification polymorphic DNA; DDGE, denaturing gradient gel electrophoresis.

Table 2.5   Selected alternative amplification techniques to the PCR. Two broad methodologies exist that either amplify the target molecules such as DNA and RNA or detect the target and amplify a signal molecule bound to it

Technique	Type of assay	Specific examples or uses
Target amplification methods		
Ligase chain reaction (LCR)	Non-isothermal, employs thermostable DNA ligase	Mutation detection
Nucleic acid sequence based amplification (NASBA)	Isothermal, involving use of RNA, RNase H/reverse transcriptase, and T7 DNA polymerase	Viral detection, e.g. HIV
Signal amplification methods		
Branched DNA amplification (b-DNA)	Isothermal microwell format using hybridisation or target/capture probe and signal amplification	Mutation detection

HIV, human immunodeficiency virus.

2.13.5 General applications of the PCR

There are a number of molecular biological methods where the PCR has been used to great effect. The labelling of gene probes is one such area which has traditionally been undertaken by techniques such as nick translation (Section 2.12.3). The nature of the PCR makes it an ideal method for gene probe production and labelling. PCR products may be labelled at the 5′ and 3′ ends using the methods indicated in Sections 2.13.1 and 2.13.2. This may be undertaken before the PCR by labelling the oligonucleotide primers or the resulting PCR product. However, since the PCR is essentially two primer extension reactions it allows the incorporation of nucleotides that have been labelled either radioactively or with a non-radioactive label such as biotin. The advantage of the PCR as a gene probe and labelling system is the fact that it offers great flexibility and may be rapidly produced.

A further important modification of the PCR is termed quantitative PCR. This allows the PCR to be used as a means of identifying the initial concentrations of template DNA and is very useful for the measurement of, for example, a virus or an mRNA for a protein expressed in abnormal amounts in a disease process. Early quantitative PCR methods involved the comparison of a standard or control DNA template amplified with separate primers at the same time as the specific target DNA. These types of quantification rely on the reaction being exponential and so any factors affecting this may also affect the result. Other methods involve the incorporation of a radiolabel through the primers or nucleotides and their subsequent detection following purification of the PCR product. An alternative automated method of great promise is the 5′-exonuclease detection system or TaqMan assay. Here, an oligonucleotide probe is labelled with a fluorescent reporter and quencher molecule at each end. When the primers bind to their target sequence, the 5′-exonuclease activity of Taq polymerase degrades and releases the reporter from the quencher. A signal is thus generated that increases in direct proportion to the number of starting molecules. Thus a detection system is able to induce and detect fluorescence in real time as the PCR proceeds. This has important implications in, for example, the rapid detection of bacterial and viral sequences in clinical samples.

One of the most useful general applications of the development of the PCR is direct PCR sequencing. This traditionally involved the cloning of sequences into vectors developed for chain termination sequencing. However, the rapid accumulation of PCR products allows nucleotide sequence information to be obtained very quickly. A number of methods for direct PCR sequencing are indicated in Section 2.14.2. Further applications of the PCR are described in the respective sections in Chapter 3.

2.14 **NUCLEOTIDE SEQUENCING OF DNA**

The determination of the order or sequence of bases along a length of DNA is one of the central techniques in molecular biology. Although it is now possible to derive amino acid sequence information with a degree of reliability (Chapter 6), it is frequently more convenient and rapid to analyse the DNA coding information. The precise usage of codons, information regarding mutations and polymorphisms and the identification of gene regulatory control sequences can only be elucidated by analysing DNA sequences. Two techniques have been developed for this, one based on an enzymic method frequently termed Sanger sequencing after its developer and a chemical method, Maxam and Gilbert sequencing, named for the same reason. At present Sanger sequencing is by far the most popular method and many commercial kits are available for its use; however, there are certain occasions such as the sequencing of short oligonucleotides where the Maxam and Gilbert method is more appropriate.

One absolute requirement for Sanger sequencing is that the DNA to be sequenced is in a single-stranded form. Traditionally, this demanded that the DNA fragment of interest be inserted and cloned into a specialised bacteriophage vector, M13, which is naturally single stranded (Section 3.3.3). Although M13 is still universally used, the advent of the PCR has provided the means not only to amplify a region of any genome or cDNA but also very quickly to generate the corresponding nucleotide sequence. This has led to an explosion in the accumulation of DNA sequence information and has provided much impetus for gene discovery and genome mapping (Section 3.9).

The Sanger method is simple and elegant and in many ways mimics the natural ability of DNA polymerase to extend a growing nucleotide chain on the basis of an existing template. Initially, the DNA to be sequenced is allowed to hybridise with an oligonucleotide primer, which is complementary to a sequence adjacent to the 3′ side of DNA within a vector such as M13 or in a PCR product. The oligonucleotide will then act as a primer for the synthesis of a second strand of DNA, catalysed by DNA polymerase. Since the new strand is synthesised from its 5′ end, virtually the first DNA to be made will be complementary to the DNA to be sequenced. One of the deoxyribonucleoside triphosphates (dNTPs) that must be provided for DNA synthesis is radioactively labelled with ^{32}P or ^{35}S and so the newly synthesised strand will be labelled with these isomers.

2.14.1 Dideoxynucleotide chain terminators

The reaction mixture is then divided into four aliquots, representing the four dNTPs A, C, G and T. In addition to all of the dNTPs being present in the A tube, an analogue of dATP is added (2′,3′-dideoxyadenosine triphosphate (ddATP)) that is similar to A but has no 3′-hydroxyl group and so will terminate the growing chain, since a $5′ \rightarrow 3′$ phosphodiester linkage cannot be formed without a 3′-hydroxyl group. The situation for tube ddC is identical, except that ddCTP is added, similarly the ddG and ddT tubes contain ddGTP and ddTTP, respectively (Fig. 2.36).

Since the incorporation of ddNTP rather than dNTP is a random event, the reaction will produce new molecules varying widely in length, but all terminating at the same type of base. Thus four sets of DNA sequence are generated, each terminating at a different type of base, but all having a common 5′-end (the primer). The four labelled and chain-terminated samples are then denatured by heating and loaded next to each other on a polyacrylamide gel for electrophoresis. Electrophoresis is performed at approximately 70 °C in the presence of urea, to prevent renaturation of the DNA, since even partial renaturation alters the rates of migration of DNA fragments. Very thin, long gels are used for maximum resolution over a wide range of fragment lengths (Section 12.4.2). After electrophore-

Fragment to be sequenced, cloned in M13 phage

3′ – – – AG – – – CTGCTCGCAT – – – 5′
         TC – – – GA
         ⎵⎵⎵⎵⎵⎵
             Primer

         │ DNA polymerase
         │ 4 dNTPs (radioactive)
         ↓ ddGTP

Synthesis of complementary second strands:

5′ TC – – – GACddG 3′
5′ TC – – – GACGAddG 3′
5′ TC – – – GACGAGCddG 3′

Denature to give single strands

Run on sequencing gel alongside products of
ddCTP, ddATP and ddTTP reactions

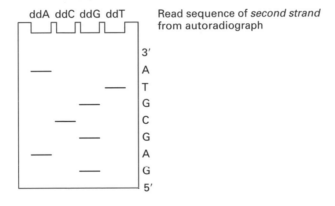

Read sequence of *second strand*
from autoradiograph

Fig. 2.36. Sanger sequencing of DNA.

sis, the positions of radioactive DNA bands on the gel are determined by autoradiography (Chapter 14.2.3). Since every band in the track from the dideoxya-
denosine triphosphate sample must contain molecules that terminate at
adenine, and those in the ddCTP terminate at cytosine, etc., it is possible to read
the sequence of the newly synthesised strand from the autoradiograph, provided
that the gel can resolve differences in length equal to a single nucleotide (Fig.
2.37). Under ideal conditions, sequences up to about 400 bases in length can be
read from one gel.

2.14.2 Direct PCR sequencing

It is possible to undertake nucleotide sequencing from double-stranded molecules
such as plasmid cloning vectors and PCR products but the double-stranded DNA

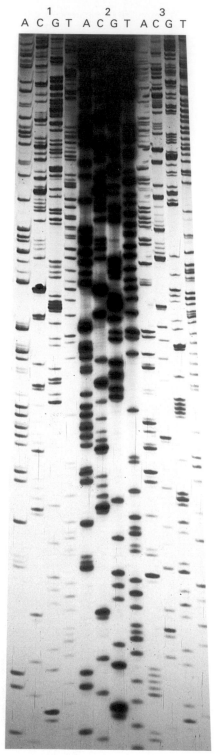

Fig. 2.37. Autoradiograph of a DNA sequencing gel. Samples were prepared using the Sanger dideoxy method of DNA sequencing. Each set of four samples was loaded into adjacent tracks, indicated by A, C, G and T, depending on the identity of the dideoxyribonucleotide used for that sample. Two sets of samples were labelled with ^{35}S (1 and 3) and one was labelled with ^{32}P (2). It is evident that ^{32}P generates darker but more diffuse bands than does ^{35}S, making the bands nearer the bottom of the autoradiograph easy to see. However, the broad bands produced by ^{32}P cannot be resolved near the top of the autoradiograph, making it impossible to read a sequence from this region. The much sharper bands produced by ^{35}S allow sequences to be read with confidence along most of the autoradiograph and so a longer sequence of DNA can be obtained from a single gel.

Direction of electrophoretic movement

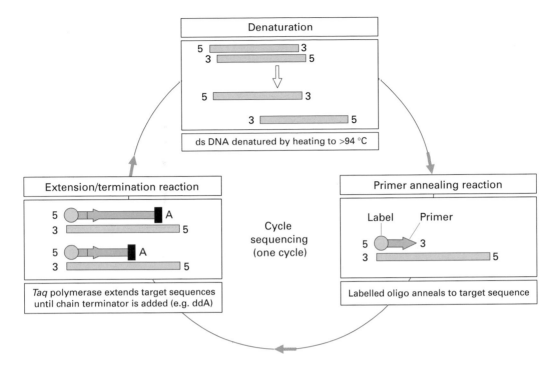

Fig. 2.38. Simplified scheme of cycle sequencing. Linear amplification takes place with the use of labelled primers. During the extension and termination reaction, the chain terminator dideoxynucleotides are incorporated into the growing chain. This takes place in four separate reactions (A, C, G, and T). The products are then run on a polyacrylamide gel and the sequence analysed. The scheme indicates the events that take place in the A reaction only. ds, double-stranded.

must be denatured prior to annealing with primer. In the case of plasmids, an alkaline denaturation step is sufficient; however, for PCR products this is more problematic and a focus of much research. Unlike plasmids, PCR products are short and reanneal rapidly, so preventing the reannealing process or biasing the amplification towards one strand by using a primer ratio of 100:1 can overcome this problem to a certain extent. Denaturants such as formamide or dimethylsulphoxide (DMSO) have also been used with some success in preventing the reannealing of PCR strands after their separation.

It is possible to physically separate and retain one PCR strand by incorporating a molecule such as biotin into one of the primers. After PCR, the strand with the biotin molecule may be removed by affinity chromatography with strepavidin, leaving the complementary PCR strand. This affinity purification provides single-stranded DNA derived from the PCR product and, although this is somewhat time consuming, does provide high quality single-stranded DNA for sequencing.

One of the most useful methods of sequencing PCR products is termed PCR cycle sequencing. This is not strictly a PCR, since it involves linear amplification with a single primer. Approximately 20 cycles of denaturation, annealing and extension take place. Radiolabelled or fluorescent-labelled dideoxynucleotides are then introduced into the final stages of the reaction to generate the chain-terminated extension products (Fig. 2.38). Automated direct PCR sequencing is increasingly being refined, allowing greater lengths of DNA to be analysed in one sequencing run and providing a very rapid means of analysing DNA sequences.

2.14.3 Automated fluorescent DNA sequencing

Recent advances in dye terminator chemistry have led to the development of automated sequencing methods that involve the use of dideoxynucleotides labelled with different fluorochromes. The label is incorporated into the ddNTP and this is used to carry out chain termination, as in the standard reaction indicated in Section 2.14.1. The advantage of this modification is that, since a different label is incorporated with each ddNTP, it is unnecessary to perform four separate reactions. Therefore the four chain-terminated products are run on the same track of a denaturing electrophoresis gel. Each product, with their base-specific dye, is excited by a laser and the dye then emits light at its characteristic wavelength. A diffraction grating separates the emissions, which are detected by a charge-coupled device (CCD) and the sequence interpreted by a personal computer. In addition to real-time detection, the lengths of sequence that may be analysed are in excess of 500 bp (Fig. 2.39). Further improvements are likely to be made not in the sequencing reactions themselves but in the electrophoresis of the chain-terminated products. Here, capillary electrophoresis may be used where liquid polymers in thin capillary tubes would substantially decrease the electrophoresis run times. The consequence of automated sequencing and the incorporation of PCR cycle sequencing has substantially decreased the time needed to undertake sequencing projects. This has given rise to the use of banks of automated robotic sequencing systems in factory style units that are now in operation in various laboratories throughout the world, especially those undertaking work for the various genome-sequencing projects (Section 3.9).

2.14.4 Maxam and Gilbert sequencing

The chemical cleavage method of DNA sequencing developed by Maxam and Gilbert is often used for sequencing small fragments of DNA such as oligonucleotides. A radioactive label is added to either the 3′ or the 5′ end of a double-stranded DNA preparation (Fig. 2.40). The strands are then separated by electrophoresis under denaturing conditions, and analysed separately. DNA labelled at one end is divided into four aliquots; each is treated with chemicals that act on specific bases by methylation or removal of the base. Conditions are chosen so that, on average, each molecule is modified at only one position along its length; every base in the DNA strand has an equal chance of being modified. After the modification reactions, the separate samples are cleaved by piperidine, which breaks phosphodiester bonds exclusively at the 5′ side of nucleotides whose base has been modified. The result is similar to that produced by the Sanger method, since each

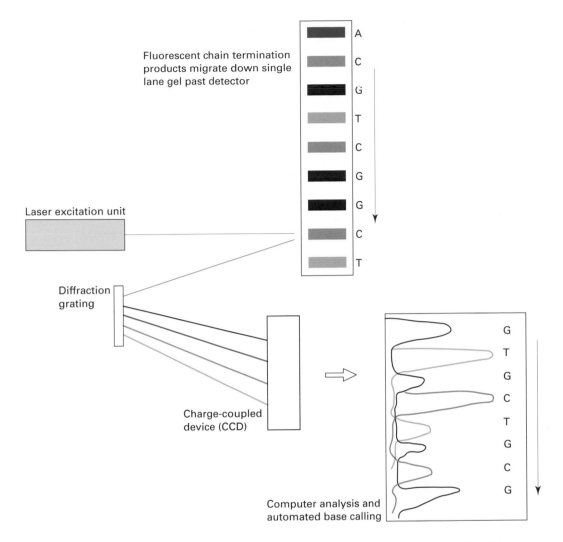

Fig. 2.39. Automated fluorescent sequencing detection using single-lane gel and charge-coupled device.

sample now contains radioactively labelled molecules of various lengths, all with one end in common (the labelled end), and with the other end cut at the same type of base. Analysis of the reaction products by electrophoresis is as described for the Sanger method.

2.15 BIOINFORMATICS AND THE INTERNET

Sequencing technology has now reached such a level of sophistication that it is quite common for a large stretch of DNA to be sequenced and for that sequence to be manipulated or stored in a computer database. This has given rise to a whole

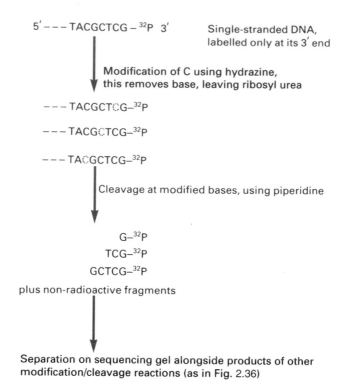

Fig. 2.40. Maxam and Gilbert sequencing of DNA. Only modification and cleavage of deoxycytidine is shown, but three more portions of the end-labelled DNA would be modified and cleaved at G, G + A, and T + C, and the products would be separated on the sequencing gel alongside those from the C reactions.

new area or molecular biology termed bioinformatics. A number of large sequence facilities are now fully automated and download sequences automatically to those databases from robotic work station servers. This increase in genetic information has luckily been matched by developments in computer hardware and software. There are now a large number of genetic databases that have sequence information representing a variety of organisms. The largest include GenBank at the National Institutes of Health (NIH) in the USA, EMBL at the European Bioinformatics Institute (EBI) at Cambridge, UK, and the DNA database of Japan (DDBJ) at Mishima in Japan. There are also many other databases within which specialist DNA and protein sequences are stored, all of which may be accessed over the Internet. A number of these important databases and World Wide Web resources are listed in Table 2.6.

It is possible once a nucleotide sequence has been deduced to search an existing database for similar, homologous, sequences and for generic gene or protein coding sequences. Thus it is possible to search for open reading frames, for example sequences beginning with a start codon (ATG) and continuing with a significant number of 'coding' triplets before a stop codon is reached. There are a

Table 2.6	Nucleic acid and protein database resources available on the World Wide Web	
Database or resource		URL (uniform resource locator)

General DNA sequence databases

EMBL	European genetic database	http://www.ebi.ae.uk
GenBank	US genetic database	http://ncbi.nlm.nih.gov
DDBJ	Japanese genetic database	http://ddbj.nig.ac.jp

Protein sequence databases

Swiss-Prot	European protein sequence database	http://expasy.hcuge.ch/sprot/sprot-top.html
TREMBL	European protein sequence database	http://www.ebi.ac.uk/pub/databases/trembl
PIR	US protein information resource	http://www.nbrf.georgetown.edu/pir

Protein structure databases

PDB	Brookhaven protein database	http://www.pdb.bnl.gov
NRL-3D	Protein structure database	http://www.gdb.org/Dan/proteins/nrl3d.html

Genome project databases

Human Mapping Database, Johns Hopkins, USA	http://gdbwww.gdb.org
dbEST (cDNA and partial sequences)	http://www.ncbi.nih.gov
Généthon Genetic maps based on repeat markers	http://www.genethon.fr
Whitehead Institute (YAC and physical maps)	http://www-genome.wi.mit.edu

number of other sequences that may be used to define coding sequences, these include ribosome binding sites, splice site junctions, poly(A) polymerase sequences and promoter sequences that lie outside the coding regions (Section 3.9.2). It is now relatively straightforward to use sequence analysis software to search a new sequence for identity within a chosen database. Software programs such as BLAST and FASTA provide the means to align sequences, and as such homology searching provides important clues to the potential structure and function of a given DNA sequence. It is further possible in some cases to generate a graphic three-dimensional model of a putative protein encoded by a DNA sequence (Fig. 2.41). The atomic coordinates of protein structures generated from X-ray crystallography or nuclear magnetic resonance (NMR) data are also held in databases. The largest of these is the protein databank (PDB) held at Brookhaven in the USA. It is possible, although difficult at present, to predict secondary protein structures from translated nucleotide sequences. Such predicted molecular models are very complex to produce, requiring sophisticated numerical processing; however, they do provide important insights into protein structure and function and are constantly being refined. Another exciting future possibility is that molecular modelling could be combined with virtual reality systems allowing real-time interaction of proteins and ligands to be observed. Whatever the means of displaying modelled proteins, there is no doubt that even now they are extremely important in the rational design and modification of proteins and enzymes (Section 3.6.2).

The main development in computing that has allowed the explosion in sequence analysis is the Internet. This is a worldwide system that links numerous

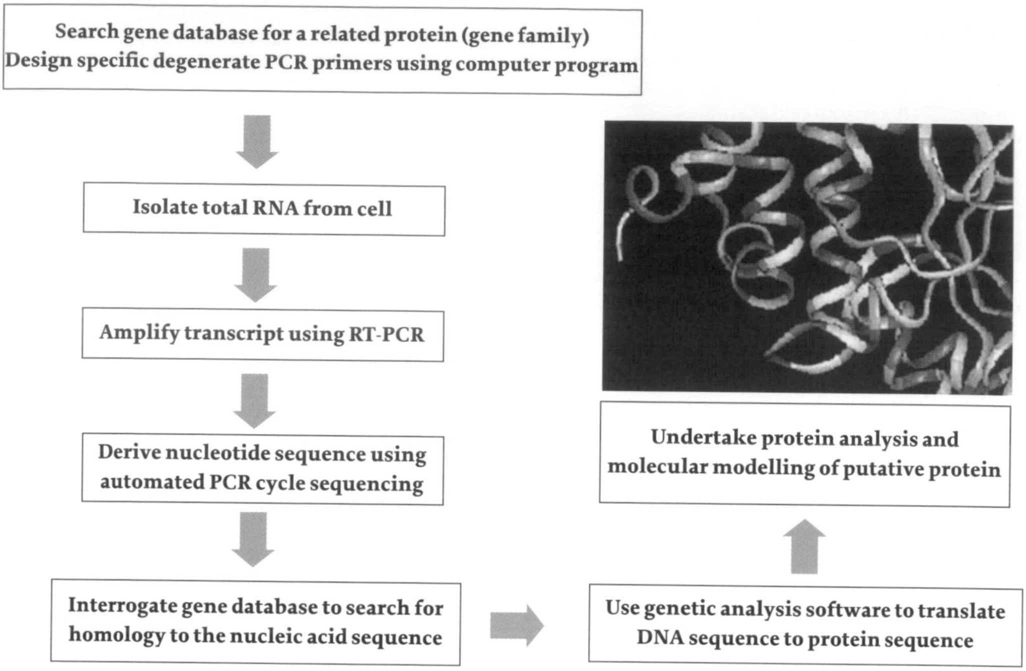

Fig. 2.41. Possible generalised scheme of work using bioinformatics to generate protein information.

computers, local networks, research, commercial and government institutions and establishments, and the World Wide Web (WWW). DNA databases and other nucleic acid sequence and protein analysis software may all be accessed over the Internet, given the relevant software and authority. This is now relatively straightforward with so-called Web browsers, which provide a user-friendly graphical interface for sequence manipulation. Consequently the new, expanding and exciting areas of bioscience research are those that analyse genome and cDNA sequence databases (genomics) and also their protein counterpart (proteomics). This is sometimes referred to as in silico research. Nowadays there is no doubt that it is just as important to have internet and database access as it is to have equipment and reagents for practical molecular biology.

2.16 KEY TERMS

3′-end labelling	aminoacyl tRNA	base-stacking
3′-hydroxyl	annealing	bioinformatics
5′-end labelling	anticodon	cap
5′-hydroxyl	antiparallel	CAT box
adenine	automated sequencing	charging
allele	autoradiography	chromatin
alternative splicing	B-DNA	chromosomal DNA

classical satellite DNA
clover leaf secondary structure
codon
cohesive-ended
complementary
Cot curve
cytosine
dam system
degeneracy
denature
deproteinised
dideoxynucleotide chain terminators
direct PCR sequencing
DNA ligase
DNA methylase
double helix
double-stranded
downstream
electroelution
elongation
enhancer
exons
exonuclease
gene
gene probe
gene synthesisers
genetic databases
genetic fingerprinting
genome
genomics
guanine
heterogeneous nuclear RNA
heterozygous
histones
homology searching
homozygous
housekeeping genes
hybrid molecules
hybridisation
hyperchromic effect
hypochromic effect
hypomethylated
in silico research
Initiation
intercalation
introns
isoschizomers

karyotype
Klenow fragment
lactose operon
lagging strand
leading strand
ligase chain reaction
locus
Maxam and Gilbert sequencing
melting temperature
messenger RNA (mRNA)
microsatellite DNA
minisatellite DNA
minus strand
molecular modelling
nick translation
non-radioactive labels
northern blotting
nucleoside
nucleosome
nucleotide
Okazaki fragments
oligonucleotide primers
oligonucleotide probe
oligonucleotide
open reading frames
operons
origin of replication
PCR cycle sequencing
peptidyl transferase
plus strand
poly(A) tail
polarity
polymerase chain reaction
polymorphism
post-transcriptional processing
post-translational modifications
preinitiation complex
primer
probe
promoter
proteomics
purine
pyrimidine
quantitative PCR
rapid amplification of polymorphic
    DNA
rate of renaturation

reading frame
renaturation
repetitive DNA
restriction endonuclease
restriction enzymes
restriction mapping
reverse transcriptase–PCR
ribosomal RNA
ribosome binding site
ribosomes
Sanger sequencing
self-complementary
semi-conservative replication
Shine–Dalgarno sequence
single-stranded DNA-binding pro-
    teins
slot or dot blotting
small nuclear RNA
SOS response
Southern blot
spliced
spliceosome
Start codon
Stop codon
stringency
structural gene
TaqMan assay
target DNA
template DNA
termination
termination codon
terminator region
TFIID
thermal cyclers
thymine
transcription
transcription factors
transfer RNA
triplet
upstream
upstream promoter elements
uracil
urr system
World Wide Web
Z-DNA
zoo blotting

2.17 CALCULATIONS

Question 1 The analysis of a gene reveals that 30% of the nucleotides are G residues. Calculate the percentage values for the following.

  (i)   C
 (ii)   A and T
(iii)   T
 (iv)   A

Answer   (i) 30%
          (ii) 40%
          (iii) 20%
          (iv) 20%

If 25% G residues are present, then the same is necessary for C residues, therefore the
A + T percentage must be 100% − 60% = 40%. The ratio of A to T is 1 : 1 and so the
respective amounts are 20%.

Question 2
Gene probe labelling using random priming uses combinations of oligonucleotides
6 bp in length. Calculate the number of possible random combinations if all four
nucleotides are included.

Answer 4^6 = 4096 possible oligonucleotides.

Question 3
Calculate the possible number of amino acids that may be encoded if only two bases
defined a codon. Comment on why this is not the case.

Answer   If two bases defined a codon, only 16 amino acids would be encoded (4^2 = 16). Twenty
naturally occurring amino acids exist and so three bases are necessary.

Question 4
If a hypothetical peptide has the sequence Phe-Tyr-Met-Pro-His :

(i) Indicate why more than one nucleotide sequence is possible,
(ii) Calculate the number of possible nucleotide sequences.

Answer   (i) There is more than one possible combination because of the degeneracy of the
          genetic code.
          (ii) 32

Pheylalanine, tyrosine and histidine have two possible codon combinations, proline
has four and methionine only one. Thus every combination results in 32 possible
nucleotide sequences.

2.18 SUGGESTIONS FOR FURTHER READING

ALPHEY, L. (1997). *DNA Sequencing*. Bios Scientific, Oxford. (A very good introduction to DNA
   sequencing and bioinformatics analysis.)
BROWN, T.A. (1997). *Genetics: A Molecular Approach*, 3rd edn. Chapman & Hall, London. (A very
   good introduction to genetics and molecular biology.)
HARWOOD, A. (1996). *Basic DNA and RNA Protocols*. Humana Press, Totowa, NY. (An extensive
   collection of practical methods for DNA and RNA analysis.)
JONES, P., QIU, J. and RICKWOOD, D. (1994). *RNA Isolation and Analysis*. Bios Scientific, Oxford.
   (A very useful text explaining the principles and techniques of RNA analysis.)

NEWTON, C.R. and GRAHAM, A. (1997). *PCR*, 2nd edn. Bios Scientific, Oxford. (An excellent introduction to the methods and application of the PCR.)

RAPLEY, R. and WALKER, J.M. (1998). *Molecular Biomethods Handbook.* Humana Press, Totowa, NY. (A collection of key nucleic acid and protein analysis techniques.)

VOET, D. and VOET, J.G. (1995). *Biochemistry*, 2nd edn. John Wiley and Sons, Chichester. (An excellent general biochemistry textbook with excellent illustrations.)

Chapter 3

Molecular cloning and gene analysis

3.1 INTRODUCTION

The discovery of restriction endonucleases in the early 1970s led not only to the possibility of analysing DNA more effectively but also to the ability to cut different DNA molecules so that they could later be joined together to create new recombinant DNA fragments. The newly created DNA molecules heralded a new era in the manipulation, analysis and exploitation of biological molecules. This process termed gene cloning has enabled numerous discoveries and insights into gene structure function and regulation. Since their initial use methods for the production of gene libraries have been steadily refined and developed. Although the polymerase chain reaction, or PCR, has provided shortcuts to gene analysis there are still many cases where gene cloning methods are not only useful but are an absolute requirement. The following provides an account of the process of gene cloning and other methods based on recombinant DNA technology.

3.2 CONSTRUCTING GENE LIBRARIES

3.2.1 Digesting genomic DNA molecules

After genomic DNA has been isolated and purified (Section 2.8.1), it is digested with restriction endonucleases. These enzymes are the key to molecular cloning because of the specificity they have for particular DNA sequences. It is important to note that every copy of a given DNA molecule from a specific organism will give the same set of fragments when digested with a particular enzyme. DNA from different organisms will, in general, give different sets of fragments when treated with the same enzyme. By digesting complex genomic DNA from an organism it is possible to reproducibly divide its genome into a large number of small fragments, each approximately the size of a single gene. As indicated in Section 2.9, some enzymes cut straight across the DNA to give flush or blunt ends. Other restriction enzymes make staggered single-strand cuts, producing short single-stranded projections at each end of the digested DNA. These ends are not only identical but complementary and will base-pair with each other; they are therefore known as cohesive or sticky ends. In addition the 5′-end projection of the DNA always retains the phosphate groups.

Table 3.1 Numbers of clones required for representation of DNA in a genome library

Species	Genome size (kb)	No. of clones required	
		17 kb fragments	35 kb fragments
Bacteria (*E. coli*)	4000	700	340
Yeast	20 000	3500	1700
Fruit fly	165 000	29 000	14 500
Man	3 000 000	535 000	258 250
Maize	15 000 000	2 700 000	1 350 000

Over 500 restriction enzymes, recognising more than 200 different sites, have been characterised. The choice of which enzyme to use depends on a number of factors. For example, the recognition sequence of 6 bp will occur, on average, every 4096 (4^6) bases, assuming a random sequence of each of the four bases. This means that digesting genomic DNA with *Eco*RI, which recognises the sequence 5′-GAATTC-3′, will produce fragments each of which is, on average, just over 4 kb. Enzymes with 8 bp recognition sequences produce much longer fragments. Therefore very large genomes, such as human DNA, are usually digested with enzymes that produce long DNA fragments. This makes subsequent steps more manageable, since a smaller number of those fragments need to be cloned and subsequently analysed (Table 3.1).

3.2.2 Ligating DNA molecules

The DNA products resulting from restriction digestion to form sticky ends may be joined to any other DNA fragments treated with the same restriction enzyme. Thus, when the two sets of fragments are mixed, base-pairing between sticky ends will result in the annealing of fragments that were derived from different starting DNA. There will, of course, also be pairing of fragments derived from the same starting DNA molecules, termed reannealing. All these pairings are transient, owing to the weakness of hydrogen bonding between the few bases in the sticky ends, but they can be stabilised by use of an enzyme, DNA ligase, in a process termed ligation. This enzyme, usually isolated from bacteriophage T4 and called T4 DNA ligase, forms a covalent bond between the 5′-phosphate at the end of one strand and the 3′-hydroxyl of the adjacent strand (Fig. 3.1). The reaction, which is ATP dependent is often carried out at 10 °C to lower the kinetic energy of the molecules, and so reduce the chances of base-paired sticky ends parting before they have been stabilised by ligation. However, long reaction times are needed to compensate for the low activity of DNA ligase in the cold. It is also possible to join blunt ends of DNA molecules, although the efficiency of this reaction is much lower than in sticky-ended ligations.

Since ligation reconstructs the site of cleavage, recombinant molecules produced by ligation of sticky ends can be cleaved again at the 'joins', using the same

Fragments produced by cleavage with *Bam*H I

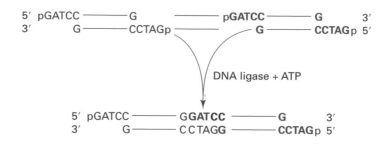

Fig. 3.1. Ligation molecules with cohesive ends. Complementary cohesive ends base-pair, forming a temporary link between two DNA fragments. This asscociation of fragments is stabilised by the formation of $3' \rightarrow 5'$ phosphodiester linkages between cohesive ends, a reaction catalysed by DNA ligase.

restriction enzyme that was used to generate the fragments initially. In order to propagate digested DNA from an organism it is necessary to join or ligate that DNA with a specialised DNA carrier molecule termed a vector (Section 3.3). Each DNA fragment is inserted by ligation into the vector DNA molecule, which allows the whole recombined DNA to then be replicated indefinitely within microbial cells (Fig. 3.2). In this way a DNA fragment can be cloned to provide sufficient material for further detailed analysis or for further manipulation. Thus, all of the DNA extracted from an organism and digested with a restriction enzyme will result in a collection of clones. This collection of clones is known as a gene library.

3.2.3 Aspects of gene libraries

There are two general types of gene library: a genomic library, which consists of the total chromosomal DNA of an organism; and a cDNA library, which represents the mRNA from a cell or tissue at a specific point in time (Fig. 3.3). The choice of the particular type of gene library depends on a number of factors, the most important being the final application of any DNA fragment derived from the library. If the ultimate aim is understanding the control of protein production for a particular gene or its architecture, then genomic libraries must be used. However, if the goal is the production of new or modified proteins, or the determination of tissue-specific expression and timing patterns, cDNA libraries are more appropriate. The main consideration in the construction of genomic or cDNA libraries is therefore the nucleic acid starting material. Since the genome of an organism is fixed, chromosomal DNA may be isolated from almost any cell type in order to prepare genomic DNA. In contrast, however, cDNA libraries represent only the mRNA being produced from a specific cell type at a particular time in the cell's development. Thus, it is important to consider carefully the cell or tissue type from which the mRNA is to be derived in the construction of cDNA libraries.

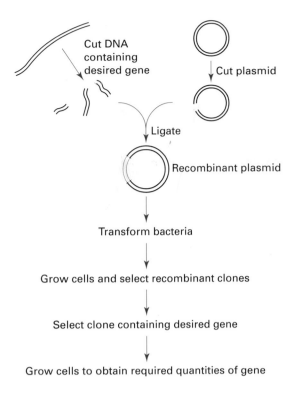

Cut DNA
containing
desired gene

Cut plasmid

Ligate

Recombinant plasmid

Transform bacteria

Grow cells and select recombinant clones

Select clone containing desired gene

Grow cells to obtain required quantities of gene

Fig. 3.2. Outline of gene cloning.

There are a variety of cloning vectors available, many based on naturally occurring molecules such as bacterial plasmids or bacteria-infecting viruses. The choice of vector also depends on whether a genomic library or cDNA library is constructed. The various types of vector are explained in more detail in Section 3.3.

3.2.4 **Genomic DNA libraries**

Genomic libraries are constructed by isolating the complete chromosomal DNA from a cell, and digesting it into fragments of the desired average length with restriction endonucleases. This can be achieved by partial restriction digestion with an enzyme that recognises tetranucleotide sequences. Complete digestion with such an enzyme would produce a large number of very short fragments, but, if the enzyme is allowed to cleave only a few of its potential restriction sites before the reaction is stopped, each DNA molecule will be cut into relatively large fragments. Average fragment size will depend on the relative concentrations of DNA and restriction enzyme and, in particular, on the conditions and duration of incubation (Fig. 3.4). It is also possible to produce fragments of DNA by physical shearing, although the ends of the fragments may need to be repaired to make them flush ended. This is achieved by using a modified DNA polymerase termed Klenow polymerase. This is prepared by cleavage of DNA polymerase with subtilisin,

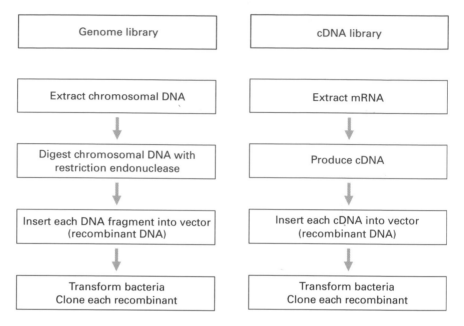

Fig. 3.3. Comparison of the general steps involved in the construction of genomic and complementary DNA (cDNA) libraries.

giving a large enzyme fragment which has no $5' \rightarrow 3'$ exonuclease activity, but which still acts as a $5' \rightarrow 3'$ polymerase. Using the appropriate dNTPs, this will fill in any recessed 3' ends on the sheared DNA.

The mixture of DNA fragments is then ligated with a vector, and subsequently cloned. If enough clones are produced there will be a very high chance that any particular DNA fragment such as a gene will be present in at least one of the clones. To keep the number of clones to a manageable size, fragments about 10 kb in length are needed for prokaryotic libraries, but the length must be increased to about 40 kb for mammalian libraries. It is possible to calculate the number of clones that must be present in a gene library to give a probability of obtaining a particular DNA sequence. This formula is:

$$N = \frac{\ln(1-P)}{\ln(1-f)}$$

where N is the number of recombinants, P is the probability and f is the fraction of the genome in one insert. For the *Escherichia coli* DNA chromosome of 5×10^6 bp and with an insert size of 20 kb, the number of clones needed (N) would therefore be 1×10^3, with a probability of 0.99.

3.2.5 cDNA libraries

There may be several thousand different proteins being produced in a cell at any one time, all of which have associated mRNA molecules. To identify any one of

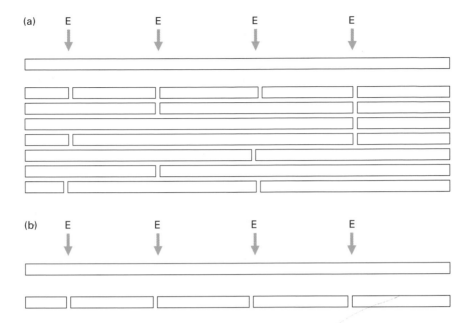

Fig. 3.4. Comparison of (a) partial and (b) complete digestion of DNA molecules at restriction enzymes sites (E).

those mRNA molecules, clones of each individual mRNA have to be synthesised. Libraries that represent the mRNA in a particular cell or tissue are termed cDNA libraries. mRNA cannot be used directly in cloning as it is too unstable. However, it is possible to synthesise complementary DNA molecules (cDNAs) to all the mRNAs from the selected tissue. The cDNA may be inserted into vectors and then cloned. The production of cDNA is carried out using an enzyme termed reverse transcriptase, which is isolated from RNA-containing retroviruses.

Reverse transcriptase is an RNA-dependent DNA polymerase and will synthesise a first-strand DNA complementary to an mRNA template, using a mixture of the four dNTPs. There is also a requirement (as with all polymerase enzymes) for a short oligonucleotide primer to be present (Fig. 3.5). With eukaryotic mRNA bearing a poly(A) tail, a complementary oligo(dT) primer may be used. Alternatively random hexamers may be used, which randomly anneal to the mRNAs in the complex. Such primers provide a free 3′-hydroxyl group that is used as the starting point for the reverse transcriptase. Regardless of the method used to prepare the first-strand cDNA, one absolute requirement is high quality undegraded mRNA (Section 2.8.2). It is usual to check the integrity of the RNA by gel electrophoresis (Section 2.8.3). Alternatively, a fraction of the extract may be used in a cell-free translation system, which, if intact mRNA is present, will direct the synthesis of proteins represented by the mRNA molecules in the sample (Section 3.7).

Following the synthesis of the first DNA strand, a poly(dC) tail is added to its 3′ end, using terminal transferase and dCTP. This will also, incidentally, put a

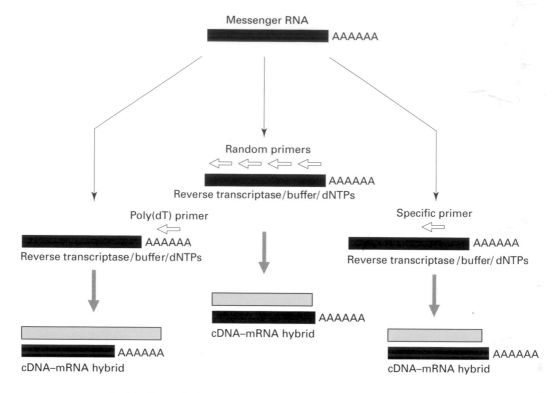

Fig. 3.5. Strategies for producing first-strand cDNA from mRNA.

poly(dC) tail on the poly(A) of mRNA. Alkaline hydrolysis is then used to remove the RNA strand, leaving single-stranded DNA that can be used, like the mRNA, to direct the synthesis of a complementary DNA strand. The second-strand synthesis requires an oligo(dG) primer, base-paired with the poly(dC) tail, which is catalysed by the Klenow fragment of DNA polymerase I. The final product is double-stranded DNA, one of the strands being complementary to the mRNA. One further method of cDNA synthesis involves the use of RNase H. Here, synthesis of the first-strand cDNA is carried out as above with reverse transcriptase but the resulting mRNA–cDNA hybrid is retained. RNase H is then used at low concentrations to nick the RNA strand. The resulting nicks expose 3′-hydroxyl groups, which are used by DNA polymerase as a primer to replace the RNA with a second strand of cDNA (Fig. 3.6).

3.2.6 Treatment of blunt cDNA ends

Ligation of blunt-ended DNA fragments is not as efficient as ligation of sticky ends, therefore with cDNA molecules additional procedures are undertaken before ligation with cloning vectors. One approach is to add to the cDNA small, double-stranded molecules with one internal site for a restriction endonuclease; these are termed nucleic acid linkers. Numerous linkers are commercially available with

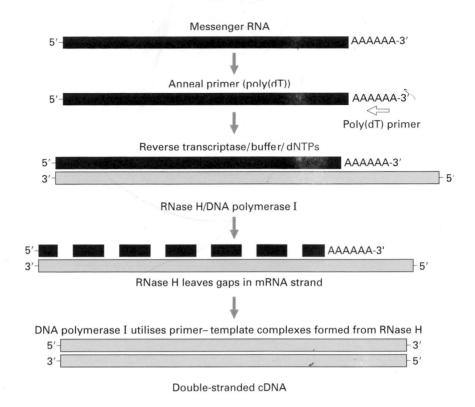

Fig. 3.6. Second-strand cDNA synthesis using the RNase H method.

internal restriction sites for many of the most commonly used restriction enzymes. Linkers are blunt end ligated to the cDNA but, since they are added much in excess of the cDNA, the ligation process is reasonably successful. Subsequently the linkers are digested with the appropriate restriction enzyme, which provides the sticky ends for efficient ligation to a vector digested with the same enzyme. This process may be made easier by the addition of adaptors rather than linkers, which are identical except that the sticky ends are preformed and so there is no need for restriction digestion following ligation (Fig. 3.7).

3.2.7 Enrichment methods for RNA

Frequently an attempt is made to isolate the mRNA transcribed from a desired gene within a particular cell or tissue that produces the protein in high amounts. If the cell or tissue produces a major protein of the cell, a large fraction of the total mRNA will code for the protein. An example of this is the B cells of the pancreas, which contain high levels of proinsulin mRNA. In such cases it is possible to precipitate polysomes, which are actively translating the mRNA, by using antibodies to the ribosomal proteins; mRNA can then be dissociated from the precipitated ribosomes. More usually, the mRNA required is only a minor component of the

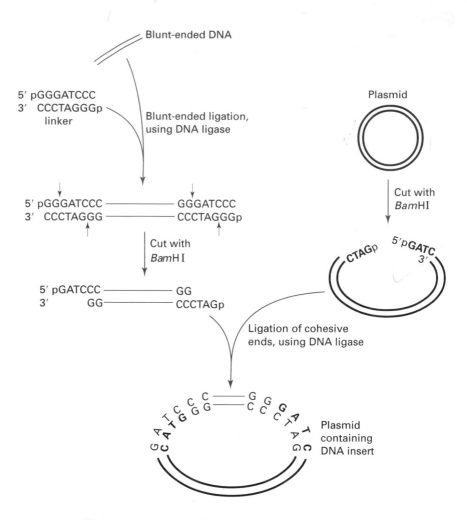

Fig. 3.7. Use of linkers. In this example, blunt-ended DNA is inserted into a specific restriction site on a plasmid, after ligation to a linker containing the same restriction site.

total cellular mRNA. In such cases total mRNA may be fractionated by size using sucrose density gradient centrifugation (Section 5.7.2). Then each fraction is used to direct the synthesis of proteins using an *in vitro* translation system (Section 3.7).

3.2.8 **Subtractive hybridisation**

It is often the case that genes are transcribed in a specific cell type or differentially activated during a particular stage of cellular growth, often at very low levels. It is possible to isolate those mRNA transcripts by subtractive hybridisation. Usually the mRNA species common to the different cell types are removed, leaving the cell type or tissue-specific mRNAs for analysis (Fig. 3.8). This may be undertaken by isolating the mRNA from the so called subtractor cells and producing a first strand

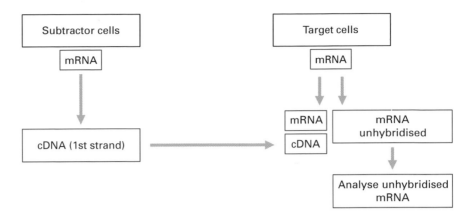

Fig. 3.8. Scheme of analysing specific mRNA molecules by subtractive hybridisation.

cDNA (Section 3.2.5). The original mRNA from the subtractor cells is then degraded and the mRNA from the target cells isolated and mixed with the cDNA. All the complementary mRNA–cDNA molecules common to both cell types will hybridise, leaving the unbound mRNA, which may be isolated and further analysed. A more rapid approach for analysing the differential expression of genes has been developed using the polymerase chain reaction (PCR). This technique, differential display, is explained in greater detail in Section 3.8.1.

3.2.9 Cloning PCR products

While PCR has to some extent replaced cloning as a method for the generation of large quantities of a desired DNA fragment, there is, in certain circumstances, still a requirement for the cloning of PCR-amplified DNA. For example, certain techniques such as *in vitro* protein synthesis are best achieved with the DNA fragment inserted into an appropriate plasmid or phage cloning vector (Section 3.7.1). Cloning methods for PCR follow closely the cloning of DNA fragments derived from the conventional manipulation of DNA. This may be achieved through one of two ways: blunt-ended or cohesive-ended cloning. Certain thermostable DNA polymerases such as *Taq* DNA polymerase and *Tth* DNA polymerase give rise to PCR products having a 3' overhanging A residue. It is possible to clone the PCR product into dT vectors, termed dA:dT cloning. This makes use of the fact that the terminal additions of A residues may be successfully ligated to vectors prepared with T residue overhangs to allow efficient ligation of the PCR product (Fig. 3.9). The reaction is catalysed by DNA ligase, as in conventional ligation reactions (Section 3.2.2)

It is also possible to carry out cohesive-ended cloning with PCR products. In this case, oligonucleotide primers are designed with a restriction endonuclease site incorporated into them. Since the complementarity of the primers needs to be absolute at the 3' end, the 5' end of the primer is usually the region for the location of the restriction site. This needs to be designed with care, since the efficiency of

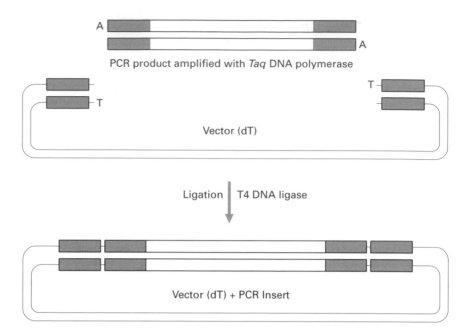

Fig. 3.9. Cloning of PCR products using dA:dT cloning.

digestion of certain restriction endonucleases decreases if extra nucleotides not involved in recognition are absent at the 5'-end. In this case the digestion and ligation reactions are the same as those undertaken for conventional reactions (Section 3.2.1)

3.3 **CLONING VECTORS**

For the cloning of any molecule of DNA it is necessary for that DNA to be incorporated into a cloning vector. These are DNA elements that may be stably maintained and propagated in a host organism for which the vector has replication functions. A typical host organism is a bacterium, such as *Escherichia coli*, that grows and divides rapidly. Any vector with a replication origin in *E.coli* will replicate efficiently (together with any incorporated DNA). Thus, any DNA cloned into a vector will enable the amplification of the inserted foreign DNA fragment and also allow any subsequent analysis to be undertaken. In this way the cloning process resembles the PCR, although there are some major differences between the two techniques. By cloning, it is possible not only to store a copy of any particular fragment of DNA but also to produce unlimited amounts of it (Fig. 3.10).

The vectors used for cloning vary in their complexity, ease of manipulation, selection and the amount of DNA sequence they can accommodate (the insert capacity). Vectors have in general been developed from naturally occurring molecules such as bacterial plasmids, bacteriophages or combinations of the elements that make them up, such as cosmids (Section 3.3.4). For gene library constructions

Table 3.2 Comparison of vectors generally available for cloning DNA fragments

Vector	Host cell	Vector structure	Insert range (kb)
M13	*E. coli*	Circular virus	1–4
Plasmid	*E. coli*	Circular plasmid	1–5
Phage λ	*E. coli*	Linear virus	2–25
Cosmids	*E. coli*	Circular plasmid	35–45
BACs	*E. coli*	Circular plasmid	50–300
YACs	*S. cerevisiae*	Linear chromosome	100–2000

BAC, bacterial artificial chromosome; YAC, yeast artificial chromosome.

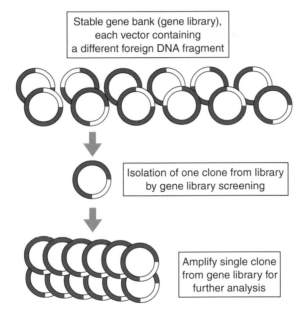

Fig. 3.10. Production of multiple copies of a single clone from a stable gene bank or library.

there is a choice and trade-off between various vector types, usually related to the ease of the manipulations needed to construct the library and the maximum size of foreign DNA insert of the vector (Table 3.2). Thus vectors with the advantage of large insert capacities are usually more difficult to manipulate, although there are many more factors to be considered, which are indicated in the following treatment of vector systems.

3.3.1 Plasmids

Many bacteria contain an extrachromosomal element of DNA, a plasmid, which is a relatively small, covalently closed circular molecule, carrying genes for antibiotic

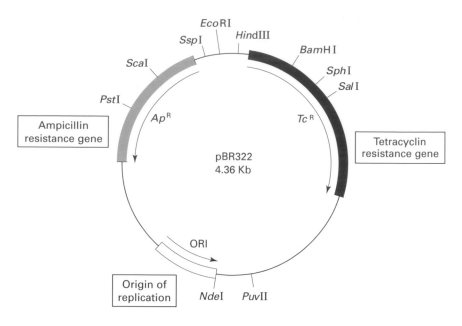

Fig. 3.11. Map and important features of pBR322.

resistance, conjugation or the metabolism of 'unusual' substrates. Some plasmids are replicated at a high rate by bacteria such as *E. coli* and so are excellent potential vectors. In the early 1970s a number of natural plasmids were artificially modified and constructed as cloning vectors by a complex series of digestion and ligation reactions. One of the most notable plasmids, termed pBR322 after its developers *B*olivar and *R*odriguez (pBR), was widely adopted and illustrates the desirable features of a cloning vector, as indicated below (Fig. 3.11).

(i) The plasmid is much smaller than a natural plasmid, which makes it more resistant to damage by shearing, and increases the efficiency of uptake by bacteria, a process termed transformation.

(ii) A bacterial origin of DNA replication ensures that the plasmid will be replicated by the host cell. Some replication origins display stringent regulation of replication, in which rounds of replication are initiated at the same frequency as cell division. Most plasmids, including pBR322, have a relaxed origin of replication, whose activity is not tightly linked to cell division, and so plasmid replication will be initiated far more frequently than chromosomal replication. Hence a large number of plasmid molecules will be produced per cell.

(iii) Two genes coding for resistance to antibiotics have been introduced. One of these allows the selection of cells which contain plasmid: if cells are plated on medium containing an appropriate antibiotic, only those that contain plasmid will grow to form colonies. The other resistance gene can be used, as described below, for detection of those plasmids that contain inserted DNA.

(iv) There are single recognition sites for a number of restriction enzymes at various points around the plasmid, which can be used to open or linearise the circular plasmid. Linearising a plasmid allows a fragment of DNA to be inserted and the circle closed. The variety of sites not only makes it easier to find a restriction enzyme that is suitable for both the vector and the foreign DNA to be inserted, but, since some of the sites are placed within an antibiotic resistance gene, the presence of an insert can be detected by loss of resistance to that antibiotic. This is termed insertional inactivation.

Insertional inactivation is a useful selection method for identifying recombinant vectors with inserts. For example, a fragment of chromosomal DNA digested with *Bam*H1 would be isolated and purified. The plasmid pBR322 would also be digested at a single site, using *Bam*HI, and both samples would then be deproteinised to inactivate the restriction enzyme. *Bam*HI cleaves to give sticky ends, and so it is possible to obtain ligation between the plasmid and digested DNA fragments in the presence of T4 DNA ligase. The products of this ligation will include plasmid containing a single fragment of the DNA as an insert, but there will also be unwanted products, such as plasmid that has recircularised without an insert, dimers of plasmid, fragments joined to each other, and plasmid with an insert composed of more than one fragment. Most of these unwanted molecules can be eliminated during subsequent steps. The products of such reactions are usually identified by agarose gel electrophoresis (Section 2.8.3).

The ligated DNA must now be used to transform *E. coli*. Bacteria do not normally take up DNA from their surroundings, but can be induced to do so by prior treatment with Ca^{2+} at 4 °C; they are then said to be competent, since DNA added to the suspension of competent cells will be taken up during a brief increase in temperature termed heat shock. Small, circular molecules are taken up most efficiently, whereas long linear molecules will not enter the bacteria.

After a brief incubation to allow expression of the antibiotic resistance genes, the cells are plated onto medium containing an antibiotic, for example ampicillin. Colonies that grow on these plates must be derived from cells containing plasmid, since this carries the gene for resistance to ampicillin. It is not, at this stage, possible to distinguish between those colonies containing plasmids with inserts and those which simply contain recircularised plasmids. To do this, the colonies are replica plated, using a sterile velvet pad, onto plates containing tetracycline in their medium. Since the *Bam*HI site lies within the tetracycline resistance gene, this gene will be inactivated by the presence of insert, but will be intact in those plasmids which have merely recircularised (Fig. 3.12). Colonies that grow on ampicillin but not on tetracycline must therefore contain plasmids with inserts. Since replica plating gives an identical pattern of colonies on both sets of plates, it is straightforward to recognise the colonies with inserts, and to recover them from the ampicillin plate for further growth. This illustrates the importance of a second gene for antibiotic resistance in a vector.

Although recircularised plasmid can be selected against, its presence decreases the yield of recombinant plasmid containing inserts. If the digested plasmid is

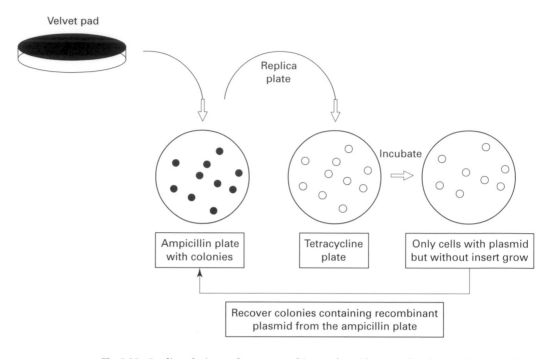

Velvet pad

Replica
plate

Incubate

| Ampicillin plate with colonies | Tetracycline plate | Only cells with plasmid but without insert grow |

Recover colonies containing recombinant
plasmid from the ampicillin plate

Fig. 3.12. Replica plating to detect recombinant plasmids. A sterile velvet pad is pressed
onto the surface of an agar plate, picking up some cells from each colony growing on that
plate. The pad is then pressed on to a fresh agar plate, thus inoculating it with cells in a
pattern identical with that of the original colonies. Clones of cells that fail to grow on the
second plate (e.g. owing to the loss of antibiotic resistance) can be recovered from their
corresponding colonies on the first plate.

treated with the enzyme alkaline phosphatase prior to ligation, recircularisation
will be prevented, since this enzyme removes the 5'-phosphate groups essential
for ligation. Links can still be made between the 5'-phosphate of the insert and the
3'-hydroxyl of the plasmid, so only recombinant plasmids and chains of linked
DNA fragments will be formed. It does not matter that only one strand of the
recombinant DNA is ligated, since the nick will be repaired by bacteria transformed with these molecules.

The valuable features of pBR322 have been enhanced by the construction of a
series of plasmids termed pUC (produced at the University of California) (Fig. 3.13).
There is an antibiotic resistance gene for tetracycline and origin of replication for E.
coli. In addition the most popular restriction sites are concentrated into a region
termed the multiple cloning site (MCS). In addition the MCS is part of a gene in its
own right and codes for a portion of a polypeptide called β-galactosidase. When the
pUC plasmid has been used to transform the host cell E. coli, the gene may be
switched on by adding the inducer isopropyl-β-D-thiogalactopyranoside (IPTG). Its
presence causes the enzyme β-galactosidase to be produced (Section 2.6.5). The functional enzyme is able to hydrolyse a colourless substance called 5-bromo-4-chloro-3-
indolyl-β-galactopyranoside (X-gal) to a blue insoluble material (Fig. 3.14).

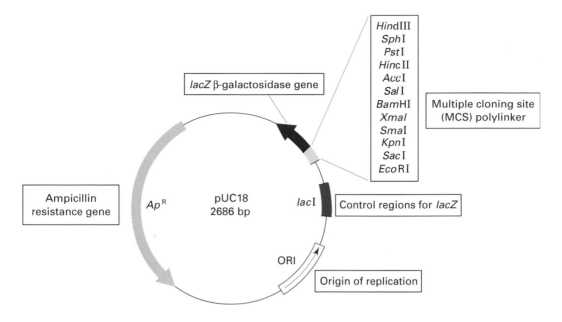

Fig. 3.13. Map and important features of pUC18

However, if the gene is disrupted by the insertion of a foreign fragment of DNA, a non-functional enzyme results that is unable to carry out hydrolysis of X-gal. Thus, a recombinant pUC plasmid may be easily detected, since it is white or colourless in the presence of X-gal, whereas an intact non-recombinant pUC plasmid will be blue, since its gene is fully functional and not disrupted. This elegant system termed blue/white selection allows the initial identification of recombinants to be undertaken very quickly and has been included in a number of subsequent vector systems. This selection method and insertional inactivation of antibiotic resistance genes do not, however, provide any information on the character of the DNA insert, merely the status of the vector. To screen gene libraries for a desired insert, hybridisation to gene probes is required and this is explained in Section 3.5.

3.3.2 **Virus-based vectors**

A useful feature of any cloning vector is the amount of DNA it may accept or have inserted before it becomes unviable. Inserts greater than 5 kb increase plasmid size to the point at which efficient transformation of bacterial cells decreases markedly, and so bacteriophages (bacterial viruses) have been adapted as vectors in order to propagate larger fragments of DNA in bacterial cells. Cloning vectors derived from λ bacteriophage are commonly used, since they offer an approximately 16-fold advantage in cloning efficiency in comparison with the most efficient plasmid cloning vectors.

Bacteriophage λ, is a linear, double-stranded phage, approximately 49 kb in

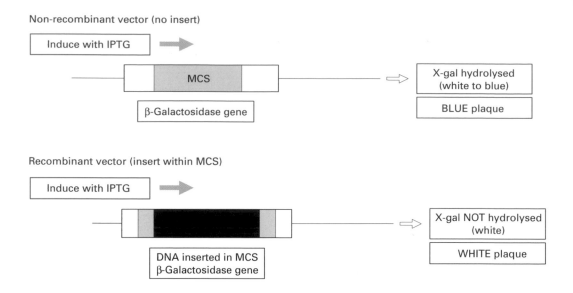

Fig. 3.14. Principle of blue/white selection for the detection of recombinant vectors.

length (Fig. 3.15). It infects *E. coli* with great efficiency by injecting its DNA through the cell membrane. In the wildtype phage λ the DNA follows one of two possible modes of replication. It may become stably integrated into the *E. coli* chromosome, where it lies dormant until a signal triggers its excision. This is termed the lysogenic life cycle. Alternatively, it may follow a lytic life cycle, where it is replicated upon entry to the cell, phage head and tail proteins are synthesised rapidly and new functional phage assembled. The phage are subsequently released from the cell by lysing of the cell membrane to infect further *E. coli* cells nearby. At the extreme ends of phage λ are 12 bp sequences termed cos (*cohesive*) sites. Although they are asymmetric, they are similar to restriction sites and allow the phage DNA to be circularised. Phage may be replicated very efficiently in this way, the result being concatemers of many phage genomes which are cleaved at the cos sites and inserted into newly formed phage protein heads.

Much use has been made of phage λ in the production of gene libraries, mainly because of its efficient entry into *E. coli* cells and the fact that larger fragments of DNA may be stably integrated. For the cloning of long DNA fragments, up to approximately 25 kb, much of the non-essential λ DNA that codes for the lysogenic life cycle is removed and replaced by the foreign DNA insert. The recombinant phage is then assembled into preformed viral protein particles, a process termed *in vitro* packaging. These newly formed phage are used to infect bacterial cells which have been plated out on agar (Fig. 3.16).

Once inside the host cells, the recombinant viral DNA is replicated. All the genes needed for normal lytic growth are still present in the phage DNA, and so multiplication of the virus takes place by cycles of cell lysis and infection of surrounding cells, giving rise to plaques of lysed cells on a background, or lawn, of

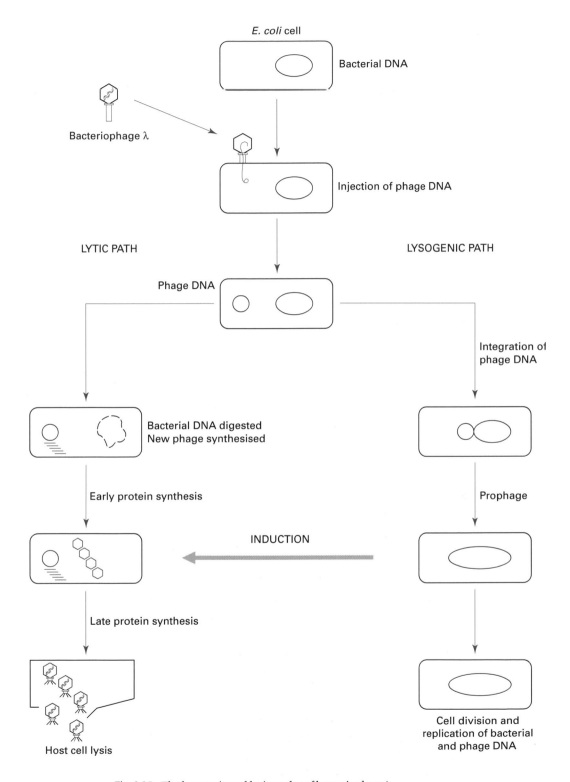

Fig. 3.15. The lysogenic and lytic cycles of bacteriophage λ.

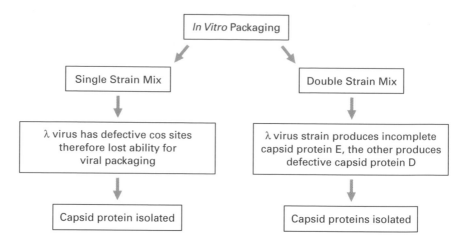

Fig. 3.16. Two strategies for producing *in vitro* packaging extracts for bacteriophage λ.

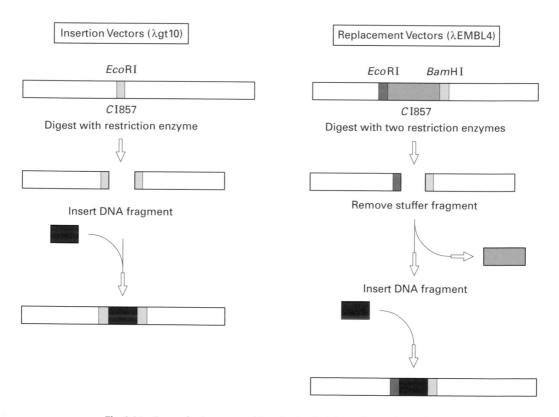

Fig. 3.17. General schemes used for cloning in λ insertion and λ replacement vectors. *C*I857 is a temperature-sensitive mutation that promotes lysis at 42 °C after incubation at 37 °C.

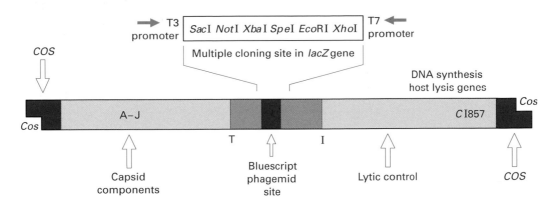

Fig. 3.18. General map of λZap cloning vector, indicating important areas of the vector. The multiple cloning site is based on the *lacZ* gene, providing blue/white selection based on the β-galactosidase gene. In between the initiator (I) site and terminator (T) site lies sequences encoding the phagemid Bluescript.

bacterial cells. The viral DNA including the cloned foreign DNA can be recovered from the viruses from these plaques and analysed further by restriction mapping (Section 2.9) and agarose gel electrophoresis (Section 2.8.3).

In general two types of λ phage vectors have been developed, λ insertion vectors and λ replacement vectors (Fig. 3.17). λ insertion vectors accept less DNA than the replacement type, since the foreign DNA is merely inserted into a region of the phage genome with appropriate restriction sites; common examples are λgt10 and λcharon16A. With a replacement vector a central region of DNA not essential for lytic growth is removed (a stuffer fragment) by a double digestion with, for example, *Eco*RI and *Bam*HI. This leaves two DNA fragments termed right and left arms. The central stuffer fragment is replaced by inserting foreign DNA between the arms to form a functional recombinant λ phage. The most notable examples of λ replacement vectors are λEMBL and λZap.

λZap is a commercially produced cloning vector that includes unique cloning sites clustered into an MCS (Fig. 3.18). Furthermore the MCS is located within a *lacZ* region, enabling a blue/white screening system based on insertional inactivation. It is also possible to express foreign cloned DNA from this vector. This is a very useful feature of some λ vectors, since it is then possible to screen for protein product rather than for the DNA inserted into the vector. This screening is therefore undertaken with antibody probes directed against the protein of interest (Section 3.5.4). Other features that make this a useful cloning vector are the ability to produce RNA transcripts termed cRNA or riboprobes. This is possible because two promoters for RNA polymerase enzymes exist in the vector, a T7 and a T3 promoter which flank the MCS (Section 3.4.2).

One of the most useful features of λZap is that it has been designed to allow automatic excision *in vivo* of a small 2.9 kb colony-producing vector termed a pha gemid, pBluescript SK (Section 3.3.3). This technique is sometimes termed single stranded DNA rescue and occurs as the result of a process called superinfection

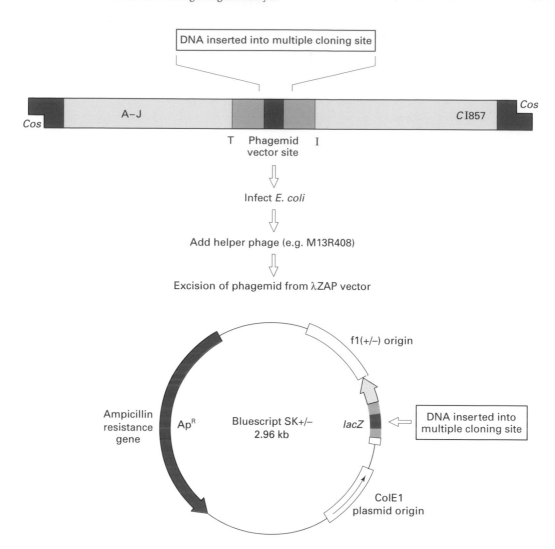

Fig. 3.19. Single-stranded DNA rescue of phagemid from λZap. The single-stranded phagemid pBluescript SK may be excised from λZap by addition of helper phage. This provides the necessary proteins and factors for transcription between the I and T sites in the parent phage to produce the phagemid with the DNA cloned into the parent vector.

where helper phage are added to the cells which are then grown for an additional period of approximately 4 h (Fig. 3.19).

The helper phage displace a strand within the λZap that contains the foreign DNA insert. This is circularised and packaged as a filamentous phage similar to M13 (Section 3.3.3). The packaged phagemid is secreted from the *E. coli* cell and may be recovered from the supernatant. Thus the λZap vector allows a number of diverse manipulations to be undertaken without the necessity of recloning or subcloning foreign DNA fragments. The process of subcloning is sometimes necessary when the manipulation of gene fragment cloned a general purpose vector needs to be inserted into a more specialised vector for the application of techniques such as *in vitro* mutagenesis or protein production (Section 3.6).

3.3.3 M13 and phagemid-based vectors

Much use has been made recently of single-stranded bacteriophage vectors such as M13 and vectors that have the combined properties of phage and plasmids, termed phagemids. M13 is a filamentous coliphage with a single-stranded circular DNA genome (Fig. 3.20). Upon infection of *E. coli*, the DNA replicates initially as a double-stranded molecule but subsequently produces single-stranded virions for infection of further bacterial cells (lytic growth). The nature of these vectors makes them ideal for techniques such as chain termination sequencing (Section 3.6.1) and *in vitro* mutagenesis (Section 3.6.2), since both require single-stranded DNA.

M13 or phagemids such as pBluescript SK infect *E. coli* harbouring a male-specific structure termed the F pillus (Fig. 3.21). They enter the cell by adsorption to this structure and, once inside, the phage DNA is converted to a double-stranded replicative form or RF DNA. Replication then proceeds rapidly until some 100 RF molecules are produced within the *E. coli* cell. DNA synthesis then switches to the production of single strands and the DNA is assembled and packaged into the capsid at the bacterial periplasm. The bacteriophage DNA is then encapsulated by the major coat protein, gene VIII protein, of which there are approximately 2800 copies, with three to six copies of the gene III protein at one end of the particle. The extrusion of the bacteriophage through the bacterial periplasm results in decreased growth rate of the *E. coli* cell rather than host cell lysis and is visible on a bacterial lawn as a clear area. Approximately 1000 packaged phage particles may be released into the medium in one cell division.

In addition to producing single-stranded DNA, the coliphage vectors have a number of other features that make them attractive as cloning vectors. Since the bacteriophage DNA is replicated as a double-stranded RF DNA intermediate, a number of regular DNA manipulations may be performed such as restriction digestion, mapping and DNA ligation. RF DNA is prepared by lysing infected *E. coli* cells and purifying the supercoiled circular phage DNA with the same methods used for plasmid isolation. Intact single-stranded DNA packaged in the phage protein coat located in the supernatant may be precipitated with reagents such as polyethylene glycol, and the DNA purified with phenol/chloroform (Section 2.8.1). The bacteriophage may thus act as a plasmid under certain circumstances and at other times produce DNA in the fashion of a virus. A family of vectors derived from M13, termed M13mp8/9, mp18/19 etc, is currently widely used and has a number of highly useful features. All contain a synthetic MCS which is located in the *lacZ* gene without disturbing the reading frame of the gene. This allows efficient selection to be undertaken on the basis of blue/white screening (Section 3.3.1). As the series of vectors was developed, the number of restriction

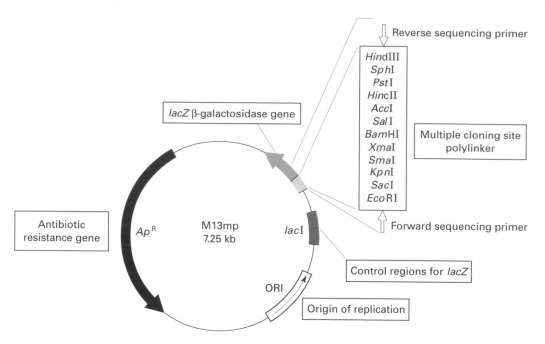

Fig. 3.20. Genetic map and important features of bacteriophage vector M13.

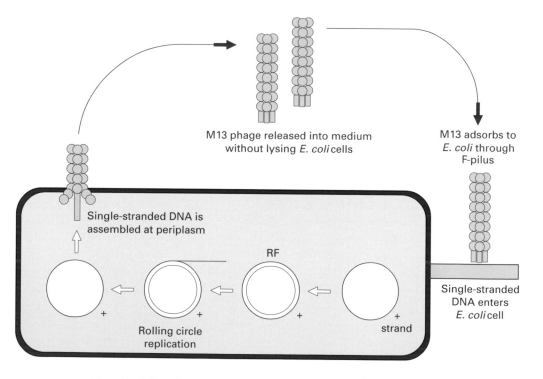

Fig. 3.21. Life cycle of bacteriophage M13. The bacteriophage virus enters the *E. coli* cell through the F pillus. It then enters a stage where the circular single strands are converted to double strands. Rolling-circle replication then produces single strands, which are packaged and extruded through the *E. coli* cell membrane.

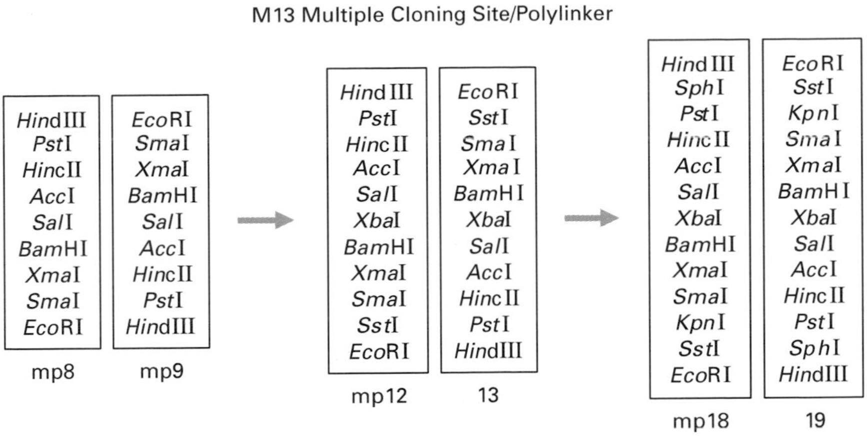

M13 Multiple Cloning Site/Polylinker

*Hind*III	*Eco*RI
*Pst*I	*Sma*I
*Hinc*II	*Xma*I
*Acc*I	*Bam*HI
*Sal*I	*Sal*I
*Bam*HI	*Acc*I
*Xma*I	*Hinc*II
*Sma*I	*Pst*I
*Eco*RI	*Hind*III
mp8	mp9

→

*Hind*III	*Eco*RI
*Pst*I	*Sst*I
*Hinc*II	*Sma*I
*Acc*I	*Xma*I
*Sal*I	*Bam*HI
*Xba*I	*Xba*I
*Bam*HI	*Sal*I
*Xma*I	*Acc*I
*Sma*I	*Hinc*II
*Sst*I	*Pst*I
*Eco*RI	*Hind*III
mp12	13

→

*Hind*III	*Eco*RI
*Sph*I	*Sst*I
*Pst*I	*Kpn*I
*Hinc*II	*Sma*I
*Acc*I	*Xma*I
*Sal*I	*Bam*HI
*Xba*I	*Xba*I
*Bam*HI	*Sal*I
*Xma*I	*Acc*I
*Sma*I	*Hinc*II
*Kpn*I	*Pst*I
*Sst*I	*Sph*I
*Eco*RI	*Hind*III
mp18	19

Fig. 3.22. Design and orientation of polylinkers in M13 series. Only the main restriction enzymes are indicated.

sites was increased in an asymmetric fashion. Thus M13mp8, mp12, mp18 and sister vectors that have the same MCS but in reverse orientation, M13mp9, mp13 and mp19, respectively, have more restriction sites in the MCS, making these vectors more useful since there is a greater choice of restriction enzymes (Fig. 3.22). However, one problem frequently encountered with M13 is the instability and spontaneous loss of inserts greater then 6 kb.

Phagemids are similar to M13 and replicate in a similar fashion. One of the first phagemid vectors, pEMBL, was constructed by inserting a fragment of another phage, f1, containing a phage origin of replication and elements for its morphogenesis, into a pUC8 plasmid. After superinfection with helper phage, the f1 origin is activated, allowing single-stranded DNA to be produced. The phage is assembled into a phage coat, extruded through the periplasm and secreted into the culture medium in a way similar to that of M13. Without superinfection, the phagemid replicates as a pUC-type plasmid and the RF DNA isolated is double stranded. This allows further manipulations such as restriction digestion, ligation and mapping analysis to be performed. The pBluescript SK vector is also a phagemid and can be used in its own right as a cloning vector and manipulated as if it were a plasmid. It may, like M13, be used in nucleotide sequencing and site-directed mutagenesis, and it is also possible to produce RNA transcripts that may be used in the production of labelled cRNA probes or riboprobes (Section 3.4.2)

3.3.4 Cosmid-based vectors

The way in which bacteriophage λ DNA is replicated is of particular interest in the development of larger insert cloning vectors termed cosmids (Fig. 3.23). These are especially useful for the analysis of highly complex genomes and are an important part of various genome mapping projects (Section 3.9).

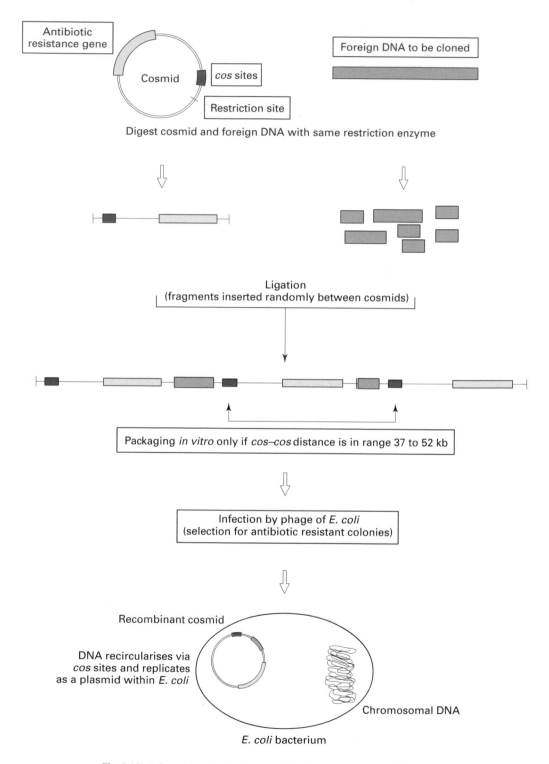

Fig. 3.23. Scheme for cloning foreign DNA fragments in cosmid vectors.

The upper limit of the insert capacity of bacteriophage λ is approximately 21 kb. This is because of the requirement for essential genes and the fact that the maximum length between the cos sites is 52 kb. Consequently, cosmid vectors have been constructed that incorporate the *cos* sites from bacteriophage λ and also the essential features of a plasmid, such as the plasmid origin of replication, a gene for drug resistance, and several unique restriction sites for insertion of the DNA to be cloned. When a cosmid preparation is linearised by restriction digestion, and ligated to DNA for cloning, the products will include concatamers of alternating cosmid vector and insert. The only requirement for a length of DNA to be packaged into viral heads, therefore, is that it should contain *cos* sites spaced the correct distance apart; in practice this spacing can range between 37 and 52 kb. Such DNA can be packaged *in vitro* if bacteriophage head precursors, tails and packaging proteins are provided. As the cosmid is very small, inserts of about 40 kb in length will be most readily packaged. Once inside the cell, the DNA recircularises through its *cos* sites, and from then onwards behaves exactly like a plasmid.

3.3.5 Large insert capacity vectors

The advantage of vectors that accept fragments of DNA larger than phage λ or cosmids means that fewer clones need to be screened when one is searching for the foreign DNA of interest. Cosmids have also had an enormous impact in the mapping of the genomes of organisms such as the mouse and are used extensively in the human genome mapping project (Section 3.9.3). Recent developments have allowed the production of large-insert capacity vectors based on bacterial (BACs), mammalian (MACs) and virus P1 (PACs), artificial chromosomes. However, perhaps the most significant development is vectors based on yeast artificial chromosomes or YACs.

3.3.6 Yeast artificial chromosome (YAC) vectors

YACs are linear molecules composed of a centromere, telomere and a replication origin termed an ARS element (autonomous replicating sequence). The YAC is digested with restriction enzymes at the SUP4 site (a suppressor tRNA gene marker) and *Bam*HI sites separating the telomere sequences (Fig. 3.24). This produces two arms, and the foreign genomic DNA is ligated to produce a functional YAC construct. YACs are replicated in yeast cells; however, the external cell wall of the yeast needs to be removed to leave a spheroplast. This is osmotically unstable and also needs to be embedded in a solid matrix such as agar. Once the yeast cells are transformed, only correctly constructed YACs with associated selectable markers are replicated in the yeast strains. DNA fragments with repeated sequences, which are sometimes difficult to clone in bacteria-based vectors may also be cloned in YAC systems. The main advantage of YAC-based vectors, however, is the ability to clone very large fragments of DNA. The stable maintenance and replication of foreign DNA fragments of up to 2000 kb have been

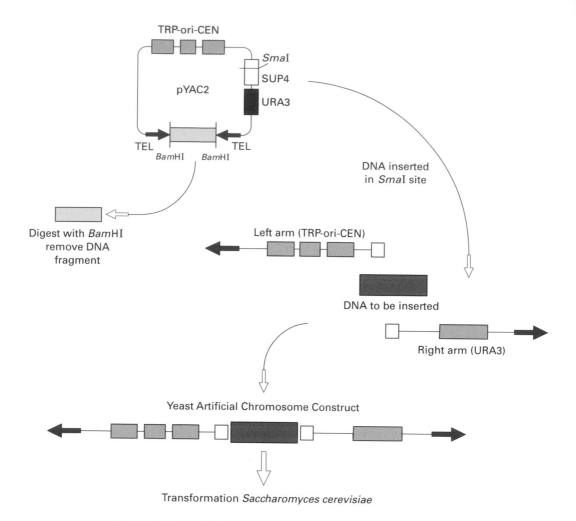

Fig. 3.24. Scheme for cloning large fragments of DNA into YAC vectors.

carried out in YAC vectors and they are the main vector of choice in the various genome mapping and sequencing projects (Section 3.9)

3.3.7 **Vectors used in eukaryotes**

The use of *E. coli* for general cloning and manipulation of DNA is well established; however, numerous developments have been made in cloning from eukaryotic cells. Plasmids used for cloning DNA in eukaryotic cells require a eukaryotic origin of replication and marker genes that will be expressed by eukaryotic cells. At present the two most important applications of plasmids to eukaryotic cells are cloning in yeast and in plants.

Although yeast has a natural plasmid called the 2μ circle, this is too large for use in cloning. Plasmids such as the the yeast episomal plasmid (YEp) have been created by genetic manipulation using replication origins from the 2μ circle, and by incorporating a gene that will complement a defective gene in the host yeast cell. If, for example, a strain of yeast is used that has a defective gene for the biosynthesis of an amino acid, an active copy of that gene on a yeast plasmid can be used as a selectable marker for the presence of that plasmid. Yeast, like bacteria, can be grown rapidly, and it is therefore well suited for use in cloning. Of particular use has been the creation of shuttle vectors which have origins of replication for yeast and bacteria such as *E. coli*. This means that constructs may be prepared rapidly in the bacteria and delivered into yeast for expression studies.

The bacterium *Agrobacterium tumefaciens* infects plants that have been damaged near soil level, and this infection is often followed by the formation of plant tumours in the vicinity of the infected region. It is now known that *A. tumefaciens* contains the Ti plasmid, part of which is transferred into the nuclei of plant cells that are infected by the bacterium. Once in the nucleus, plasmid DNA is maintained by integration into the chromosomal DNA. The integrated DNA carries genes for the synthesis of opines (which are metabolised by the bacteria but not by the plants) and for tumour induction (hence 'Ti'). DNA inserted into the correct region of the Ti plasmid will be transferred to infected plant cells, and in this way it has been possible to clone and express foreign genes in plants (Fig. 3.25). This is a prerequisite for the genetic engineering of crops.

3.3.8 Delivery of vectors into eukaryotes

Following the production of a recombinant molecule, the so-called constructs are subsequently introduced into cells to enable it to be copied a large number of times as the cells replicate. Initial recombinant DNA experiments were performed in bacterial cells because of the latter's ease of growth and short doubling time. Gram-negative bacteria such as *E. coli* can be made 'competent' for the introduction of extraneous plasmid DNA into cells (Section 3.3.1). The natural ability of bacteriophage to introduce DNA into *E. coli* has also been well exploited and results in 10- to 100-fold higher efficiency for the introduction of recombinant DNA compared to transformation of competent bacteria with plasmids. These well-established and traditional approaches are the reason why so many cloning vectors have been developed for *E. coli*. The delivery of cloning vectors into eukaryotic cells is, however, not as straightforward as that for the prokaryote *E. coli*.

It is possible to deliver recombinant molecules into animal cells by transfection. The efficiency of which can be increased by first precipitating the DNA with Ca^{2+} or making the membrane permeable with divalent cations or high molecular weight polymers such as DEAE–dextran or polyethylene glycol (PEG). The technique is rather inefficient although a selectable marker that provides resistance to a toxic compound such neomycin can be used to monitor the success. Alternatively, DNA can be introduced into animal cells by electroporation. In this process the cells are subjected to pulses of a high voltage gradient, causing many of them to take up DNA from the surrounding solution. This technique has proved to be useful with cells from a range of animal, plant and microbial sources. More

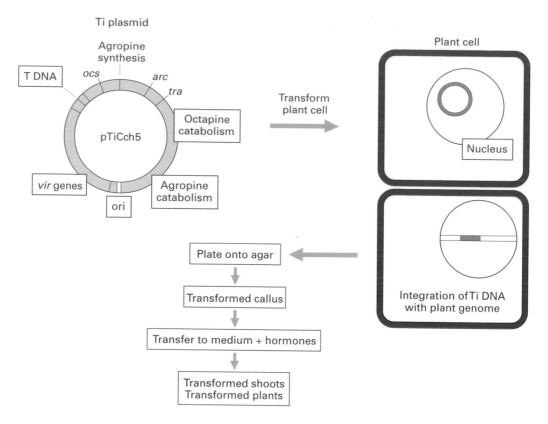

Fig. 3.25. Scheme for cloning in plant cells using the Ti plasmid.

recently the technique of lipofection has been used as the delivery method. The recombinant DNA is encapsulated in a core of lipid-coated particles that fuse with the lipid membrane of cells and thus release the DNA into the cell. Microinjection of DNA into cell nuclei of eggs or embryos has also been performed successfully in many mammalian cells.

The ability to deliver recombinant molecules into plant cells is not without its problems. Generally the outer cell wall of the plant must be stripped, usually by enzymic digest, to leave a protoplast. The cells are then able to take up recombinants from the supernatant. The cell wall can be regenerated by providing appropriate media. In cases where protoplasts have been generated, transformation may also be achieved by electroporation. An even more dramatic transformation procedure involves propelling microscopically small titanium or gold pellet microprojectiles, coated with the recombinant DNA molecule, into plant cells in intact tissues. This biolistic technique involves the detonation of an explosive charge, which is used to propel the microprojectiles into cells at a high velocity. The cells then appear to reseal themselves after the delivery of the recombinant molecule. This is a particularly promising technique for use with plants whose protoplasts will not regenerate whole plants.

3.4 HYBRIDISATION AND GENE PROBES

3.4.1 Cloned DNA probes

The ready availability of custom synthesis of oligonucleotides and the PCR have contributed to the rapid production of gene probes. These are usually designed from gene databases or gene family related sequences as indicated in Section 2.11. However, there are many gene probes that have been derived from cDNA or from genomic sequences and which have been cloned into plasmid and phage vectors. These require manipulation before they may be labelled and used in hybridisation experiments. Gene probes may vary in length from 100 bp to a number of kilobases although this is dependent on their origin. Many are short enough to be cloned into plasmid vectors and are useful in that they may be manipulated easily and are relatively stable both in transit and in the laboratory. The DNA sequences representing the gene probe are usually excised from the cloning vector by digestion with restriction enzymes and purified. In this way vector sequences that may hybridise non-specifically and cause high background signals in hybridisation experiments are removed. There are various ways of labelling DNA probes and these are described in Section 2.12.

3.4.2 RNA gene probes

It is also possible to prepare cRNA probes or riboprobes by *in vitro* transcription of gene probes cloned into a suitable vector. A good example of such a vector is the phagemid pBluescript SK, since at each end of the MCS where the cloned DNA fragment resides are promoters for T3 or T7 RNA polymerase (Section 3.3.3). The vector is then made linear with a restriction enzyme, and T3 or T7 RNA polymerase is used to transcribe the cloned DNA fragment. Provided a labelled dNTP is added in the reaction, a riboprobe labelled to a high specific activity will be produced (Fig. 3.26). One advantage of riboprobes is that they are single stranded and their sensitivity is generally regarded as superior to cloned double stranded probes, as indicated in Section 3.4.1. They are used extensively in *in situ* hybridisation and for identifying and analysing mRNA and are described in more detail in Section 3.8.

3.5 SCREENING GENE LIBRARIES

3.5.1 Colony and plaque hybridisation

Once a cDNA or genomic library has been prepared, the next task requires the identification of the specific fragment of interest. In many cases this may be more problematic than the library construction itself, since many hundreds of thousands of clones may be in the library. One clone containing the desired fragment needs to be isolated from the library and therefore a number of techniques, based mainly on hybridisation, have been developed.

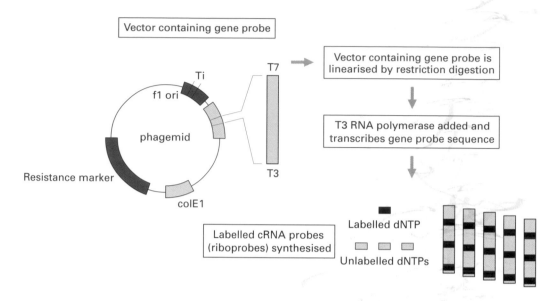

Fig. 3.26. Production of cDNA (riboprobes) using T3 RNA polymerase and phagemid vectors.

Colony hybridisation is one method used to identify a particular DNA fragment from a plasmid gene library (Fig. 3.27). A large number of clones are grown up to form colonies on one or more plates, and these are then replica plated onto a nylon membrane placed on solid agar medium. Nutrients diffuse through the membranes and allow colonies to grow on them. The colonies are then lysed, and liberated DNA is denatured and bound to the membrane, so that the pattern of colonies is replaced by an identical pattern of bound DNA. The membrane is then incubated with a prehybridisation mix containing non-labelled non-specific DNA such as salmon sperm DNA to block non-specific sites. Following this, denatured labelled gene probe is added. Under hybridising conditions the probe will bind only to cloned fragments containing at least part of its corresponding gene (Section 2.11). The membrane is then washed to remove any unbound probe and the binding detected by autoradiography of the membrane. If non-radioactive labels have been used then alternative methods of detection must be employed (Section 2.12). By comparison of the patterns on the autoradiograph with the original plates of colonies, those which contain the desired gene (or part of it) can be identified and isolated for further analysis. A similar procedure is used to identify desired genes cloned into bacteriophage vectors. In this case the process is termed plaque hybridisation. It is the DNA contained in the bacteriophage particles found in each plaque that is immobilised onto the nylon membrane. This is then probed with an appropriately labelled complementary gene probe and the detection undertaken as for colony hybridisation.

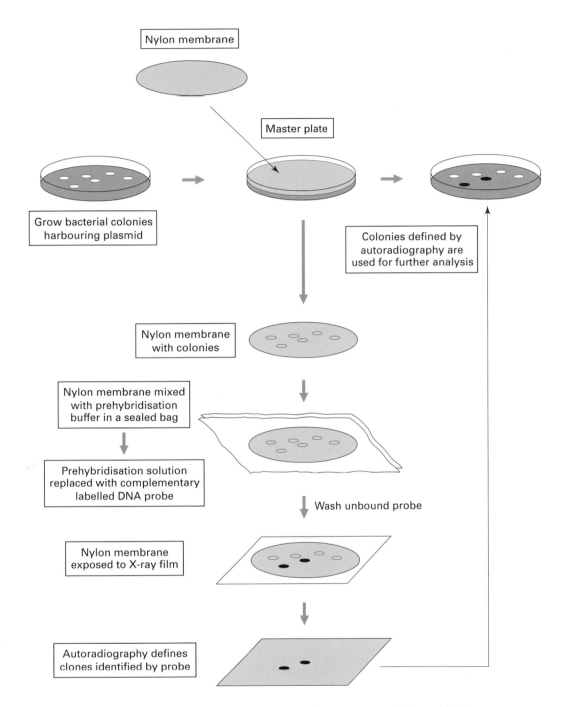

Fig. 3.27. Colony hybridisation technique for locating specific bacterial colonies harbouring recombinant plasmid vectors containing desired DNA fragments. This is achieved by hybridisation to a complementary labelled DNA probe and autoradiography.

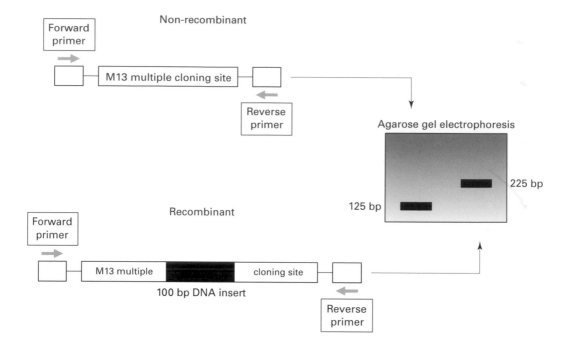

Fig. 3.28. PCR screening of recombinant vectors. In this figure, the M13 non-recombinant has no insert and so the PCR undertaken with forward and reverse sequencing primers gives rise to a product 125 bp in length. The M13 recombinant with an insert of 100 bp will give rise to a PCR product of 125 bp + 100 bp = 225 bp and thus may be distinguished from the non-recombinant by analysis on agarose gel electrophoresis.

3.5.2 PCR screening of gene libraries

In many cases it is now possible to use the PCR to screen cDNA or genomic libraries constructed in plasmids or bacteriophage vectors. This is usually undertaken with primers that anneal to the vector rather than the foreign DNA insert. The size of an amplified product may be used to characterise the cloned DNA and subsequent restriction mapping is then carried out (Fig. 3.28). The main advantage of the PCR over traditional hybridisation-based screening is the rapidity of the technique: PCR screening may be undertaken in 3 to 4 h whereas it may be several days before detection by hybridisation is achieved. The PCR screening technique gives an indication of the size of the cloned inserts rather than their sequence; however, PCR primers that are specific for a foreign DNA insert may also be used. This allows a more rigorous characterisation of clones from cDNA and genomic libraries.

3.5.3 Hybrid select/arrest translation

The difficulty of characterising clones and detecting a desired DNA fragment from a mixed cDNA library may be made simpler by two useful techniques termed hybrid select (release) translation or hybrid arrest translation. After preparation of a cDNA library in a plasmid vector, the plasmid is extracted from part of each colony, and each preparation is then denatured and immobilised on a nylon membrane (Fig. 3.29). The membrane is soaked in total cellular mRNA, under stringent conditions, usually a temperature only a few degrees below T_m, in which hybridisation will occur only between complementary strands of nucleic acid. Hence, each membrane will bind just one species of mRNA, since it has only one type of cDNA immobilised on it. Unbound mRNA is washed off the membrane, and then the bound mRNA is eluted and used to direct *in vitro* translation (Section 3.7). By immunoprecipitation or electrophoresis of the protein, the mRNA coding for a particular protein can be detected, and the clone containing its corresponding cDNA is isolated. This technique is known as hybrid release translation. In a related method called hybrid arrest translation a positive result is indicated by the absence of a particular translation product when total mRNA is hybridised with excess cDNA. This is a consequence of the fact that mRNA cannot be translated when it is hybridised to another molecule.

3.5.4 Screening expression cDNA libraries

In some cases the protein for which the gene sequence is required is partially characterised and in these cases it may be possible to produce antibodies to that protein. This allows immunological screening to be undertaken rather than gene hybridisation. Such antibodies are useful, since they may be used as the probe if little or no gene sequence is available. In these cases it is possible to prepare a cDNA library in a specially adapted vector termed an expression vector, which transcribes and translates any cDNA inserted into it. The protein is usually synthesised as a fusion with another protein such as β-galactosidase. Common examples of expression vectors are those based on bacteriophage, such as λgt11 and λZap or plasmids such as pEX. The precise requirements for such vectors are identical with vectors that are dedicated to producing proteins *in vitro* and are described in Section 3.7.1. In some cases, expression vectors incorporate inducible promoters that may be activated by, for example, increasing the temperature and allowing stringent control of expression of the cloned cDNA molecules (Fig. 3.30).

The cDNA library is plated out and a nylon membrane filter prepared as for colony/plaque hybridisation. A solution containing the antibody to the desired protein is then added to the membrane. The membrane is then washed to remove any unbound protein and a further labelled antibody, which is directed to the first antibody, is applied. This allows visualisation of the plaque or colony that contains the cloned cDNA for that protein and this may then be picked from the agar plate and pure preparations grown for further analysis.

3.6 APPLICATIONS OF GENE CLONING

3.6.1 Sequencing cloned DNA

DNA fragments cloned into plasmid vectors may be subjected to the chain termination sequencing method detailed in Section 2.14. However, since plasmids are

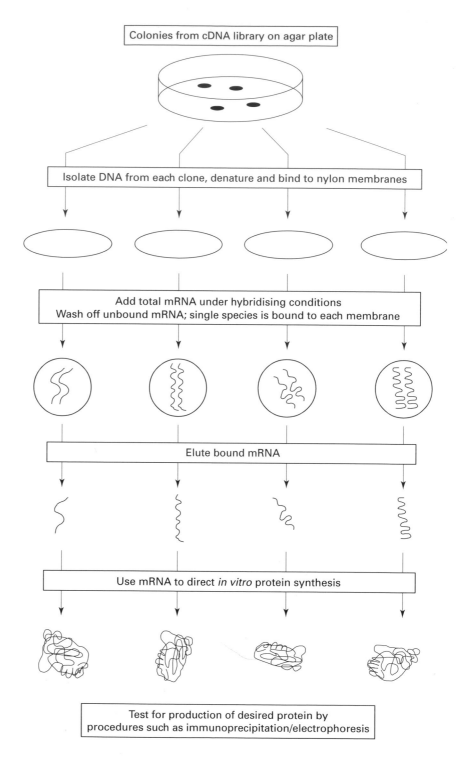

Colonies from cDNA library on agar plate

Isolate DNA from each clone, denature and bind to nylon membranes

Add total mRNA under hybridising conditions
Wash off unbound mRNA; single species is bound to each membrane

Elute bound mRNA

Use mRNA to direct *in vitro* protein synthesis

Test for production of desired protein by
procedures such as immunoprecipitation/electrophoresis

Fig. 3.29. General principles involved in the technique of a hybrid select translation.

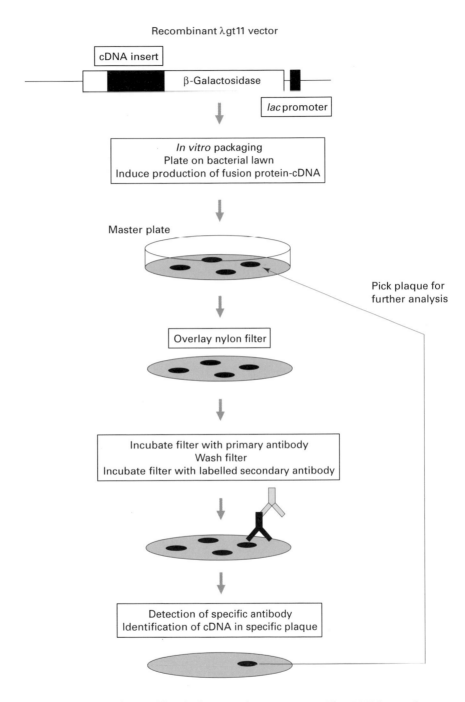

Fig. 3.30. Screening of cDNA libraries in expression vector λgt11. The cDNA inserted upstream from the gene for β-galactosidase will give rise to a fusion protein under induction (e.g. with IPTG). The plaques are then blotted onto a nylon membrane filter and probed with an antibody specific for the protein coded for by the cDNA. A secondary labelled antibody directed to the specific antibody can then be used to identify the location (plaque) of the cDNA.

double stranded, further manipulation needs to be undertaken before this may be attempted. In these cases the plasmids are denatured, usually by alkali treatment. Although the plasmids containing the foreign DNA inserts may reanneal, the kinetics of the reaction are such that the strands are single stranded for a long enough period of time to allow the sequencing method to succeed. It is also possible to include denaturants such as formamide to the reaction mixture to further prevent reannealing. In general however the superior results gained with sequencing single-stranded DNAs from M13 or single-stranded phagemids means that cloned DNAs of interest are usually subcloned into such vectors.

M13 vectors are the traditional choice for chain termination sequencing because of the single-stranded nature of their DNA (Section 2.14). A further modification that makes M13 useful in chain termination sequencing is the placement of universal priming sites at -20 or -40 bases from the start of the MCS. This allows any gene to be sequenced by using one universal primer, since annealing of the primer prior to sequencing occurs outside the MCS and so is M13 specific rather than gene specific. This obviates the need to synthesise new oligonucleotide primers for each new foreign DNA insert. A further, reverse, priming site is also located at the opposite end of the polylinker, allowing sequencing in the opposite orientation to be undertaken.

3.6.2 *In vitro* mutagenesis and rational design

One of the most powerful developments in molecular biology has been the ability to artificially create defined mutations in a gene and analyse the resulting protein following *in vitro* expression. Numerous methods are now available for producing site-directed mutations, many of which now involve the PCR, and are commonly termed protein engineering. It is possible to undertake a logical sequence of analytical and computational techniques centred around a protein design cycle. This involves the biochemical preparation and analysis of proteins, the subsequent identification of the gene encoding the protein and its modification. The production of the modified protein and its further biochemical analysis completes the concept of rational redesign to improve a protein's structure and function (Fig. 3.31).

The use of design cycles and rational design systems are exemplified by the study and manipulation of subtilisin. This is a serine protease of broad specificity and considerable industrial importance, being used in soap powder and in the food and leather industries. Approximately 600 tonnes per annum are produced for the cleaning industry. Protein engineering has been used to alter the specificity, pH profile and stability to oxidative, thermal and alkaline inactivation. Analysis of homologous thermophiles and their resistance to oxidation has also been improved. Engineered subtilisins of improved bleach resistance and wash performance are now used in many brands of washing powders.

3.6.3 Oligonucleotide-directed mutagenesis

The traditional method of site-directed mutagenesis demands that the gene be already cloned or subcloned into a single-stranded vector such as M13.

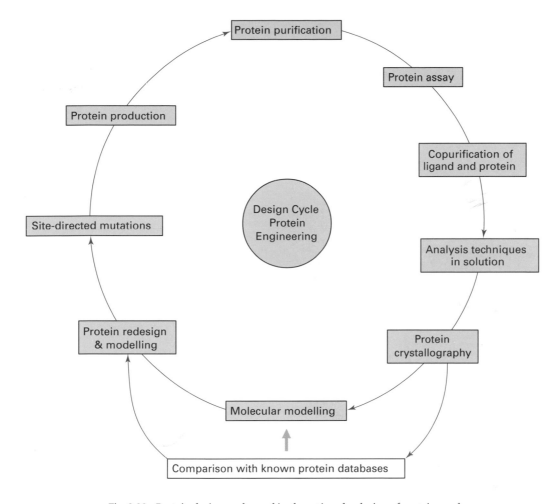

Fig. 3.31. Protein design cycle used in the rational redesign of proteins and enzymes.

Complete sequencing of the gene is essential to identify a potential region for mutation. Once the precise base change has been identified, an oligonucleotide is designed that is complementary to part of the gene but has one base difference. This difference is designed to alter a particular codon, which, after translation, gives rise to a different amino acid and hence may alter the properties of the protein.

The oligonucleotide and the single-stranded DNA are annealed and DNA polymerase is added together with the dNTPs. The primer for the reaction is the 3′ end of the oligonucleotide. The DNA polymerase produces a new DNA strand complementary to the existing one but incorporating the oligonucleotide with the base mutation. The subsequent cloning of the recombinant produces multiple copies, half of which contain a sequence with the mutation and the other half the wild-type sequence. Plaque hybridisation using the oligonucleotide as the probe is then used at a stringency that allows only those plaques containing a mutated sequence

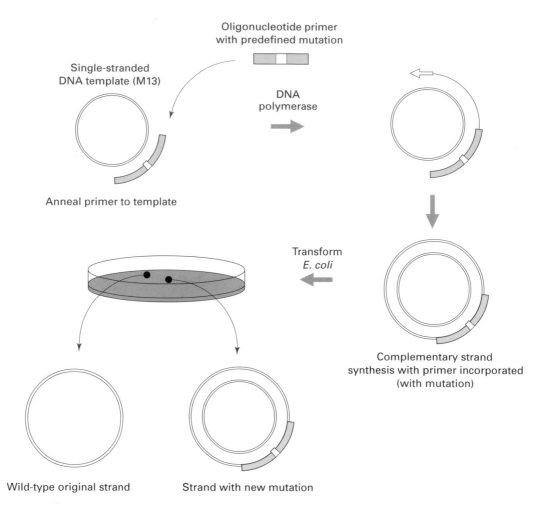

Fig. 3.32. Oligonucleotide-directed mutagenesis. This technique requires a knowledge of nucleotide sequence, since an oligonucleotide may then be synthesised with the base mutation. Annealing of the oligonucleotide to complementary (except for the mutation) single-stranded DNA provides a primer for DNA polymerase to produce a new strand and thus incorporates the primer with the mutation.

to be identified (Fig. 3.32). Further methods have also been developed that simplify the process of detecting the strands with the mutations.

3.6.4 PCR-based mutagenesis

The PCR has been adapted to allow mutagenesis to be undertaken and this relies on single bases mismatched between one of the PCR primers and the target DNA becoming incorporated into the amplified product after thermal cycling.

The basic PCR mutagenesis system involves the use of two primary PCR reactions to produce two overlapping DNA fragments both bearing the same mutation

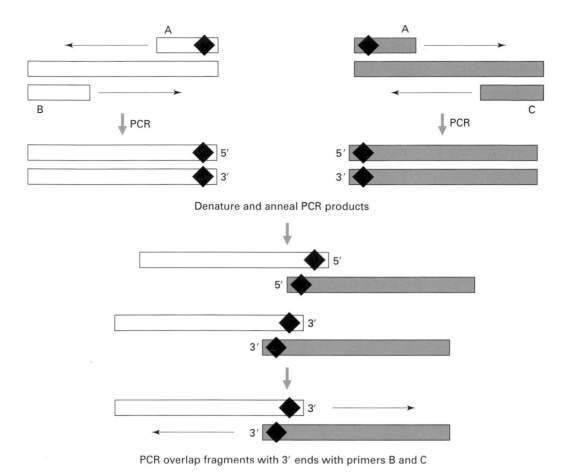

Fig. 3.33. Construction of a synthetic DNA fragment with a predefined mutation using overlap PCR mutagenesis.

in the overlap region. The technique is termed overlap extension PCR. The two separate PCR products are made single stranded and the overlap in sequence allows the products from each reaction to hybridise. Following this, one of the two hybrids bearing a free 3′-hydroxyl group is extended to produce a new duplex fragment. The other hybrid with a 5′-hydroxyl group cannot act as substrate in the reaction. Thus the overlapped and extended product will now contain the directed mutation (Fig. 3.33). Deletions and insertions may also be created with this method, although the requirements of four primers and three PCR reactions limit the general applicability of the technique. A modification of the overlap extension PCR may also be used to construct directed mutations, this is termed megaprimer PCR. This method utilises three oligonucleotide primers to perform two rounds of PCR. A complete PCR product, the megaprimer, is made single stranded and this is used as a large primer in a further PCR reaction with an additional primer.

The above are all methods for creating rational, defined mutations as part of a design cycle system. However, it is also possible to introduce random mutations into a gene and select for enhanced or new activities of the protein or enzyme it encodes. This accelerated form of artificial molecular evolution may be undertaken using error-prone PCR, where deliberate and random mutations are introduced by a low fidelity PCR amplification reaction. The resulting amplified gene is then translated and its activity assayed. This has already provided novel evolved enzymes such as a *p*-nitrobenzyl esterase, which exhibits an unusual and surprising affinity for organic solvents. This accelerated evolutionary approach to protein engineering has been useful in the production of novel phage-displayed antibodies and in the development of antibodies with enzymic activities (catalytic antibodies) (Section 7.3.6).

3.7 EXPRESSION OF FOREIGN GENES

One of the most useful applications of recombinant DNA technology is the ability to artificially synthesise large quantities of natural or modified proteins in a host cell such as bacteria or yeast. The benefits of these techniques have been enjoyed for many years since the first insulin molecules were cloned and expressed in 1982 (Table 3.3). Contamination of other proteins such as the blood product factor VIII with infectious agents has also increased the need to develop effective vectors for *in vitro* expression of foreign genes. In general the expression of foreign genes is carried out in specialised cloning vectors (Fig. 3.34). However, it is possible to use cell-free transcription and translation systems that direct the synthesis of proteins without the need to grow and maintain cells. *In vitro* translation is carried out with the appropriate amino acids, ribosomes, tRNA molecules and isolated mRNA fractions. Wheatgerm extracts or rabbit reticulocyte lysates are usually the systems of

Table 3.3   **A number of recombinant DNA-derived human therapeutic reagents**

Therapeutic area	Recombinant product
Drugs	Erythropoetin
	Insulin
	Growth hormone
	Coagulation factors (e.g. factor VIII)
	Plasminogen activator
Vaccines	Hepatitis B
Cytokines/growth factors	GM-CSF
	G-CSF
	Interleukins
	Interferons

GM-CSF, granulocyte–macrophage colony-stimulating factor; G-CSF, granulocyte colony-stimulating factor.

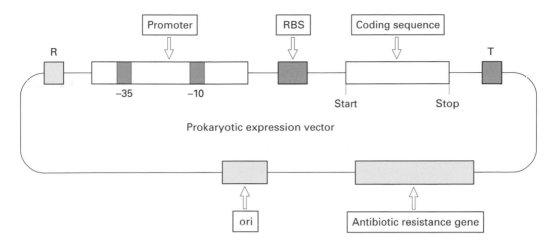

Fig. 3.34. Components of a typical prokaryotic expression vector. To produce a transcript (coding sequence) and translate it, a number of sequences in the vector are required. These include the promoter and ribosome-binding site (RBS). The activity of the promoter may be modulated by a regulatory gene (R), which acts in a way similar to that of the regulatory gene in the *lac* operon. T indicates a transcription terminator.

choice for *in vitro* translation. The resulting proteins may be detected by polyacrylamide gel electrophoresis or by immunological detection using western blotting (Section 12.3.9). Recently oligonucleotide PCR primers have been designed to incorporate a promoter for RNA polymerase and a ribosome binding site. When the so-called expression PCR (E-PCR) is carried out, the amplified products are denatured and transcribed by RNA polymerase, after which they are translated *in vitro*. The advantage of this system is that large amounts of specific RNA are synthesised, thus increasing the yield of specific proteins (Fig. 3.35).

3.7.1 Production of fusion proteins

For a foreign gene to be expressed in a bacterial cell, it must have particular promoter sequences upstream from the coding region, to which the RNA polymerase will bind prior to transcription of the gene. The choice of promoter is vital for correct and efficient transcription, since the sequence and position of promoters are specific to a particular host such as bacteria (Section 2.6.5). It must also contain a ribosome binding site, placed just before the coding region. Unless a cloned gene contains both of these sequences, it will not be expressed in a bacterial host cell. If the gene has been produced via cDNA from a eukaryotic cell, then it will certainly not have any such sequences. Consequently, expression vectors have been developed that contain promoter and ribosome binding sites positioned just before one or more restriction sites for the insertion of foreign DNA. These regulatory sequences, such as that from the *lac* operon of *E. coli*, are usually derived from genes which, when induced, are strongly expressed in bacteria. Since the mRNA

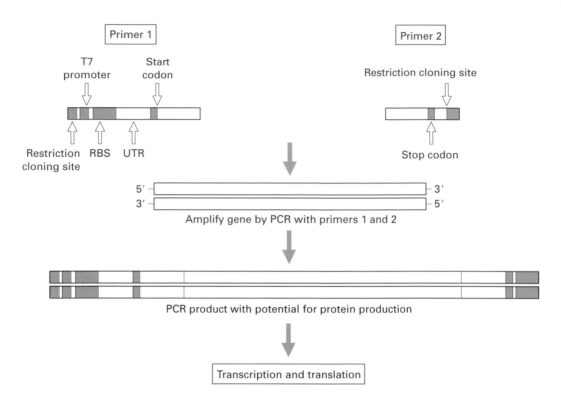

Fig. 3.35. Expression PCR (E-PCR). This technique amplifies a target sequence with one primer that contains a transcriptional promoter, ribosome binding site (RBS), untranslated leader region (UTR) and start codon. The other primer contains a stop codon. The amplified PCR products may be used in transcription and translation to produce a protein.

produced from the gene is read as triplet codons, the inserted sequence must be placed so that its reading frame is in phase with the regulatory sequence. This can be ensured by the use of three vectors that differ only in the number of bases between promoter and insertion site, the second and third vectors being, respectively, one and two bases longer than the first. If an insert is cloned in all three vectors then, in general, it will subsequently be in the correct reading frame in one of them. The resulting clones can be screened for the production of a functional foreign protein (Section 3.5.4).

In some cases the protein is expressed as a fusion with a general protein such as β-galactosidase or glutathione S-transferase (GST) to facilitate its recovery (Section 6.3.5). It may also be tagged with a moiety such as a polyhistidine (6 × His-tag) which binds strongly to a nickel-chelate-nitrilotriacetate (Ni-NTA) chromatography column (Section 13.9.6). The usefulness of this method is that the binding is independent of the three-dimensional structure of the 6 × His-tag and so recovery is efficient, even under the strong denaturing conditions often required for membrane proteins and inclusion bodies (Fig. 3.36). The tags are

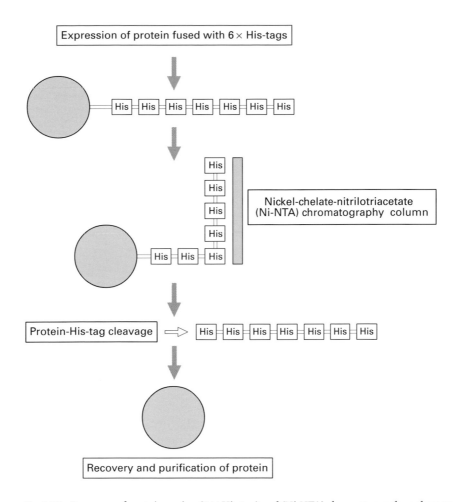

Fig. 3.36. Recovery of proteins using (6 × His-tag) and (Ni-NTA) chromatography columns.

subsequently removed by cleavage with a reagent such as cyanogen bromide and the protein of interest purified by protein biochemical methods such as chromatography and polyacrylamide gel electrophoresis (Chapter 6).

It is not only possible but usually essential to use cDNA instead of a eukaryotic genomic DNA to direct the production of a functional protein by bacteria. This is because bacteria are not capable of processing RNA to remove introns, and so any foreign genes must be preprocessed as cDNA if they contain introns. A further problem arises if the protein must be glycosylated, by the addition of oligosaccharides at specific sites, in order to become functional. Although the use of bacterial expression systems is somewhat limited for eukaryotic systems, there are a number of eukaryotic expression systems based on plant, mammalian, insect and yeast cells. These types of cell can perform such post-translational modifications, producing a correct glycosylation pattern and in some cases the correct removal of introns. It is also possible to include a signal or address sequence at the 5′ end of the mRNA that directs the protein to a particular cellular compartment or even out of the cell altogether into the supernatant. This makes the recovery of expressed recombinant proteins much easier, since the supernatant may be drawn off while the cells are still producing protein.

One useful eukaryotic expression system is based on the monkey COS cell line. These cells each contain a region derived from a mammalian monkey virus, simian virus 40 (SV40). A defective region of the SV40 genome has been stably integrated into the COS cell genome. This allows the expression of a protein called the large T antigen, which is required for viral replication. When a recombinant vector having the SV40 origin of replication and carrying foreign DNA is inserted into the COS cells, viral replication takes place. This results in a high level of expression of foreign proteins. The disadvantage of this system is the ultimate lysis of the COS cells and limited insert capacity of the vector. Much interest is also currently focused on other modified viruses, vaccinia virus and baculovirus. These have been developed for high level expression in mammalian cells and insect cells, respectively. The vacinnia virus in particular has been used to correct defective ion transport by introducing a wild-type cystic fibrosis gene into cells bearing a mutated cystic fibrosis gene (CFTR). There is no doubt that the development of these vector systems will enhance eukaryotic protein expression in the future.

3.7.2 **Phage display techniques**

As a result of the production of phagemid vectors and as a means of overcoming the problems of screening large numbers of clones generated from genomic libraries of antibody genes, a method for linking the phenotype or expressed protein with the genotype has been devised. This is termed phage display, since a functional protein is linked to a major coat protein of a coliphage, whilst the single-stranded gene encoding the protein is packaged within the virion. The initial steps of the method rely on the PCR to amplify gene fragments that represent functional domains or subunits of a protein such as an antibody. These are then cloned into a phage display vector which is an adapted phagemid vector (Section 3.3.3) and used to transform *E. coli*. A helper phage is then added to provide accessory proteins for new phage molecules to be constructed. The DNA fragments representing the protein or polypeptide of interest are also transcribed and translated, but linked to the major coat protein gIII. Thus, when the phage is assembled, the protein or polypeptide of interest is incorporated into the coat of the phage and displayed, whilst the corresponding DNA is encapsulated (Fig. 3.37).

There are numerous applications for the display of proteins on the surface of bacteriophage virus, and commercial organisations have been quick to exploit this technology. One major application is the analysis and production of engineered antibodies from which the technology was mainly developed. In general, phage-based systems have a number of novel applications in terms of ease of selection rather than screening of antibody fragments, allowing analysis by methods

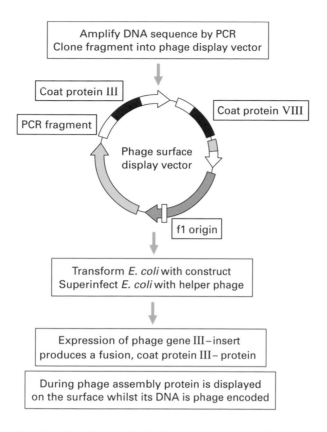

Fig. 3.37. Flow diagram indicating the main steps in the phage display technique.

such as affinity chromatography (Section 13.9). In this way it is possible to generate large numbers of genes for antibody heavy and light chains by PCR amplification and mix them in a random fashion. This recombinatorial library approach may provide new or novel partners to be formed as well as naturally existing ones. This strategy is not restricted to antibodies and vast libraries of peptides may be used in this combinatorial chemistry approach to identify novel compounds of use in biotechnology and medicine.

Phage-based cloning methods also offer the advantage of allowing mutagenesis to be performed with relative ease. This may allow the production of antibodies with affinities approaching that derived from the human or mouse immune system. This may be brought about by using an error-prone DNA polymerase in the initial steps of constructing a phage display library. It is possible that these types of library may provide a route to high affinity recombinant antibody fragments that are difficult to produce by more conventional hybridoma fusion techniques (Section 4.2.4). Surface display libraries have also been prepared for the selection of ligands, hormones and other polypeptides in addition to allowing studies on protein–protein or protein–DNA interactions, or determining the precise binding domains in these receptor–ligand interactions.

3.8 ANALYSING GENES AND GENE EXPRESSION

3.8.1 Identifying and analysing mRNA

A number of very useful techniques have been developed that allow the fine structure of a particular mRNA to be analysed and the relative amounts of an RNA quantified. This is not only important for gene regulation studies but may also be used as a marker for certain clinical disorders. Traditionally the northern blot has been used for detection of particular RNA transcripts by the blotting of extracted mRNA and immobilisation of it on a nylon membrane (Section 2.10). Subsequent hybridisation with labelled gene probes allows precise determination of the size and nature of a transcript. However, recently much use has been made of a number of nucleases that digest only single-stranded nucleic acids and not double-stranded molecules. In particular the ribonuclease protection assay (RPA) has allowed much information to be gained regarding the nature of mRNA transcripts (Fig. 3.38). In the RPA, single-stranded mRNA is hybridised to a labelled single-stranded RNA probe, which is in excess. The hybridised part of the complex becomes protected whereas the unhybridised part of the probe made from RNA is digested with RNase A and RNase T1. The protected fragment may then be analysed on a high resolution polyacrylamide gel. This method may give valuable information regarding the mRNA in terms of the precise structure of the transcript (transcription start site, intron/exon junctions, etc.). It is also quantitative and requires less RNA than does a northern blot. A related technique, S1 nuclease

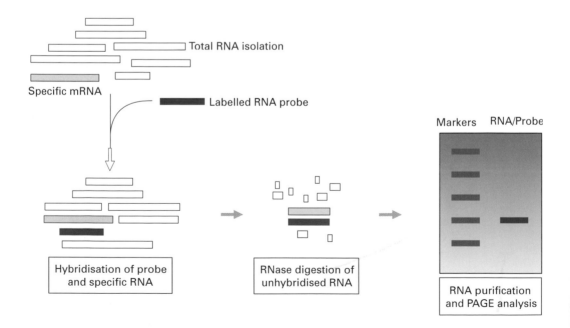

Fig. 3.38. Steps involved in the ribonuclease protection assay (RPA).

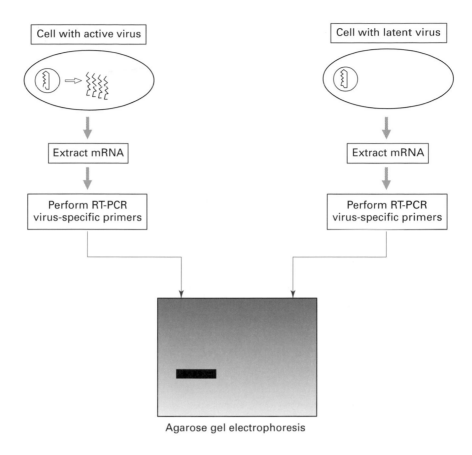

Fig. 3.39. Representation of the detection of active viruses using RT–PCR.

mapping, is similar, although the unhybridised part of a DNA probe, rather than an RNA probe, is digested, this time with the enzyme S1 nuclease.

The PCR has also had an impact on the analysis of RNA by the development of a technique known as reverse transcriptase-PCR (RT-PCR). Here, the RNA is isolated and a first-strand cDNA synthesis undertaken with reverse transcriptase; the cDNA is then used in a conventional PCR (Section 3.2.5). Under certain circum stances a number of thermostable DNA polymerases have reverse transcriptase activity that obviates the need to separate the two reactions and allows the RT–PCR to be carried out in one tube. One of the main benefits of RT–PCR is the ability to identify rare or low levels of mRNA transcripts with great sensitivity. This is especially useful when detecting, for example, viral gene expression and furthermore enables the means of differentiating between latent and active virus (Fig. 3.39). The level of mRNA production may also be determined by a modification of the PCR termed quantitative PCR (Section 2.13.4)

In many cases the analysis of tissue-specific gene expression is required and again the PCR has been adapted to provide a solution. This technique, differential display, is also an RT–PCR based system requiring that isolated mRNA be first converted into

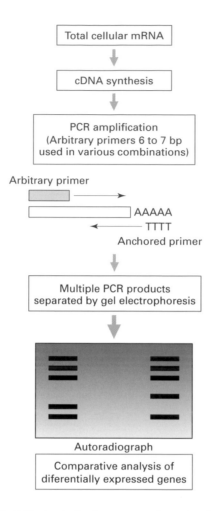

Fig. 3.40. Analysis of gene expression using differential display PCR.

cDNA. Following this, one of the PCR primers, designed to anneal to a general mRNA element such as the poly(A) tail in eukaryotic cells is used in conjunction with a combination of arbitrary 6–7 bp primers that bind to the 5′-end of the transcripts. Consequently, this results in the generation of multiple PCR products with reproducible patterns (Fig. 3.40). Comparative analysis by gel electrophoresis of PCR products generated from different cell types therefore allows the identification and isolation of those transcripts that are differentially expressed. As with many PCR-based techniques, the time to identify such genes is dramatically reduced, from the weeks that are required to construct and screen cDNA libraries to a few days.

3.8.2 Analysing genes *in situ*

Gross chromosomal changes are often detectable by microscopic examination of the chromosomes within a karyotype (Section 2.3). Single or restricted numbers of

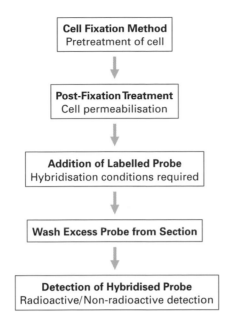

Fig. 3.41. General scheme for *in situ* hybridisation.

base substitutions, deletions, rearrangements or insertions are far less easily detectable but may induce similarly profound effects on normal cellular biochemistry. *In situ* hybridisation makes it possible to determine the chromosomal location of a particular gene fragment or gene mutation. This is carried out by preparing a radiolabelled DNA or RNA probe and applying this to a tissue or chromosomal preparation fixed to a microscope slide. Any probe that does not hybridise to complementary sequences is washed off and an image of the distribution or location of the bound probe is viewed by autoradiography (Fig. 3.41). Using tissue or cells fixed to slides it is also possible to carry out *in situ* PCR. This is a highly sensitive technique where PCR is carried out directly on the tissue slide with the standard PCR reagents. Specially adapted thermal cycling machines are required to hold the slide preparations and allow the PCR to proceed. This allows the localisation and identification of, for example, single copies of intracellular viruses.

An alternative labelling strategy used in karyotyping and gene localisation is fluorescent *in situ* hybridisation (FISH). This method, sometimes termed chromosome painting, is based on *in situ* hybridisation where different gene probes are labelled with different fluorochromes, each specific for a particular chromosome. The advantage of this method is that separate gene regions may be identified and comparisons made within the same chromosome preparation. The technique is also likely to be highly useful in genome mapping for ordering DNA probes along a chromosomal segment (Section 3.9).

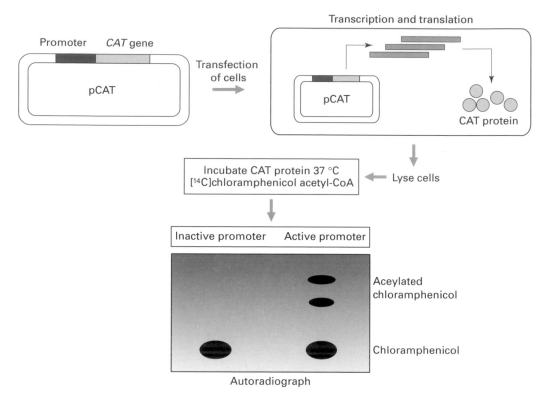

Fig. 3.42. Assay for promoters using the reporter gene for chloramphenicol acetyl transferase (CAT).

3.8.3 Analysing promoter–protein interactions

To determine potential transcriptional regulatory sequences, genomic DNA fragments may be cloned into specially devised promoter probe vectors. These contain sites for insertion of foreign DNA that lie upstream from a reporter gene. A number of reporter genes are currently used, including the *lacZ* gene (encoding β-galactosidase), the *CAT* gene (encoding chloramphenicol acetyl transferase (CAT)) and the *lux* gene, which produces luciferase and is determined by means of a bioluminescent assay (Section 9.8). Fragments of DNA potentially containing a promoter region are cloned into the vector and the constructs transfected into eukaryotic cells. Any expression of the reporter gene will be driven by the foreign DNA, which must therefore contain promoter sequences (Fig. 3.42). These plasmids and other reporter genes such as those using the firefly luciferase gene allow quantification of gene transcription in response to transcriptional activators.

The binding of a regulatory protein or transcription factor to a specific DNA site results in a complex that may be analysed by the technique termed gel retardation. Under gel electrophoresis the migration of a DNA fragment bound to a protein of a relatively large mass will be retarded in comparison to the DNA fragment alone.

For gel retardation to be useful, the region containing the promoter DNA element must be digested or mapped with a restriction endonuclease before it is complexed with the protein. The location of the promoter may then be defined by finding the position on the restriction map of the fragment that binds to the regulatory protein and therefore is retarded during electrophoresis. One potential problem with gel retardation is the ability to define the precise nucleotide-binding region of the protein, since this depends on the accuracy and detail of the restriction map and the convenience of the restriction sites. However, it is a useful first step in determining the interaction of a regulatory protein with a DNA-binding site.

DNA footprinting relies on the fact that the interaction of a DNA-binding protein with a regulatory DNA sequence will protect that DNA sequence from degradation by an enzyme such as DNase I. The DNA regulatory sequence is first labelled at one end with a radioactive label and then mixed with the DNA-binding protein (Fig. 3.43). DNase I is added and conditions favouring a partial digestion are then carried out. This limited digestion ensures that a number of fragments are produced where the DNA is not protected by the DNA binding protein. The protected region will remain undigested. All the fragments are then separated on a high resolution polyacrylamide gel alongside a control digestion where no DNA-binding protein is present. The autoradiograph of a gel will contain a ladder of bands representing the partially digested fragments. Where DNA has been protected, no bands appear; this region or hole is termed the DNA footprint. The position of the protein-binding sequence within the DNA may be elucidated from the size of the fragments on either side of the footprint region. Footprinting is a more precise method of locating a DNA protein interaction than gel retardation; however, it is unable to give any information on the precise interaction with, or the contribution of, individual nucleotides.

In addition to the detection of DNA sequences that contribute to the regulation of gene expression, an ingenious way of detecting the protein transcription factors has been developed. This is termed the yeast two-hybrid system. Transcription factors have two domains, one for DNA binding and the other to allow binding to further proteins (activation domain). These occur as part of the same molecule in natural transcription factors, for example TFIID (Section 2.4.6). They may also be formed from two separate domains. Thus a recombinant molecule is formed encoding the protein under study as a fusion with the DNA-binding domain. It cannot, however, activate transcription. Genes from a cDNA library are expressed as a fusion with the activator domain, this also cannot initiate transcription. When the two fractions are mixed together, transcription is initiated if the domains are complementary (Fig. 3.44). This is indicated by the transcription of a reporter gene such as the *CAT* gene (Section 3.8.3). The technique is not confined merely to transcription factors and may be applied to any protein system where interaction occurs.

3.8.4 **Transgenics and gene targeting**

In many cases it is desirable to analyse the effect of certain genes and proteins in an organism rather than in the laboratory. Furthermore the production of

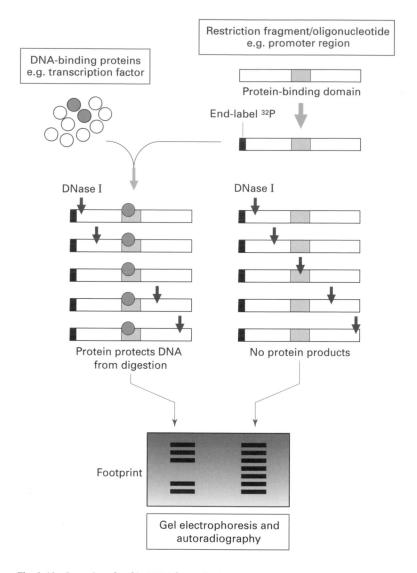

Fig. 3.43. Steps involved in DNA footprinting.

pharmaceutical products and therapeutic proteins is also desirable in a whole organism. This also has important consequences for the biotechnology and agricultural industries (Table 3.4) (Section 3.10). The introduction of foreign genes into germline cells and the production of an altered organism is termed transgenics. There are two broad strategies for transgenesis. The first is direct transgenesis in mammals, whereby recombinant DNA is injected directly into the male pronucleus of a recently fertilised egg. This is then raised in a foster mother animal, resulting in offspring that are all transgenic. Selective transgenesis is where the recombinant DNA is transferred into embryo stem cells (ES cells). The cells are then cultured in the laboratory and those expressing the desired protein selected

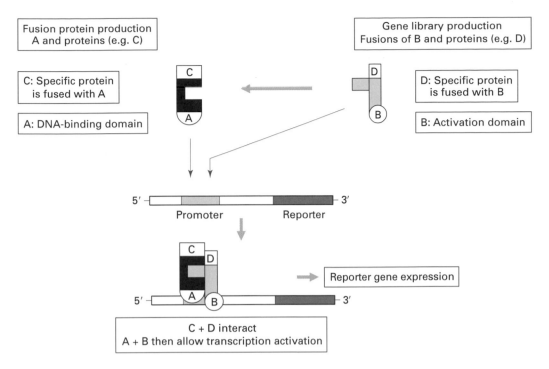

Fig. 3.44. Yeast two-hybrid system (interaction trapping technique). Transcription factors have two domains, one for DNA biding (A) and the other to allow binding to further proteins (B). Thus, a recombinant molecule is formed from a protein (C) as a fusion with the DNA-binding domain. It cannot, however, activate transcription alone. Genes from a cDNA library (D) are expressed as a fusion with the activator domain (B) but also cannot initiate transcription alone. When the two fractions are mixed together, transcription is initiated if the domains are complementary and expression of a reporter gene takes place.

and incorporated into the inner cell mass of an early embryo. The resulting trans-genic fetus develops in a foster mother, but in this case the transgenic animal is a mosaic or chimaeric, since only a small proportion of the cells will be expressing the protein. The initial problem with both approaches is the random nature of the integration of the recombinant DNA into the genome of the egg or embryo stem cells. This may produce proteins in cells where it is not required or disrupt genes necessary for correct growth and development.

A refinement of this, however, is gene targeting, which involves the production of an altered gene in an intact cell, a form of *in vivo* mutagenesis as opposed to *in vitro* mutagenesis (Section 3.6.2). The gene is inserted into the genome of, for example, an ES cell by specialised viral-based vectors. The insertion is non-random, since identical sequences exist on the vector to the gene and on the gene to be targeted. Thus, homologous recombination may introduce a new genetic property to the cell, or inactivate an existing one; this is termed gene knockout. Perhaps the most important aspect of these techniques is that they allow animal models of human diseases to be created. This is useful, since the physiological and

Table 3.4 Use of transgenic mice for investigation of selected human disorders

Gene/protein	Genetic lesion	Disorder in humans
Tyrosine kinase (TK)	Constitutive expression of gene	Cardiac hypertrophy
HIV transactivator	Expression of HIV *tat* gene	Kaposi's sarcoma
Angiotensinogen	Expression of rat angiotensinogen gene	Hypertension
Cholesterol ester transfer protein (CET protein)	Expression of *CET* gene	Atherosclerosis
Hypoxanthine-guanine phosphoribosyl transferase (HPRT)	Inactivation of *HPRT* gene	HPRT deficiency

biochemical consequences of a disease are often complex and difficult to study, impeding the development of diagnostic and therapeutic strategies.

3.8.5 Analysing genetic mutations

There are several types of mutation that can occur in nucleic acids, either transiently or when stably incorporated into the genome. During evolution, mutations may be inherited in one or both copies of a chromosome, resulting in polymorphisms within the population (Section 2.3). Mutations may potentially occur at any site within the genome; however, there are several instances whereby mutations occur in limited regions. This is particularly obvious in prokaryotes, where elements of the genome (hypervariable regions) undergo extensive mutations to generate large numbers of variants, by virtue of the high rate of replication of the organisms. Similar hypervariable sequences are generated in the normal antibody immune response in eukaryotes. Mutations may have several effects upon the structure and function of the genome. Some mutations may lead to undetectable effects upon normal cellular functions, termed conservative mutations. An example of these are mutations that occur in intron sequences and therefore play no part in the final structure and function of the protein or its regulation. Alternatively, mutations may result in profound effects upon normal cell function such as altered transcription rates or changes in the sequence of mRNAs necessary for normal cellular processes.

Mutations occurring within exons may alter the amino acid composition of the encoded protein by causing amino acid substitution or by changing the reading frame used during translation. These point mutations have been detected traditionally by Southern blotting or, if a convenient restriction site is available, by restriction fragment length polymorphism (RFLP) (Section 2.9). However, the PCR has been used to great effect in mutation detection, since it is possible to use allele-specific oligonucleotide PCR (ASO-PCR), where two competing primers and one general primer are used in the reaction (Fig. 3.45). One of the primers is directly complementary to the known point mutation whereas the other is a wild-type

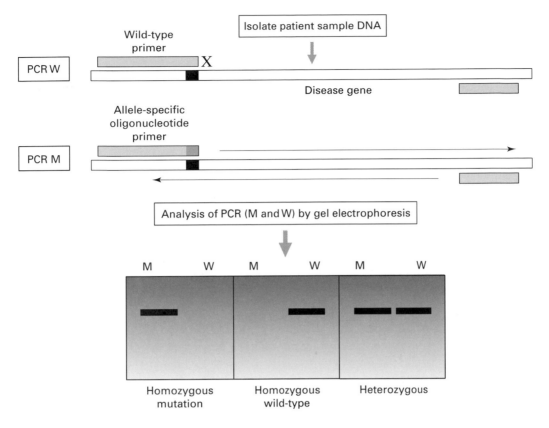

Fig. 3.45. Point mutation detection using allele-specific oligonucleotide PCR (ASO–PCR).

primer; that is, the primers are identical except for the terminal 3′-end base. Thus, if the DNA contains the point mutation, only the primer with the complementary sequence will bind and be incorporated into the amplified DNA, whereas if the DNA is normal the wild-type primer is incorporated. The results of the PCR are analysed by agarose gel electrophoresis. A further modification of ASO-PCR has been developed where the primers are each labelled with different fluorochrome. Since the primers are labelled differently, a positive or negative result is produced directly without the need to examine the PCRs by gel electrophoresis.

Various modifications now allow more than one PCR to be carried out at a time (multiplex PCR), and hence the detection of more than one mutation is possible at the same time. Where the mutation is unknown it is also possible to use a PCR system with a gel-based detection method termed denaturing gradient gel electrophoresis (DGGE). In this technique, a sample DNA heteroduplex containing a mutation is amplified by the PCR, which is also used to attach a G + C-rich sequence to one end of the heteroduplex. The mutated heteroduplex is identified by its altered melting properties through a polyacrylamide gel that contains a gradient of denaturant such as urea. At a certain point in the gradient, the heteroduplex will denature relative to a perfectly matched homoduplex and thus may be

Table 3.5 **Main methods of detecting mutations in DNA samples**

Technique	Basis of method	Main characteristics of detection
Southern blotting	Gel based	Labelled probe hybridisation to DNA
Dot/slot blotting	Sample application	Labelled probe hybridisation to DNA
Allele-specific oligo-PCR (ASO)-PCR)	PCR based	Oligonucleotide matching to DNA sample
Denaturing gradient gel electrophoresis (DGGE)	Gel/PCR based	Melting temperature of DNA strands
Single-stranded conformation polymorphism (SSCP)	Gel/PCR based	Conformation difference of DNA strands
Ligase chain reaction (LCR)	Gel/automated	Oligonucleotide matching to DNA sample
DNA sequencing	Gel based	Nucleotide sequence analysis of DNA
DNA microchips	Glass chip based	Sample DNA hybridisation to oligo arrays

identified. The GC 'clamp' maintains the integrity of the end of the duplex on passage through the gel (Fig. 3.46). The sensitivity of this and other mutation detection methods has been substantially increased by the use of PCR, and further mutation techniques used to detect known or unknown mutations are indicated in Table 3.5.

3.8.6 Detecting DNA polymorphisms

Polymorphisms are particularly interesting elements of the human genome and as such may be used as the basis for differentiating between individuals. All humans carry repeats of sequences known as minisatellite DNA, of which the number of repeats varies between unrelated individuals. Hybridisation of probes that anneal to these sequences in Southern blotting provides the means to type and identify these unrelated individuals (Section 2.3).

DNA fingerprinting is a collective term for two distinct genetic testing systems that use either 'multilocus' probes or 'single-locus' probes. Initially described DNA fingerprinting probes were multilocus, so termed because they detect hypervariable minisatellites throughout the genome, i.e at multiple locations within the genome. In contrast, several single-locus probes were discovered, which under specific conditions detect only the two alleles at a single locus and generate what have been termed DNA profiles because, unlike multilocus probes, the two-band pattern result is in itself insufficient to uniquely identify an individual.

Techniques based on the PCR have been coupled to the detection of minisatellite loci. The inherent larger size of such DNA regions were not best suited to PCR amplification; however, new PCR developments are beginning to allow this to take place. The discovery of polymorphisms within the repeating sequences of minisatellites has led to the development of a PCR-based method that distinguishes an individual on the basis of the random distribution of repeat types along

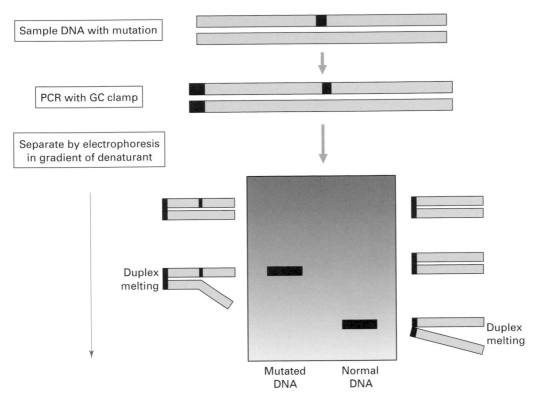

Fig. 3.46. Detection of mutations using denaturing gradient gel electrophoresis (DGGE).

the length of a person's two alleles for one such minisatellite. Known as minisatellite variant repeat (MVR) analysis or digital DNA typing, this technique can lead to a simple numerical coding of the repeat variation detected. Potentially, this combines the advantages of PCR sensitivity and rapidity with the discriminating power of minisatellite alleles. Thus, for the future there are a number of interesting identification systems under development and evaluation. The genetic detection of polymorphisms has been used in many cases of paternity testing and immigration control and is becoming a central factor in many criminal investigations. It is also a valuable tool in plant biotechnology for cereal typing and in the field of pedigree analysis and animal breeding.

3.8.7 Microarrays and DNA microchips

One of the most exciting genetic analysis techniques in the last few years has been the development of microarrays or DNA microchips. These provide a radically different approach to large-scale analysis and quantification of genes and gene expression. A microarray consists of an ordered arrangement of hundreds or thousands of DNA sequences such as oligonucleotides or cDNAs deposited onto a solid surface approximately $1.2\,cm \times 1.2\,cm$. The solid support is usually glass, although silicon wafers have also been used successfully. Currently the arrays are synthesised on or off the glass and require complex fabrication methods similar to that used in producing microchips. They may also be spotted by robotic ultrafine microarray deposition instruments, which dispense volumes as low as 30 picolitres.

The arrays may represent mRNA produced in a particular cell type (cDNA expression arrays) or may alternatively represent coding and regulatory regions of a particular gene or group of genes. One currently developed commercial example uses a 50 000 oligonucleotide array that represents known mutations in a tumour suppressor gene called *p53*, the product of which is known to be mutated in many human cancers. Thus, a sample of the patients DNA is incubated on the array and any unhybridised DNA washed off. The array is then analysed and scanned for patterns of hybridisation. Any mutations in the *p53* gene may be rapidly analysed by computer interpretation of the resulting hybridisation pattern and the mutation defined. The potential of microarrays appears to be limitless and a number of arrays have been developed for the detection of various genetic mutations including the cystic fibrosis *CFTR* gene (cystic fibrosis transmembrane regulator), recently discovered breast cancer genes *BRCA1* and *BRCA2* and for the human immunodeficiency virus (HIV).

At present, microarrays require DNA to be highly purified, which limits their applicability. However, as DNA purification becomes automated and microarray technology develops, it is not difficult to envisage numerous laboratory tests on a single DNA microchip. This could be used for analysing not only single genes but for large numbers of genes or DNA representing microorganisms, viruses etc. Since the potential for quantification of gene transcription exists, microarrays could also be used in defining a particular disease status. The capacity for a DNA microarray to contain numerous sequences has given rise to the possibility of performing DNA sequencing by hybridisation. This technique, which is currently under development, may be very significant as it will allow large amounts of sequence information to be gathered very rapidly and assist in many fields of molecular biology, especially in large genome-sequencing projects.

3.9 ANALYSING WHOLE GENOMES

Perhaps the most ambitious projects in the biosciences are the initiatives to map and completely sequence a number of genomes from various organisms. At present initiatives are underway for the mapping and sequencing of a number of organisms indicated in Table 3.6. A number have been completed already such as the bacterium *E. coli* and the yeast *S. cerevisiae* and some such as the *C. elegans* are near completion. The mouse and the ultimate challenge, the human genome, are also both currently in progress. The demands of such large-scale mapping and sequencing have provided the impetus for the development and refinement of even the most standard of molecular biological techniques such as DNA sequencing. It has also led to new methods of identifying the important coding sequences that represent proteins and enzymes.

Table 3.6	Current selected genome-sequencing projects	
Organism		Genome size (Mb)
Bacteria	*Escherichia coli*	4.6
Yeast	*Saccharomyces cerevisiae*	14
Roundworm	*Caenorhabditis elegans*	100
Fruit fly	*Drosophila melanogaster*	165
Puffer fish	*Fugu rubripes rubripes*	400
Mouse	*Mus musculus*	3000

3.9.1 Physical genome mapping

In terms of genome mapping a physical map is the primary goal. Genetic linkage maps have also been produced by determining the recombination frequency between two particular loci. YAC-based vectors essential for large-scale cloning contain DNA inserts that are on average 300 000 bp in length, which is longer by a factor of 10 than the longest inserts in the clones used in early mapping studies. The development of vectors with large insert capacity has enable the production of contigs. These are continuous, overlapping, cloned fragments that have been positioned relative to one another. From these maps, any cloned fragment may be identified and aligned to an area in one of the contig maps. In order to position cloned DNA fragments, resulting from the construction of a library, in a YAC or cosmid it is necessary to detect overlaps between the cloned DNA fragments. Overlaps are created because of the use of partial digestion conditions with a particular restriction endonuclease when the libraries are constructed. This ensures that when each DNA fragment is cloned into a vector it has overlapping ends that theoretically may be identified and the clones positioned or ordered so that a physical map may be produced (Fig. 3.47).

In order to position the overlapping ends it is preferable to undertake DNA sequencing, however due to the impracticality of this approach, a fingerprint of each clone is carried out using restriction enzyme mapping. Although this is not an unambiguous method of ordering clones it is useful when one is also applying statistical probabilities of the overlap between clones. In order to link the contigs, techniques such as *in situ* hybridisation may be used or a probe generated from one end of a contig in order to screen a different disconnected contig. This method of probe production and identification is termed 'walking', and has been used successfully in the production of physical maps of *E. coli* and yeast genomes. This cycle of clone to fingerprint to contig is amenable to automation; however, the problem of closing the gaps between contigs remains very difficult.

In order to define a common way for all research laboratories to order clones and connect physical maps together an arbitrary molecular technique based on the PCR has been developed using sequence tagged sites (STS). An STS is a small unique sequence of between 200 and 300 base-pairs that is amplified by PCR

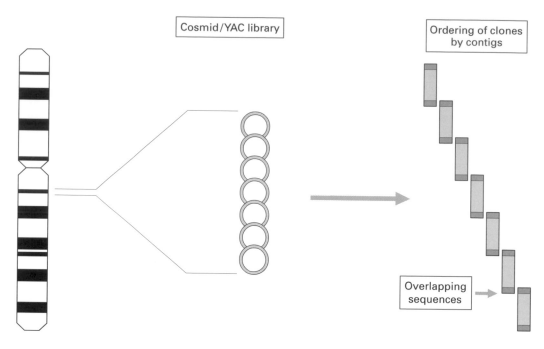

Fig. 3.47. Physical mapping using continuous overlapping cloned fragments (contigs). In order to assign the position of cloned DNA fragments resulting from the construction of a library in a YAC or cosmid vector, overlaps are detected between the clone fragments. These are created because of the use of partial digestion conditions when the libraries are constructed.

(Fig. 3.48). The uniqueness of the STS is defined by the PCR primers that flank the STS. A PCR with those primers is performed and if the PCR results in selected amplification of the target region it may be defined as a potential STS marker. In this way defining STS markers that lie approximately 100 000 bases apart along a contig map allows the ordering of those contigs. Thus, all research groups working with clones have definable landmarks with which to order clones produced in their genomic libraries.

An STS that occurs in two clones will overlap and may therefore be used to order the clones in a contig. Clones containing the STS are usually detected by Southern blotting, where the clones have been immobilised on a nylon membrane. Alternatively a library of clones may be divided into pools and and each pool screened by PCR. This is usually a more rapid method of identifying an STS within a clone and further refinements of the PCR-based screening method allows the identification of a particular clone within a pool (Fig. 3.49). STS elements may also be generated from variable regions of the genome to produce a polymorphic marker that may be traced through families along with other DNA markers and located on a genetic linkage map. These polymorphic STSs are useful, since they may serve as markers on both a physical map and a genetic linkage map for each chromosome and therefore provide a useful marker for aligning the two types of map.

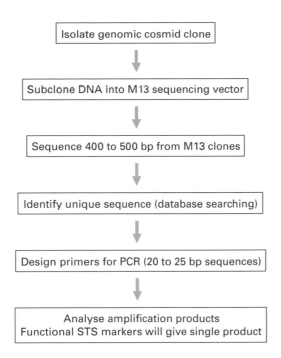

Fig. 3.48. General scheme of the production of a functional STS marker.

3.9.2 **Gene discovery and localisation**

A number of disease loci have been identified and localised to certain chromosomes. This has been facilitated by the use of *in situ* mapping techniques such as FISH (Section 3.8.2). In fact a number of genes have been identified, and the protein determined, where little was initially known about the gene except for its location. This method of gene discovery is known as positional cloning and was instrumental in the isolation of the *CFTR* gene responsible for the disorder cystic fibrosis (Fig. 3.50).

The genes that are actively expressed in a cell at any one time are estimated to comprise as little as 10% of the total DNA. The remaining DNA is packaged and serves an as yet unknown function. Recent investigations have found that certain active genes may be identified by the presence of so-called HTF (*Hpa*II *tiny frag-ments*) islands often found at the 5′-end of genes. These are C + G-rich sequences that are not methylated and form tiny fragments on digestion with the restriction enzyme *Hpa*II. A further gene discovery method that has been used extensively in the past few years is a PCR-based technique giving rise to a product termed an expressed sequence tag (EST). This represents part of a putative gene for which a function has yet to be assigned. It is carried out on cDNA by using primers that bind to an anchor sequence such as a poly(A) tail and primers that bind to sequences at the 5′-end of the gene. Such PCRs may subsequently be used to map the putative gene to a chromosomal region or be used as probes to search a

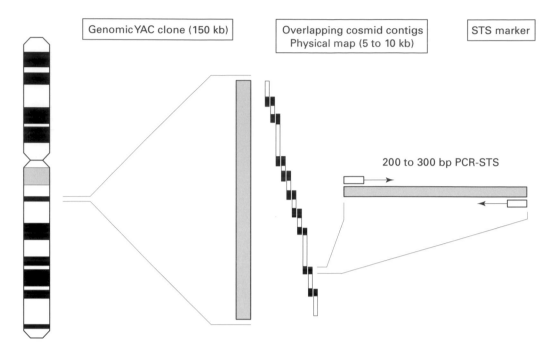

Genomic YAC clone (150 kb)

Overlapping cosmid contigs
Physical map (5 to 10 kb)

STS marker

200 to 300 bp PCR-STS

Fig. 3.49. The derivation of an STS marker. An STS is small unique sequence of between 200 and 300 bp that is amplified by PCR and allows ordering along a contig map. Such sequences are definable landmarks with which to order clones produced in genome libraries and usually lie approximately 100 000 bp apart.

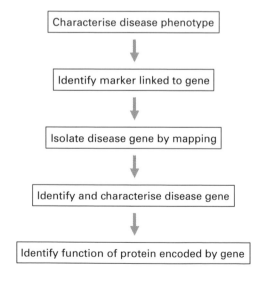

Characterise disease phenotype

Identify marker linked to gene

Isolate disease gene by mapping

Identify and characterise disease gene

Identify function of protein encoded by gene

Fig. 3.50. The scheme of identification of a disease gene by positional cloning.

Table 3.7	Techniques used to determine putative gene encoding sequences
Identification method	Main details
Zoo blotting (cross-hybridisation)	Evolutionary conservation of DNA sequences that suggest functional significance
Homology searching	Gene database searching to gene family-related sequences
Identification of CpG islands	Regions of hypomethylated CpG frequently found 5′ to genes in vertebrate animals
Identification of open reading frames (ORF) promoters/splice sites/RBS	DNA sequences scanned for consensus sequences by computer
Northern blot hybridisation	mRNA detection by binding to labelled gene probes
Exon trapping technique	Artificial RNA splicing assay for exon identification
Expressed sequence tags (ESTs)	cDNAs amplified by PCR that represent part of a gene

RBS, ribosome binding site; cDNA, complementary DNA.

genomic DNA library for the remaining parts of the gene. Much interest currently lies in ESTs, since they may represent a shortcut to gene discovery.

A further gene isolation system that uses adapted vectors, termed exon trapping or exon amplification, may be used to identify exon sequences. Exon trapping requires the use of a specialised expression vector that will accept fragments of genomic DNA containing sequences for splicing reactions to take place. Following transfection of a eukaryotic cell line a transcript is produced that may be detected by using specific primers in an RT–PCR. This indicates the nature of the foreign DNA by virtue of the splicing sequences present. A list of further techniques that aid in the identification of a potential gene encoding sequence is given in Table 3.7.

3.9.3 Human genome mapping project

There is no doubt that the mapping and sequencing of the human genome is one of the most ambitious projects in current science. It will certainly bring new insights into gene function and gene regulation, provide a means of identifying DNA mutations or lesions found in current genetic disorders and point to new ways of potential therapy. It is also a multicollaborative effort that has engaged many scientific research groups around the world and given rise to many scientific, technical, financial and ethical debates. One interesting issue is the sequencing of the whole genome in relation to the coding sequences. Much of the human genome appears to be non-coding and composed of repetitive sequences. Only a small portion of the genome appears to encode enzymes and other proteins. Nevertheless this still corresponds to approximately 90 000 genes, and their mapping and sequencing are exciting prospects. The study further aims to understand and possibly provide the eventual means of treating some of the 4000 known genetic diseases in addition to other diseases whose inheritance is multifactorial. The diversity of the human genome is also an area of great interest and is currently under study. Despite some initial reservations, the sequence is predicted to be completed by the year 2005 at the earliest; after this the equally difficult task of decoding and interpreting the complete sequence will be required.

3.10 **MOLECULAR BIOTECHNOLOGY AND APPLICATIONS**

It is a relatively short period of time since the early 1970s, when the first recombinant DNA experiments were carried out. However, huge strides have been made not only in the development of molecular biological techniques but also in their practical application. The molecular basis of disease and the new areas of genetic analysis and gene therapy hold great promise. In the past, medical science relied on the measurement of protein and enzyme markers which reflected disease states. It is possible now not only to detect such abnormalities at an earlier stage using mRNA techniques but also in some cases to predict such states using genome analysis. The complete mapping and sequencing of the human genome and the development of techniques such as DNA microchips will certainly accelerate such events. Perhaps even more difficult is the elucidation of diseases that are multifactorial and involve a significant contribution from environmental factors. One of the best-studied examples of this type of disease is cancer. Molecular genetic analysis has defined a discrete set of cellular genes, oncogenes, which play key roles in the disease. These genes and their proteins have major functions in the cell cycle and are intimately involved in cell regulation. A number of these are indicated in Table 3.8. In a number of cancers, well-defined molecular events have been correlated with mutations in these oncogenes and therefore in the corresponding protein. It is already possible to screen for and predict the fate of some disease processes at an early stage, a point which itself raises significant ethical dilemmas. In addition to understanding cellular processes both in normal and disease states great promise is also held in drug discovery and molecular gene therapy. A number of genetically engineered therapeutic proteins and enzymes have been developed and are already having an impact on disease management. In addition, the correction of disorders at the gene level (gene therapy) is also under way and perhaps is one of the most impressive applications of molecular biology to date. A number of these developments are indicated in Table 3.9.

The production of modified crops and animals for farming and as sources of important therapeutic proteins is also one of the most exciting and controversial developments of molecular biology. Modified crops now have improved resistance to environmental factors and greater stability (Table 3.10). Transgenic animals hold great promise for improving livestock quality, low cost production of pharmaceuticals and disease-free or disease-resistant strains. In the future this

Table 3.8 General classification of oncogenes and their cellular and biochemical functions

Oncogene	Example	Main details
G-proteins	H-K- and N-*ras*	GTP-binding protein/GTPase
Growth factors	*sis, nt-2, hst*	β-chain of PDGF (platelet-derived growth factor)
Growth factor receptors	*erbB*	Epidermal growth factor receptor (EGFR)
	fms	Colony-stimulating factor-1 receptor
Protein kinases	*abl, src*	Protein tyrosine kinases
	mos, ras	Protein serine kinases
Nucleus-located transcription factors	*myc*	DNA-binding protein
	myb	DNA-binding protein
	jun, fos	DNA-binding protein

Table 3.9 A number of selected examples of targets for gene therapy

Disorder	Defect	Gene target	Target cell
Emphysema	Deficiency (α1-AT)	α1-Antitrypsin (α1-AT)	Liver cells
Gaucher disease (storage disorder)	GC deficiency	Glucocerebrosidase	GC fibroblasts
Haemoglobinpathies	Thalassaemia	β-Globin	Fibroblasts
Lesch-Nyhan syndrome	Metabolic deficiency	Hypoxanthine guanine phosphoribosyl (HPRT)	HPRT cells
Immune system disorder	Adenosine deaminase deficiency	Adenosine deaminase (ADA)	T,B cells

Table 3.10 Current selected plant/crops modified by genetic manipulation

Crop or plant	Genetic modification
Canola (oil seed rape)	Insect resistance, seed oil modification
Maize	Herbicide tolerance, resistance to insects
Rice	Modified seed storage protein, insect resistance
Soybean	Tolerance to herbicide, modified seed storage protein
Tomato	Modified ripening, resistance to insects and viruses
Sunflower	Modified seed storage protein

may overcome such factors as contamination with agents such as bovine spongioform encephalitis (BSE). There is no doubt that improved methods of producing livestock by whole-animal cloning will be a also be of major benefit. All of these developments do, however, require debate and the many ethical considerations that arise from them require careful consideration.

3.11 **KEY TERMS**

2μ circle
5-bromo-4-chloro-3-indolyl-β-
   galactopyranoside
6 × His-tag
activation domain
adaptors
address sequence
agrobacterium tumefaciens
allele-specific oligonucleotide–PCR
autonomous replicating sequence
bacterial artificial chromosomes
bacteriophage vectors
bacteriophages
baculovirus
biolistic
blue/white selection
blunt ends
catalytic antibodies
cDNA library
cell-free translation system
chain termination sequencing
cloned DNA
cohesive or sticky ends
colony hybridisation
combinatorial chemistry
competent cells
complementary DNA
conservative mutations
contig maps
contigs
cohesive *cos* sites
COS cell line
cosmids
cRNA
dA:dT cloning
denaturing gradient gel
   electrophoresis
differential display
digital DNA typing
direct transgenesis
DNA binding domain
DNA fingerprinting
DNA footprinting
DNA microchip
electroporation
embryo stem cells
error-prone PCR
exon amplification
exon trapping
expressed sequence tag
expression PCR
expression vector
first-strand cDNA
fluorescent *in situ* hybridisation
GC clamp
gel retardation

gene cloning
gene knockout
gene library
gene probes
gene targeting
gene therapy
genome mapping
genomic library
glycosylated proteins
heat shock
homologous recombination
HTF islands
human genome mapping project
hybrid arrest translation
hybridisation
hypervariable regions
immunological screening
in situ hybridisation
in situ PCR
in vitro expression
in vitro packaging
in vitro transcription
in vitro translation
insert capacity
insertional inactivation
Klenow polymerase
lac operon
λ insertion vectors
λ replacement vectors
lawn
ligation
linkers
lipofection
Lysogenic life cycle
lytic life cycle
M13
Mammalian artificial chromosomes
megaprimer PCR
microinjection
microprojectiles
minisatellite variant repeat
molecular evolution
multiple cloning site
multiplex PCR
northern blot
oncogenes
overlap extension PCR
P1 artificial chromosomes
partial restriction digestion
pBR322
PCR mutagenesis
PCR screening
pEMBL
phage display
phagemid
physical map

plaque hybridisation
plaques
plasmid
polymerase chain reaction
polysomes
positional cloning
post-translational modifications
prehybridisation mix
promoter probe vectors
protein design cycle
protein engineering
protoplast
pUC
quantitative PCR
random hexamers
rational design
reading frame
reannealing
recombinant DNA
recombinatorial library
relaxed origin of replication
replica plating
replication origin
replicative form
reporter gene
reverse transcriptase
reverse transcriptase – PCR
ribonuclease protection assay
riboprobes
ribosome binding site
RNase H
S1 nuclease mapping
second-strand synthesis
selective transgenesis
sequence-tagged sites
shuttle vectors
single-stranded DNA rescue
single-strand DNA digestion
spheroplast
stringent
stuffer fragment
subcloning
subtractive hybridisation
superinfection
transfection
transformation
transgenics
tumour induction
vaccinia virus
vector
western blotting
yeast artificial chromosomes
yeast episomal plasmid
yeast two-hybrid system

3.12 **SUGGESTIONS FOR FURTHER READING**

BROWN, T.A. (1997). *Genetics: A Molecular Approach*, 3rd edn. Chapman & Hall, London. (A very good introduction to genetics and molecular biology.)

HARWOOD, A. (1996). *Basic DNA and RNA Protocols*. Humana Press, Totowa, NY. (An extensive collection of practical methods for DNA and RNA analysis.)

NEWTON, C.R. and GRAHAM, A. (1997). *PCR*. 2nd edn. Bios Scientific, Oxford,. (An excellent introduction to the methods and application the PCR.)

OLD, R.W. and PRIMROSE, S.B. (1994). *Principles of Gene Manipulation*, 5th edn. Blackwell Science, Oxford. (An advanced text on methods of genetic manipulation.)

PRIMROSE, S.B. (1998) *Principles of Genome Analysis*, 2nd edn. Blackwell Science, Oxford. (A well-written text on current methods of genome analysis.)

RAPLEY, R. and WALKER, J.M. (1998). *Molecular Biomethods Handbook*. Humana Press, Totowa, NY. (A collection of key nucleic acid and protein techniques.)

STRACHEN T. and READ, A.P. (1996). *Human Molecular Genetics*. Bios Scientific, Oxford. (An excellent and very comprehensive textbook with excellent illustrations.)

Chapter 4

Immunochemical techniques

4.1 INTRODUCTION

The immune system of animals is responsible for mounting immune responses against molecules recognised as being foreign (non-self). The science of immunology studies such responses and the immune system responsible for them.

The immune system provides protection for animals against infectious microorganisms (viruses, bacteria, mycoplasmas, fungi and protozoa) and also helps in the elimination of parasites and toxins. It combats tumours and neoplastic cells and can reject transfused cells and transplanted organs from genetically non-identical animals. Its physiological role is to ensure that the animal is free from life-threatening life forms and biological substances (the derivation of the word 'immunology' is from the Latin *immunitas* = freedom from). Inappropriate (i.e. undesirable) immune responses can cause clinical problems such as allergies, graft-versus-host disease and autoimmune disorders. Immune responses can be classified as either innate or aquired. Innate immunity does not require prior exposure to the foreign substance and is mediated mainly by cells of the monocytic lineage (e.g. macrophages) and polymorphonuclear leukocytes. Innate immunity is relatively non-specific, although it clearly normally distinguishes between self and non-self. It constitutes a potent, rapid-reacting, first-line defence against invasion and unwanted infection. Laboratory procedures based on innate immunity are limited in usefulness in general application to biochemical methodology.

Acquired immunity requires exposure ('priming') to the non-self material. It is primarily mediated by lymphocytes and may be further divided into cell-mediated and humoral immune responses. Cell-mediated immunity can be attributed mainly to the activity of T lymphocytes, which interact with foreign substances (antigens) in a specific manner and mediate a diverse array of immunobiological processes; for example, cytotoxic T cells specifically 'kill' unwanted cells or microorganisms. Methodology based on cell-mediated immune mechanisms can be useful for the study of cellular immunology and some aspects of clinical immunology, but its application to biochemistry is neither easy nor (usually) useful.

Humoral immunity is mediated primarily by soluble proteins known as antibodies, which circulate in blood and permeate most body organs. They can also be present on cell surfaces, where they function as antigen receptors and binding proteins. Antibodies are produced and secreted by B lymphocytes, but this is influenced by the activity of cells of other types (especially lymphocytes of the T-helper type). Terminally differentiated B cells known as plasma cells are the most potent natural secretors of antibodies. The study of antibodies (and some other Immunologically important molecules such as complement components) is known as immunochemistry. Such antibodies can show exquisite specificity and sensitivity for antigens, although this is not always the case, and many procedures and methods have been devised which exploit these properties. Such methods are known as immunochemical techniques. They are obviously very important for studying aspects of immunology itself but are invaluable methods for carrying out investigations in just about every biological science (especially biochemistry). Definitions of some commonly used immunochemical terms are given in Table 4.1.

4.1.1 **Antibodies**

Antibodies are a group of globular proteins known as immunoglobulins. These consist of monomers or multimers of a basic four-chain, bilaterally symmetrical structure containing two light and two heavy chains (Fig. 4.1). Five varieties of heavy chain (known as γ, μ, α, δ and ϵ chains) occur in higher vertebrates and these determine the class of the immunoglobulin (known as IgG, IgM, IgA, IgD and IgE, respectively; Table 4.2). All classes can bind antigen but the immunobiological functions mediated by the immunoglobulin molecules vary. In mammals, the IgG and IgA classes are divided into subclasses, which reflect different heavy chain amino acid sequences (but less different than the sequences of the different classes). The number of subclasses found differs between species. The light chains do not mediate significant immunobiological activity, but do contribute to antigen binding and the stability and higher structure of the immunoglobulin molecule. IgG, IgE and IgD are predominantly monomers of the basic four-chain structure, but IgA is often dimeric and IgM is pentameric, at least in mammals. Multimeric IgA and IgM contain an additional small protein known as the J chain, which is necessary for polymerisation, and IgA present in secretions also contains a protein known as the secretory component.

Immunoglobulin molecules can be cleaved by some proteolytic enzymes to yield fragments that are useful for immunochemical procedures and also reveal important aspects of antibody structure and function. The plant protease papain cleaves human IgG to yield three fragments of approximately the same size (about 50 000 M_r). Two of the fragments are identical and one is different; the former can be separated from the latter using ion-exchange chromatography. The two identical fragments are able to bind antigen in a monovalent manner, but cannot precipitate antigen from solution or in gel. They are known as fragment–antigen binding or Fab in immunochemical terminology. The third fragment does not bind antigen, but early biochemical studies showed it to be more easy to crystallize than the Fab fragments (this reflects a greater homogeneity in structure). It is known as fragment crystallisable or Fc by immunochemists. The mammalian protease pepsin cleaves human IgG at low pH to produce one large fragment, a smaller fragment and some small peptides. The large fragment (100 000 M_r) can

Table 4.1 Glossary of immunochemical terms

Antigen
A substance which is recognised and bound by an antibody.

Antigenic determinant
See epitope.

Antiserum
Serum from an animal containing antibodies reacting with particular antigens. Sometimes known as an immune serum.

Autoantibodies
Antibodies that react with self antigen(s). These are not normally present in blood or body fluids, but, if present, are often associated with pathological conditions known as autoimmune diseases, e.g. rheumatoid arthritis, systemic lupus erythematosus, primary biliary cirrhosis, insulin-dependent diabetes mellitus.

Clone
A growing population of cells, derived from a single progenitor cell. The clone is derived asexually by continued division and all cells are genetically identical unless mutation occurs during growth.

Divalent
Able to bind two molecules of ligand. A divalent antibody is thus able to bind two molecules of antigen.

Epitope
A site on the antigen that is recognised and bound by an antibody. It is normally about six amino acids or carbohydrate residues in size. Epitopes on protein antigens may not be continuous in structure. Sometimes also called an antigenic determinant.

Lymphocytes
Cells associated with functions responsible for development and maintenance of specific immunity. They are a subdivision of leukocytes and are the main constituents of lymphoid tissues.

Immunogen
A substance or mixture of substances used to induce an immune response.

Microtitre plate
Plastic plate containing many (usually 96) wells in which many types of imunoassay may be carried out more conveniently than in individual tubes. The wells may be flat-bottomed for use in ELISA, U-shaped for use in RIA or V-shaped for haemagglutination tests. They may be flexible or rigid.

Monovalent
Able to bind only one molecule of ligand.

Multivalent
Able to bind more than one molecule of ligand.

Myeloma cells
Tumour cells of plasma cell lineage. Sometimes also called plasmacytoma cells.

Paraprotein
Monoclonal immunoglobulin secreted by myeloma cells (see above). Such molecules closely resemble immunoglobulins produced by 'normal' plasma cells/lymphocytes. They are sometimes called myeloma proteins.

Peptide
A molecule consisting of a number of amino acid residues linked by peptide bonds. Large peptides are sometimes called polypeptides and/or proteins.

Plasma
Fluid obtained from uncoagulated blood after removal of cellular components. Differs from serum (see below) in containing all components of the coagulation system. Its preparation necessitates the use of an anticoagulant, e.g. heparin, citrate.

Serum
Fluid derived from coagulated blood after removal of the clot and cell components.

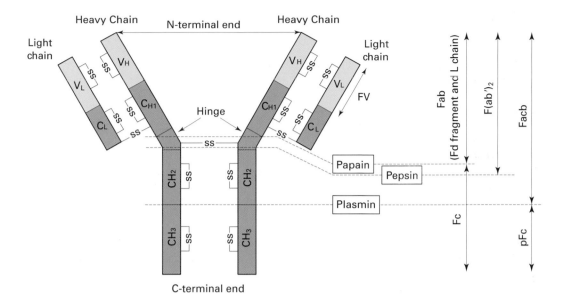

Fig. 4.1. General structure of IgG showing enzyme cleavage sites and resulting fragments. Note that the number of −S−S− bonds in the hinge area varies according to subclass and species.

bind antigen divalently (as long as the antigen is relatively small), can cross-link antigen and can form antigen complexes that precipitate. It is structurally very similar to a dimer of the Fab fragment produced by papain digestion and is known as F(ab′)₂. Similarly, the smaller fragment is a truncated version of the Fc fragment and is known as Fc′. Both papain and pepsin cleave the IgG molecule in the hinge region, but the former enzyme cuts next to the hinge on the N-terminal side whereas the latter enzyme acts on the C-terminal side of the hinge (see Fig. 4.1). This explains the production of monovalent Fab fragments by papain, but divalent dimeric antigen-binding F(ab′)₂ fragments by pepsin; the two Fab′ components comprising F(ab′)₂ are linked via the disulphide bridges that make up the hinge region. Other enzymes can also be used to derive immunoglobulin fragments, but papain and pepsin are the most commonly used. Similar fragments can be produced from non-human IgG, but there is considerable species variation in susceptibility to digestion. Enzyme-derived fragments of other immunoglobulin classes can also be produced (see Suggestions for further reading, Section 4.13).

For most immunochemical procedures, IgG is by far the most useful immunoglobulin reagent.

4.1.2 Immunoglobulin structure, immunoglobulin genes and the generation of antibody diversity

Immunoglobulin chains of particular classes or types contain distinct regions that are either very constant in sequence or more variable. The chains are built up of

Table 4.2 Polypeptide chain composition of human immunoglobulins

Class/subclass	Normal serum concentration (mg ml⁻¹)	M_r (×10⁻³)	H chains domains	Chain compositions	M_r (×10⁻³) Total	M_r (×10⁻³) Peptide	% Carbohydrate of chains (no. of groups)	Hinge amino acids	Intra-heavy chain disulphide bonds
IgG1	5–10	146	4	2γ1	51	49	3–4 (1)	15	2
				2L(κ:λ 2:1)	23	23	<0.5		
IgG2	1.8–3.5	146	4	2γ2	51	49	3–4 (1)	12	4
				2L(κ:λ 2:1)	23	23	<0.5		
IgG3	0.6–1.2	170	4	2γ3	60	57	3–4 (1)	62	11
				2L(κ:λ 1:1)	23	23	<0.5		
IgG4	0.3–0.6	146	4	2γ4	51	49	3–4 (1)	12	2
				2L(κ:λ 1:1)	23	23	<0.5		
IgM	0.5–2.0	900	5	10μ	67	57	12–16 (5)	0	1[a]
				2L(κ:λ 3:1)	23	23	<0.5		
				1J[f]	15	14	7.5		
IgA1[b]	0.8–3.4	160	4	2α1	56	50	10–15 (5)	20	2[c]
				2L(κ:λ 1:1)	23	23	<0.5		
IgA2[b]	0.2–0.6	160	4	2α2	53	48	10–15 (2)	7	2[c]
				2L(κ:λ 1:1)	23	23	<0.5		
Secretory IgA1 or IgA2[d]	–	390	4	4α	53–56	48–50	10–15		
				4L	23	23	<0.5		
				1J	15	14	7.5		
				ISC[e]	75	63	15–16		
IgD	0.003–0.3	165	4	2δ	60	51	14–71 (3)	64	1
				2L(κ:λ 1:10)	23	23	<0.5		
IgE	0.0001–0.0007	185	5	2ε	70	59	13–16 (6)	0	2
				2L	23	23	<0.5		

[a] There is one intra-heavy chain disulphide bond linking cysteines between C_H2 and C_H3 domains; there are further disulphide bonds between monomer units.

[b] Data are given for the monomeric form which predominates in human sera. Polymeric forms also exist (up to pentamer); these contain one molecule of J chain per polymer in addition to α and L chains.

[c] There is an additional disulphide bond from the cysteine in the tailpiece to either the corresponding cysteine in the other heavy chain or to a cysteine in J chain or secretory component in secretory IgA.

[d] Data are given for the dimer; a tetrameric form is also common in humans.

[e] SC, secretory component, derived from a membrane-bound poly(Ig)receptor used to transport the IgA through epithelial cells during its secretion.

Source: Reproduced from M. A. Kerr and R. Thorpe, *Immunochemistry Labfax* (1994), Bios Scientific, Oxford.

domains which exhibit a similar three-dimensional structure (Fig. 4.1). The heavy chains are made up of three (γ-, α- and δ-chains) or four (μ- and ϵ-chains) constant domains and one variable domain, whereas light chains have one constant and one variable domain (Fig. 4.1 and Table 4.2). The constant regions of antibodies are important for immunoglobulin three-dimensional structure, are responsible for most immunobiological functions such as complement fixation and interact with the immunoglobulin receptors found on many types of cells. The variable regions are responsible for binding antigen. Within the variable regions are relatively short sequences that show particularly high variability in sequence and these are responsible for direct interaction with the antigen. These are known as hypervariable regions or complementarity-determining regions *(CDRs)*, and there are three of these per heavy or light chain. The less variable portions of the variable regions are important for maintenance of the appropriate structure of the antibody molecule, especially for efficient antigen binding.

Immunoglobulins are clear exceptions to the normal rule that one gene codes for one protein chain, and several germline genes are involved in coding for each of the heavy and light chains. The constant regions of heavy chains are coded for by single genes, one for each class or subclass, known as C_H genes, which are distinct in the germline from genes for the heavy chain variable region (V_H genes). Relatively large numbers of variable region genes occur in clusters (for human heavy chains there are about 100 V_H genes) and between these and the constant region genes there are additional short genes that code for joining (*J*; six for human heavy chain genes) and diversity-associated (*D*; four for human heavy chain genes) sequences. A similar gene organization exists for the light chains (known as V_L, J_L and C_L gene segments), except that D sequence light chain genes do not occur; there are about 70 V_L and 4 *J* genes for human κ light chains. Early in B cell maturation, translocation of the genes occurs such that a linear assembly of a particular *V* gene with a *J* gene, a *D* gene (only for heavy chains) and a *C* gene occurs; this codes for a complete immunoglobulin chain. This results in the ability of an animal to produce a range of immunoglobulin molecules that differ particularly in their hypervariable region sequences and thus the part of the molecule that binds antigen. This diversity can be increased by use of variable amounts of the D region (for heavy chains) and by somatic mutation during maturation of the immune response. All of these combinations are responsible for the ability of at least higher vertebrates to produce a very large number of different antibodies (theoretical considerations suggest that humans can produce an estimated 10^8 different antibodies), and accounts for the differing specificity and affinity of immunoglobulin molecules for antigen. It also allows production of antibodies that recognise virtually *any* foreign antigen of appropriate size. These properties of antibodies are exploited in immunochemical methods.

4.2 **PRODUCTION OF ANTIBODIES**

Virtually all immunochemical techniques rely on the use of antibodies and their effectiveness is dependent on the quality of the antibody or antibodies employed.

The nature of the antibody affects both the specificity of the methods (i.e. the ability to discriminate between the desired analyte and other substances that may be present) and the sensitivity of the procedure (i.e. its ability to detect/measure low concentrations of the analyte). The avidity of the antibody for antigen is important for the latter (see Section 4.9). Although some antibodies that can be useful in immunochemical methods occur 'naturally', for example some autoantibodies, it is normally necessary to stimulate their production by immunising animals (but see Section 4.2.6 for an an important exception to this). Many different procedures for this have been developed.

4.2.1 **The immune response; polyclonal and monoclonal antibodies**

All vertebrates can produce antibodies against foreign antigens. However, responses in lower vertebrates are very limited (although even the most primitive animals, such as hagfish and lampreys, can mount immune responses against some non-self proteins) and normally antibodies derived from such species are not useful for immunochemical methods. Mammals mount the most useful humoral immune responses and mammalian antibodies are normally used in immunochemical techniques. However, avian antibodies can also be employed in special cases. In most cases IgG antibodies are the most useful for immunochemical techniques, but IgM and IgA can be used for some procedures. IgE is limited to studies relating to allergic and anaphylactic phenomena and IgD is not normally useful. No specific functions have been identified for secreted IgD.

It is now clear that each mature B lymphocyte secretes an antibody with a single immunoglobulin sequence. The humoral response to antigen results in activation of a heterogeneous population of B cells that secretes different immunoglobulins. Maturation of the response results in clonal expansion of these initially primed cells to derive populations of plasma cells that secrete an array of antigen-binding immunoglobulins, often of different classes and subclasses. In the antigen-binding fraction of antibodies, immunoglobulins showing variable specificity and avidity for the immunogen will be present. Usually, many different antibodies, recognising several different epitopes on each antigen are present. Such a response is described as polyclonal, as antibody is derived from more than one clone of B lymphocytes and shows heterogeneity in the amino acid sequences of the antigen-binding immunoglobulins present. Preparations of such polyclonal antibodies, either unpurified as immune sera or purified (see Section 4.3) are often used for immunochemical techniques. However, more recently, methods have been developed for deriving monoclonal antibodies, which are derived from a single B cell clone and show identical amino acid sequence. Monoclonal antibody preparations show homogeneous characteristics (including specificity and avidity for antigen, i.e. they recognise a single epitope) and can be advantageous for immunochemical purposes, if carefully selected and characterised. Production of monoclonal antibodies is considered in Section 4.2.3.

4.2.2 **Production of polyclonal antibodies (antisera)**

It is possible to produce antibodies that bind to proteins, peptides, carbohydrates and nucleic acids, but the latter show little if any specificity for sequence and so are usually of little use for immunochemical techniques. Antibodies against carbohydrate can be used for analytical work, but can show limited specificity, except in some special cases. In general, most immunochemical methods are devised for use with antibodies that recognise proteins and peptides.

Most higher vertebrates will produce a humoral immune response against a 'foreign' protein. However, the magnitude of the antibody response depends on a number of variables. Of particular importance are the size of the protein/peptide and the phylogenetic distance between the source of the antigen and the animal used to produce antibody. For the latter it is generally the case that the greater the phylogenetic difference, the better. However, choice of species for antibody production also depends on the amount of antigen available, the amount of antiserum required and the quality of antiserum desired. In some cases use of closely related species or even different strains of a single species for derivation of antigen and production of antibodies can provide antibodies with particular properties/specificities. The most important consideration for immunogenicity is the difference in amino acid sequence (and therefore structure) of the antigen used as immunogen and the equivalent antigen (if present) in the animal used to produce antibody. It is generally the case that the greater this difference, the more immunogenic the antigen will be. In some cases, particular parts of the antigen produce very potent immune responses and such epitopes are known as immunodominant.

Peptides with an M_r of less than about 2000 are normally poorly or non-immunogenic. Immunogenicity tends to increase with size; proteins with $M_r > 10\,000$ are usually immunogenic as long as they are recognised as foreign in responding animals.

Antibodies that bind small peptides (and other small, non-immunogenic molecules such as steroids and drugs) can be produced by linking (conjugating) these substances to larger proteins (known as carrier proteins). The antisera produced will contain antibodies that recognise the carrier as well as others that bind to the small molecule. Some proteins are particularly effective as carriers (such as keyhole limpet haemocyanin and thyroglobulin) and some produce a restricted anti-carrier humoral response, such as purified protein derivative (PPD) from Bacille, Calmette, Guérin (BCG). Substances that are not immunogenic alone, but are when conjugated, are known as haptens.

For production of potent antibodies that perform well in immunochemical techniques, it is usually necessary to use an adjuvant as part of the immunogen. Such substances potentiate the immune reponse by forming a slow-release depot of antigen, by stimulating T cell help or by aiding antigen presentation. Some adjuvants function by more than one of these effects (see Table 4.3 for some adjuvants commonly used for immunochemical purposes). Although a single immunisation with antigen will usually result in production of antibodies, such antisera

Table 4.3	Some commonly used adjuvants
Adjuvant	Composition and use
Freund's complete adjuvant (FCA)	Mineral oil containing heat-killed mycobacteria (*Mycobacterium tuberculosis* or *M. butyricum*) Used as emulsion with aqueous antigen
Freund's incomplete adjuvant (FIA)	Mineral oil Used as emulsion with aqueous antigen
Alum	Complex aluminium salts. There are various versions of the adjuvant: some can be purchased ready for use (e.g. Alhydrogel); others can be prepared in the laboratory by mixing various salts, e.g. $NaHCO_3$, and aluminium potassium sulphate. Aqueous antigen is absorbed to gel
Bentonite	Wyoming sodium bentonite (Montmorillonite) as gel. Aqueous antigen adsorbed to surface
Quil A	Saponin derived from *Quillaja saponana* Molina (South American tree). Mixed to form a complex with aqueous antigen
Muramyl dipeptide (MDP)	*N*-Acetylmuramyl-L-alanyl-D-isoglutamine. Mixed with aqueous antigen. Various derivations of MDP are also used as adjuvants
Monophosphoryl lipid A (MPL)	Used in various formulations, often as an emulsion with oils. Antigen included in emulsion
Bacillus pertussis	Killed organisms mixed with aqueous antigen

FCA is probably the most potent adjuvant but may be inappropriate for some purposes.
Source: Reproduced from M. A. Kerr and R. Thorpe, *Immunochemistry Labfax* (1994), Bios Scientific, Oxford

are usually suboptimal, containing antibodies of low avidity and a high proportion of IgM, which can be of limited use for immunochemical methods. It is usual practice to use several subsequent immunisations, spaced such that the immune response is boosted to produce a hyperimmune animal, with a high concentration of avid antibodies specific for antigen in its blood. Such 'hyperimmune sera' (really antisera from hyperimmunised animals) are usually the polyclonal reagents of choice for immunochemical techniques. Precise details of amount of antigen used and spacing of 'boosting' immunisations vary enormously according to antigen and species used; for some general principles see Table 4.4. In general, the larger the animal, the more antigen is required; however, larger animals contain more blood (and therefore serum/plasma). Thus larger animals will require the availability of greater quantities of immunogen for antibody production, but will generate larger amounts of antiserum (mice will produce only a few millilitres whereas sheep and horses can yield several litres).

Table 4.4 Examples of immunisation protocols that have been used successfully

Species	Priming	Rest period (weeks)	First boost	Rest period (weeks)	Subsequent boosts
Mice, rats and guinea pigs	5–100 μg antigen in FCA (or other adjuvant), s.c. or i.m.	2–3	50–100 μg antigen in FIA, other adjuvant or PBS, i.m. or s.c.	3	5–100 μg antigen in FIA or PBS, i.p., s.c., i.m. or i.v.
Rabbits	50–250 μg antigen in FCA or other adjuvant, i.d., i.m. or s.c.	3–4	50–250 μg antigen in FIA or other adjuvant or PBS, i.m., or s.c.	4 or longer	50–250 μg antigen in FIA or PBS, i.m., s.c. or i.v.
Sheep and goats	250 μg–10 mg antigen in FCA or other adjuvant, i.m., s.c. or i.d.	4	250 μg–10 mg antigen in FIA or other adjuvant, i.m. or s.c..	4–8 or longer	250 μg–10 mg antigen in FIA or other adjuvant, i.m., s.c. or i.v.
Horses and donkeys	250 μg–50 mg antigen in FCA or other adjuvant, i.m., s.c. or i.d.	4	250 μg–50 mg antigen in FIA or other adjuvant, i.m. or s.c.	4–8 or longer	250 μg–50 mg antigen in FIA or other adjuvant, i.m. or s.c.
Primates	50 μg–1 mg antigen in adjuvant, i.m. or s.c.		50 μg–1 mg antigen in adjuvant, or PBS, i.m., s.c. or i.v.	4–8 or longer	50 μg–1 mg antigen in adjuvant or PBS, i.m., s.c. or i.d.
Chickens	30–200 μg antigen in FCA or other adjuvant, i.m.	2–3	30–200 μg antigen in FIA or other adjuvant, i.m.	3 or longer	30–200 μg in FIA or other adjuvant or PBS, i.m.

FCA Freund's complete adjuvant; FIA, Freund's incomplete adjuvant; PBS, phosphate-buffered saline; i.p., intraperitoneally; s.c., subcutaneously; i.m., intramuscularly; i.v., intravenously; i.d., intradermally.
Source: Reproduced from M. A. Kerr and R. Thorpe., *Imunochemistry Labfax* (1994), Bios Scientific, Oxford.

4.2.3 **Monoclonal antibodies**

Monoclonal antibodies can be especially useful for immunochemical methods. Such antibodies are secreted by cloned, i.e. monoclonal cells. Mature, antibody-secreting lymphocytes from immunised animals can be cloned, but these survive for only a very short period in culture, and therefore do not provide useful amounts of antibody. However, procedures have been developed to allow production of large quantities of monoclonal antibodies by producing continuously growing (immortal) cell lines that secrete antibody efficiently. These involve generation of hybrid cells, transformation of lymphocytes with a virus, or recombinant DNA procedures.

4.2.4 **Hybridoma production**

In 1975, Köhler and Milstein devised a procedure for producing hybrid cells that secrete antibody and grow continuously in culture (Fig. 4.2). This involves fusing lymphocytes from immune mice with mouse myeloma cells. Such hybrid fused cells, known originally as fusomas but later as hybridomas inherit the ability to secrete antibody from the lymphocyte parent and the ability to grow continuously from the myeloma cell. Myeloma cell lines that no longer secrete immunoglobulin paraprotein have been derived and are advantageous for hybridoma technology (the hybridomas derived do not secrete the paraprotein).

Lymphocytes and myeloma cells are mixed together at high density and treated with a fusing agent (nowadays polyethylene glycol, although Sendai virus was originally used). Under such conditions, fused cells are produced but unfused lymphocytes and myeloma cells predominate and the latter will overgrow and overwhelm the hydridomas if they are not removed. This is normally achieved by the use of a selective medium in which the myeloma cells die, but hybridomas survive. The most widely used selective system involves the inclusion of the antibiotic aminopterin in growth medium. This inhibits the *de novo* nucleotide synthesis pathway, in which nucleotides (and thus eventually nucleic acids) are produced from small molecules. Normal cells survive in this medium as they are able to use the salvage pathway for nucleic acid synthesis, in which nucleotides produced by breakdown of nucleic acid are recycled. But, if cells are unable to produce the enzyme hypoxanthine–guanine phosphoribosyl transferase (HGPRT), they are unable to utilise the salvage pathway and therefore die in aminopterin-containing medium. Such cells can be produced by culture in 8-azaguanine and numerous HGPRT-negative mouse myeloma cell lines have been established.

After fusion of lymphocytes with HGPRT-negative myeloma cells, aminopterin-containing medium, supplemented with hypoxanthine and thymidine to ensure an adequate supply of substrates for the salvage pathway (HAT medium) is added, which kills myeloma cells but allows hybridomas to survive as they inherit HGPRT from the lymphocyte parent. Residual unfused lymphocytes die after a short period in culture, which results in a pure preparation of hybridomas that can be cloned using one of three procedures:

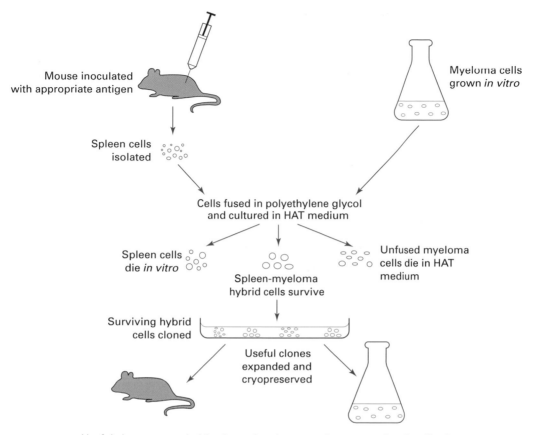

Useful clones expanded *in vitro* or in mice to produce monoclonal antibodies

Fig. 4.2. A schematic representation of a typical procedure for production of murine monoclonal antibodies.

(i) *Limiting dilution cloning*, in which a single hybridoma cell suspension is diluted and dispensed into culture plate wells to approximate one cell per well (and numbers surrounding this). Wells are inspected to assess clonality and, after culture, cell supernatant is assessed for the presence of appropriate antibody. This procedure is normally repeated (often more than once) to obtain a monoclonal hybridoma line.

(ii) *soft agar cloning*, in which a single cell suspension is diluted in approximately 0.25% molten agar, overlayed on solid 0.5% agar and allowed to set. Clones grow in culture as foci that can be located visually (using an inverted microscope). When of appropriate size, the resulting clumps of cells are 'picked' from the agar using a fine Pasteur pipette, cultured in medium and the supernatant assessed for antibody content.

(iii) *cloning using fluorescence-activated cell sorting*, in which cells are fluorescently labelled for appropriate antibody secretion (e.g. using fluorescein isothlocyanate-labelled antigen) and then individually isolated using flow cytometry via a fluorescence-activated cell sorter (FACS) machine. Appropriate cells are cultured and supernatants screened for antibody content.

All cloning methods are designed to produce cultures of monoclonal hybridomas but do not guarantee this. Repeating the cloning techniques will obviously increase the chance of cells being monoclonal, but cloning checks need to be used if assurance of monoclonality is to be obtained. For this, 'subclones' of the hybridoma lines are prepared (as above) and the percentage of cells secreting antibody of appropriate defined specificity assessed. If the parental line is monoclonal, this should be close to 100%. If not, the hybridoma line either is not monoclonal or is unstable in respect to secretion of monoclonal antibody.

Such monoclonal cell lines can be grown in culture to produce supernatant containing monoclonal antibody (industrial-scale fermenters or hollow fibre culture supports can be used that yield kilograms of antibody) or grown in the peritoneal cavities of mice to produce ascitic fluid containing high concentrations (about 5 to 10 mgml^{-1}) of antibody. The cell lines can be cryopreserved to provide an everlasting source of monoclonal antibody.

A similar approach can be used for the production of rat monoclonal antibodies, except O-diazoacetyl-L-serine (azaserine) is sometimes substituted for aminopterin in the selective medium. This inhibits a range of amination reactions, some of which are essential for *de novo* purine synthesis. Hamster heterohybridomas can also be produced by fusing hamster lymphocytes with mouse HGPRT-deficient myeloma cells. Hybridoma technology is generally less successful with higher mammals, owing to the lack of suitable myeloma cell lines for fusion and the instability of mouse/higher species lymphocyte heterohybridomas. A rabbit myeloma cell line suitable for production of rabbit hybridomas has been described.

4.2.5 Transformation of lymphocytes with virus; production of human monoclonal antibodies

In some cases, it it desirable or even essential to use human rather than rodent monoclonal antibodies. For example, human antibodies are generally better for *in vivo* therapeutic use in humans as they are much less immunogenic and mediate immunobiological functions, and it can be very difficult if not impossible to produce rodent monoclonal antibodies against some antigens, for example the human Rh D blood group antigen. A few hybridoma-derived human monoclonal antibodies have been produced (almost always from heterohybridomas), but this approach is difficult and inefficient. However, infection of human B lymphocytes with Epstein–Barr virus results in transformation of a subpopulation of cells and allows the production of continuously growing cell lines that can be cloned. Some of these clones secrete monoclonal antibody, which can be used for therapeutic and immunochemical purposes. A relatively high proportion of such cell lines secrete IgM antibody, but lines secreting immunoglobulin of all classes and sub-classes can be produced. Some cell lines show instability and low level immuno-globulin secretion that can sometimes be resolved by fusion with stable non-antibody-secreting heterohybridomas or myeloma lines.

4.2.6 **Engineered antibodies**

Although mouse or rat monoclonal antibodies with the desired antigen-binding properties can be produced from deliberately immunised laboratory animals, a problem with their clinical use in humans, for example in cancer patients, is that they can elicit an immune response in the recipient as they are recognised as being 'foreign'. Also, some potential applications of monoclonal antibodies may require particular effector functions (mediated by the Fc portion of particular subclasses) combined with a particular specificity (determined by the variable portion), which may not be readily produced simply by immunisation. Small antibody frag-ments rather than the relatively large intact molecule may be preferable for other clinical applications, for example where tissue penetration is desired. Genetic engineering methods have therefore been developed to attempt to overcome these limitations. Genes encoding antibody heavy and light chains can be amplified using the polymerase chain reaction (PCR) and cloned into suitable vectors for expression and manipulation, for example splicing the variable region from one antibody to the constant region of another. Mammalian cells are usually used for expression of whole antibodies (to ensure glycosylation and correct chain folding and assembly) whereas antibody fragments can be expressed in *Escherichia coli*. It has also become possible to mimic the *in vivo* antibody response *in vitro* by express-ing antibody fragments derived from gene repertoires on the surface of bacterio-phage (phage display) to allow selection of particular specificities.

Polymerase chain reaction amplification of antibody genes

Antibody genes may be readily amplified by PCR. This amplification involves repeated cycles of extension between two oligonucleotide primers that hybridise to the 5′ and 3′ ends of the gene sequence. The steps involve: (i) preparation of a cell lysate and extraction of the RNA (this fraction will contain the mRNA which encodes the antibody heavy and light chains); (ii) synthesis of single-stranded complementary DNA (cDNA) using the enzyme reverse transcriptase, the RNA/cDNA hybrid then being used as a template for the PCR; and (iii) specific amplification of the antibody gene(s) present in the RNA/cDNA template using oligonucleotide primers that anneal to sequences outside the region for which sequence information is required (usually the variable region; Fig. 4.3). Primers can be designed for PCR amplification of most families of variable region genes as the nucleotide sequences flanking the variable region genes are relatively con-served. The incorporation of restriction endonuclease sites in the primers allows subsequent cloning of the amplified gene(s).

The starting material may be a hybridoma secreting a monoclonal antibody to allow, for example, genetic manipulations. Alternatively, RNA prepared from

(a)

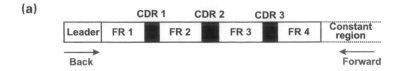

(b)

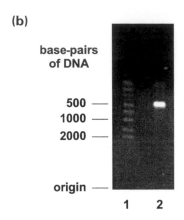

Fig. 4.3. PCR amplification of a heavy chain variable region gene. (a) The position of the forward and back primers relative to the variable region. FR, framework region; CDR, complementarity-determining region. (b) Photograph showing agarose gel electrophoretic analysis of the product of PCR amplification of the heavy chain variable region gene (track 2). Track 1 shows DNA markers. The gel was stained with ethidium bromide (a fluorescent dye that binds to nucleic acid) and viewed under ultraviolet illumination.

human peripheral blood lymphocytes can be used to prepare repertoires of heavy and light chain variable region genes to allow the creation of antibody fragment gene repertoires and phage display (see below).

Gene repertoires and phage display

Amplified heavy and light variable region (V_H and V_L, respectively) gene repertoires can be spliced together using a stretch of synthetic DNA that encodes a peptide 'linker' to form single-chain (sc) Fv antibody fragment gene repertoires (Fv fragments are the smallest antibody fragments that still contain the intact antigen-binding site; Fig. 4.4b). The use of a linker prevents the otherwise non-covalently attached V_H and V_L portions from dissociating. The scFv repertoire is then reamplified with flanking primers containing appropriate restriction endonuclease sites which allow subsequent digestion with the appropriate enzymes and ligation into a suitable phage display vector, for example pHEN-1, which is then expressed in *E. coli*. Thus, a phage antibody 'library' can be created. The phage display vector allows the scFv fragments to be expressed at the surface of the phage as a fusion product with a phage coat protein. This allows phage-encoding fragments to be selected by screening against antigen bound to a solid support.

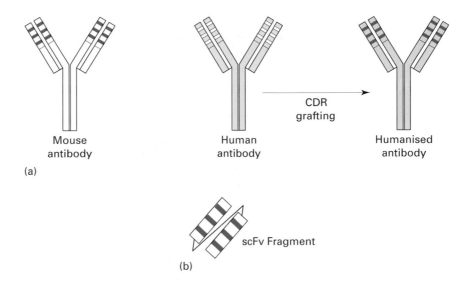

(a)

(b)

Fig. 4.4. Genetically engineered antibodies and fragments. (a) CDR (complementarity-determining region) grafting to produce humanised antibody; (b) single-chain Fv fragment.

Alternatively, soluble scFv fragments can be expressed (depending on the strain of *E. coli* used as host). A potential advantage of the above technology is the production of antibodies from non-immunised individuals. This depends on the creation of a vast number of antibody gene repertoires, phage display, and selection using the antigen of interest.

The use of antibody fragments may be advantageous for certain clinical applications, for example their small size should increase tumour penetration. However, their use in the laboratory as reagents can be problematical as they tend to have relatively low functional affinity.

Strategies for reducing immunogenicity

Several approaches have been developed to render antibodies less immunogenic, whilst retaining their antigen-binding properties. In chimaeric antibodies, the constant domains of the mouse or rat antibody are substituted with those of human sequence. This also confers effective Fc-mediated properties for *in vivo* use in humans and human-based *in vitro* methods. The constant domains may even be substituted with a non-antibody protein such as a toxin or enzyme. An alternative approach is to humanise the mouse or rat antibody by grafting the mouse CDR into human variable region genes (Fig 4.4a). These antibodies need to be expressed in mammalian cells. Amino acid residues may also have to be changed or added to ensure correct conformation of the variable region.

Sequencing monoclonal antibodies

PCR cloning of antibody variable region genes has greatly facilitated elucidation of the encoded amino acid sequences, since it is much easier to sequence the nucleic acid encoding the antibody, and then translate this into protein sequence, than to carry out amino acid sequencing by Edman degradation (see Section 6.4.3) of immunoglobulin protein. The latter method of sequencing requires relatively large amounts of pure antibody preparations and is limited to relatively short stretches of sequence, which necessitates sequencing many overlapping peptides to obtain a complete sequence. Determining the amino acid sequence of antibodies allows their structure to be correlated with their immunological properties, for example antigen-binding properties, and prediction of their three-dimensional shape. The nucleotide sequence also gives information on the use of germline genes in a given antibody response (remember that the antibody-encoding genes are formed from the joining of different germline gene segments during lymphocyte maturation; Section 4.1) and the process of affinity maturation (somatic mutation).

Amplified antibody genes can be sequenced directly; alternatively, to avoid any spurious sequences present in the PCR product, the amplified material can be cloned into a bacteriophage vector and used to transform *E. coli* to provide more reliable and reproducible sequence data. The chain termination method of sequencing is described in Section 2.14.

4.3 PURIFICATION AND FRAGMENTATION OF IMMUNOGLOBULINS

Many immunochemical techniques can be carried out using unpurified antibody in the form of antisera, monoclonal antibody-containing culture supernatant or rodent ascites, for example agar gel methods or immunohistochemistry (Sections 4.4 and 4.8). However, other methods require partial or complete purification of specific antibodies or at least isolation of the total immunoglobulin fraction, for example if they are to be labelled (Section 4.5), immobilised for use in immunoaffinity chromatography (Section 4.3.4), or analysed by isoelectric focusing (Section 12.3.4) or high performance liquid chromatography (HPLC) (Section 10.4). There are a variety of procedures available for purifying immunoglobulins, the optimal method and experimental details depend on the class/subclass, the species in which the antibody was produced, the intended use, and the type of starting material, for example serum in the case of polyclonal antibodies or culture supernatant or ascites in the case of monoclonal antibodies. Methods of immunoglobulin purification from the mixtures of proteins found in serum, culture supernatant and ascites include precipitation techniques that exploit differential solubility characteristics of antibodies and other proteins: ion-exchange chromatography (exploits charge differences between immunoglobulins and other proteins), gel filtration (separates proteins according to size) and affinity chromatography (exploits a specific interaction between antibody and a molecule which it binds – termed the 'ligand' from the Latin *ligare* = to tie or bind). It may be necessary to combine two or more of these procedures to achieve the required purity. However, only affinity chromatography using immobilised antigen is normally capable of purifying antibodies of a single specificity unless the starting material contains a monoclonal antibody.

4.3.1 **Precipitation techniques**

Certain salts, organic solvents and organic polymers cause immunoglobulin molecules to precipitate from solution to form visible, insoluble aggregates that can be collected by centrifugation, and then resolubilised in an appropriate buffer (see Section 6.3.4). Immunoglobulin molecules in solution are surrounded by a tightly bound hydration shell, and precipitation techniques work by perturbing this hydration layer. Immunoglobulins are soluble within a certain salt concentration range, but become insoluble at both high and low extremes. High concentrations of salts attract the hydration layer away from the protein as the ions become solvated, encouraging hydrophobic areas on the immunoglobulin molecule to interact with similar areas on other molecules causing 'clumping' of molecules. This is called 'salting out' and results in reversible precipitation of the antibody. Multiply charged anions with monovalent cations are most effective at salting out; ammonium and sodium sulphate are most commonly used. However, the solubility of some immunoglobulins also decreases as the salt concentration is lowered because there are insufficient ions to maintain hydration of the immunoglobulin protein. This is called euglobulin precipitation, and is particularly useful for preliminary purification of IgM, although it usually does not work well for IgG. Water-miscible organic solvents can also be used to precipitate immunoglobulins by decreasing the solvating power of water. Ethanol precipitation is used on an industrial scale for fractionation of immunoglobulin from other plasma proteins. Polyethylene glycol is a high molecular weight, water-soluble organic polymer that can be used to separate immunoglobulins from other plasma proteins by precipitation, in a similar way to organic solvents.

Precipitation of immunoglobulin tends to be most effective at its isoelectric point (the pH at which the immunoglobulin has no net charge), since electrostatic repulsion between molecules is minimised. Precipitation techniques are cheap and easy to carry out but are often used only as a preliminary step in multistep purification schedules as the product is usually not sufficiently pure.

4.3.2 **Gel filtration**

Gel filtration separates molecules according to size (Section 13.8). Since IgM is considerably larger than other immunoglobulin subclasses and most other serum proteins, conventional or HPLC gel filtration is commonly used for IgM purification. Although gel filtration alone is not very good for IgG purification, it can be used in combination with other methods such as ion-exchange chromatography for IgG purification.

4.3.3 **Ion-exchange chromatography**

Conventional or HPLC or fast protein liquid chromatography (FPLC) ion-exchange chromatography systems make use of the surface charge of immunoglobulins to separate them from other components (Section 13.7). At neutral pH,

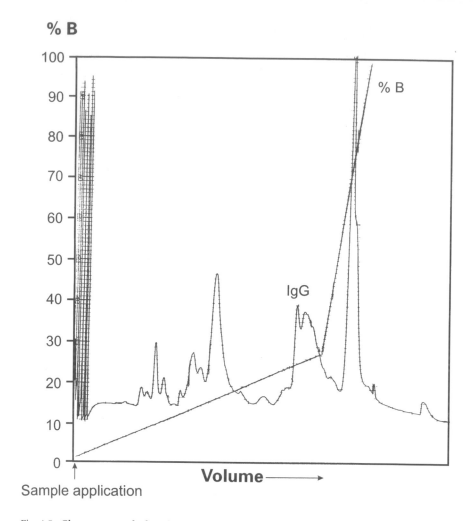

Fig. 4.5. Chromatograph showing purification of mouse IgG from ascites using fast protein liquid chromatography ion-exchange chromatography. A preliminary IgG purification step was carried out using ammonium sulphate precipitation from the ascites (Section 4.3.1). The precipitate was redissolved and equilibrated in 20 mM triethanolamine pH 7.7 (A). The anion-exchanger was also equilibrated in A. Following application of the sample, a salt gradient formed by using increasing amounts of B (A + 1 M NaCl) was used to elute the immunoglobulin. The peak corresponding to IgG is indicated.

most immunoglobulins are negatively charged and will bind to positively charged anion-exchange matrices. Increasing the salt concentration or changing the pH of the buffer will then elute the immunoglobulin from the matrix (Fig. 4.5).

4.3.4 Affinity chromatography

Affinity chromatography exploits a specific but reversible interaction between a ligand that is covalently attached to an inert support and the antibody to be purified

Table 4.5 Ligands for affinity chromatography

Ligand type	Example(s)	Antibody purification
Hapten	DNP	Antibodies that bind hapten
Antigen	Haemoglobin, factor VIII	Antibodies of a single specificity
Bacterial immunoglobulin binding protein	Protein A, protein G	Most IgG subclasses from many species
	Protein L	Some κ chains from many species
Anti-immunoglobulin antibodies	Goat anti-human IgG antibodies	Class and/or species-specific immunoglobulin fraction
Lectins	Jacalin	Human IgA
	Mannan-binding protein	Mouse IgM

DNP, dinitrophenol.

(Section 13.9). The ligand may be, for example, an antigen for purification of antibodies of a particular specificity, an anti-immunoglobulin antibody for purification of antibodies from a particular species, class or subclass, or an immunoglobulin-binding protein: several strains of bacteria produce such proteins that bind immunoglobulin with high affinity (Table 4.5). The most commonly used bacterial immunoglobulin-binding proteins are called protein A and protein G; they bind the constant region of IgG (depending on species and subclass). A light-chain-binding protein has also been described (protein L), but this binds only some light chain types. Affinity chromatography using immobilised protein A or G is often the method of choice for purification of IgG monoclonal antibodies from culture supernatants. The inert support can be agarose, sepharose, polyacrylamide, polystyrene or high pressure stable acrylic polymer for use in HPLC. Alternatively, ligand can be attached to magnetic beads, which can then be isolated using a magnetic attractor. Many different immobilised ligands are available commercially; alternatively, ligands can be coupled, via primary amine, carboxyl or thiol groups, to activated supports in the laboratory (for examples, see Fig. 4.6). When the solution containing the antibody is brought into contact with the immobilised ligand, the antibody binds to the ligand and is thus also immobilised (Fig. 4.7). The non-bound material can then be washed away. The specific interaction between antibody and ligand is then disrupted to elute the antibody (see below), whilst the ligand remains immobilised. Conditions for dissociating the specific ligand–antibody interaction commonly disrupt the electrostatic interactions and/or hydrophobic bonding (due to van der Waals' interactions) involved in antibody-ligand binding (Table 4.6).

Lectins are glycoproteins of non-immune origin, isolated from plants and animals, which bind specific carbohydrates such as galactose or fucose. For example, mannan-binding protein (MBP) is a mannose- and *N*-acetylglucosamine-binding lectin found in mammalian sera. When coupled to an inert support, it can be used to

(a)   Mechanism of activation of Sepharose by CNBr to allow subsequent coupling of proteins via amine groups

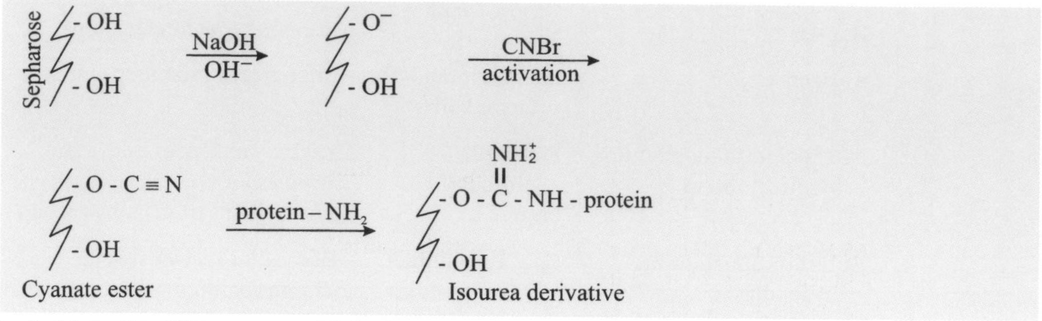

At high pH, CNBr reacts with hydroxyl groups on the Sepharose to form cyanate esters. These react with the amine groups of proteins to form covalent linkages.

(b)   Mechanism of ligand immobilisation via commercially available *N*-hydroxy succinamide ester coupling

(i) Affi-Gel 10 (used for basic protein coupling)

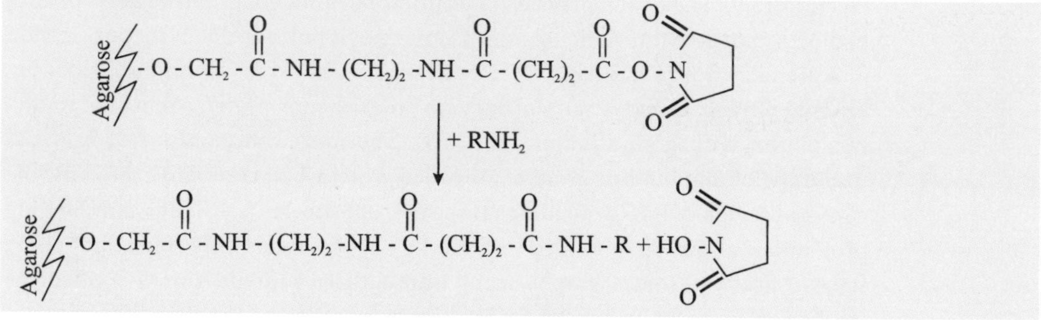

(ii) Affi-Gel 15 (used for acidic protein coupling)

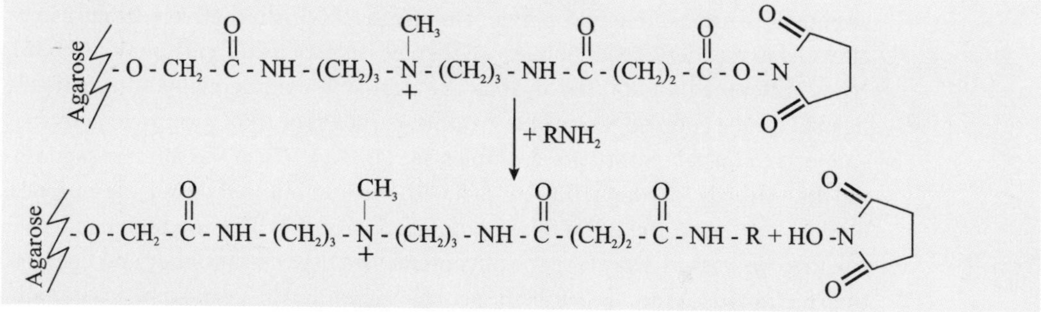

Fig. 4.6. Coupling of ligands to supports to prepare affinity columns.

Table 4.6	Conditions for elution of antibodies from affinity columns
Elution conditions	Mode of action
Glycine-HC1, pH 2.2–2.8 1 M propionic acid 0.05 M diethylamine, pH 11.5 1 M ammonia, pH 11.0	Change conformation and disrupt electrostatic interactions
2–8 M urea 5–6 M guanidine hydrochloride	Strongly denaturing
3.5 M sodium thiocyanate 4 M potassium thiocyanate 2–5 M MgCl₂, KI, NaI	Chaotropic agents
50% ethylene glycol, pH 11.5 10% (v/v) dioxane at acid pH	Disrupt hydrophobic interactions

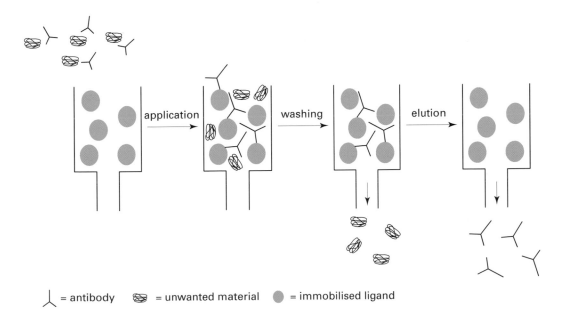

= antibody   = unwanted material   = immobilised ligand

Fig. 4.7. Diagrammatic representation of antibody purification by affinity chromatography.

purify mouse IgM, which contains 12% to 16% mannose-containing carbohydrate. Jacalin is a galactose-binding lectin that can be used to purify human IgA1.

Affinity chromatography techniques using immobilised antibodies are widely used to purify antigens.

4.3.5 Fragmentation and dissociation of immunoglobulins

Some applications of antibodies require the use of antibody fragments rather than the intact molecule (see Section 4.1.1). For example, removing the antibody Fc

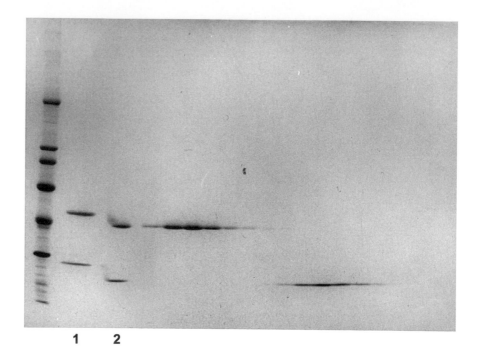

1   2

Fig. 4.8. Analysis of separated heavy and light chains of IgG using sodium dodecyl sulphate – polyacrylamide gel electrophoresis (SDS-PAGE). IgG was reduced and alkylated and the heavy and light chains were separated by gel filtration in propionic acid. The fractions were analysed by SDS-PAGE under non-reducing conditions. Lanes 1 and 2 show the reduced and alkylated IgG before gel filtration, analysed under reducing and non-reducing conditions, respectively. Note the apparent increase in size of the chains (lane 1) when analysed under conditions that reduce the intra-chain disulphide bonds. Molecular weight markers are on the left.

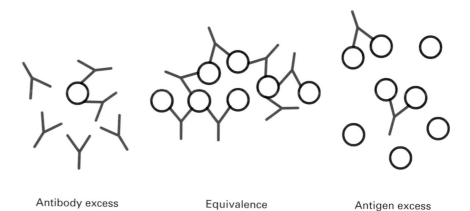

Antibody excess   Equivalence   Antigen excess

Fig. 4.9. Diagrammatic representation of immune complexes formed at varying antigen : antibody ratios. Immunoprecipitation occurs only when an insoluble antigen–antibody lattice is formed at the equivalence point.

portion will prevent binding of antibodies to Fc receptors present on leukocytes and other cells. This may be necessary if cell surface antigens recognised by the antibody are to be evaluated by, for example, immunofluorescence microscopy. The preparation of antibody fragments normally involves the use of proteolytic enzymes to cleave peptide bonds. Different enzymes can be used to cleave the heavy chain in specific places to give rise to different fragments. The most commonly used fragments are those produced by papain, pepsin and plasmin; their cleavage sites on IgG are shown in Fig. 4.1, with fragment nomenclature. These enzymes are available commercially either in soluble form or covalently coupled to Sepharose (an inert support), which facilitates removal of the enzyme when digestion is completed (the Sepharose and immobilised enzyme can be removed simply by centrifugation). Antibodies can also be dissociated into their constitutive chains. The heavy and light chains are joined by disulphide bridges that can be easily broken by a reducing agent such as dithiothreitol under conditions that leave the intrachain disulphide bonds intact. An alkylating agent such as iodoacetamide can then be used to ensure that the bonds do not reform. However, the heavy and light chains will still associate non-covalently unless a dissociating agent such as propionic acid is added. The chains can be separated on the basis of differing size by gel filtration (Fig. 4.8). Isolated immunoglobulin chains usually bind antigen less avidly than do the intact molecule and fragments such as Fab and $F(ab')_2$.

4.4 IMMUNOPRECIPITATION

An important property of many antibodies is their ability to precipitate antigens from solution. Antibodies are divalent (IgG) or multivalent (IgM), and if the antigen is also multivalent, the antibody–antigen interactions give rise to a molecular lattice that is too large to remain in solution, so precipitation occurs. The formation of an insoluble antibody–antigen complex is very dependent on antibody and antigen concentration, and occurs within a narrow concentration range known as the zone of equivalence. This represents the conditions under which macromolecular antigen/antibody complexes are formed that are sufficiently large to be precipitated. Outside the equivalence concentration, conditions known as antigen or antibody excess occur, which result in the formation of small, soluble complexes (see Fig. 4.9). However, precipitation never occurs with some monoclonal antibodies that recognise a single epitope on an antigen (i.e. a monovalent antigen) because a lattice is not formed.

Immunoprecipitation can be exploited in both agar techniques and in solution.

4.4.1 Agar and agarose immunoprecipitation

Agar is a high molecular weight polysaccharide derived from seaweed; agarose is a purified linear galactan hydrocolloid isolated from the same substance. Both dissolve in aqueous solutions upon heating and, upon cooling, form gels with a large pore size that allows most proteins, including antibodies, to diffuse through. If antibody migrating through the gel encounters antigen, an insoluble precipitate is commonly formed at equivalence. The precipitate can often be visualised as an opaque line in the gel (precipitin line); the use of a protein stain such as Coomassie Brilliant Blue allows visualisation of weak (invisible) precipitin lines. Protein antigens that are insoluble in physiological buffers (e.g. membrane or cytoskeletal proteins) can be solubilised in non-ionic detergents for analysis in detergent-containing gels without adversely affecting the formation of the precipitin line.

Precipitation techniques in agar are typically carried out using gels 2 to 3 mm thick, cast on glass (e.g. microscope) slides (warm agar solution is simply poured onto the slide and allowed to set). Wells are then cut into the gel using, for example, a large bore pipette. In diffusion techniques, antibody and/or antigen migrate through the gel by simple diffusion. In double diffusion, separate wells cut in the agar are filled with antibody and antigen, respectively (Fig. 4.10). Both diffuse into and through the agar, automatically forming concentration gradients. Provided these cover the equivalence concentrations, a precipitin line is formed at the equivalence point. The technique can be used to give information on antigenic (and hence structural) similarities or differences between antigens (Fig. 4.11).

In single radial immunodiffusion (SRID), antigen is loaded into wells cut in an agar gel containing a fixed concentration of antibody (Fig. 4.10). A precipitin ring around the well is formed at equivalence. The diameter of the ring at equivalence is related to the antigen concentration. Two relationships have been determined: (i) the square of the ring diameter is proportional to the antigen concentration (Mancini method; Fig. 4.12); (ii) the diameter of the ring is proportional to the log of the antigen concentration (Fahey and McKelvey method). This technique is useful for determining concentrations of antigens such as serum proteins. For example, if the agar contains specific antibodies against human IgG, and wells cut into the gel are loaded with test samples containing unknown quantities of human IgG (e.g. serum samples) together with calibrator samples containing known concentrations of human IgG, precipitin rings will form around the wells at equivalence. By measuring the ring diameters produced by the calibrator samples of known IgG concentration, a standard curve can be constructed by plotting the square of the diameter of the precipitin ring against the IgG concentration. The square of the ring diameters of the test samples can then be read off the standard curve to give the IgG concentration in the test samples (see Fig. 4.12).

In immunoelectrophoresis, a mixture of proteins containing the antigen are first separated by agar gel electrophoresis. Antibody is then allowed to diffuse through the gel from a trough cut in the gel parallel to the direction of electrophoresis (Fig. 4.10). Precipitin arcs are then formed where antibody meets antigen at equivalence. A disadvantage of this technique is the relatively poor resolution of antigen mixtures using agar gel electrophoresis, but it can be useful for detecting precipitating antibodies. Clinically, the technique is carried out on samples of patient's serum, concentrated urine or spinal fluid to detect abnormalities in

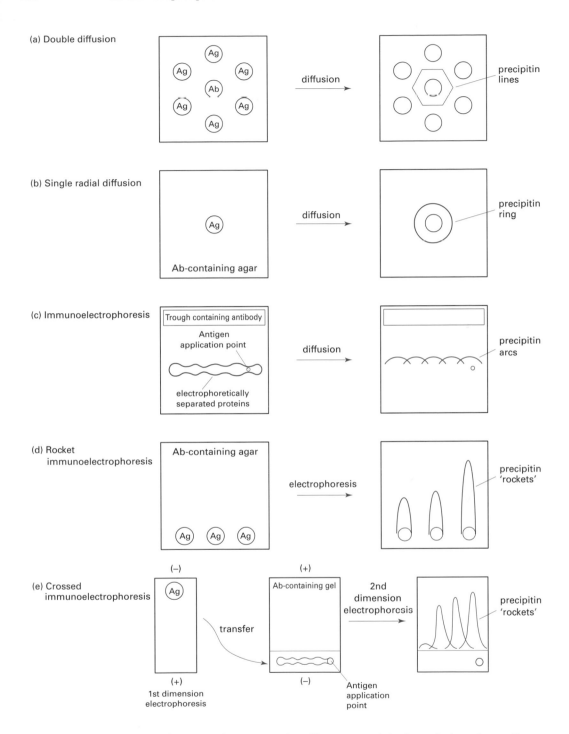

Fig. 4.10. Diagrammatic representation of immunoprecipitation techniques in agar. For details, see the text. Ag, antigen; Ab, antibody.

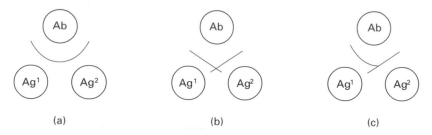

Fig. 4.11. Interpretation of precipitin lines following double immunodiffusion. Fusion of immunoprecipitin lines (a) infers immunochemical identity of antigens (Ag) 1 and 2, whereas crossing of the lines (b) shows their non-identity. Partial fusion or spur formation (c) suggests partial identity, i.e. antigen 2 has some determinants that are not shared by antigen 1, but all the determinants recognised by these antibodies (Ab) that are present on antigen 1 are also present on antigen 2.

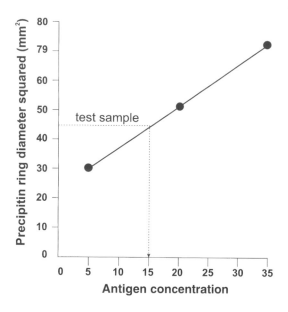

Fig. 4.12. The use of single radial immunodiffusion to measure antigen concentrations in test samples. The standard curve was constructed from the square of the precipitin ring diameters given by calibrator samples containing known amounts of antigen. The square of the precipitin ring diameters of the test samples can then be read from the standard curve to give the antigen concentration in the samples.

concentrations of antigens and/or the presence of abnormal proteins relative to normal control samples analysed at the same time.

Rocket immunoelectrophoresis is an adaption of single radial immunodiffusion and involves electrophoretic migration of antigen from wells cut in antibody-containing gel (Fig. 4.10). At equivalence, rocket-shaped precipitin lines are formed, the area under which is proportional to the antigen concentration. The technique can be used to determine antigen concentrations in unknown samples (e.g. serum protein levels) by reference to a standard curve as in RID, or to investigate immunochemical relationships between different samples if these are placed in adjacent wells close together (see Fig. 4.11 for interpretation of precipitin line patterns).

In crossed immunoelectrophoresis, proteins are first separated by agar gel electrophoresis, after which they are electrophoresed into an antibody-containing gel at right angles to the direction of the first electrophoresis (Fig. 4.10). The technique can be used for analysis of serum proteins.

The sensitivity of precipitation techniques in agar varies enormously depending on the antibodies and antigens involved.

4.4.2 Immunoprecipitation in solution

An antibody can be used specifically to immunoprecipitate its antigen from a mixture of proteins in solution, for example a cell lysate. If the immunoprecipitate is insoluble, it can be sedimented by centrifugation for analysis; soluble antibody–antigen complexes can be isolated by precipitation with an immunoglobulin-binding protein such as protein A or G, or an anti-immunoglobulin antibody, or those reagents covalently bound to an insoluble support such as agarose (see Section 4.3.4). This basic method forms the basis of classical radioimmunoassays (RIA) (see Section 4.7.1). It also allows the isolation of an unknown antigen from a mixture of proteins. For the latter, it may be necessary to label the mixture of proteins, for example cell lysate, with ^{125}I prior to immunoprecipitation. The immunoprecipitate can then be analysed by SDS-PAGE (Section 12.3.1) and autoradiography (Section 14.2.3) to give information on the antigen. Alternatively, non-radiolabelled immunoprecipitate can be analysed by SDS–PAGE and immunoblotting with antibodies of known specificity (Section 4.6), which can allow positive identification of immunoprecipitated proteins. Immunoprecipitation is commonly carried out on radiolabelled intact cells or cell membranes to give information on cell surface antigens (Fig. 4.13).

Although an antibody can be used to analyse individual proteins in a mixture separated by SDS–PAGE using immunoblotting procedures (Section 4.6), immunoprecipitation in solution has the advantage that the antibody is allowed to react with native rather than partially denatured antigen as is the case in immunoblots. Some antigens lose their immunoreactivity following electrophoresis and immunoblotting, or even (especially for cell surface antigens) solubilisation. This occurs when epitopes are conformation dependent or arise through the interaction of several protein subunits/components.

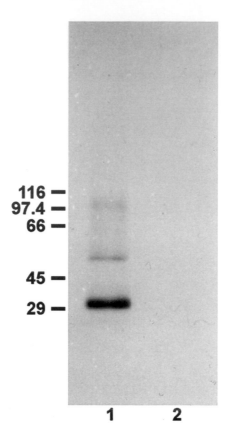

Fig. 4.13. Autoradiograph of monoclonal anti-Rh D immune precipitates from ^{125}I-labelled Rh D-positive and Rh D-negative erythrocyte membranes after analysis by SDS-PAGE. Human erythrocytes positive or negative for the Rh D blood group antigen were surface labelled with[125] I. The cells were lysed by hypotonic shock and the membranes incubated with monoclonal anti-Rh D. After being washed to remove unbound antibody, the membranes were solubilised and the antibody–antigen complexes isolated using protein A–Sepharose. The antibody–antigen complexes were then analysed by SDS-PAGE and autoradiography. The molecular weight of the major protein immunoprecipitated from Rh D-positive membranes is approximately 31 000 (lane 1) and corresponds to the Rh D polypeptide. No protein was immunoprecipitated from the Rh D-negative membranes (lane 2). The relative positions of the molecular weight markers are shown ($M_r \times 10^{-3}$).

4.5 LABELLING ANTIBODIES

The specificity of antibodies makes them powerful analytical tools. Although immunoprecipitation techniques in agar (see Section 4.4) result in visible precipitated antibody–antigen complexes, in most immunochemical assays binding of antibody to antigen can only be visualised by labelling the antibody (or sometimes antigen) or (more commonly) an antibody against immunoglobulin (see Section 4.5.1) with a marker that can be qualitatively and sometimes quantitatively detected. Thus an antibody can be labelled with a radioactive isotope for use

Table 4.7	**Common antibody labels for immunochemical techniques**	
Label	Examples	Main use(s)
Fluorochromes	Fluorescein	Immunohisto/cytochemistry; flow cytofluorimetry; fluorimetric assays
	Rhodamine	Immunohisto/cytochemistry; flow cyotfluorimetry
	Phycoerythrin	Flow cytofluorimetry
	Texas Red	Flow cytofluorimetry
	7-amino-4-methylcoumarin 3-acetate (AMCA)	Flow cytofluorimetry
	a BODIPY derivatives	Flow cytofluorimetry
	a Cascade Blue	Flow cytofluorimetry
Enzymes	AP	Immunohistochemistry; EIA; immunoblotting
	β-Galactosidase	As above
	HRP	As above; immunoelectron microscopy
	Glucose oxidase	Immunohistochemistry
	Urease	EIA
Radioisotope	^{125}I	Competitive and non-competitive RIA
Electron dense	Gold	Immunoelectron microscopy
	Ferritin	As above

BODIPY, 4,4-difluoro-4-bora-3a,4a–diaza-s-indacene; AP, alkaline phosphatase; EIA, enzyme immunometric assay; HRP, horseradish peroxidase.
a Trademark of Molecular Probes Inc.

in radioimmunoassays, or an enzyme which gives a coloured product for use in enzyme-linked immunosorbent assay (ELISA), or a fluorochrome which emits visible fluorescence for use in immunohistochemistry (Table 4.7). Binding of unlabelled antibody to antigen in these techniques would be undetectable. Antibodies labelled with fluorochromes or enzymes are commonly referred to as conjugates.

4.5.1 **Direct and indirect immunochemical procedures**

In simple, direct immunochemical procedures, the antibody against the antigen of interest (the 'primary' antibody) is conjugated with the label. In the more commonly used indirect procedures, binding of unlabelled primary antibody to the antigen is detected using a labelled antibody against immunoglobulin (or less commonly, a labelled bacterial immunoglobulin-binding protein such as protein A or protein G). This secondary antibody is usually raised against the immunoglobulin from the animal species in which the primary antibody was produced, and may also be class or subclass specific. Direct and indirect procedures are illus-

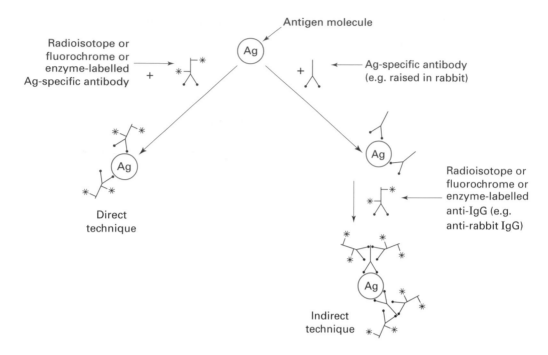

Fig. 4.14. Diagrammatic representation of direct and indirect immunochemical methodology. Ag, antigen.

trated diagrammatically in Fig. 4.14. Indirect methods utilising labelled anti-immunoglobulin antibodies have several advantages over direct procedures: they are more sensitive, since several labelled anti-immunoglobulin molecules can bind to each unlabelled primary antibody, resulting in a stronger signal; each primary antibody does not have to be labelled individually as, for example, labelled rabbit anti-mouse IgG antibodies will recognise all mouse IgG monoclonal antibodies; and there is no risk of loss of reactivity of the primary antibody as a result of direct labelling. However, there are cases that necessitate the use of directly labelled antibodies (see Sections 4.8.3 and 4.8.5). A semi-direct procedure takes advantage of the high affinity specific interaction between biotin and avidin/streptavidin (see Section 4.5.5) and involves the use of biotinylated primary antibody and labelled avidin/streptavidin preparations.

4.5.2 **Radiolabelling**

Radioiodination

The most commonly used radioisotope for radiolabelling antibodies is [125]I. This isotope is readily available as Na[125]I, is relatively inexpensive and has a high specific activity. It emits γ-radiation, which can be easily and directly detected and quantified using a γ-counter, and is good for autoradiography. However, suitable

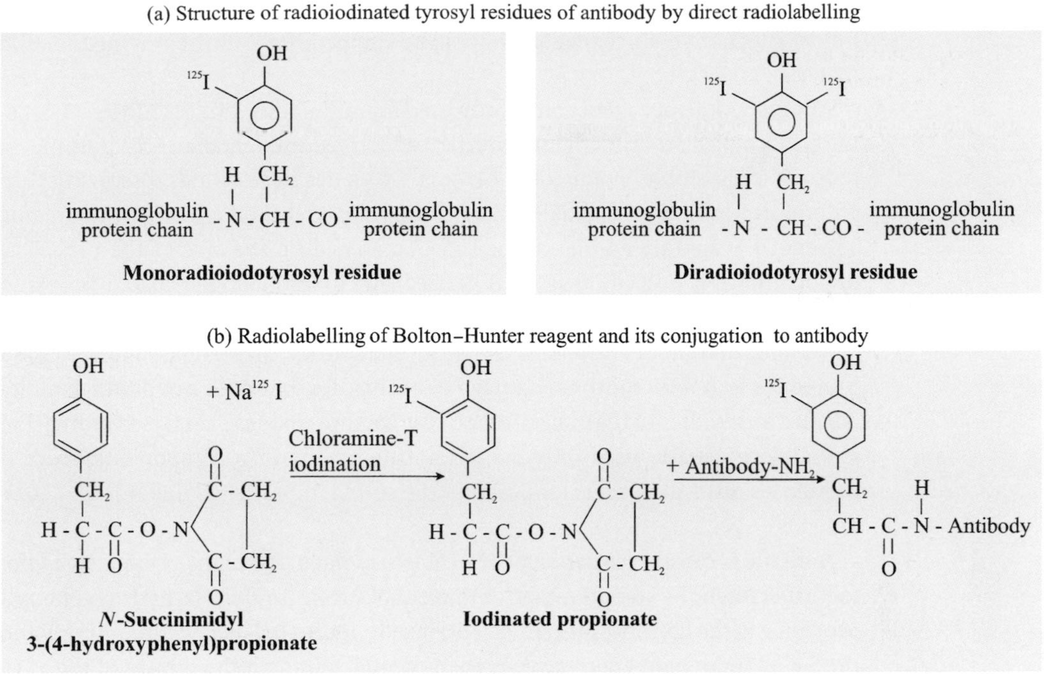

(a) Structure of radioiodinated tyrosyl residues of antibody by direct radiolabelling

Monoradioiodotyrosyl residue

Diradioiodotyrosyl residue

(b) Radiolabelling of Bolton–Hunter reagent and its conjugation to antibody

N-Succinimidyl
3-(4-hydroxyphenyl)propionate

Iodinated propionate

Fig. 4.15. Direct and indirect radiolabelling of antibodies with ^{125}I.

precautions must be taken to minimise exposure of workers to radiation and to prevent contact, contamination and ingestion (the thyroid is particularly susceptible). Covalent labelling of proteins directly with ^{125}I involves oxidative generation of cationic iodine (I$^+$) and its spontaneous electrophilic addition to tyrosine residues, and, to a lesser extent, to tryptophan and histidine residues. The major substitution is a monoiodotyrosyl residue, although di-iodotyrosyl residues may also be formed (Fig. 4.15). The concentrations of reagents should allow for only one or two tyrosine residues per antibody molecule to be ^{125}I-labelled otherwise loss of immunoreactivity and/or radiation damage may occur.

There are several established methods for radioiodination, which differ in the choice of oxidising agent used to generate I$^+$. Since strong oxidising agents can destroy the immunoreactivity of antibodies, there must be a compromise between efficient generation of I$^+$ and preservation of antigen-binding capacity.

Chloramine T (*N*-chloro-*p*-toluene sulphonamide) is an aromatic oxidising agent commonly used for high specific activity iodination of antibodies and other proteins. Chloramine T iodination is very rapid (45 s), but it can denature antibodies and lead to loss of antigen-binding capacity. The reaction must be stopped quickly after appropriate iodination, by adding a reducing agent such as sodium metabisulphite or an excess of tyrosine to 'mop up' iodine as iodotyrosine. Following radioiodination, the antibody needs to be separated from free (i.e. non-antibody bound) ^{125}I. This can be achieved either by gel filtration, or if IgG antibody has been radiolabelled, a strongly basic anion exchanger can be used to adsorb iodotyrosine. The use of chloramine T immobilised on beads offers a milder alternative, since the reaction can be stopped simply by removing the solid material.

Another oxidising agent commonly used for radioiodination is iodogen (1,3,4,6-tetrachloro-3α, 6α-diphenylglycoluril), which is milder than chloramine T. Iodogen is insoluble in aqueous solvents, so its use necessitates dissolving it in chloroform or benzene, usually in a plastic tube, and then allowing the organic solvent to evaporate and leave the iodogen coated on the side of the tube. The radioiodination procedure is then carried out in the iodogen-coated tube and stopped by taking the solution out of the tube.

Radioiodination of antibodies using the enzyme lactoperoxidase is a very mild procedure that does minimal damage to antibodies, but does not produce radio-labelled antibodies of high specific activity. Lactoperoxidase-catalysed iodination is therefore usually used only for iodinating cell surface components, since it minimises diffusion of reactants across the cell membrane to label internal components.

Antibodies can also be conjugated with low molecular weight, previously radio-iodinated phenolic compounds. Commonly, N-succinimidyl 3-(4-hydroxyphenyl) propionate (the Bolton–Hunter reagent) is radioiodinated using chloramine T and the 5-[^{125}I] iodophenyl derivative is then conjugated to amino groups of the antibody (Fig. 4.15). The advantage of indirectly radiolabelling antibodies in this way is that there is no risk of oxidative damage, but, as with direct labelling, only one or two residues per antibody molecule should be conjugated with the iodophenyl derivative.

4.5.3 Labelling with fluorochromes

Fluorochromes emit fluorescent light under ultraviolet illumination. The fluorescence of fluorochrome-labelled antibody in solution can be quantified using a fluorimeter. However, the greatest use of fluorochrome-labelled antibodies is in immunohisto/cytochemistry where binding of fluorochrome-labelled antibodies to tissue sections or cells is visualised using a microscope equipped with fluorescence optics (Section 4.8.3). Antibodies labelled with fluorochromes are used extensively in flow cytometric techniques (Section 4.8.5).

Many fluorochromes are available with different excitation and emission spectra, but the ones most commonly used for microscopy are fluorescein, which emits green fluorescence, and tetramethylrhodamine, which emits red fluorescence. For conjugation, fluorescein and tetramethylrhodamine isothiocyanate are usually used, they readily form covalent linkages with primary amine groups on lysine residues in the antibody molecule (Fig. 4.16), although iodoacetamido derivatives of fluorescein and rhodamine are also available for coupling via sulphydryl groups. Other fluorochromes, mostly used in flow cytofluorimetry, and which can be coupled to amine (or sulphydryl groups) include Texas Red (sulphorhodamine; Fig. 4.16), 7-amino-4-methylcoumarin 3-acetate (AMCA; fluoresces blue) and BODIPY (4,4-difluoro-4-bora-3a,4a-diaza-s-indacene).

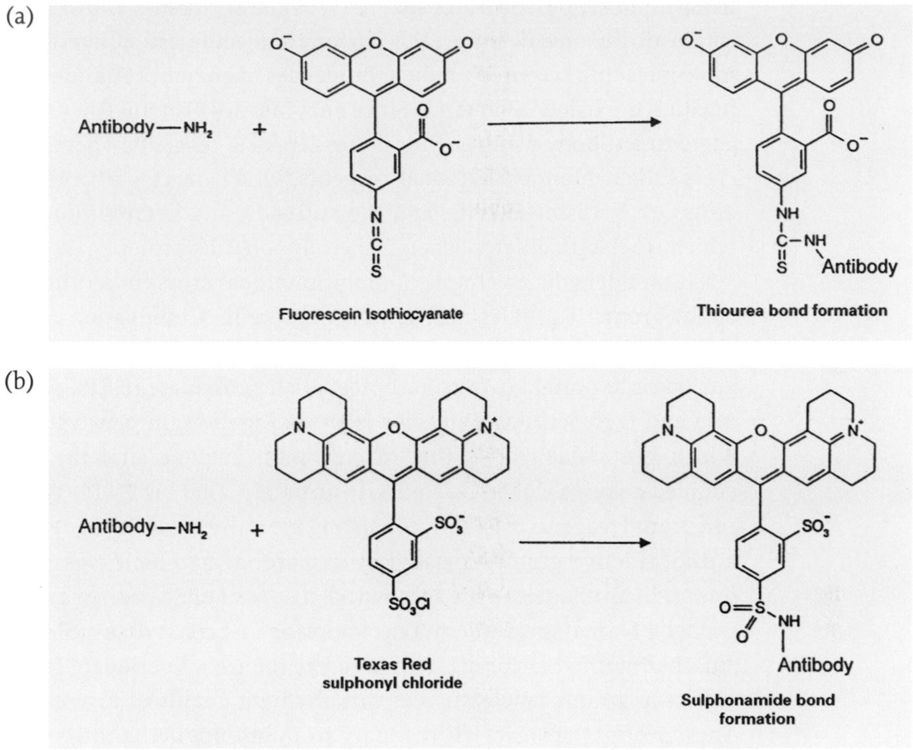

(a)

(b)

Fig. 4.16. Conjugation of (a) fluorescein isothiocyanate and (b) Texas Red (sulphorhodamine) to amine groups of antibody.

Phycobiliproteins are a group of intensely fluorescent proteins found in algae and cyanobacteria and widely used in flow cytofluorimetry. They include B- and R-phycoerythrin (M_r 240 000), C-phycocyanin (M_r 72 000) and allophycocyanin (M_r 110 000). Phycobiliproteins can be attached via their amine groups to the thiol groups of the antibody, using chemical heterobifunctional cross-linking agents (Section 4.5.4).

4.5.4 Labelling with enzymes

Enzyme-labelled antibodies are widely used in immunoassays (e.g. ELISA), immunoblotting and immunohisto/cytochemistry. In each case, direct or indirect binding (Section 4.5.1) of the enzyme-labelled antibody to antigen (which may be in tissue sections or on blots or on the wells of a microtitre plate) is visualised by carrying out the enzyme reaction in which a colourless substrate is converted to a coloured product. In enzyme immunoassays, the product needs to be soluble to allow spectrophotometric quantification; in immunoblotting and immunohistochemical procedures, the product must be insoluble to allow precise localisation of the initial antigen–antibody interaction and visible either directly by eye or using microscopy. The use of enzyme-labelled antibodies allows catalytic amplification of the signal, since each enzyme molecule can convert many substrate molecules into coloured product. Properties of enzymes commonly used for conjugation are listed in Table 4.8. Since enzymes are proteins, they have to be conjugated to antibody using chemical cross-linking reagents. There are two types of cross-linker: homobifunctional reagents, which react with the same chemical group on both the enzyme and the antibody, and heterobifunctional reagents, which react with different chemical groups on each protein.

Glutaraldehyde is a simple homobifunctional cross-linker that cross-links the amine groups (e.g. of lysine; Fig. 4.17) of proteins. Conjugation can be carried out either in a one-step procedure in which the glutaraldehyde is added to a mixture of enzyme and protein (works for horseradish peroxidase (HRP), alkaline phosphatase and β-galactosidase), or, for HRP conjugation, in a two-step procedure in which glutaraldehyde is first reacted with enzyme, and the glutaraldehyde-coupled enzyme is then reacted with antibody. There is a wide range of heterobifunctional reagents available, consisting typically of an amine-reactive group and a thiol-reactive group separated by a spacer arm, which cross-links the amine groups of antibodies to the sulphydryl groups of enzymes. An example is succinimidyl-4-(N-maleimidomethyl)cyclohexane 1-carboxylate (SMCC; Fig. 4.17). Another method of conjugation involves the use of periodate to generate active aldehyde groups by cleavage of carbohydrate chains of glycoprotein enzymes. These groups then react with primary amine groups in the antibody to form Schiff bases, which are then reduced to produce stable bonds.

4.5.5 Biotinylation of antibodies

The very high affinity interaction (affinity constant $> 10^{15}$ M^{-1}) between biotin (vitamin H; M_r 244) and avidin (a protein from egg white) or streptavidin (a protein from the bacterium *Streptomyces avidinii*) can be exploited in immunochemical techniques by conjugating biotin to antibodies for use with fluorochrome- or enzyme-conjugated or radiolabelled avidin/streptavidin (Fig. 4.18). Antibodies can be conjugated easily with biotin derivatives, most commonly N-hydroxysuccinimidobiotin or analogues incorporating a spacer arm. The latter reduces steric hinderance by increasing the distance between the biotin and the antibody. Most of these biotin derivatives react with primary amine groups, although there are some which are reactive with thiol groups or carbohydrate residues on the immunoglobulin.

4.6 IMMUNOBLOTTING

In many cases it is informative to establish the specificity of antibodies by investigating their ability to recognise components present in complex mixtures. Specific antibodies can also be used to identify such components and establish cross-reactivities that may occur with immunochemically related molecular species. For such methods it is clearly necessary to separate the antigenic

Table 4.8 Properties of enzymes used for conjugation to antibodies

Enzyme	Source	Structure	Reaction catalysed
Peroxidase	Horseradish	Monomeric glycoprotein M_r 40 000	H_2O_2 + oxidisable substrate $\rightarrow$ oxidised product + $2H_2O$
Alkaline phosphatase	Calf intestine (usually)	Zn^{2+}-containing glycoprotein	R-O-P + H_2O $\rightarrow$ R-OH + P_i orthophosphoric monoester substrate alcohol inorganic phosphate
β-Galactosidase	*E. coli*	Multimeric protein (4 subunits) M_r 540 000	β-D-Galactoside + H_2O $\rightarrow$ galactose + alcohol
Glucose oxidase	*Aspergillus niger*	Flavo-glycoprotein	β-D-glucose + O_2 $\rightarrow$ H_2O_2 + gluconic acid
Urease	Jack bean	M_r 480 000	$(NH_2)_2CO$ + $3H_2O$ $\rightarrow$ CO_2 + $2NH_4OH$

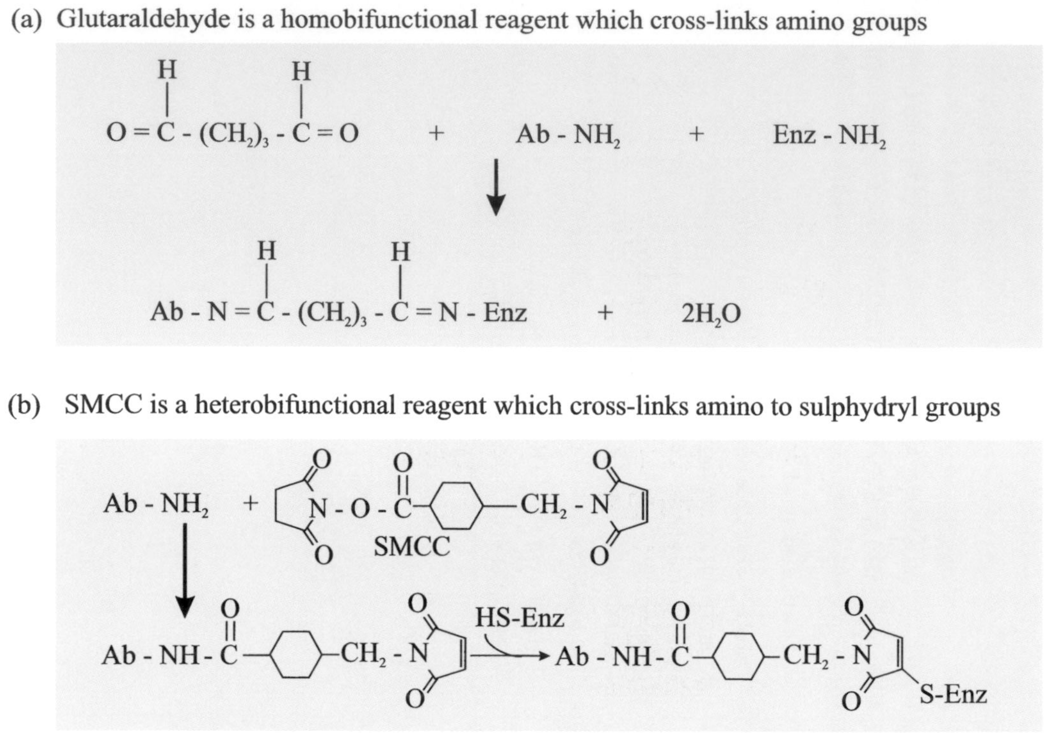

(a) Glutaraldehyde is a homobifunctional reagent which cross-links amino groups

$$O = \overset{\overset{\displaystyle H}{|}}{C} - (CH_2)_3 - \overset{\overset{\displaystyle H}{|}}{C} = O \quad + \quad Ab - NH_2 \quad + \quad Enz - NH_2$$

$$Ab - N = \overset{\overset{\displaystyle H}{|}}{C} - (CH_2)_3 - \overset{\overset{\displaystyle H}{|}}{C} = N - Enz \quad + \quad 2H_2O$$

(b)   SMCC is a heterobifunctional reagent which cross-links amino to sulphydryl groups

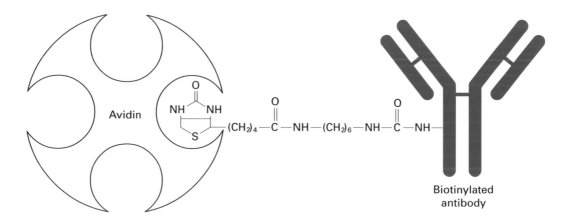

Fig. 4.17. (a) and (b) Structure and mode of action of cross-linking reagents. Ab, antibody; Enz, enzyme.

Fig. 4.18. The interaction of biotin-conjugated IgG with avidin. The binding is very strong and each avidin molecule has four biotin binding sites. For the structure shown, coupling of biotin to immunoglobulin has been carried out using biotinamidocaproate N-hydroxysuccinimide ester.

(a)   (b)

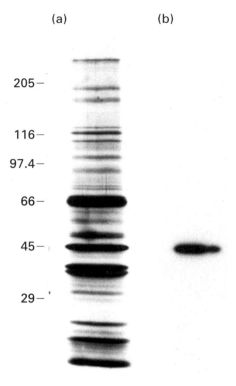

205—

116—

97.4—

66—

45—

29—

Fig. 4.19. Use of immunoblotting to show how specific antibodies can be used to identify their antigens in complex mixtures. Components of smooth muscle homogenate were separated using SDS-PAGE in duplicate tracks. One track was protein-stained to allow visualisation of all the components present in the homogenate (lane A); components in the second track were electrophoretically transferred to nitrocellulose and incubated with mouse monoclonal antibody against smooth muscle α-actin followed by ^{125}I-labelled anti-mouse IgG. Following autoradiography, one protein band is immunostained (lane B) corresponding to smooth muscle α-actin. The relative positions of molecular weight markers ($\times 10^{-3}$) are shown.

components using an analytical method. In theory, any biochemical technique can be used for this, but the high resolving power of polyacrylamide gel electro-phoretic methods (especially SDS–PAGE and isoelectric focusing; see Sections 12.3.1 and 12.3.4) makes these ideal for such purposes. The most commonly used technique involves transferring separated proteins from polyacrylamide gels to a porous membrane and probing this 'blot' with antibody (antibody can be applied directly to the gel, but the very limited permeability of polyacrylamide gel makes this inefficient and time-consuming). Antibody–antigen complexes are then detected either by the use of labelled anti-immunoglobulin reagent or by labelling the antibody directly with radioisotope (^{125}I is usually employed for this) or enzyme (see Section 4.5). Antigens recognised by antibody thus appear as 'bands' on autoradiographs or substrate-developed blots and comparison of these with protein-stained gels allows identification of antigens recognised by antibody (Fig. 4.19). This process shows some similarity to Southern and northern blotting used with nucleic acid and is known as immunoblotting or 'western' blotting (see also Section 12.3.9).

Nitrocellulose is normally employed as the porous membrane for immunoblotting, but other materials are also occasionally used. Increased sensitivity with immunoblotting can be obtained by the use of enhanced chemiluminescence (ECL) development. In ECL-linked immunoblotting, peroxidase-conjugated anti-immunoglobulin is used to detect antigen–antibody complexes (cf. ELISA; Section 4.7.3). This enzyme is used to generate a peracid by cleavage of hydrogen peroxide and this in turn oxidises a substrate to yield light, which is detected using X-ray film (as for autoradiography). The substrate is normally luminol, and phenolic 'enhancer' compounds are included to increase photon yield. Other ECL systems have been developed for use with alkaline phosphatase conjugates. ECL detection is sensitive and fast compared to direct use of enzyme or radioisotope conjugates. Other chemiluminiscence amplification systems suitable for use in immunoblotting involving different enzymes, substrates and enhancers are also available.

4.7 IMMUNOASSAYS

Many immunochemical techniques provide quantitative assessment of the concentration of analyte in pure solutions or complex mixtures, for example single radial immunodiffusion and rocket immunoelectrophoresis (Section 4.4.1). However, the great potential of the application of immunochemistry to sensitive and specific assay of a diverse range of chemical and biological molecules has led to very considerable effort being focused in this area. Many versions of basic immunochemical assay principles now exist; such methodologies are termed immunoassays to emphasise their quantitative aspect.

Refinements to immunoassay methodology for research purposes have been driven mainly by the need for ever greater specificity and particularly sensitivity. Immunoassays are widely used for routine diagnostic/prognostic purposes and other applications (e.g. measuring levels of enviromental contaminants such as pesticides and toxic by-products of industrial processes); techniques that allow high sample throughput, ease of automation (robotic processing is often used), economy, robustness, precision and accuracy have been developed and are being sought. A thorough description of all alternative immunoassay techniques and formats would occupy several volumes, but the general principles and some of the more frequently employed options are described below.

4.7.1 Competitive binding immunoassays

In competitive binding immunoassays, antigen present in the samples to be assayed competes with a fixed amount of labelled antigen in the presence of a limiting quantity of antibody. When the system has reached equilibrium, free antigen is separated from antibody-bound antigen and the amount of labelled antigen present in the latter determined by scintillation (for β emission) or γ counting.

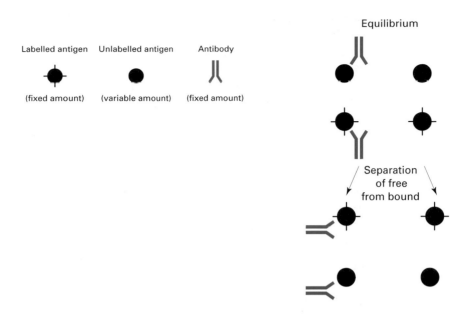

Fig. 4.20. Diagrammatic representation of competitive binding (inhibition) immunoassay.

This is inversely proportional to the concentration of antigen present in the samples (see Fig. 4.20). Inclusion of a number of dilutions of a standard solution of known antigen content allows the construction of a dose–response curve (often known as a standard curve), which can be used, by comparison, to derive antigen concentrations in samples. The earliest immunoassays were of this type, and the most common label used was a radioisotope (^{3}H, ^{125}I). Such assays are normally known as radioimmunoassays (RIAs), although they should be called competitive binding radioimmunoassays to distinguish them from radiobinding assays (Section 4.7.3). The first RIA described was for insulin, and similar approaches using binding proteins rather than antibodies were also developed at this time, for example for vitamin B12. The sensitivity of such assays varies considerably and depends on several factors, such as the label used. RIAs using ^{125}I labels can theoretically reach a sensitivity of 10^{-14}M, but in practice this is usually $\leq 10^{-12}$M. In developing an RIA, it is initially necessary to derive an antibody versus labelled antigen binding curve to select appropriate antibody and labelled antigen concentrations for the assay. Normally, conditions at which 50% to 70% of the labelled antigen is bound by antibody are selected for the competitive RIA. Numerous procedures have been developed for separating free from bound antigen (see Table 4.9).

RIAs have been produced for a wide range of analytes from small molecules (e.g. steroids, peptide hormones in human or animal serum/plasma) to large proteins (e.g. serum levels of α_2-macroglobulin, immunoglobulins). They can be precise, accurate and economical (very small amounts of antibody are required). However,

Table 4.9 Methods for separating bound and free labeled ligand in radio-immunoassays

Method	Principle
Coated charcoal	Adsorption of bound or free fraction
Florisil	
S. aureus – protein A	
Polyethylene glycol	Fractional precipitation of bound fraction
Ethanol	
Ammonium sulphate	
Second antibody	Precipitation of bound fraction
soluble	
solid phase – cellulose	
– magnetic particles	
First antibody	Precipitation of bound fraction
solid phase – coated disks and tubes	
– cellulose	
– magnetic particles	

they are difficult to automate, take a relatively long time and the dose–response curve usually covers only a relatively narrow range of analyte concentration. They can be less sensitive than some other immunoassays. It is also necessary to establish systems for containment and disposal of radioactive reagents and for medical surveillance of staff involved in use of RIA methods. This bureaucracy has resulted in a reduction in use of RIA technology.

As the antibody concentrations used are limiting, competitive binding assays are sometimes called reagent (antigen) excess immunoassays (cf. immunometric assays; Section 4.7.2). Competitive immunoassays using non-radioisotope labels have been developed, but this approach is rather disappointing. Use of enzyme labels often results in insensitive assays and other labelling options can produce non-robust, imprecise and insensitive assays. The reason for this is not always clear, but labelling antigen with relatively bulky enzyme molecules (rather than the small atoms used in RIA) can alter antibody recognition of labelled compared with unlabelled antigen species, causing assay problems. This limitation has resulted in decreasing use of competitive immunoassay technology.

4.7.2 **Immunometric assays**

Immunometric assays differ from competitive immunoassays in several ways, although they provide similar quantitative information concerning antigen concentration. In the first-described immunometric assays, a fixed amount of labelled antibody was allowed to react with variable amounts of antigen. Unbound labelled antibody was then removed by washing and the labelled antibody remaining measured to provide an estimate of the antigen content (see Fig. 4.21). This approach is rarely used nowadays, but the concept of using an excess of

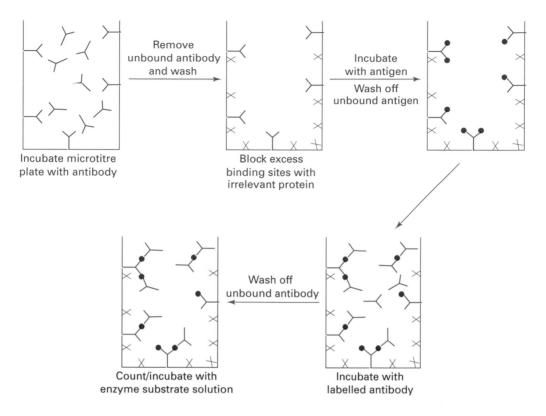

Fig. 4.21. Diagrammatic representation of a two-site immunometric assay (IRMA or two-site ELISA) for estimation of antigens. This particular format uses 96-well microtitre plates.

labelled antibody, i.e. antibody excess immunoassays, rather than excess of labelled antigen (antigen excess immunoassays, i.e. competitive immunoassays) has numerous advantages and a few disadvantages (see below).

In most recently devised immunometric assays, antigen is allowed to react with insoluble or immobilised antibody, i.e. is 'captured' from solution, and the bound antigen is then detected using an excess of another (or in some special cases the same) antibody specific for the antigen. Captured antibody can be immobilised by covalent attachment to agarose microbeads, or by electrostatic binding to plastic or glass beads or the surfaces of plastic tubes or microtitre plates (see Fig. 4.22). The latter option is most often used, and special plates are available that have been treated to optimise antigen binding. Some methods use immobilised anti-Fc immunoglobulin to ensure the captured antibody is immobilised in the correct orientation to interact optimally with antigen.

The detecting antibody can be directly labelled or can be indirectly measured using labelled anti-immunoglobulin reagent or other approaches, for example the avidin–biotin interaction (Section 4.5.5). Immunometric assays are usually relatively fast to carry out, can be very sensitive, and cover a wider range of analyte concentration than competitive assays. However, they require more antibody

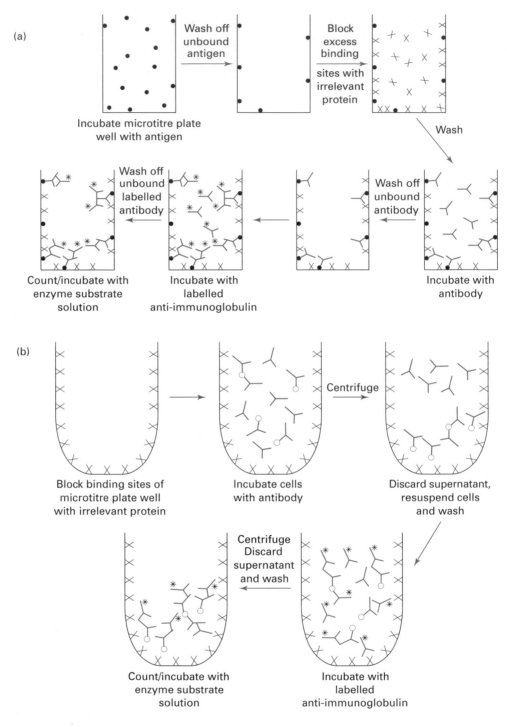

Fig. 4.22. Diagrammatic representation of microtitre plate format solid-phase binding immunoassays: (a) for antibodies directed against soluble antigens; (b) for antibodies directed against cell surface antigens.

than competitive assays and normally two antibodies that recognise different determinants on the antigen are needed. Some immunometric assay formats (especially those employing microtitre plate layouts; see Fig. 4.21) can be automated and performed and controlled robotically to enable very high sample throughput.

Immunometric assays using radiolabelled antibody have been developed for a wide range of analytes and the first such assays were of this type. They are known as immunoradiometric assays (IRMAs). Even more immunometric assays using enzyme-labelled antibodies have been produced and these should be referred to as enzyme immunometric assays (EIAs or EIMAs). However, they are often unfortunately called ELISAs, which confuses them with enzyme-linked immunobinding assays (Section 4.7.3). To try to distinguish them from 'real' ELISAs, they are often called sandwich ELISAs or two-site ELISAs. Most enzyme immunometric assays use a colorimetric substrate that is measured spectrophotometrically to determine antigen concentration. However, fluorescent substrates can be used for some enzymes (such as β-galactosidase) that have been claimed to increase assay sensitivity. An ever-increasing range of other labelling systems have been devised for immunometric assays and some of these are described in Section 4.7.4. All immunometric assays require calibration using dilutions of a standard solution of analyte of known concentration (cf. competitive immunoassays). The requirement that immunometric assay theory requires antibodies recognising different epitopes on antigen limited their application until the advent of monoclonal antibody technology (Section 4.2). Polyclonal antibodies can be used for immunometric assays, but unless the antigen is polymeric this approach is of limited use owing to occupation, by the capture antibody, of the antibody-binding sites recognised by the detecting antibody. The use of two monoclonal antibodies recognising different antigenic epitopes that do not display steric hindrance for binding of either antibody allows optimisation of immunometric assays. Combination of the use of a monoclonal antibody (for capture) with polyclonal detecting antibody can provide sensitive and specific immunoassays. Selection of appropriate antibodies and producing antibody preparations of appropriate quality are crucial for successful immunometric assays.

4.7.3 Solid-phase immunobinding assays (for estimation of antibody)

Immunobinding assays are solid phase assays using immobilised antigen for assessing the antibody content of samples. They are often regarded as immunoassays, although their value for accurate quantification of antibody concentration can be questioned (if accuracy is important it is usually better to use an immunometric or competitive binding assay; Sections 4.7.1 and 4.7.2). However, immunobinding assays are very easy, quick, cheap and simple, and are ideal for checking the comparative antibody content of sera and other biological fluids and especially for screening sera from immunised animals, hybridoma culture supernatants, ascitic fluid and pathological samples. Antigen-containing solution is simply incubated in plastic tubes or (more often) in the wells of plastic microtitre plates, which allows a (small) proportion of the protein to coat the surfaces of the tubes or wells. After unbound antigen(s) has been washed away, the samples of known or unknown antibody content are incubated in the antigen-coated tubes/wells. Antibody (if present) binds to the immobilised antigen(s) and, after washing, can be detected using labelled anti-immunoglobulin or immunoglobulin-binding protein (see Fig. 4.22). Such assays, which use radiolabelled antibody or antibody-binding protein are nomally called solid-phase radiobinding assays, but most assays used nowadays employ enzyme-labelled detecting reagent. They are usually called enzyme-linked immunosorbent assays (ELISAs) but can be referred to as solid-phase enzyme immunobinding assays. Unfortunately, enzyme immunometric assays are also often called ELISAs (Section 4.7.2) and to try to avoid confusion, the immunometric version is sometimes called two-site ELISA whereas the binding assay type is known as one-site ELISA. As antigen is simply captured onto tube or well surfaces by non-specific binding, such assays are occasionally known as sticky plate assays or (especially when complex impure antigen solution is used) as dirty plate techniques.

Quantification can be achieved by comparison with a standard solution of known antibody content, but this can be difficult largely due to the heterogeneity of immunoglobulin molecules present. It is very common to express comparative results as a titre derived from dose–response curves generated using different samples. Mid-point titres, i.e. the dilution at which 50% maximal binding is achieved, are the usual way of calculating the titre, but this requires the maximal value of the dose–response curve to be the same for all samples. The use of end-point titres, i.e. the minimal dilution at which no signal is generated, is unreliable and very often invalid.

A variant of conventional solid-phase immunobinding assays, usually known as dot blot assays are occasionally encountered. For these techniques, antigen-containing solution is spotted, dried onto nitrocellulose filters and then incubated with samples with suspected antibody content. Any antigen-specific antibodies are then detected by using an enzyme-labelled or radiolabelled anti-immunoglobulin or antibody-binding protein. Advantages of the method are that antigen can be concentrated by repeat spotting at a single location on the filter, and that many antigen samples can be incubated with a single antibody sample. A major disadvantage is that valid quantification of results is virtually impossible. The name of the technique is misleading as no blotting actually occurs at any stage of the assay; it probably relates to many technical similarities with immunoblotting (see Section 4.6). A possibly better name is dot immunobinding assay, but this is not often used.

4.7.4 Enhanced Immunoassays

The quest for evermore sensitive immunoassays has resulted in the design of amplification systems to enhance the signal derived from the immunoassay (cf. immunoblotting; Section 4.6). Most of these are based on the enzyme immunometric assay (two-site ELISA) format and are carried out in microtitre plates. Several different amplification systems have been developed but a commonly

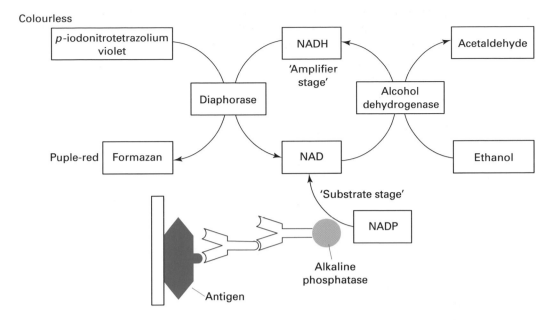

Fig. 4.23. Substrate amplification system for the detection of alkaline phosphatase.

encountered system is enzyme-linked, and is added as a 'cassette' to a conventional alkaline phosphatase-based two-site immunometric assay. In this, the alkaline phosphatase is used to dephosphorylate NADP + to produce NAD+. The NAD+ comprises the limiting concentration reagent of an alcohol dehydrogenase cata-lysed loop in which the NAD+ is reduced to NADH and this in turn generates a coloured formazan by reduction from the oxidised leukoformazan (see Fig. 4.23). The additional enzyme-catalysed loop amplifies the original signal considerably compared to that which could be produced from the alkaline phosphatase conju-gate alone. Another popular amplification system, known as the ELISA amplifica-tion system or ELAST (see Fig. 4.24) uses a standard peroxidase-based immunometric assay, but involves incorporation of a biotinylated tyramine reagent that, when oxidised (by the peroxidase conjugate), binds covalently to tyrosine or tryptophan residues present on the excess of blocking protein used to coat antigen-unoccupied sites on the microtitre plate surface. The immobilised biotin is then detected using labelled streptavidin (Section 4.5.5). The amplifica-tion system results in a far greater number of immobilised biotin molecules than would arise from the use of a simple biotin-labelled antibody.

Amplification systems almost always result in enhanced signal, but this often affects both the 'real' analyte-derived output and the assay background. At worst, this can simply increase the total assay signal but not improve sensitivity. Unless care is shown, use of potent amplification systems can result in less robust assays, with increased chance of assay artefacts.

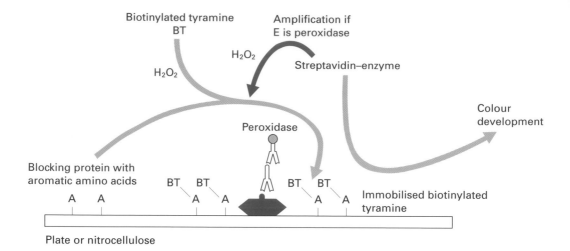

Fig. 4.24. Principles of the ELAST amplification system.

4.7.5 Peptide-based immunobinding assays (peptide mapping, epitope mapping)

Synthetic peptides can be substituted for antigen in solid-phase immunobinding assays. This allows detection of antibodies with known epitope specificity and also the determination of the epitope specificity of new antibodies (peptide mapping or epitope mapping). For the latter, a series of overlapping sequence peptides are made, covering the entire primary structure of the antigen and used sequentially to coat the wells of microtitre plates. Incubation with either labelled antibody or antibody followed by labelled anti-immunoglobulin allows the identification of peptides recognised by the antibody and therefore elucidation of the epitope(s) recognised by the antibody(s). This approach is especially useful with monoclonal antibodies. Usually peptides of 10 to 18 residues length are used, with an overlap of about 5 to 8 residues. The procedure is simple and valuable, but is limited to detection of 'linear' antigenic determinants and care must be taken to ensure that all the peptides bind efficiently to microtitre plate well surfaces. Coating the wells with polylysine can improve peptide binding (it produces a relatively strong positively charged surface) or they can be synthesised with biotin end-residues and captured with streptavidin-coated plates (this also optimises orientation on binding). It is also possible to synthesise peptides on 'pins' formed in the wells of special plates and use these for mapping (the pepscan procedure). The 'pin' heads are chemically activated to ensure binding of activated amino acid residues to be added sequentially thus building the required peptide sequence.

4.7.6 Fluorescence- and photoluminescence-based immunoassays

In attempts to increase assay sensitivity and ease, a variety of adaptions of the basic competitive and especially immunometric immunoassay methods have

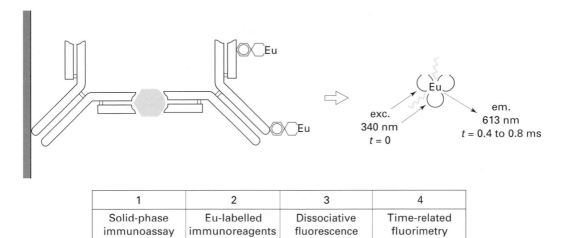

1	2	3	4
Solid-phase immunoassay	Eu-labelled immunoreagents	Dissociative fluorescence enhancement	Time-related fluorimetry

Fig. 4.25. The dissociative fluorescence enhancement principle exemplified in a two-site sandwich assay. exc., excitation; em., emission.

been developed and involve fluorescence or luminescence readouts. At their simplest, these substitute fluorescent or luminiscent substrates for the colorimetric substrates normally used for two-site ELISAs. These are called fluorimetric EIAs or enzyme-linked fluorescence immunoassays (ELFIAs) and luminoimmunoassays (LIAs) or enzyme-linked chemiluminescence immunoassays (ECLIAs), respectively. However, some assays use sufficiently different approaches to be considered separately (see below).

4.7.7 Delayed enhanced lanthanide fluorescence immunoassay

Most delayed enhanced lanthanide fluorescence immunoassays (DELFIAs) use the standard two-site immunometric assay principle and are carried out in microtitre plates. The detecting antibody (see Fig. 4.25) is labelled directly with a lanthanide (these are 4f transition metals – europium is usually used in DELFIA) that is non-covalently coupled via a chelating agent such as diethylenetriaminepenta-acetic anhydride (DTPA) or diethylenetriaminetetra-acetic anhydride (DTTA). After carrying out the immunometric assay, the lanthanide is released from the antibody by lowering the pH to about 3.2 (the chelates are unstable at this pH) and free lanthanide is then captured using a soluble diketone. This is complexed into micelles, which prevents subsequent quenching of fluorescence (the so-called enhancer step). The antibody–lanthanide chelates are not fluorescent, but the captured, micelle-bound lanthanide ion is, and this permits its detection. The peak fluorescence emission of miscelle-complexed lanthanides is relatively slow and this allows delayed measurement of light output after addition of the enhancing reagents. By this means, artefactual immediate autofluorescence due to sample components etc. can be distinguished from the later 'real' lanthanide signal.

Because of this, such assays are often called time-resolved immunofluorimetric assays (TRIFMA). In such assays, the fluorescence is proportional to the amount of antigen present in samples. DELFIAs can be sensitive, fast, accurate, robust, cover a relatively wide analyte concentration range and run using robots to allow very high sample throughput.

4.7.8 Homogeneous substrate-labelled fluorescence immunoassay

Substrate-labelled fluorescence immunoassays (SLFIAs) use principles similar to competitive immunoassays, but do not require separation of free from bound antigen. They require the synthesis of antigen conjugates containing a chemical structure that is not fluorescent per se, but is cleaved by an enzyme to yield an intensely fluorescent compound. They also need an antibody that binds the antigen conjugate such that the enzyme is prevented from cleaving it and liberating the fluorochrome. In SLFIA, samples containing known and unknown amounts of antigen are incubated with a fixed amount of antigen conjugate in the presence of a limiting concentration of antibody. Under such conditions, the antigen in the samples competes for antibody with the conjugated antigen. After equilibrium has been reached, enzyme is added to liberate the fluorochrome from non-antibody-bound antigen conjugate. The fluorescence measured is therefore proportional to the amount of antigen in the samples. A combination of the enzyme β-galactosidase and conjugates prepared by coupling antigen to a galactosyl 4-methylumbelliferyl residue is often employed for SLFIA. The β-galactosidase hydrolyses the conjugate to liberate free 4-methylumbelliferone, which is readily measured using fluorimetry. A major difficulty encountered with the general application of this type of assay is producing the appropriate antibody, i.e. an antibody that effectively inhibits the enzyme-catalysed reaction. It is usually only successful for relatively small analytes, for example morphine and other opiates.

4.8 IMMUNOHISTO/CYTOCHEMISTRY

To understand cell structure, organisation and function, and cell or tissue development and differentiation in health and disease, it is often necessary to be able to determine the distribution of an antigen *in situ*. Immunohistochemical and immunocytochemical techniques exploit the specific interaction of an antibody with its antigen to locate or to determine the distribution of the antigen *in situ* in tissues or cells, respectively. Alternatively, these procedures can be carried out using tissues or cells known to contain a particular antigen to investigate the specificity of antibodies or antisera. The principle of immunohisto/cytochemistry is analagous to solid-phase immunobinding (Section 4.7.3) and immunoblotting (Section 4.6), except that the antibody is incubated with thin sections of solid tissue mounted on glass slides or cell preparations containing the antigen rather than with antigen immobilised on microtitre plates or nitrocellulose membranes. In immunohisto/cytochemistry, the antibody (or anti-immunoglobulin antibody; Section 4.5.1) must be conjugated with a fluorescent or enzyme label that gives an

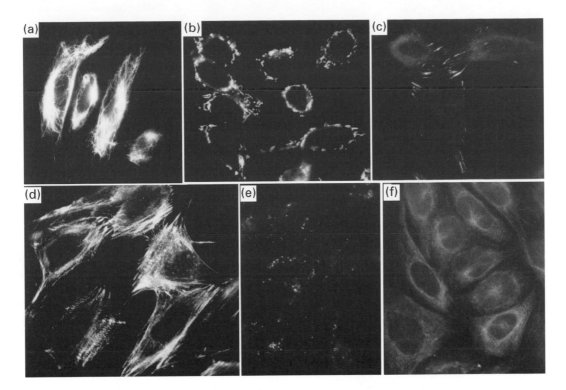

Fig. 4.26. Immunofluorescence photomicrographs showing immunostaining of cellular organelles: (a) intermediate filaments; (b) mitochondria; (c) microspikes; (d) stress fibres; (e) granules; (f) cytoplasmic component(s). Monolayers of the rat glioma cell line C6 were incubated with human IgM monoclonal antibodies and then fluorescein-labelled anti-human IgM.

intense signal to allow visualisation when the sections or cells are examined using immunoenzyme microscopy. The location of the label reveals the site of the antibody–antigen interaction, which can be localised to, for example, particular cell types or cellular organelles (an example is shown in Fig. 4.26).

All immunohisto/cytochemical procedures need stringent positive and negative control antibodies for comparison with the test antibody to ensure that the immunostaining is specific. Although it is common for the binding of labelled antibody to a specific tissue or cellular antigen to be referred to as immunostaining, this term should not be confused with the differential staining of tissue constituents by routine chemical stains such as haematoxylin and eosin for histology and pathology.

4.8.1 Immunoenzyme microscopy

The main advantage of enzyme labels (usually horseradish peroxidase (HRP) or alkaline phosphatase (AP); Section 4.5.4) for immunohisto/cytochemical procedures is that an ordinary white light microscope can be used for viewing the sections or cells, and the use of chemical counterstains such as haematoxylin (stains nuclei blue) aids in identification of morphology. The main disadvantages are the presence of endogenous tissue enzymes (which can give high background staining) and the extra step involved in carrying out the enzyme reaction.

4.8.2 The peroxidase–anti-peroxidase technique

The PAP technique is a modification of the indirect enzyme immunohisto/cytochemical procedure for amplifying the signal (Fig. 4.27). In this method, unlabelled anti-rabbit or anti-mouse immunoglobulin forms a bridge between rabbit or mouse primary antibody, respectively, and a peroxidase–(rabbit or mouse)–anti-peroxidase complex. Alkaline phosphatase–anti-alkaline phosphatase complexes are also available. An advantage of this procedure is that no possible destruction of antibody and/or enzyme can occur during chemical coupling. Specially developed commercial systems that exploit both anti-immunoglobulin and biotin–avidin reactions are also available. Such amplification systems are many times more sensitive than standard indirect procedures.

4.8.3 Immunofluorescence techniques

Immunohistochemistry was originally developed using fluorochrome-labelled antibodies (see Section 4.5.3). Their use has dramatically increased in recent years with the expansion of flow cytofluorimetric techniques, which allow analysis of single cells in suspension according to the expression of cell surface antigens (Section 4.8.5), and the advent of confocal microscropy in which laser light sources replace the standard light sources to allow analysis of images at different depths through the tissue section or cell to build up a three-dimensional picture. A unique application of fluorochrome-labelled antibodies for immunohisto/cytochemistry is that, because different fluorochromes emit different wavelengths of ultraviolet light, the use of appropriate filters on a fluorescence microscope allows the same tissue section or cell sample to be immunostained with two, three or even four different antibodies, each of which is used in conjunction with a different fluorochrome. Such double or triple staining procedures sometimes necessitate the use of directly conjugated primary antibodies, as, for example, fluorescein conjugated rabbit anti-mouse immunoglobulin antibodies will not distinguish between primary mouse monoclonal antibodies of differing specificity.

The choice of fluorochrome depends on the light source, detection system available and personal preference. Light sources include tungsten, quartz-halogen or mercury arc lamps for fluorescence microscopes, argon ion or krypton–argon lasers for flow cytometry.

Fluorochrome-labelled antibodies are quick and easy to use, and offer good sensitivity. Their main disadvantage is the requirement for a microscope equipped with fluorescence optics, and that the fluorescence, particularly that of fluorescein, fades during prolonged viewing of individual microscopic fields unless a powerful reducing agent such as 1,4-bicyclo-2,2,2-octane is included in the

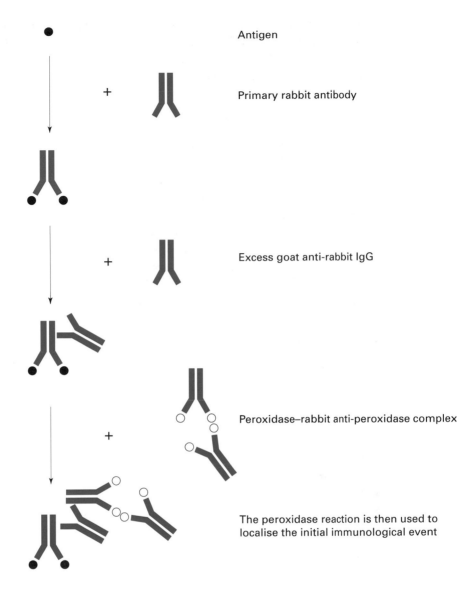

Antigen

Primary rabbit antibody

Excess goat anti-rabbit IgG

Peroxidase–rabbit anti-peroxidase complex

The peroxidase reaction is then used to localise the initial immunological event

Fig. 4.27. Diagrammatic representation of the peroxidase–anti-peroxidase technique. •, antigen; ○, peroxidase.

mountant. Such agents are thought to suppress a destructive reaction of the fluorescein in its excited state with protein. Autofluorescence of some tissue components, i.e. their intrinsic fluorescence, can also be a problem.

4.8.4 Capping

An important feature of immunostaining viable cells, particularly lymphocytes, is the aggregation of cell surface antigens due to cross-linkage by intact antibodies.

Such patches eventually form a cap over one pole of the cell, which is subsequently shed or endocytosed. Capping can be visualised using fluorochrome-labelled antibodies and provides information on the association of molecules carrying different antigenic markers if double or triple immunofluorescence labelling is carried out. It can be prevented by immunostaining at 4 °C or in the presence of sodium azide, which prevents modulation of cell surface molecules, or by the use of monovalent Fab fragments, in order to study the initial binding of antibody to cell surface antigen.

4.8.5 Flow cytometry

A disadvantage of assessment of immunocytochemical staining using conventional microscopy is that it is very difficult to quantify the intensity of the immunostaining. Although it is possible to estimate the proportion of cells that are immunostained in a population by performing manual cell counts, the accuracy of the estimate is dependent on the total number of cells that are counted and the proportion of positive cells.

These limitations are overcome in flow cytofluorimetric analysis. In this technique, cells that have been labelled with fluorochrome-conjugated antibody in suspension are introduced into a liquid jet and passed individually through the beam of a laser. As each cell passes through it emits a flash of fluorescence and scattered light. The signals are collected and converted by the flow cytofluorimeter to give quantitative information on the intensity of fluorescence and the light-scattering properties of each cell. Forward light scatter is related to cell size; the amount of side scatter is related to the granularity of the cell (presence of intracellular granules, pronounced organelles and/or nucleus). Examples of data displays are shown in Fig. 4.28. Many thousands of cells can be quickly analysed in this way, for example with respect to the proportion of cells that are immunostained or the intensity of fluorescence. Flow cytofluorimeters are also able to sort cells according to specified parameters such as intensity of fluorescence and size (cells usually remain viable after immunostaining with fluorochrome-labelled antibody). Many fluorochromes are available for flow cytofluorimetric analysis that allow simultaneous monitoring for several colours, provided the emission spectra do not overlap. This allows the use of several antibodies, conjugated with different fluorochromes, at the same time. Directly conjugated monoclonal antibodies are often used in flow cytofluorimetric techniques. This permits simultaneous labelling with several fluorochromes (see Sections 4.8.3 and 4.5.3). Also the anti-immunoglobulin conjugates used in indirect immunocytochemical techniques can either bind directly to lymphocytes that express cell surface immunoglobulin or bring about agglutination of primary antibody-coated cells. (IgG is divalent and can bind two primary antibody molecules, each of which is bound to a separate cell, thus bringing the cells together.) A wide range of directly conjugated monoclonal antibodies against different cell surface markers such as the CD (cluster of differentiation) series of antigens, which are characteristic of different populations of blood cells, are

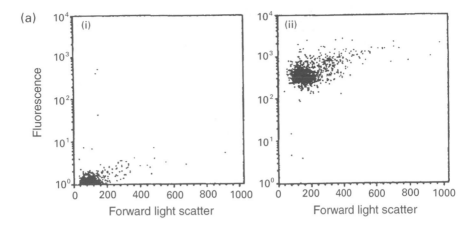

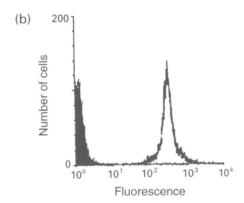

Fig. 4.28. Examples of flow cytometry displays. (a) Dot plots of erythrocytes (red blood cells) stained with a fluorescently labelled mouse monoclonal anti-haemoglobin antibody (ii) or a fluorescently labelled irrelevant mouse monoclonal antibody (i). Each dot represents an erythrocyte. The intensity of fluorescence is on the y-axis; forward light scatter (i.e. size) is on the x-axis. The erythrocytes are not fluorescently stained with the irrelevant antibody (i), but virtually all the cells are stained with the anti-haemoglobin antibody (ii). (b) The same data displayed as a profile histogram with number of cells on the y-axis and intensity of fluorescence on the x-axis.

available commercially. These allow analysis of cell sets and subsets involved in biological systems to be evaluated, for example T and B lymphocyte populations. If immunostaining of surface antigens of viable cells for flow cytometric analysis is being carried out, steps may have to be taken to prevent non-antigen-specific binding of antibody to Fc receptors that are present on, for example, leukocytes. This can be achieved either by blocking these sites with non-immune serum that contains high levels of immunoglobulin, or by the use of antibody F(ab')$_2$ fragments.

4.8.6 **Immuno-electron microscopy**

Subcellular detail that is not discernible by conventional microscopy can be resolved using electron microscopy since electrons have a shorter wavelength than white or ultraviolet light. Antibodies labelled with electron-dense reagents such as gold or ferritin (an iron-containing protein) or with HRP, which can yield an electron-dense product with an appropriate substrate, are used in immunoelectron microscopy to immunostain ultrathin sections of tissue or cells.

4.9 **AFFINITY AND AVIDITY**

Determining the affinity of an antibody can be important for predicting and/or explaining its immunochemical characteristics. Affinity is defined as the equilibrium constant when 'a monovalent antibody reacts with (binds) a monovalent antigen, i.e. an antigenic determinant'. As antibodies are usually di- or multivalent, and antigens usually have more than one antigenic determinant, this concept is relatively rarely encountered. The term avidity is normally used to describe the equilibrium constant applicable to whole antibody–antigen interactions and this includes the affinity component plus additive factors due to multiple valency of binding and other considerations. The terms affinity and avidity are sometimes replaced by intrinsic affinity and functional affinity, respectively, and these are certainly more descriptive.

4.9.1 **Measurement of affinity and avidity**

The affinity of monovalent antibody for its epitope can be expressed arithmetically as the equilibrium association constant using the following relationship:

$$K_a = \frac{[AgAb]}{[Ag][Ab]}$$

where K_a is the equilibrium association constant, [Ag] is the concentration of antigen, [Ab] is the concentration of antibody, and [AgAb] is the concentration of the antigen–antibody complex.

Practically, this requires that all components are absolutely pure and relate to equilibrium in homogeneous solution. Such conditions rarely apply to most immunochemical techniques as applied to biochemical methodology. However, calculating the relative affinity of antibodies can be useful in predicting their use in immunochemical techniques (see also Section 8.2).

4.10 **IMMUNOCHEMICAL USE OF SURFACE PLASMON RESONANCE**

Surface plasmon resonance (Section 8.2.3) uses the optical properties at the surface of a thin gold-film-coated glass 'chip' to study binding phenomena. The physical principles of the method are as follows. A beam of polarised light will be internally reflected by the chip (mounted on a glass prism). The angle of reflection is changed if material binds to the surface of the chip and the alteration in the angle of reflection is proportional to the *mass* of substance bound to the chip surface. Instruments for the application of surface plasmon resonance technology to immunochemistry are commercially available. The Biacore™ biosensor system is probably most appropriate for general immunochemical use, can be programmed for a variety of differing applications and is automated. In this system, the chip is coated with a dextran matrix to which antigen or antibody can be chemically coupled, and thus immobilised. Samples to be analysed for antigen (if antibody has been immobilised) or antibody (if antigen has been immobilised) are allowed to flow over the chip surface, and binding is continuously detected by measuring the alteration in the angle of reflection of light incident on the prism side of the chip. The measurements are directly proportional to the mass of substance binding and can be used to compare the antigen or antibody content of samples and also for calculation of kinetic parameters related to antigen–antibody interaction, for example association and dissociation affinity constants.

Surface plasmon resonance is a rapid procedure (measurements are made in a few minutes), does not require labelling of antibodies or antigens or the use of anti-immunoglobulin reagents and can be adapted for a wide range of purposes. It is not usually particularly sensitive, for example compared with immunoassays, but can be used to allow detection of very low affinity interactions.

4.11 **KEY TERMS**

acquired immunity	Fc	immunogen
affinity	flow cytofluorimetric techniques	immunoglobulin
antibody	flow cytometry	immunoprecipitation
antigen	hapten	innate immunity
avidity	humanised antibody	monoclonal antibody
capping	hybridoma	plasma cell
chimaeric antibodies	hyperimmune	polyclonal response
competitive binding assays	hypervariable region	radioimmunoassay
conjugate	immunoaffinity chromatography	sensitivity
constant region	immunoassays	single-chain antibody fragment
double diffusion	immunobinding assays	single radial immunodiffusion
enhanced chemiluminescence	immunoblot	specificity
enzyme immunometric assays	immunoblotting	substrate-labelled fluorescence
enzyme-linked immunosorbent	immunocytochemistry	immunoassay
assay	immunodominant	time-resolved immunofluorimetric
epitope	immunoelectrophoresis	assays
epitope mapping	immunoenzyme microscopy	variable region
Fab	immunohistochemistry	

4.12 **CALCULATION**

Question 1

Single radial diffusion for estimating the concentration of antigen. The precipitin ring diameters of an antigen calibrator at three different concentrations were:

Concentration ($\mu g\,cm^{-3}$)	Ring diameter (mm)	Ring diameter (mm^2)
10	4	16
60	7	49
100	8.7	76

Use graph paper to plot the calibrator concentration against the square of the ring diameter to give a calibration curve.

The ring diameter of the sample of unknown antigen concentration was 6 mm. Using the calibration graph, determine the concentration of the antigens in the unknown.

Answer $40\,\mu g\,cm^{-3}$.

4.13 **SUGGESTIONS FOR FURTHER READING**

HERMANSON, G. T. (1996). *Bioconjugate Techniques*. Academic Press Inc., London and New York. (A very comprehensive, detailed account of just about every procedure for congugating labels to biological molecules. Includes a large number of methods used to produce congugates employed in immunochemical techniques.)

HERMANSON, G. T., KRISHNA MALLIA, A. and SMITH, P. K. (1992). *Immobilised Affinity Ligand Techniques*. Academic Press Inc., London and New York. (Exhaustive coverage of affinity chromotography procedures including immuno-affinity methods. Deals with numerous procedures for isolation of antibodies, etc.)

HERZENBERG, L. A., HERZENBERG, L. A., WEIR, D. M. and BLACKWELL, C. (eds.) (1997). *Weir's Handbook of Experimental Immunology*, 5th edn, Blackwell Science, Oxford. (A large four-volume detailed text dealing with most immunological methods. Very good on the theoretical basis of techniques and contains considerable experimental details. Volume 1 deals specifically with immunochemistry and molecular immunology.)

JOHNSTONE, A. and THORPE, R. (1996). *Immunochemistry In Practice*, 3rd edn. Blackwell Science, Oxford. (Contains detailed protocols for many immunochemical techniques plus a resumé of their underlying scientific basis.)

JOHNSTONE, A. P. and TURNER, M. W. (eds.) (1997). *Immunochemistry – A Practical Approach*. IRL Press, Oxford. (Chapters devoted to many immunochemical procedures.)

KEMENY, D. M. and CHALLACOMBE, S. J. (eds.) (1988). *ELISA and Other Solid Phase Immunoassays*. John Wiley and Sons, Chichester. (A volume devoted to fundamental aspects of enzyme-linked immunoassays.)

KERR, M. A. and THORPE, R. (eds.) (1994). *Immunochemistry Labfax*. Bios Scientific, Oxford. (Contains much immunochemical information concerning immunoglobulins, immunochemical reagents, and other substances used in immunochemical techniques.)

LACHMANN, P. J., PETERS, D. K., ROSEN, F. S. and WALPORT, M. J. (eds.) (1993). *Clinical Aspects Of Immunology*, 5th edn. Blackwell Science, Oxford. (A large three-volume work describing most aspects of clinical immunology and much theoretical immunology.)

ROITT, I. M. (1998). *Essential Immunology*, th edn. Blackwell Science, Oxford. (An excellent general textbook on immunology.)

Chapter 5

Centrifugation techniques

5.1 INTRODUCTION

Centrifugation separation techniques are based upon the behaviour of particles in an applied centrifugal field and assume that the parameters of the molecules under investigation, such as the relative molecular mass, shape and density, may be related to the behaviour of those molecules in a gravitational field.

If a solution of large particles is left to stand, then the particles will tend to sediment under the influence of gravity. For a given particle, the rate or velocity at which it sediments is proportional to the force applied, so that the particles sediment more rapidly when the force applied is greater than the gravitational force of the earth. The basis of centrifugation separation techniques, therefore, is to exert a larger force than does the earth's gravitational field, thus increasing the rate at which the particles sediment. The particles are normally suspended in a specific liquid medium, held in tubes or bottles, which are located in a rotor. The rotor is positioned centrally on the drive shaft of the centrifuge. Particles that differ in density, shape or size can be separated because they sediment at different rates in the centrifugal field, each particle sedimenting at a rate that is directly proportional to the applied centrifugal field.

Centrifugation techniques are of two main types. Preparative centrifugation techniques are concerned with the actual separation, isolation and purification of, for example, whole cells, subcellular organelles, plasma membranes, polysomes, ribosomes, chromatin, nucleic acids, lipoproteins and viruses, for subsequent biochemical investigations. Very large amounts of material may be involved when microbial cells are harvested from culture media, plant and animal cells from tissue culture or plasma from blood. Relatively large amounts of cellular particles may also be isolated in order to study their morphology, composition and biological activity. It is also possible to isolate biological macromolecules, such as nucleic acids and proteins, from preparations that have received some measure of purification by, for example, fractional precipitation (Section 6.3.4). In contrast, analytical centrifugation techniques are devoted mainly to the study of pure, or virtually pure, macromolecules or particles. They are concerned primarily with the study of the sedimentation characteristics of biological macromolecules and molecular structures, rather than with the collection of particular fractions. They require only small amounts of material and utilise specially designed rotors and detector systems to continuously monitor the process of sedimentation of the material in the centrifugal field. Such studies yield information from which the purity, relative molecular mass and shape of the material may be deduced. Since preparative centrifugation techniques are more commonly used in undergraduate courses, this chapter concentrates on these techniques and deals only briefly with analytical centrifugation techniques.

5.2 **BASIC PRINCIPLES OF SEDIMENTATION**

The rate of sedimentation is dependent upon the applied centrifugal field (G) being directed radially outwards; this is determined by the square of the angular velocity of the rotor (ω, in radians s^{-1}) and the radial distance (r, in centimetres) of the particle from the axis of rotation, according to the equation

$$G = \omega^2 r \tag{5.1}$$

Since one revolution of the rotor is equal to 2π radians, its angular velocity, in radians s^{-1}, can be readily expressed in terms of revolutions per minute (rev min^{-1}), the common way of expressing rotor speed being

$$\omega = \frac{2\pi\ \text{rev min}^{-1}}{60} \tag{5.2}$$

The centrifugal field (G) in terms of rev min^{-1} is then

$$G = \frac{4\pi^2(\text{rev min}^{-1})^2 r}{3600} \tag{5.3}$$

and is generally expressed as a multiple of the earth's gravitational field ($g = 981$ cm s^{-2}), i.e. the ratio of the weight of the particle in the centrifugal field to the weight of the same particle when acted on by gravity alone, and is then referred to as the relative centrifugal field (RCF) or more commonly as the 'number times g'.

$$\text{Hence RCF} = \frac{4\pi^2(\text{rev min}^{-1})^2 r}{3600 \times 981} \tag{5.4}$$

which may be shortened to give

$$\text{RCF} = (1.118 \times 10^{-5})(\text{rev min}^{-1})^2 r \tag{5.5}$$

When conditions for the centrifugal separation of particles are reported, therefore, rotor speed, radial dimensions and time of operation of the rotor must all be quoted. Since biochemical experiments are usually conducted with particles dissolved or suspended in solution, the rate of sedimentation of a particle is dependent not only upon the applied centrifugal field but also upon the mass of the particle, which may be expressed as the product of its volume and density, the density and viscosity of the medium in which it is sedimenting and the extent to which its shape deviates from spherical. When a particle sediments it must displace some of the solution in which it is suspended, resulting in an apparent upthrust on the particle equal to the weight of liquid displaced. If a particle is assumed to be spherical and of known volume and density, the latter being corrected for the buoyancy due to the density of the medium, then the net outward force (F) it experiences when centrifuged at an angular velocity of ω radians s^{-1} is given by

$$F = \frac{4}{3}\pi r_p^3 (\rho_p - \rho_m)\omega^2 r \tag{5.6}$$

where $\frac{4}{3}\pi r_p^3$ is the volume of a sphere of radius r_p, ρ_p is the density of the particle, ρ_m is the density of the suspending medium, and r is the distance of the particle from the centre of rotation. Particles, however, generate friction as they migrate through the solution. If a particle is rigid and spherical and moving at a known velocity, then the frictional force (F_o) opposing motion is given by

$$F_o = vf \tag{5.7}$$

where v is the velocity or sedimentation rate of the particle, and f is the frictional coefficient of the particle in the solvent.

The frictional coefficient of a particle is a function of its size, shape and hydration, and of the viscosity of the medium, and according to the Stokes equation, for an unhydrated spherical particle, is given by

$$f = 6\pi\eta r_p \tag{5.8}$$

when η is the viscosity coefficient of the medium.

For asymmetric and/or hydrated particles, the actual radius of the particle in equation 5.8 is replaced by the effective or Stokes radius, r_{eff}. An unhydrated, spherical particle of known volume and density, and present in a medium of constant density, therefore accelerates in a centrifugal field, its velocity increasing until the net force of sedimentation equals the frictional force resisting its motion through the medium, i.e.

$$F = F_o \text{ or } \tfrac{4}{3}\pi r_p^3 (\rho_p - \rho_m)\omega^2 r = 6\pi\eta r_p v \tag{5.9}$$

In practice, the balancing of these forces occurs quickly and the particle reaches a constant velocity because the frictional resistance increases with the velocity of the particle. Under these conditions, the net force acting on the particle is zero. Hence, the particle no longer accelerates but achieves a maximum velocity, with the result that it now sediments at a constant rate. Its rate of sedimentation (v) is then given by

$$v = \frac{dr}{dt} = \frac{2r_p^2(\rho_p - \rho_m)\omega^2 r}{9\eta} \tag{5.10}$$

It can be seen from equation 5.10 that the sedimentation rate of a given particle is proportional to its size, to the difference in density between the particle and the medium and to the applied centrifugal field. It is zero when the density of the particle and the medium are equal; it decreases when the viscosity of the medium increases, and increases as the force field increases. However, since the equation involves the square of the particle radius, it is apparent that the size of the particle has the greatest influence upon its sedimentation rate. Particles of similar density, but only slightly different in size, can therefore have large differences in their sedimentation rate. Intergration of equation 5.10 yields equation 5.11, which gives the sedimentation time for a spherical particle in a centrifugal field as a function of the variables involved and in relation to the distance travelled by the particle in the centrifuge tube:

$$t = \frac{9\eta}{2\omega^2 r_p^2 (\rho_p - \rho_m)} \ln \frac{r_b}{r_t} \tag{5.11}$$

where t is the sedimentation time in seconds, r_t is the radial distance from the axis of rotation to liquid meniscus, and r_b is the radial distance from the axis of rotation to the bottom of the tube.

It is thus clear that a mixture of heterogeneous, approximately spherical, particles can be separated by centrifugation on the basis of their densities and/or their size, either by the time required for their complete sedimentation or by the extent of their sedimentation after a given time. These alternatives form the basis for the separation of biological macromolecules and of cell organelles from tissue homogenates. The order of separation of the major cell components is generally whole cells and cell debris first, followed by nuclei, chloroplasts, mitochondria, lysosomes (or other microbodies), microsomes (fragments of smooth and rough endoplasmic reticulum) and ribosomes.

Considerable discrepancies exist between the theory and practice of centrifugation. Complex variables not accounted for in equations 5.10 and 5.11, such as the concentration of the suspension, nature of the medium, and the design and handling of the centrifuge, will affect the sedimentation properties of a mixed population of particles. Moreover, aspherical particles exhibit a modified relationship between the sedimentation rate and the particle size, resulting in such particles sedimenting at a slower rate. Equation 5.10 can therefore be modified to give equation 5.12:

$$v = \frac{dr}{dt} = \frac{2r_p^2 (\rho_p - \rho_m)\omega^2 r}{9\eta(f/f_0)} \tag{5.12}$$

which now takes into account the frictional effect of varying particle shape on the sedimentation rate of a particle. The frictional ratio, f/f_0, where f is the frictional coefficient of the aspherical and/or hydrated particle, and f_0 is the theoretical frictional coefficient of an unhydrated sphere of the same relative molecular mass and density, is a function of the shape and hydration of the particle and, for spherical molecules such as native globular proteins, ranges from about 1 to 1.4. Where there is an appreciable asymmetry, however, as in the case of rod-like molecules such as DNA and proteins such as F-actin and myosin, larger values of f/f_0 are found. Clathrin, a major protein of coated vesicles, shows a frictional coefficient of 3.1, consistent with the suspected organisation of the molecule as a three-armed, branched, rod-like molecule. Frictional coefficients of globular proteins can also

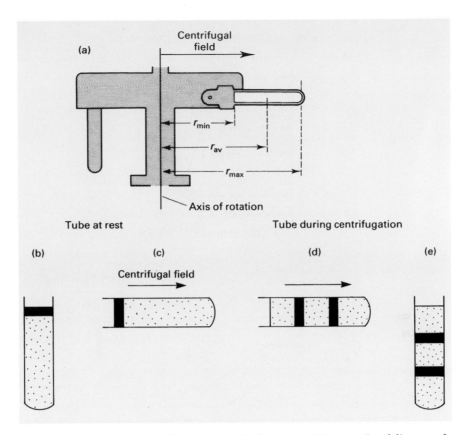

Fig. 5.1. Design and operation of the swinging-bucket rotor. (a) Cross-sectional diagram of a swinging-bucket rotor. (b) The centrifuge tube is initially loaded with gradient, the sample is then layered on top before the tube is placed in the bucket for attachment to the rotor. (c) During acceleration of the rotor the rotor bucket reorients to lie perpendicular to the axis of rotation. (d) Sedimentation and separation of the particles occur during centrifugation. (e) At the end of centrifugation the rotor decelerates, the bucket coming to rest in its original vertical position.

increase substantially with expansion to form flexible, random coils such as are brought about by unfolding of the globular protein by dissolving in concentrated solutions of urea or guanidine hydrochloride. The frictional drag increases because all parts of a random coil are in contact with the solvent, whereas a native globular protein has only its surface exposed to the solvent. Hence, particles of a given mass but different shape sediment at different rates. This point is exploited in the study of conformation of molecules by analytical ultracentrifugation (Section 5.10.3).

Although it is convenient to consider the sedimentation of particles in a uniform centrifugal field, in practice this does not occur when preparative rotors are used. Owing to the nature of rotor design (Figs. 5.1a, 5.2a, 5.3a) the effective radial dimension of a given particle will change according to its position in the sample container and will vary between r_{min} and r_{max}. Since the centrifugal field

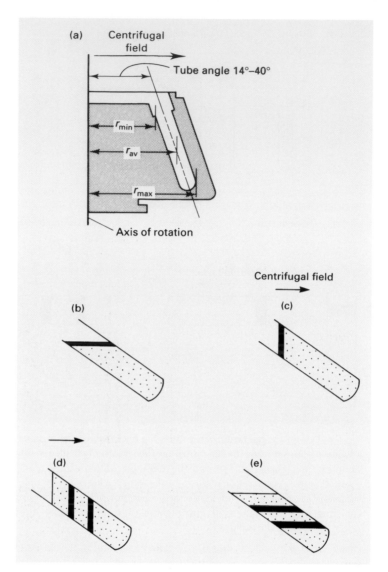

Fig. 5.2. Design and operation of the fixed-angle rotor. (a) Cross-sectional diagram of a fixed-angle rotor. (b) The centrifuge tube, after being filled with gradient, is loaded with sample and then placed in the rotor. (c) During rotor acceleration, reorientation of the sample and gradient occur. (d) Sedimentation and separation of the particles occur during centrifugation. (e) Rotor is at rest: the gradient reorients and bands of separated particles appear.

generated is proportional to $\omega^2 r$, a particle will experience a greater field the further away it is from the axis of rotation. The operative centrifugal field, in a fixed-angle rotor for example, can differ by a factor of up to 2 between the top and bottom of the centrifuge tube; thus the sedimentation rate of particles at the bottom of the tube will be twice that of identical particles near the top of the tube.

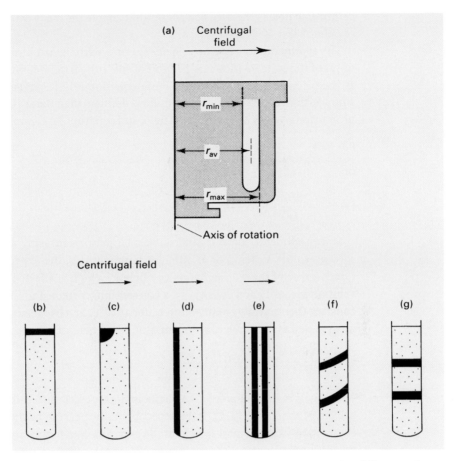

Fig. 5.3. Design and operation of the verticle tube rotor. (a) Cross-sectional diagram of a vertical tube rotor. (b) The centrifuge tube is filled with gradient; the sample is layered on top and is then placed in the rotor. (c) As the rotor accelerates, the sample and gradient begin to reorient. (d) The sample and medium reorientation is complete. (e) Sedimentation and separation of particles occur during centrifugation. (f) Reorientation of separated particles and gradient occur during the rotor deceleration. (g) Rotor is at rest: bands of separated particles and gradient are fully reoriented.

As a result, particles will tend to move faster as they sediment through a non-viscous medium. It is normal, therefore, to record the relative centrifugal field calculated from the average radius of rotation (r_{av}) of the column of liquid in the tube (i.e. the distance from the centre of rotation to the middle of the liquid column in the centrifuge tube). The average relative centrifugal field (RCF$_{av}$) is therefore the numerical average of the values exerted at r_{min} and r_{max}. If the sample container is only partially filled then, in the case of fixed-angle and swinging-bucket rotors, the minimum radius (r_{min}) is effectively increased and the particles will therefore start to sediment in a higher gravitational field and have a reduced pathlength to travel. Consequently sedimentation will be quicker. Centrifuge manuals normally provide details of the maximum permitted speed for a rotor, maximum relative centrifugal fields generated and graphs that enable the ready conversion of RCF to rev min^{-1} at r_{min}, r_{av}, and r_{max}.

The sedimentation rate or velocity (v) or a particle can also be expressed in terms of its sedimentation rate per unit of centrifugal field, commonly referred to as its sedimentation coefficient, s. From equation 5.12 it can be seen that, if the composition of the suspending medium is defined, then the sedimentation rate is proportional to $\omega^2 r$, the centrifugal field, and equation 5.12 simplifies to

$$v = s\omega^2 r \tag{5.13}$$

or

$$s = \frac{v}{\omega^2 r} = \frac{dr/dt}{\omega^2 r} \tag{5.14}$$

Since sedimentation rate studies may be performed using a wide variety of solvent–solute systems, or at different temperatures, the experimentally determined value of the sedimentation coefficient, which is affected by temperature, solution viscosity and density is, by convention, corrected to the sedimentation constant theoretically obtainable in water at 20 °C, and by means of equation 5.15, is expressed as the standard sedimentation coefficient or $s_{20,w}$.

$$s_{20,w} = s_{obs} \times \frac{\eta_{T,w}}{\eta_{20,w}} \times \frac{\eta_s}{\eta_w} \times \frac{(1 - \bar{v}\rho_{20,w})}{(1 - \bar{v}\rho_{T,s})} \tag{5.15}$$

where $s_{20,w}$ is the sedimentation coefficient expressed in terms of the standard solvent of water at 20 °C, s_{obs} is the experimentally measured sedimentation coefficient in the experimental solvent at the experimental temperature T (°C), $\eta_{T,w}$ is the viscosity of water at the experimental temperature T(°C), $\eta_{20,w}$ is the viscosity of water at 20 °C, η_s is the viscosity of the solvent at a given temperature (as near to 20 °C as possible), η_w is the viscosity of water at that temperature, $\rho_{20,w}$ is the density of water at 20 °C, $\rho_{T,s}$ is the density of the solvent at the temperature of the experiment, T(°C), and $\bar{v}$ is the partial specific volume of the solute (defined as the reciprocal of the non-hydrated density of the particle, i.e. the volume occupied by 1 kg of the particles).

For many macromolecules including nucleic acids and proteins the sedimentation coefficient usually decreases in value with increase in the concentration of solute, this effect becoming more severe with increase both in the relative molecular mass and the degree of extension of the molecule. Hence $s_{20,w}$ is usually measured at several concentrations and extrapolated to infinite dilution to obtain a value of $s_{20,w}$ at zero concentration, the $s_{20,w}^0$. The sedimentation coefficients of most biological particles are very small, and for convenience its basic unit is taken as 10^{-13} s, which is termed one Svedberg unit (S), in recognition of T. Svedberg's pioneering work in this type of analysis. Therefore, a ribosomal RNA molecule possessing a sedimentation coefficient 5×10^{-13} s is said to have a value of 5 S.

Examination of equations 5.12 and 5.14 shows that the sedimentation coefficient is influenced by such features as the shape, size and density of the particle, and hence is commonly used to characterise a particular molecule or structure.

Generally, the larger the molecule or particle, the larger is its Svedberg unit and hence the faster is its sedimentation rate. Sedimentation coefficients (in Svedberg units) for enzymes, peptide hormones and soluble proteins are 2 to 25 S, nucleic acids 3 to 100 S, ribosomes and polysomes 20 to 200 S, viruses 40 to 1000 S, lysosomes 4000 S, membranes 100 to 100×10^3 S, mitochondria 20×10^3 S to 70×10^3 S, and nuclei between 4000×10^3 S and $40\,000 \times 10^3$ S.

5.3 CENTRIFUGES AND THEIR USE

Centrifuges may be classified into four major groups: the small bench centrifuges; large capacity refrigerated centrifuges; high speed refrigerated centrifuges; and ultracentrifuges of two types, preparative and analytical.

5.3.1 Small bench centrifuges

These are the simplest and least expensive centrifuges and exist in many types of design. They are often used to collect small amounts of material that rapidly sediment (yeast cells, erythrocytes, coarse precipitates), and generally have a maximum speed of 4000 to 6000 rev min^{-1}, with maximum relative centrifugal fields of 3000 to 7000 g. Most operate at ambient temperature, the flow of air around the rotor controlling rotor temperature. Some of the latest designs, however, incorporate a refrigeration system to keep rotors cool, thus preventing denaturation of proteins. Small microfuges are available, providing virtually instant acceleration to maximum speeds of 8000 to 13 000 rev min^{-1} and developing fields of approximately 10 000 g. These centrifuges have proved extremely useful for sedimenting small volumes (250 mm^3 to 1.5 cm^3) of material very quickly (1 or 2 min). Typical applications include the rapid sedimentation of blood samples, and of synaptosomes used to study the effect of drugs on the uptake of biogenic amines.

5.3.2 Large capacity refrigerated centrifuges

These have a maximum speed of 6000 rev min^{-1} and produce a maximum relative centrifugal field approaching 6500 g. They have refrigerated rotor chambers and vary only in their maximum carrying capacity, all being capable of utilising a variety of interchangeable swinging-bucket and fixed-angle rotors enabling separation to be achieved in 10, 50 and 100 cm^3 tubes. Large total capacity (4 to 6 dm^3) centrifuges are also available that, in addition to accommodating smaller tubes, are also capable of holding bottles, each of 1.25 dm^3 capacity. In all these centrifuges, the rotors are usually mounted on a rigid suspension, hence it is extremely important that the centrifuge tubes and their contents are balanced accurately (to within 0.25 g of each other). Rotors must never be loaded with an odd number of tubes and, where the rotor is only partially loaded, the tubes must be located diametrically opposite each other in order that the load is distributed evenly around the rotor axis. These instruments are most often used to compact or collect substances that sediment rapidly, for example erythrocytes, coarse or bulky precipitates, yeast cells, nuclei and chloroplasts.

5.3.3 High speed refrigerated centrifuges

These instruments are available with maximum rotor speeds in the region of 25 000 rev min^{-1}, generating a relative centrifugal field of about 60 000 g. They generally have a total capacity of up to 1.5 dm^3, and a range of interchangeable fixed-angle and swinging-bucket rotors. These instruments are most often used to collect microorganisms, cellular debris, larger cellular organelles and proteins precipitated by ammonium sulphate. They cannot generate sufficient centrifugal force to effectively sediment viruses or smaller organelles such as ribosomes.

5.3.4 Continuous flow centrifuges

The continuous flow centrifuge is a relatively simple high speed centrifuge. The rotor, through which particles suspended in medium flow continuously (usually 1 to 1.5 dm^3 min^{-1}), is long, tubular, and non-interchangeable. As medium enters the rotating rotor, particles are sedimened against its wall and excess clarified medium overflows through an outlet port. The major application of this type of centrifuge is in the harvesting of bacteria or yeast cells from large volumes of culture medium (10 to 500 dm^3). Some high speed centrifuges can be adapted to function in the continuous flow mode by being constructed to accept a specially designed rotor (Section 5.4.5).

5.3.5 Preparative ultracentrifuges

Preparative ultracentrifuges are capable of spinning rotors to a maximum speed of 80 000 rev min^{-1} and can produce a relative centrifugal field of up to 600 000 g. The rotor chamber is refrigerated, sealed and evacuated to minimise any excessive rotor temperatures being generated by frictional resistance between the air and the spinning rotor. The temperature monitoring system is more sophisticated than in simpler instruments, employing an infrared temperature sensor that can continuously monitor rotor temperature and control the refrigeration system. An overspeed control system is also incorporated into these instruments to prevent operation of the rotor above its maximum rated speed and there are electronic circuits to detect rotor imbalance. In order to minimise vibration, caused by slight rotor imbalance that may arise due to unequal loading of the centrifuge tubes, ultracentrifuges are fitted with a flexible drive shaft system. Centrifuge tubes and their contents, however, must still be accurately balanced to within 0.1 g of each other. For safety reasons, rotor chambers of high speed and ultracentrifuges are always enclosed in heavy armour plating.

An air-driven, table-top preparative ultracentrifuge, called an airfuge, is available and is capable of accelerating a magnetically suspended 3.7 cm diameter rotor, accommodating 6 × 175 mm^3 tubes on a virtually friction-free cushion of

air in a non-vacuated chamber, to $100\,000$ rev min^{-1} ($160\,000\,g$) in approximately
$30\,s$. The airfuge has found applications in biochemical and clinical research
where there are only small volume samples requiring high centrifugal forces.
Examples include macromolecule/ligand binding–kinetic studies, steroid
hormone receptor assays, separation of the major lipoprotein fractions from
plasma, and deproteinisation of physiological fluids for amino acid analysis.

5.3.6 Analytical ultracentrifuges

These instruments are capable of operating at speeds approaching $70\,000$ rev
min^{-1} ($500\,000\,g$) and consist of a motor, a rotor contained in a protective
armoured chamber that is refrigerated and evacuated, and an optical system to
enable the sedimenting material to be observed throughout the duration of centrifugation to determine concentration distributions in the sample at any time
during centrifugation (Fig. 5.4a). Three types of optical system are available in the
analytical ultracentrifuge: a light absorption system, and the alternative Schlieren
system and Rayleigh interferometric system, both of which detect changes in the
refractive index of the solution.

The rotor is solid, with holes to hold the cells that contain the samples, and is
suspended on a wire coming from the drive shaft of a high speed motor that
allows the rotor to find its own axis of rotation. The tip of the rotor contains a
thermistor for measuring temperature. Several types of rotor are available, the
simplest type of which incorporates two cells – the analytical cell and the
counterpoise cell, which counterbalances the analytical cell. Two holes (at distances calibrated from the centre of rotation) are drilled through the counterpoise cell (Fig. 5.4b) to facilitate the calibration of distances in the analytical cell.
A wide variety of cells are available and have a capacity of between 0.4 and
$1.0\,cm^3$. Analytical cells used with the ultraviolet light absorption optical system
and the Schlieren optical system have a single $2°$ or $4°$ sector shape, to prevent
convection, and usually have a $12\,mm$ optical pathlength centrepiece, although
centrepieces of $1.5\,mm$ to $30\,mm$ are available. Double-sector cells, having two
$2.5°$ sectors and an optical pathlength that can vary from $12\,mm$ to $30\,mm$, are
used with the interference optical system, the absorption optical system when
used with the photoelectric scanner, and the Schlieren optical system when a
baseline is required. Double-sector cells allow the user to take account of absorbing components in the solvent, and to correct for the redistribution of solvent
components, particularly at high g values. Double-sector cells also facilitate
measurements of differences in sedimentation coefficients, and of diffusion
coefficients. An array of centrepieces is also available for specialised purposes.
The centrepiece is so designed that, when correctly aligned in the rotor, the walls
will be parallel to the lines of centrifugal force, behaving according to the same
principle as the swinging-bucket rotor (Section 5.4.2) to give almost ideal conditions for sedimentation. This ensures that there will be no accumulation of
material against the wall of the analytical cell during centrifugation. Analytical
cells have upper and lower plane windows of optical grade quartz or synthetic

(a)

(b)

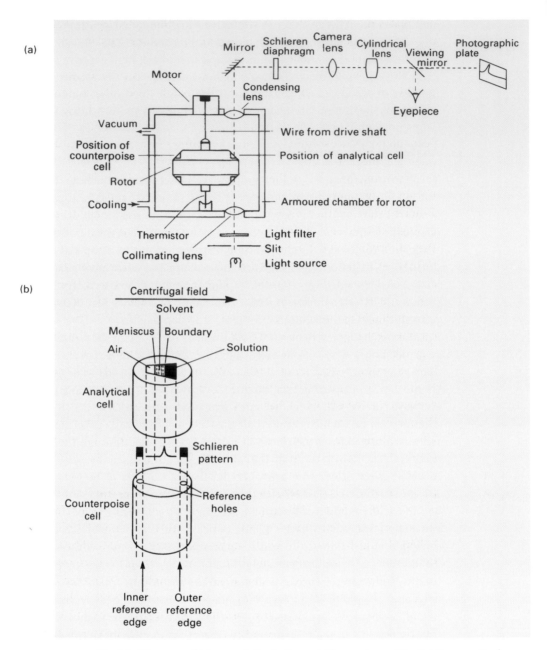

Fig. 5.4. Diagrams of (a) an analytical ultracentrifuge system with a Schlieren optical system and (b) a single-sector analytical cell and a counterpoise cell.

sapphire, the latter being used with interference optics, as they have less tendency to distort under a high gravitational field. The rotor chamber contains an upper condensing lens and a lower collimating lens; the former, together with a camera lens, focuses light on to a photographic plate, whereas the latter collimates the light so that the sample cell is illuminated by parallel light. In more advanced instruments the photographic detector system is replaced by an electronic scanning system.

In the ultraviolet light absorption system, light of a suitable wavelength is passed through the moving analytical cell containing the solution under analysis, for example protein or nucleic acid, and the intensity of the transmitted light is recorded either on a photographic plate, or by an automatic single or split-beam photoelectric scanning system. The scanner system, unlike the ultraviolet photographic method, has the advantage of allowing direct visualisation of the results during the course of the experiment and can provide a plot of the concentration of the sample at all points in the analytical cell at any particular time. Different wavelengths of light can be selected, enabling the separate movement of single components in a mixture of substances to be monitored, provided that they absorb light at different wavelengths. The Schlieren optical system makes use of the fact that, if light passes through a solution of uniform concentration, it does not deviate but, on passing through a solution having different density zones, it is refracted at the boundary between these zones. The optical system records the change in refractive index of the solution, which will vary as the concentration changes. Two Schlieren optical systems are available, differing in the way the deviated light is treated. In the Schlieren optical system the deviated light is passed through an inclined Schlieren diaphragm and a cylindrical lens. In the case of sedimenting materials in an analytical cell, a boundary is formed between the solvent, which has been cleared of particles, and the remainder of the solution containing the sedimenting material. This behaves like a refraction lens, resulting in the production of a peak in the final image on the photographic plate, which is used as the detector system. The peak is an exact record of the refractive index gradient and the area beneath it is proportional to the concentration of solute. As sedimentation proceeds, the boundary, and hence the peak, shifts, and the rate at which the peak moves gives a measure of the rate at which the material is sedimenting (Fig. 5.5). After a period of sedimentation, the peak height diminishes and the width increases, owing to radial dilution of the sample due to the sector shape of the cell. Its area, however, is unchanged. In the bright-field scanning optical system the deviated light is interrupted by a knife edge and the resultant image scanned with a photomultiplier, the resulting refractive index gradient appearing as a dark band against a bright background. The Schlieren optical system plots the refractive index gradient against distance along the analytical cell, which makes it useful for locating boundaries in sedimentation velocity measurements (Section 5.10.1). For some techniques (for example, the sedimentation equilibrium method for relative molecular mass determinations (Section 5.10.1)) the Schlieren system is not sufficiently sensitive to detect small concentration differences. Use is therefore made of the more sensitive Rayleigh interference optical system, which employs a double-sector cell, in which one sector contains the solvent and the other the solution. The optical system measures the difference in refractive index between the reference solvent and the solution by the displacement of interferences fringes caused by

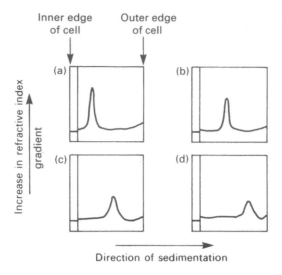

Fig. 5.5. Diagrams of the stages ((a) to (d)) of sedimentation of a macromolecule, using the technique of sedimentation velocity. Sedimentation patterns are obtained using the Schlieren optical system, which measures the refractive index gradient at each point in the cell at varying time intervals.

slits placed behind the two liquid columns, each fringe tracing a curve of the refractive index gradient against distance in the cell. Since the position of the fringes is determined by solute concentration, it is possible to measure the concentration of solute at any point along the cell.

5.4 DESIGN AND CARE OF PREPARATIVE ROTORS

5.4.1 Materials used in rotor construction

The centrifugal force created by a spinning rotor generates load or stress on the rotor material. Since rotors used for low speed centrifugation experience a much lower degree of stress in comparison to that of high speed rotors they can be made of brass, steel or Perspex. The higher stress forces generated during high speed centrifugation necessitate the use of aluminium alloy or titanium alloy. Rotors made from titanium alloy have a greater strength-to-weight ratio and are therefore capable of withstanding nearly twice the centrifugal force of rotors made from aluminium alloy. They are also more resistant to chemical corrosion and are less subject to metal fatigue. Aluminium alloy rotors, although less expensive, are far more susceptible to corrosion, being readily attacked by acids and alkalis, and high concentrations of salt solutions (e.g. NaCl and KBr used in lipoprotein fractionations, ammonium sulphate used in protein precipitation, and caesium or rubidium salts used in the preparation of density gradients). All rotors are therefore given a durable protective coating to the metal surface either by anodising in the case of aluminium rotors or by applying a black epoxy paint. Concomitant with improvements in rotor safety has been the introduction of materials in rotor construction such as carbon fibre, which is said to produce a lighter rotor with a better strength-to-weight ratio.

5.4.2 Swinging-bucket rotors

The swinging-bucket rotor (Fig. 5.1a) has buckets that start off in a vertical position but during acceleration of the rotor swing out to a horizontal position so that during centrifugation the tube, and hence the solution in the tube, is aligned perpendicular to the axis of rotation and parallel to the applied centrifugal field, the tube returning to its original position during deceleration of the rotor. Since the centrifugal field is axial, particles in a centrifugal field fan out radially from the centre of rotation rather than sedimenting in parallel lines. Some particles strike against the wall of the tube and then travel down the wall to the tube base, causing convection currents, referred to as wall effects, that disrupt the sample zones. Undesirable swirling effects that cause mixing of the tube contents are also produced during rotor acceleration and deceleration. Control of convection and swirling effects has been achieved by slowly accelerating and decelerating the rotor, and by the use of density gradient centrifugation techniques (Section 5.6.2), where the particles now sediment to form discrete bands (Fig. 5.1b to e).

5.4.3 Fixed-angle rotors

In fixed-angle rotors (Fig. 5.2a), the tubes are located in holes in the rotor body set at a fixed angle of between 14° and 40° to the vertical. Under the influence of the centrifugal field, which is exerted at an angle to the tube wall, particles move radially outwards and have only a short distance to travel before colliding with, and precipitating on, the outer wall of the centrifuge tube. A region of high concentration is formed that has a density greater than that of the surrounding medium, with the result that the precipitate sinks and collects as a small compact pellet at the outermost point of the tube. The combination of short path to the tube wall and consequent convection caused by the dense layer against the outer wall gives a rapid collection of the sample. Although the strong convective flow produced tends to have an undesirable effect when attempts are made to separate particles of similar sedimentation characteristics, the fixed-angle rotor has proved valuable for the differential separation of particles whose sedimentation rates differ by a significant order of magnitude.

Since the pocket retaining the centrifuge tube is fixed, the solution in the centrifuge tube reorients during rotor acceleration, reorienting back to its original position during deceleration of the rotor (Fig. 5.2b to e) For isopycnic centrifugation (Section 5.6.2) reorientation of the solution in the tubes has the advantage of enhancing the loading capacity of the gradient and increasing the resolution of the sample bands.

5.4.4 **Vertical tube rotors**

The vertical tube rotor (Fig. 5.3a) can be regarded as a zero-angle fixed-angle rotor in that the tubes are aligned vertically in the body of the rotor at all times. During operation of the rotor, the solution in the tube reorients through 90° during rotor acceleration to lie perpendicular to the axis of rotation and parallel to the applied centrifugal field and returns to its original position during deceleration of the rotor (Fig. 5.3b to g). Since sedimentation of particles occurs across the diameter of the tube, the vertical tube rotor presents the shortest possible pathlength for the particle. Sedimentation of particles can thus be achieved more quickly than by using either the fixed-angle rotor or the swinging-bucket rotor, and, since r_{min} is greater, due to the tubes being at the rotor's edge, a larger minimum centrifugal field is generated. In this type of rotor, however, any pellet formed is deposited along the entire length of the outer wall of the centrifuge tube, which could be a disadvantage because it tends to fall back into the solution at the end of centrifugation.

5.4.5 **Zonal rotors**

Zonal rotors may be of the batch or continuous flow type, the former being more extensively used than the latter, and are designed to minimise the wall effects that are encountered in swinging-bucket and fixed-angle rotors, and to increase sample size.

Several different types of batch-type rotor are available that differ in the method by which they are loaded and unloaded. Low speed batch rotors, designed to operate near 5000 rev min^{-1} (5000 g) are made of aluminium, having a thick transparent Perspex top and bottom to permit direct examination of particle sedimentation during the course of centrifugation. High speed batch rotors are made of aluminium or titanium alloy and can operate at speeds up to 60 000 rev min^{-1} (256 000 g). The body of a typical batch-type rotor is either a large cylindrical container or a hollow bowl, in which the rotor volume varies with the square of the radial distance from the centre of rotation. The centre of the rotor has a core to which is attached a vane assembly that divides the rotor internally into four sector-shaped compartments and minimises swirling of the rotor contents. The vanes or septa have radial ducts to allow gradient to be pumped to the periphery of the rotor from the centre core. The rotor is enclosed by a threaded lid. The capacity of batch-type rotors range from 300 cm^3 to 2000 cm^3, with the gradient material filling the entire enclosed space. The rotor core may be of two main types. The most commonly used standard core permits the loading and unloading of the rotor while it is spinning (dynamic method), whereas the second core type (the reorienting gradient core) is designed to allow the rotor to be loaded and unloaded with a reorienting gradient while it is at rest (static method).

In the dynamic mode of operation, loading of the standard core-type rotor is achieved while the rotor is revolving at approximately 2000 rev min^{-1}. The lighter end of the preformed gradient is pumped into the rotor first through a fixed or a removable seal to emerge at the periphery and form a uniform layer held in a

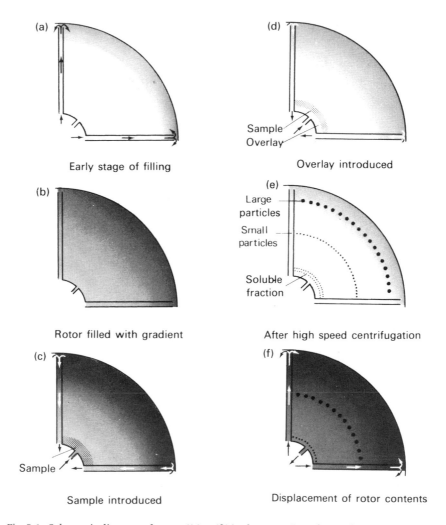

(a)

Early stage of filling

(b)

Rotor filled with gradient

(c)

Sample

Sample introduced

(d)

Sample
Overlay

Overlay introduced

(e)

Large
particles

Small
particles

Soluble
fraction

After high speed centrifugation

(f)

Displacement of rotor contents

Fig. 5.6. Schematic diagram of stages ((a) to (f)) in the operation of a zonal rotor. (Reproduced by kind permission of Measuring and Scientific Equipment Ltd.)

vertical orientation against the outer rotor wall by centrifugal force (Fig. 5.6a). The successive addition of denser gradient results in a continuous centripetal displacement of the lighter gradient towards the rotor core (Fig. 5.6b). When the gradient has been pumped into the rotor, fluid cushion, as dense as or denser than the heaviest end of the preformed gradient, is introduced into the rotor to fill it completely. The sample is then introduced by the fluid line leading to the rotor centre (Fig. 5.6c) from which it is subsequently displaced by the addition of an overlay of low density liquid (Fig. 5.6d), an equal volume of cushion being displaced from the periphery. After removal of the gradient lines to the rotor, the rotor is accelerated to the operating speed, for the required time interval, to give either rate zonal or isopycnic zonal separation (Fig. 5.6e). Recovery of the gradient and separated particles is then accomplished by decelerating the rotor to its original 2000 rev min^{-1}

and the rotor contents displaced, lighter end first, by introducing additional cushion to the periphery of the rotor (Fig. 5.6f). A modified rotor core is available that adds versatility to the operation of the zonal rotor by allowing fractions to be recovered at the rotor's edge as well as its centre. Edge loading is accomplished by the introduction of a buffer or distilled water at the rotor centre and collecting the fractions through the edge ports of the core. This modification has the advantage that it is more economic in the use of the displacing gradient.

In the static method of zonal centrifugation, using the reorienting (Reograd) gradient core, the sample solution is layered on top of a density gradient in the rotor while it is at rest (Fig. 5.7a). The rotor is then slowly accelerated to about 1000 rev min^{-1} to prevent mixing of the rotor contents, during which time the sample and gradient layers reorient under centrifugal force (Fig. 5.7b). Near operating speeds the zones approach a vertical orientation, and at very high speeds, where the ratio between the centrifugal force and the acceleration due to gravity in a downward direction is very high, the zones become vertical (Fig. 5.7c). Particle separation occurs with the rotor at its operating speed (Fig. 5.7d). At the completion of the separation the rotor is decelerated from its operating speed to 1000 rev min^{-1} and then slowly decelerated to rest. This is to prevent mixing of the rotor contents when sample and gradient layers reorient back to the horizontal position (Fig. 5.7e). With the rotor at rest, the contents can be displaced from it and recovered either by drawing the contents out of the bottom of the rotor or by displacing the gradient out through the top (Fig. 5.7f). Static loading and unloading of the rotor is most suitable for the isolation of long, fragile particles, such as DNA strands, which would otherwise be damaged by the rotating seal assembly used in the dynamic method and has become an accepted method for the separation of lipoprotein fractions from large volumes of plasma or serum. The design of all of the batch-type rotor cores enables the zones to be collected without any appreciable loss of resolution achieved during centrifugation. The static and dynamic methods give equally good resolutions. To aid zone isolation, the gradient emerging from the rotor is passed through a suitable monitoring device, for example a photocell, to determine protein content by its ultraviolet absorption at 280 nm wavelength (Section 6.3.2, or a suitable monitor to detect radioactivity (Section 14.2), and the collected into fractions to be analysed for concentration of gradient material (using a refractometer), for specific biological activity, or for some other appropriate property.

Batch-type zonal rotors have been used to remove contaminating proteins from a variety of preparations and for the separation and isolation of hormones, enzymes, macroglobulins, ribosomal subunits, viruses and subcellular organelles from animal or plant tissue homogenates.

Continuous flow zonal rotors are designed for high speed separation of relatively small quantities of solid matter from large volumes of suspension and are particularly useful for the harvesting of cells and the large-scale isolation of viruses. The rotors are similar in shape to batch-type zonal rotors, but differ in the design of the core because of the different fluid flow patterns in the rotor. In operation, the suspension is continuously fed into the rotor during centrifugation at a flow rate of up to 9 dm^3 h^{-1}. The sedimenting material moves into the rotor

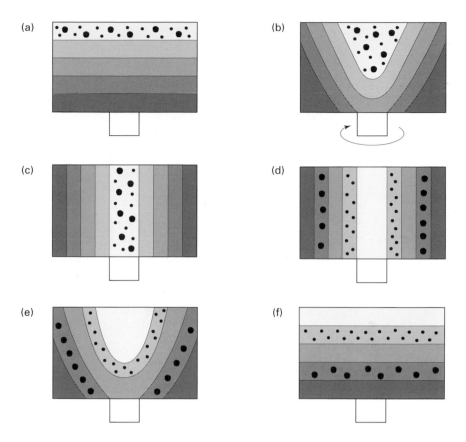

Fig. 5.7. Schematic diagram of a reorienting (Reograd) rotor system. (a) Rotor is filled at rest with density gradient and sample layer. (b) Rotor is accelerated and layers reorient under centrifugal force. (c) Layers become vertical at sufficiently high rotor speed. (d) Particles now separate through the gradient with the rotor at speed. (e) During rotor deceleration, layers containing separated particles reorient. (f) At rest, rotor contents are displaced and various zones recovered (small dots represent small-sized particles; large dots represent large-sized particles).

chamber, while the particle-free effluent leaves the rotor through an outlet line. The rotor may be operated without a density gradient, in which case the sample particles are allowed to pellet on the rotor wall and recovered after the rotor has been stopped at the conclusion of the run. Alternatively, a density gradient may be used and the particles separated according to differences in their density. The separated bands may then be recovered in a manner similar to that described for the operation of the batch-type zonal rotor using the standard core.

5.4.6 **Elutriator rotors**

The elutriator rotor (Fig. 5.8a) is a type of continuous flow rotor that contains recesses to hold a single conical-shaped separation chamber, the apex of which

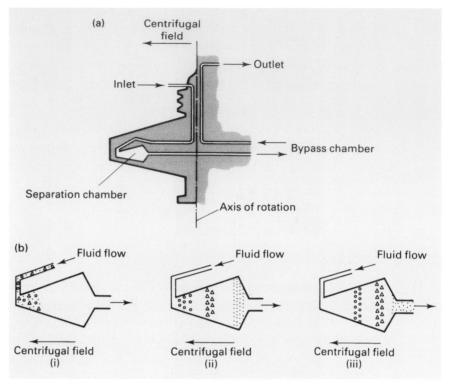

Fig. 5.8. (a) Cross-section through an elutriator rotor and (b) the separation of particles in the separation chamber of an elutriator rotor by centrifugal elutriation.

points away from the axis of rotation, and a by-pass chamber on the opposite side of the rotor that serves as a counterbalance and to provide the fluid outlet. The separation chamber may be of two types that differ in capacity and have slightly different shapes. With the aid of a windowed centrifuge door and a stroboscopic lamp, whose flash rate is synchronised with the rotor speed, apertures in the rotor allow the rotor chamber contents to be observed during centrifugation. Particles suspended in a uniform low density medium are pumped into the rotor chamber at its peripheral edge via a rotating seal assembly while the rotor is spinning at a preselected speed (usually between 1000 and 3000 rev min^{-1}). Since the separation chamber is conically shaped (Fig. 5.8b), a gradient of liquid flow velocity, which gradually decreases as the diameter of the chamber increases towards its centripetal end (i.e. towards the axis of rotation), will therefore exist in the chamber that opposes the applied centrifugal field. The tendency of particles of differing sedimentation rate to sediment in the centrifugal field (Fig. 5.8b(i)) is therefore balanced against the controlled flow of liquid being pumped through the separation chamber in the opposite direction towards its centripetal end. Particles then band in the separation chamber at a position where their sedimentation velocity, which in the uniform low density medium used will be proportional to their size, is balanced by liquid flow rate in the opposite direction (Fig. 5.8b(ii)).

Larger particles accumulate towards the centrifugal end of the chamber where the liquid flow velocity is high, while the smaller particles accumulate towards the centripetal end of the chamber where the liquid flow velocity is low. Either by a stepwise decrease in rotor speed or by a stepwise increase in liquid flow rate through the separation chamber, collection of the separated uniformly sized particles can be made centripetally in order of successively increasing diameter by elutriation from the chamber (Fig. 5.8b(iii)).

With the technique of centrifugal elutriation (Section 5.6.3) the elutriator rotor has been used successfully to separate various cell types from mammalian testis, different types of monocytes and lymphocytes from human blood, to purify Kupffer and endothelial cells from sinusoidal liver cells and fat storing cells from rat liver, and for the bulk separation of rat brain cells and the fractionation of yeast cell populations.

5.4.7 Care of rotors

The protective anodised coating on aluminium rotors is very thin (approximately 0.025 mm) and does not provide a high degree of protection against corrosion; thus rotors should always be handled with care to prevent scratching. The use of acid solutions, strong alkaline detergents (e.g. Decon 90), and salt solutions can also easily damage the protective coating, leading to corrosion and eventually failure of the rotor. After use, therefore, rotors should be thoroughly washed, preferably with deionised water and, because moisture is a potential source of corrosion, left to drain and dry upside down in a warm atmosphere; they should then be stored in a clean, dry environment. Rotor outer surfaces only can be given a protective coat of lanolin or silicone polish. Swinging-bucket rotors, however, should never be completely immersed in water because the bucket hanging mechanism is difficult to dry and can rust. Titanium rotors are essentially resistant to corrosion. However, rotors made of titanium alloy containing aluminium or ferrous compounds are prone to corrosion.

It is important to note that all rotors are designed to carry a maximum load at a maximum speed, which is based on the rotor tubes or bottles being filled with a solution whose density is no greater than $1.2 \, \text{g cm}^{-3}$. A reduction in the maximum rated speed (known as derating the rotor) is therefore required if the density of the solution exceeds this value. This reduction can be calculated from the equation

$$M_n = \sqrt{\left(\frac{1.2 \times M^2}{N} \right)} \qquad\qquad (5.16)$$

where M is the usual maximum rotor speed using a solution of density $1.2 \, \text{g cm}^{-3}$ and M_n is the new maximum rotor speed when a solution with a density of $N \, \text{g cm}^{-3}$ is used. Speed reductions are also required when stainless steel caps and/or tubes are used and to prevent recrystallisation of high density salt solutions, which could occur when the salt concentration exceeds the solubility limit of the solution.

To prevent possible damage to the drive shaft of the centrifuge due to vibration caused by rotor imbalance, sample loads should be balanced within the limits specified by the manufacturer – each opposing pair of sample containers being balanced individually, and the total load balanced symmetrically in the rotor. Swinging-bucket rotors should not be run with any buckets or caps removed or individual rotor buckets interchanged, because they form an integral part of the balance of the rotor.

During acceleration and deceleration of the rotor, cyclic stretching and relaxing of the metal can cause metal fatigue, leading to the eventual failure of the rotor. To avoid overstressing the rotor and ensure its continued safe operation, an accurate record should be kept of its total usage, i.e. the number of runs (at any speed up to its maximum number of revolutions per minute) and the time of each run, so that the rotor can either be derated after a certain number of runs (e.g. 1000) or hours of centrifugation (e.g. 2500) or replaced after a set period of time, as specified by the manufacturer.

5.5 SAMPLE CONTAINERS

Centrifuge tubes and bottles are manufactured in a range of different sizes ($100\,mm^3$ to $1\,dm^3$), in varying thickness and rigidity and from a wide variety of materials including glass, cellulose esters, polyallomer, polycarbonate, polyethylene, polypropylene, kynar (a high relative molecular mass homopolymer of vinylidene fluoride), nylon and stainless steel.

The correct choice of sample container is important in order to achieve the desired degree of separation of particles from a sample mixture. It is important before commencing centrifugation to consult manufacturers' technical literature to determine the limitations of the material from which the container is made. The type of container used will depend upon such factors as the nature and volume of the sample to be centrifuged, the type of rotor to be used, the available centrifuge, the centrifugal forces to be withstood, its chemical resistance to various solvents, upper and lower temperature limits and physical properties, i.e. whether the tube is transparent or opaque, and can be sliced or punctured for post-centrifugation analysis.

Glass centrifuge tubes are usually suitable only for centrifugation at low speeds because they disintegrate in higher centrifugal fields. Thin-walled tubes may be used in swinging-bucket rotors because the tube is protected from the forces trying to deform it by the surrounding bucket; however, thick-walled tubes are usually required when fixed-angle and vertical tube rotors are used because the large forces exerted on the tube tend to collapse it. Centrifuge tubes and bottles should always be filled to the correct level, and maximum allowable rotor speeds, depending on the particular container, observed. The need to cap bottles and tubes usually depends upon the speed at which the sample is to be centrifuged, the type of container and the nature of the sample. Ideally, tubes used in fixed-angle and vertical tube ultracentrifuge rotors should always be completely filled in order to support the tube against the very high centrifugal forces generated. It is especially important that tubes are capped and sealed with special leak-proof sealing caps when material that may be a biohazard or radioactive is being centrifuged. Capping and sealing of tubes used in vertical tube rotors and most fixed-angle rotors are also important because the tubes have to withstand the large upward hydrostatic force generated during centrifugation by the liquid in the tube.

5.6 SEPARATION METHODS IN PREPARATIVE ULTRACENTRIFUGES

5.6.1 Differential centrifugation

This method is based upon the differences in the sedimentation rate of particles of different size and density. As can be seen from equation 5.12, centrifugation will initially sediment the largest particles. For particles of the same mass but different density, the ones with the highest density (e.g. peroxisomes, $\rho = 1.23$ g cm^{-3} in sucrose solution) will sediment at a faster rate than the less dense particles (e.g. plasma membranes, $\rho = 1.16$ g cm^{-3} in sucrose solution) of similar mass. Particles having similar banding densities (e.g. most of the subcellular organelles, where $\rho = 1.1$ to 1.3 g cm^{-3} in sucrose solution) can usually be efficiently separated one from another by differential centrifugation or the rate zonal method (Section 5.6.2), provided there is about a ten-fold difference in their mass.

In differential centrifugation, the material to be separated (e.g. a tissue homogenate) is divided centrifugally into a number of fractions by increasing (stepwise) the applied centrifugal field. The centrifugal field at each stage is chosen so that a particular type of material sediments, during the predetermined time of centrifugation, to give a pellet of particles sedimented through the solution, and a supernatant solution containing unsedimented material. Any type of particle originally present in the homogenate may be found in the pellet or the supernatant or both fractions, depending upon the time and speed of centrifugation and the size and density of the particle. At the end of each stage, the pellet and supernatant are separated and the pellet washed several times by resuspension in the homogenisation medium, followed by recentrifugation under the same conditions. This procedure minimises cross-contamination, improves particle separation and eventually gives a fairly pure preparation of pellet fraction. To appreciate why the pellet is never absolutely pure (homogeneous), however, it is necessary to consider the conditions prevailing in the centrifuge tube at the beginning of each stage.

Initially all particles of the homogenate are homogeneously distributed throughout the centrifuge tube (Fig. 5.9a). During centrifugation, particles move down the centrifuge tube at their respective sedimentation rates (Fig. 5.9b to e) and start to form a pellet on the bottom of the centrifuge tube. Ideally, centrifugation is continued long enough to pellet all the largest class of particles (Fig. 5.9c), the resulting supernatant then being centrifuged at a higher speed to separate medium-sized particles and so on. However, since particles of varying sizes and densities were distributed homogeneously at the commencement of centrifugation, it is evident that the pellet will not be homogeneous but will contain a mixture of all the sedimented components, being enriched with the fastest (heaviest) sedimenting particles. In the time required for the complete sedimentation of

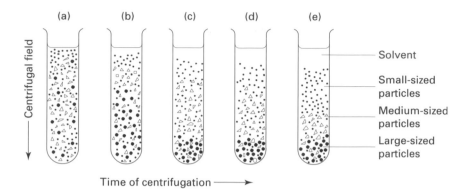

Fig. 5.9. Differential sedimentation of a particulate suspension in a centrifugal field. (a) Particles are uniformly distributed throughout the centrifuge tube. (b) to (e) Sedimentation of particles during centrifugation is dependent upon their size, shape and density.

heavier particles, some of the lighter and medium-sized particles, originally suspended near the bottom of the tube, will also sediment and thus contaminate the fraction. Pure preparations of the pellet of the heaviest particle cannot therefore be obtained in one centrifugation step. It is only the most slowly sedimenting component of the mixture remaining in the supernatant liquid after all the larger particles have been sedimented that can be purified by a single centrifugation step, but its yield is often very low.

The separation achieved by differential centrifugation may be improved by repeated (two or three times) resuspension of the pellet in homogenisation medium and recentrifugation under the same conditions as in the original pelleting, but this will inevitably reduce the yield obtained. Further centrifugation of the supernatant in gradually increasing centrifugal fields results in the sedimentation of the intermediate and finally the smallest and least dense particles. A scheme for the fractionation of rat liver homogenate into the various subcellular fractions is given in Fig. 5.10. In spite of its inherent limitations, differential centrifugation is probably the most commonly used method for the isolation of cell organelles from homogenised tissue.

5.6.2 Density gradient centrifugation

There are two methods of density gradient centrifugation, the rate zonal technique and the isopycnic (isodensity or equal density) technique, and both can be used when the quantitative separation of all the components of a mixture of particles is required. They are also used for the determination of buoyant densities and for the estimation of sedimentation coefficients.

Particle separation by the rate zonal technique is based upon differences in the size, shape and density of the particles, the density and viscosity of the medium and the applied centrifugal field. However, since similar types of biological particle are

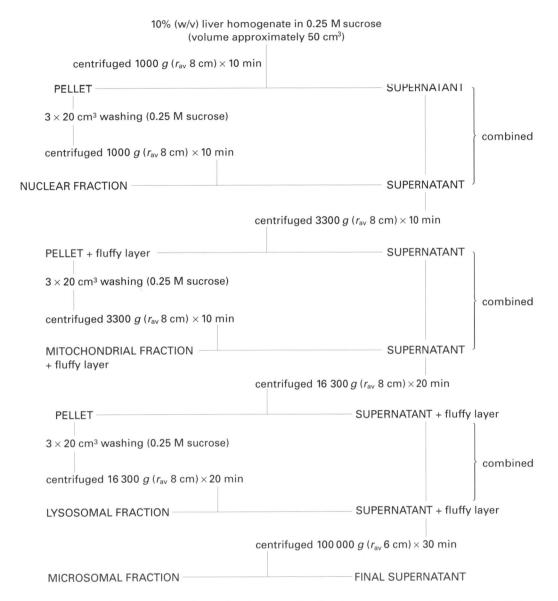

Fig. 5.10. Scheme for the fractionation of rat liver homogenate into the various subcellular fractions.

often similar in shape and their densities fall into a relatively narrow range, and the maximum density of the gradient is chosen not to exceed that of the densest particle to be separated, separation of similar types of particles by the rate zonal technique is based mainly upon differences in their size. Subcellular organelles, therefore, such as mitochondria, lysosomes and peroxisomes, which have different densities but are similar in size, do not separate efficiently using this method, but the separation of proteins of similar density and differing only three-fold in relative

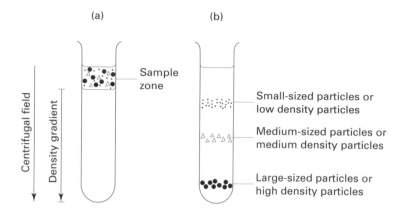

Fig. 5.11. Rate separation and isopycnic separation using a density gradient. (a) Mixture of particles layered on top of a preformed liquid density gradient prior to centrifugation; (b) centrifugation of particles. For rate separation, the required fraction does not reach its isopycnic position. For isopycnic separation, centrifugation is continued until the desired particles have reached their isopycnic position in the gradient.

molecular mass can be achieved easily. The technique involves carefully layering a sample solution on top of a preformed liquid density gradient, the highest density of which does not exceed that of the densest particles to be separated. The function of the gradient is primarily to stabilise the liquid column in the tube against movement resulting from convection currents and secondarily to produce a gradient of viscosity that helps to improve the resolution of the gradient. The sample is then centrifuged until the desired degree of separation is effected, i.e. for sufficient time for the particles to travel through the gradient to form discrete zones or bands (Fig. 5.11), which are spaced according to the relative velocities of the particles. Since the technique is time dependent, centrifugation must be terminated before any of the separated zones pellet at the bottom of the tube. The technique has been used for the separation of enzymes, hormones, RNA–DNA hybrids, ribosomal subunits, subcellular organelles, for the analysis of size distribution of samples of polysomes and lipoprotein fractionations and may be adapted for bulk preparative work using a zonal rotor (Section 5.4.5).

Isopycnic centrifugation depends solely upon the buoyant density of the particle and not its shape or size and is independent of time, the size of the particle affecting only the rate at which it reaches its isopycnic position in the gradient. The technique is used to separate particles of similar size but of differing density. Hence soluble proteins, which have a very similar density (e.g. $\rho = 1.3$ g cm^{-3} in sucrose solution), can not usually be separated by this method, whereas subcellular organelles (e.g. Golgi apparatus ($\rho = 1.11$ g cm^{-3}), mitochondria ($\rho = 1.19$ g cm^{-3}), and peroxisomes ($\rho = 1.23$ g cm^{-3}) in sucrose solution) can be effectively separated.

The methods are a combination of sedimentation and flotation and involve layering the sample on top of a density gradient that spans the whole range of the

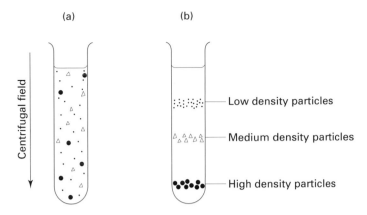

Fig. 5.12. Isopycnic centrifugation using the equilibrium isodensity method. (a) Particles distributed homogeneously throughout the tube prior to centrifugation. (b) During centrifugation the gradient is allowed to establish itself, sample particles redistribute and band in a series of zones at their respective isopycnic positions.

particle densities that are to be separated. The maximum density of the gradient, therefore, must always exceed the density of the most dense particle. While it is possible to use a discontinuous or stepwise gradient, it is preferable to use a continuous gradient (Section 5.7.1). During centrifugation, sedimentation of the particles occurs until the buoyant density of the particle and the density of the gradient are equal (i.e. where $\rho_p = \rho_m$ in equation 5.12). At this point of isodensity no further sedimentation occurs, irrespective of how long centrifugation continues, because the particles are floating on a cushion of material that has a density greater than their own. Isopycnic centrifugation, in contrast to the rate zonal technique, is an equilibrium method, the particles banding to form zones each at their own characteristic buoyant density (Fig. 5.11). In cases where, perhaps, not all the components in a mixture of particles are required, a gradient range can be selected in which unwanted components of the mixture will sediment to the bottom of the centrifuge tube while the particles of interest sediment to their respective isopycnic positions. Such a technique involves a combination of both the rate zonal and isopycnic approaches.

As an alternative to layering the particle mixture to be separated onto a preformed gradient, the sample is initially mixed with the gradient medium to give a solution of uniform density, the gradient self-forming, by sedimentation equilibrium, during centrifugation. In this method (referred to as the equilibrium isodensity method), use is generally made of the salts of heavy metals (e.g. caesium or rubidium), sucrose, colloidal silica or Metrizamide. The sample (e.g. DNA) is mixed homogeneously with, for example, a concentrated solution of caesium chloride (Fig. 5.12a). Centrifugation of the concentrated caesium chloride solution results in the sedimentation of the CsCl molecules to form a concentration gradient and hence a density gradient. The sample molecules (DNA), which were initially uniformly distributed throughout the tube, now either rise or sediment until they reach a region where the solution density is equal to their own buoyant density, i.e. their isopycnic position, where they will band to form zones (Fig. 5.12b). This technique suffers from the disadvantage that often very long centrifugation times (e.g. 36 to 48 h) are required to establish equilibrium. However, it is commonly used in analytical centrifugation to determine the buoyant density of a particle, the base composition of double-stranded DNA and to separate linear from circular forms of DNA. Many of the separations can be improved by increasing the density differences between the different forms of DNA by the incorporation of heavy isotopes (e.g. ^{15}N) during biosynthesis, a technique used by M. Meselson and F. Stahl to elucidate the mechanism of DNA replication in *Escherichia coli*, or by the binding of heavy-metal ions or dyes such as ethidium bromide. Isopycnic gradients have also been used to separate and purify viruses and analyse human plasma lipoproteins, to study the variation of buoyant density with pH for proteins and homopolypeptides and has found wide application in the analysis of nucleic acids.

5.6.3 **Centrifugal elutriation**

In this technique the separation and purification of a large variety of cells from different tissues and species can be achieved by a gentle 'washing action' using an elutriator rotor (Section 5.4.6 and Fig. 5.8). The technique is based upon differences in the equilibrium, set up in the separation chamber of the rotor, between the opposing centripetal liquid flow and applied centrifugal field being used to separate particles mainly on the basis of differences in their size. The technique does not employ a density gradient and has the advantage that any medium totally compatible with the particles can be used, for example buffered salt solutions or culture medium; because pelleting of the particles does not occur, fractionation of delicate cells or particles, between 5 and 50 μm diameter, can be achieved with minimum damage so that cells retain their viability. Separations can be achieved very quickly, giving high cell concentrations and a very good recovery yield.

5.7 **PERFORMING DENSITY GRADIENT SEPARATIONS**

5.7.1 **Formation and choice of density gradients**

All density gradient methods involve a supporting column of liquid whose density increases towards the bottom of the centrifuge tube. The function of the density gradient in rate zonal centrifugation is to stabilise the column of liquid in the centrifuge tube, prevent mixing of the separated particles due to convection currents, improve resolution of the separated components by eliminating, or largely alleviating, factors such as mechanical vibration and thermal gradients that disturb the smooth migration of particles through the suspending medium, and permit the quantitative separation of several or all components in a mixture.

However, in isopycnic centrifugation the prime function of the density gradient is to band the particles at their buoyant densities.

Density gradients of different shape (i.e. with a concentration profile of gradient medium along the tube) may be produced by techniques that fall into two major groups, the discontinuous or step gradient technique and the continuous density gradient technique.

In the discontinuous technique, two methods are available to produce the initial step gradient. In the overlayering method, known volumes of solutions of decreasing density are allowed to run slowly down the side of the centrifuge tube to form layers over each other in the centrifuge tube. Alternatively, in the under-layering method, a layer of the lightest density solution is introduced into the centrifuge tube; this is then successively underlayered, by means of a pipette placed with its tip at the bottom of the centrifuge tube, with a series of layers (corresponding to the required number of steps) of solution of increasing density, which when added displaces the less dense solution. The discontinuous gradient can be used directly by layering of the sample to be separated as a narrow zone on the top (lowest density) layer. The tube is then centrifuged under the appropriate experimental conditions. Alternatively, if the discontinous gradient is allowed to stand, the layers slowly merge by diffusion to produce a continuous linear gradient, the time required depending upon such factors as, the concentration range and viscosity of the gradient, thickness of each layer, temperature, and relative molecular mass of the solute.

The continuous density gradient technique is probably the more common of the two, and requires the use of a special piece of apparatus known as a density gradient maker, many varieties of which are commercially available and range from the simplest equipment capable of generating either linear, convex- or concave-shaped gradients to sophisticated programmable gradient makers, used mainly in centrifugation studies with zonal rotors, that are capable of producing more complex gradient shapes. Gradient makers capable of forming linear gradients, i.e. where the density of the medium in the centrifuge tube increases linearly with increasing distance from the axis of rotation, consist of two precision-bored cylindrical chambers of identical cross-sectional area that are interconnected at their base by a tube containing a control valve that allows the mixing of the contents of the two chambers to be regulated. One chamber (the mixing chamber) contains a stirrer and possesses an outlet through which the gradient is drawn off, via a length of narrow bore flexible tubing, to the centrifuge tube. If the wall of the centrifuge tube is reasonably wettable by aqueous solutions, as in the case of polypropylene, cellulose nitrate and cellulose acetate butyrate tubes, the outlet pipe from the gradient maker may be allowed to touch the wall of the centrifuge tube near to the top of the tube and the stream of liquid allowed to run slowly down the side of the tube, as it is filled, on to the top of the forming gradient.

Using this top loading method the mixing chamber of the gradient maker is filled with the most dense solution and the second chamber (the reservoir) filled with an equal amount (by weight) of a less dense solution. The hydrostatic pressures of the two liquid columns need to be equal otherwise liquid will flow through the connecting tube as soon as the control valve is opened. The dense liquid is then allowed to run slowly through the filling pipe, from the mixing chamber and down the wall of the centrifuge tube, and is immediately replaced in the mixing chamber, as a result of hydrostatic pressure, by an equivalent amount of less dense solution via the control valve. This re-establishes hydrostatic equilibrium. As a result the concentration and density of the solution in the mixing chamber, which is maintained homogeneous by constant stirring, constantly and linearly decreases as the device empties. The concentration of the gradient in the centrifuge tube will therefore decrease in a linear manner as the tube is filled.

The top loading method, however, is not suitable for use with centrifuge tubes made from materials that are hydrophobic and not wettable by aqueous solutions, such as polycarbonate or polyallomer, because the gradient material tends to gather in large droplets at the exit of the filling pipe from the gradient maker and then fall into, and disturb, the forming gradient. This problem may be overcome by bottom loading the gradient into the centrifuge tube. In this method, the less dense solution is now placed in the mixing chamber of the gradient maker and the more dense solution placed in the reservoir. By way of a probe that now leads to the bottom of the centrifuge tube less dense solution is allowed to enter the centrifuge tube first and is then displaced by solution of increasing density. Non-linear gradients (i.e. either convex or concave in concentration as a function of volume) may be produced by choosing chambers with varying cross-sectional areas. Alternatively, two mechanically driven syringes containing solutions of different densities may be used. In this case the shape of the gradient may be varied by altering the speed of pumping of one syringe with respect to that of the other.

Gradients of different shape are designed for specific purposes and are important in achieving the desired separation and purification and for the determination of such properties as the buoyant density and sedimentation coefficient of a particle. Discontinuous and continuous gradients are used in isopycnic centrifugation but discontinuous gradients are not often used in rate zonal centrifugation because artefactual bands of material can collect at the interfaces. Discontinuous gradients have been found to be the most suitable for the separation of whole cells or subcellular organelles from plant or animal tissue homogenates and for purification of some viruses. For most purposes linear gradients are used, because the gradual change in density along the gradient has been found to yield a much higher resolution of components such as ribosomal subunits, proteins, enzymes, hormones, and some plant viruses. In general, the greater the slope of the gradient, the better the resolution obtained, because tighter bands are formed due to increasing viscosity. However, for some applications better resolution is achieved using non-linear gradients. Thus, concave gradients can be used to separate light particles by flotation (e.g. serum lipoproteins), whereas heavier particles in the mixture quickly sediment through the less dense upper regions of the gradient to be banded in the region of high viscosity near the bottom of the centrifuge tube. Large particles such as ribosomal subunits, polyribosomes and some viruses usually require steep gradients and long gradient columns to enhance separation.

This may be achieved by using rotors with long slender tubes that provide the longer gradient columns, and linear-log gradients in which the logarithm of the gradient column depth is a linear function of the logarithm of the sedimentation coefficient of the particle.

Isokinetic gradients are a specialised type of continuous gradient, generally convex and exponential in shape, and are so designed that the increase in density and viscosity of the gradient balances the increase in the centrifugal field along the tube so that at a constant rotor speed all particles of equal density will move at a constant velocity at all distances along the tube, the distance travelled by each particle being proportional to the relative centrifugal force applied, the time of centrifugation and the sedimentation coefficient of the particle. Hence, if the sedimentation coefficient of a single reference marker particle is known then the sedimentation coefficients of other particles in the same gradient may be calculated, provided each particle has the same density as the particle used as the sedimentation marker.

Most gradient shapes used in zonal rotors are the same as those used in swinging-bucket rotors. However, when preparing gradients for use in zonal rotors, an allowance must be made for the fact that, whereas the parallel walls of the test tube used in swinging-bucket rotors maintain a linear volume-to-radius relationship, the bowl-shaped cavity of a zonal rotor will alter this relationship, since its value varies with the square of the radial distance from the centre of rotation. A gradient will therefore change its shape when loaded into a zonal rotor. Gradients that are prepared linear or convex in concentration with respect to rotor volume will therefore become concave and linear in shape, respectively, when introduced into the zonal rotor.

5.7.2 Sample application to the gradient

Each gradient has a defined sample capacity, which is a function of its density slope and if exceeded will result in a poor resolution of the sample; therefore, before the sample is applied to the density gradient, its optimum volume and concentration should be determined. The volume of the sample that can be applied to a centrifuge tube is a function of the cross-sectional area of the gradient exposed to the sample. Thus, sample volumes in the range 0.2 to 0.5 cm^3 may be added to tubes 1.0 to 1.6 cm in diameter, and sample volumes of up to 1 cm^3 to tubes having a diameter of approximately 2.5 cm. Effective separation of particles in a multi-component sample would not be achieved with larger sample volumes due to insufficient radial distance in the centrifuge tube. Equally, if the sample concentration on the gradient is too high or too low then either the gradient may become overloaded, resulting in a broadening of the separated zones and loss of resolution, or difficulty may be encountered in the identification of the separated bands. For proteins and nucleic acids, sample concentrations of between 1 $\mu g\ cm^{-3}$ and 1 mg cm^{-3} are recommended in sucrose gradients.

For rate zonal separations the correct method of application of the sample to the gradient is of paramount importance, because the resolving power of the gradient is greater the narrower the initial sample zone. The sample is therefore applied, usually using a narrow-bore pipette, as slowly and as gently as possible to reduce mixing with the gradient. The tip of the pipette is touched against the meniscus at the wall of the tube. The pipette is moved slightly upward to leave a thin channel of liquid between the pipette and the meniscus. In order to minimise mixing with the gradient the sample is allowed to run slowly out of the pipette and gently on to the surface of the gradient to form a sharply defined sample layer. The separation achieved in isopycnic separation is independent of the initial distribution of the sample. The volume of the sample and its initial distribution through the gradient are therefore unimportant and the sample can be carefully layered on top of a pre-formed gradient, mixed with the gradient medium in the case of self-forming gradients, or mixed with a dense solution of the gradient medium and layered under the density gradient.

5.7.3 Recovery and monitoring of gradients from centrifuge tubes

After particle separation has been achieved, it is usually necessary to remove the gradient solution in order to isolate the bands of separated material. If, however, the bands can be visually detected, recovery from the gradient can be achieved without having to unload the gradient by placing a Pasteur pipette into the band and slowly withdrawing the required material from the band. Alternatively, the band may be recovered through the side of the centrifuge tube using a hypodermic syringe. Removal of gradients from centrifuge tubes can be achieved by a number of techniques. A method of choice for most applications, however, is that of upward displacement. Either a denser solution of the gradient medium, or, for example, a solution that is marketed especially for displacement unloading of gradients (such as Maxidens, an inert, non-viscous, water-immiscible organic liquid with a density of 1.9 g cm^{-3} that does not react with the gradient medium) is either pumped through a long needle passing through the gradient to the bottom of the centrifuge tube or introduced via a hollow needle piercing the bottom of the tube. The gradient is displaced upwards and the fractions removed in sequence using a syringe or pipette, or preferably by being channelled out through an unloading cap to which is attached a collection pipe leading either to a fraction collector or directly into a flow cell of an ultraviolet spectrophotometer. A variation of this method is to fit a cap to the top of the centrifuge tube and pump either air or a less dense solution of the gradient medium into the top of the tube, the gradient then being displaced through a tube that leads from the bottom of the tube.

Alternatively, provided a pellet of cells is not present, the centrifuge tube may be punctured at its base by using a fine hollow needle. As the drops of gradient pass from the tube through the needle they may be collected by using a fraction collector, and further analysed. Analysis of the displaced gradient, in order to identify and locate the separated components, can be achieved by ultraviolet spectrophotometry (Section 9.4), refractive index measurements, scintillation counting (Section 14.2), and enzymic (Section 7.4) or chemical analysis.

5.7.4 **Nature of gradient materials and their use**

There is no ideal all-purpose gradient material; the choice of solute depends upon the nature of the particles to be fractionated. The gradient material should:

permit the desired type of separation;

be stable in solution;

be inert towards biological materials and not react with the centrifuge, rotor, tubes or caps;

not absorb light at wavelengths appropriate for spectrophotometric monitoring (visible or ultraviolet range), or otherwise interfere with assaying procedures;

be sterilisable, non-toxic or flammable;

have negligible osmotic pressure and cause minimum changes in ionic strength, pH and viscosity;

be inexpensive and readily available in pure form and capable of forming a solution covering the density range needed for a particular application without overstressing the rotor;

allow easy separation of the sample material from the gradient medium without loss of the sample or its activity.

Gradient-forming materials that provide the densities required for the separation of subcellular particles include salts of alkali metals (e.g. caesium and rubidium chloride), small neutral hydrophilic organic molecules (e.g. sucrose), hydrophilic macromolecules (e.g. proteins and polysaccharides), and a number of miscellaneous compounds such as colloidal silica (e.g. Percoll and Ludox), and non-ionic iodinated aromatic compounds (e.g. Metrizamide, Nycodenz and Renograffin).

Sucrose solutions, while suffering from the disadvantages of being very viscous at densities greater than 1.1. to 1.2 g cm^{-3} and exerting very high osmotic effects even at very low concentrations (i.e. at approximately 10% (w/v) concentration), have been found to be the most convenient gradient material for rate zonal separations. In some instances, however, glycerol is used, particularly for the separation of enzymes, or alternative media such as Ficoll (a copolymer of sucrose and epichlorohydrin), Metrizamide or Percoll gradients may be utilised. Non-ionic media, such as sucrose, glycerol, Metrizamide, Ficoll and Percoll are generally considered to be more gentle than ionic salts, such as caesium chloride and potassium bromide, and require lower centrifugal fields to achieve an adequate separation of particles. In the case of isopycnic separations, no one medium has proved satisfactory for the isolation of all types of biological particles. Hence a wide range of gradient media has been used for different types of biological sample. Ficoll has been successfully used instead of sucrose for the separation of whole cells and subcellular organelles by rate zonal and isopycnic centrifugation, but, although it is relatively inert osmotically at low concentrations, both osmolarity and viscosity rise sharply at higher concentrations (i.e. above 20% (w/v)). Caesium and rubidium salts are used exclusively for isopycnic separations and have been used most frequently for the separation of high density solutes such as nucleic acids. However, at high concentrations their high ionic strength and osmolarity tend to disrupt intra- and intermolecular bonds. Generally, ionic media have been used for the separation of nucleic acids, proteins and viruses, sucrose gradients for the isolation of organelles and viruses, and non-ionic iodinated aromatic compounds, because of their increased versatility, have been used for a much wider variety of applications. Some of the more commonly used gradient-forming materials and their applications are listed in Table 5.1.

5.8 SELECTION, EFFICIENCY AND APPLICATIONS OF PREPARATIVE ROTORS

The selection of a suitable rotor for a particular separation will depend upon such considerations as the capacity and resolving power of the rotor, the quantity and sample type, the time required for the separation, and the centrifugation technique to be used.

In practice, the swinging-bucket rotor is frequently used for rate zonal sedimentation analysis, because the long tube pathlength and minimal wall effects are advantageous in optimising particle separation, particularly with multicomponent samples. It is relatively inefficient, however, for differential centrifugation, due to the relatively long centrifugation time required because of the long pathlength of the tubes. Fixed-angle rotors have proved to be most effective when the rapid, total sedimentation of particles is required by differential centrifugation. Fixed-angle rotors, although giving good sample resolution in isopycnic centrifugation because components are banded over a larger cross-sectional area and also significantly reducing centrifugation time because of their reduced sedimentation pathlength, are seldom used for rate zonal centrifugation because undesirable wall effects can disrupt the sedimentation of the zones, thus limiting particle separation.

Vertical tube rotors are unsuitable for pelleting of particles by differential centrifugation because the pellet is distributed along the entire outer wall of the centrifuge tube and may be disturbed during deceleration of the rotor. They can, however, be used for the rate zonal separation of whole cells and subcellular organelles, but do not achieve the quality of separation obtained when the swinging-bucket rotor is used to separate macromolecules with a relative molecular mass of less than approximately 2×10^5. The main advantage of the vertical tube rotor for rate zonal centrifugation and isopycnic centrifugation is the speed of separation, because particles have a very short sedimentation pathlength across the width of the tube rather than down the length; also the minimum centrifugal field will be higher than in comparable fixed-angle rotors and swinging-bucket rotors because the tubes are located near the edge of the rotor. Although the swinging-bucket rotor, fixed-angle rotor and vertical tube rotor may be used for isopycnic centrifugation, the fixed-angle rotor and vertical tube rotor have been found to be of more use and are often used in preference to the swinging-bucket rotor because larger volumes can be handled and a better degree of resolution achieved in shorter times.

Table 5.1 Commonly used gradient materials and their application

Material	Ionic strength of solution	Maximum density of aqueous solution at 20 °C (g cm^{-3})	Ultra violet absorbance	Osmotic effect	Common uses
Caesium chloride	+++	1.91	+	+++	Banding of DNA, nucleoproteins, viruses, plasmid isolation
Caesium sulphate	+++	2.01	+	+++	Banding of DNA and RNA, purification of protecglycans
Sodium bromide	+++	1.53	+	+++	Fractionation of lipoproteins
Sodium iodide	+++	1.90	+++	+++	Banding of DNA and RNA
Glycerol	–	1.26	+	+++	Banding of membrane fragments, protein separation
Sucrose	–	1.32	+	+++	Separation of subcellular particles, proteins, viruses, and membranes
Ficoll (Pharmacia)	–	1.17	+	+(-)	Separation of whole cells, subcellular particles, viruses
Dextran	–	1.13	+	+(-)	Separation of whole cells, banding of microsomes
Bovine serum albumin	–	1.35	+++	+	Separation of whole cells
Percoll (Pharmacia)	–	1.30	+++	+	Separation of whole cells and subcellular particles
Metrizamide (Nyegaard)	–	1.46	+++	++(∗)	Separation of whole cells, subcellular particles, nuclei, ribonucleoprotein particles, membranes
Nycodenz (Nyegaard)	–	1.42	+++	++(∗)	Separation of whole cells, subcellular particles, nucleoproteins, membranes, viruses

+++, High; ++, medium; +, low; −, non-ionic. (∗) Osmotic effect increases almost linearly with concentration. (-) Very low osmotic effect below 20% (w/v) concentration; increasing almost exponentially above 30% (w/v) concentration.

| Table 5.2 | Preparative rotor types and their applications |

Rotor type	Centrifugation technique			
	Differential	Rate zonal	Isopycnic zonal	Elutriation
Swinging-bucket	−	++	+	0
Fixed-angle	+++	−	++	0
Vertical tube	−	+	+++	0
Batch zonal	−	+++	++	0
Continuous flow zonal	+++	−	++	0
Elutriator	0	0	0	+++

Use: +++, excellent; ++, good; +, reasonable; −, poor; 0, not applicable

Batch-type zonal rotors do not differ significantly from conventional rotors in their ability to separate particles, but holding large volumes of gradient make them especially useful for large-scale preparative separations and analytical separations where a number of tests may be required on the separated samples. The continuous flow zonal rotor gives a poor separation with the rate zonal technique, owing to the very short sedimentation pathlength (approximately 1 cm) but can be used for pelleting and isolation by isopycnic banding of particles that might otherwise be damaged by the pelleting technique.

The elutriator rotor provides a means for the rapid, high resolution, large capacity separation of whole cells and larger subcellular organelles, without the need either to use a gradient or to form a pellet. It is, however, of limited use in general teaching laboratories, owing to the requirement for expensive equipment, specialist accessories and an experienced user. The various types of rotor together with their applications are summarised in Table 5.2.

In order to determine the suitablility of a preparative rotor for particle sedimentation, use can be made of the k, k' and $k*$ factors that are related to the dimensions and speed of the rotor and provide a measure of the efficiency of the rotor for the material that is under investigation. The k factor provides an estimate of the time (in hours) that will be required to sediment a particle of known sedimentation coefficient, s (in Svedberg units), at the maximum speed of the rotor and is calculated on the basis that the particles are suspended in a liquid medium with a density and viscosity similar to that of water. The k' and $k*$ factors are applied to rate zonal separations in a density gradient and provide an estimate of the time required to move a band of particles of known sedimentation coefficient to the bottom of a centrifuge tube through a linear 5% to 20% (w/w) sucrose gradient at 5 °C at the maximum speed of the rotor, the k' factor being calculated on the known density of the particle and the $k*$ factor calculated on the assumption that the density of the particle in sucrose solution is 1.3 g cm^{-3}.

The k factor for the rotor can be either obtained from the manufacturers' data sheets or calculated from the equation

$$k = 2.53 \times 10^{11} \times \frac{[\ln(r_{max}) - \ln(r_{min})]}{(\text{rev min}^{-1})^2_{max}} \tag{5.17}$$

Therefore, if the k factor for the rotor and the sedimentation coefficient, s (in Svedberg units), of the particle are known, it is possible to estimate the time, in hours, to sediment a particle at the maximum speed of the rotor since

$$t = \frac{k}{s_{20,w}} \tag{5.18}$$

When the rotor is operated below its maximum speed, the k factor is increased to

$$k_{revised} = k \times \frac{(\text{rev min}^{-1})^2_{max}}{(\text{rev min}^{-1})^2_{selected}} \tag{5.19}$$

The k' factor (or $k*$ factor if the particle density is assumed to be 1.3 g cm^{-3} in sucrose solution) is calculated from the equation

$$k' = 2.53 \times 10^{11} \times \frac{[I_{Z_2} - I_{Z_1}]}{(\text{rev min}^{-1})^2_{max}} \tag{5.20}$$

where Z_1 is the minimum % (w/w) of the sucrose gradient, Z_2 is the maximum % (w/w) of the sucrose gradient, and I is the time integral value for Z_1 and Z_2 for a particle of known density (or an assumed density of 1.3 g cm^{-3} for calculation of the $k*$ factor) and obtained from tables (supplied by the instrument manufacturer) after determining Z_0 from the equation

$$Z_0 = \frac{Z_1 r_{max} - Z_2 r_{min}}{r_{max} - r_{min}} \tag{5.21}$$

where Z_0 is the solute concentration corresponding to extrapolation of a linear gradient distribution to zero radius and the time taken, in hours, for the particles to sediment through the gradient calculated from

$$t = \frac{k'}{s_{20,w}} \tag{5.22}$$

If the time required to achieve a desired degree of separation of particles using a certain rotor (A) is known, then use of equation 5.23 makes it possible to estimate the sedimentation time, in hours, needed to reproduce these results using an alternative rotor (B) if rotor (A) is unavailable:

$$t_1 = t_2(k_1/k_2) \tag{5.23}$$

where t_1 is the sedimentation time using rotor B, t_2 is the sedimentation time using rotor A, $k_1 = k$, k' or $k*$ factor for rotor B at its maximum speed, and $k_2 = k$, k' or $k*$ factor for rotor A at its maximum speed.

Since the k, k' and $k*$ factors are computed from equations (i.e. 5.17, 5.20 and 5.21) that use the r_{min} and r_{max} of a rotor, a new r_{min} has to be determined and hence a revised k, k' and $k*$ factor calculated should the sedimentation be performed using partially filled tubes.

5.9 ANALYSIS OF SUBCELLULAR FRACTIONS

5.9.1 Assessment of homogeneity

It is only when an isolation technique leads to preparations of subcellular particles completely free from contamination by other particles that the properties of
the preparations may be attributed to the particles themselves. The evaluation of
purity is therefore essential. Light and electron microscopic examination have
been used as a means of analysing the success of a particular homogenisation technique and degree of contamination of a fraction after centrifugation. Absence
of visible contamination, however, is not conclusive proof of purity because it
is often difficult to detect low levels of contaminating material. Quantitative
determination of purity has to be obtained by chemical analyses, for example
protein, DNA, assay of enzyme activity, and possibly immunological properties.
Organelles and molecules lacking assayable enzyme activities can be located
either by their light absorption or by radioactive labelling techniques.

As a basis for the interpretation of patterns of enzyme distribution in tissue fractionation studies, two general postulates have been put forward. The first presupposes that all members of a given subcellular population have the same enzyme
composition. The second assumes that each enzyme is entirely restricted to a
single site within the cell. If valid, these postulates would enable enzymes to be
used as markers for their respective organelles, for example cytochrome oxidase
and succinic dehydrogenase as mitochondrial marker enzymes, acid hydrolases as
lysosomal marker enzymes, catalase as a marker for peroxisomes and glucose 6-
phosphatase as a marker enzyme for microsomal membranes. However, it has
been demonstrated that some enzymes are located in more than one fraction, for
example malate dehydrogenase, β-glucuronidase, NADPH cytochrome c reductase. Caution must therefore be used in the selection of an enzyme as a marker for
a particular subcellular fraction. Further, the absence of marker enzymes cannot
be taken as proof of the absence of a particular organelle. It is possible that
enzymes released from their respective organelles may have been inhibited or
inactivated in some manner during the fractionating process; hence, it is normal
practice to assay for at least two marker enzymes in each fraction.

5.9.2 Presentation of results

Enzyme activity and protein content are determined both in the whole homogenate
and in each subcellular fraction isolated. The sum of the enzyme activity and
protein content of the respective fractions should not differ appreciably from that in
the initial homogenate and hence should represent the total recovery. Calculations
are then made (Table 5.3) of enzyme activity and protein content in each fraction as
a percentage of the total recovery. For this reason there is no need to convert absorbance readings into precise units of enzyme activity or milligrams of protein.

The results obtained from tissue fractionation studies may also be represented
graphically, where enzyme distribution patterns, presented in the form of

Table 5.3 Distribution pattern of a liver lysosomal enzyme as established by differential centrifugation

A. Enzyme assay

Fraction	Volume (cm³)	Total dilutions	Absorbance (660 nm)	Enzyme activity in fraction (arbitrary units)	% recovered activity in fraction
Whole homogenate	120	1:30	0.50	1800	—
Nuclear	30	1:20	0.22	132	7.4
Mitochondrial	20	1:100	0.33	660	36.9
Lysosomal	16	1:100	0.34	544	30.4
Microsomal	20	1:25	0.44	220	12.3
Supernatant	290	1:20	0.04	232	13.0
				1788	100.0

B. Protein assay

Fraction	Volume (cm³)	Total dilutions	Absorbance (540 nm)	Protein in fraction (arbitrary units)	% recovered protein in fraction
Whole homogenate	120	1:100	0.16	1920	—
Nuclear	30	1:80	0.13	312	16.4
Mitochondrial	20	1:200	0.13	520	27.4
Lysosomal	16	1:100	0.08	128	6.7
Microsomal	20	1:100	0.18	360	19.0
Supernatant	290	1:25	0.08	580	30.5
				1900	100.0

C. Relative specific activity calculations

$$\text{Relative specific activity} = \frac{\% \text{ enzyme activity in fraction}}{\% \text{ protein in fraction}}$$

Nuclear $\dfrac{7.4}{16.4} = 0.45$ 　　　 Mitochondrial $\dfrac{36.9}{27.4} = 1.35$

Lysosomal $\dfrac{30.4}{6.7} = 4.53$ 　　　 Microsomal $\dfrac{12.3}{19.0} = 0.65$

Supernatant $\dfrac{13.0}{30.5} = 0.43$

histograms, provide a visual appreciation of the results. In the histogram, each fraction is then presented separately on the ordinate scale, by its own relative specific activity, which is a measure of the degree of purification achieved. On the abscissa, each fraction is represented cumulatively, from left to right, in the order in which it is isolated, by its percentage of total protein. The area of each rectangle is then equal to the percentage of the enzyme activity in that fraction.

5.10 SOME APPLICATIONS OF THE ANALYTICAL ULTRACENTRIFUGE

The analytical ultracentrifuge has found many applications in biology, especially in the fields of protein chemistry and nucleic acid chemistry, yielding information from which the sedimentation coefficient, relative molecular mass, purity and shape of the particle may be deduced.

5.10.1 Determination of relative molecular mass

Two main approaches are available using the analytical ultracentrifuge to determine relative molecular mass of a macromolecule. These are sedimentation velocity and sedimentation equilibrium.

In the sedimentation velocity method the sedimentation coefficient of the molecule is initially determined either by boundary sedimentation or band (zonal) sedimentation. In the boundary sedimentation method, the particles are uniformly distributed through the solution in the analytical cell at the start of the experiment. The ultracentrifuge is operated at high speeds, which cause the randomly distributed particles to migrate through the solvent radially outwards from the centre of rotation. A sharp boundary, called the plateau region, is formed between the solvent that has been cleared of particles and the solvent still containing the sedimenting material. The movement of the boundary with time, which is a measure of the rate of sedimentation of the particle, is given by equation 5.14, and is followed using either the ultraviolet absorption optical system or the Schlieren optical system (Section 5.3.6). In the alternative band sedimentation method a small amount of material (about 15 mm³) is layered on top of a denser solvent, which generates its own density gradient during centrifugation, thus stabilising the solute band against convective disturbances. The movement of the migrating band is then followed using the absorption optical system using a special band-forming centrepiece in the analytical cell.

Rearrangement of equation 5.14 gives

$$s\omega^2 dt = dr/r \tag{5.24}$$

which, on integration, gives

$$s\omega^2 t = \ln r \tag{5.25}$$

Therefore, if the logarithm of the distance moved by the boundary (r) is plotted against the time taken in seconds, the sedimentation coefficient (s) for the particle may be calculated from the slope of the line divided by ω^2. The relative molecular mass of the particle may then be determined using the Svedberg equation:

$$M_r = \frac{RTs}{D(1 - \bar{v}\rho)} \tag{5.26}$$

where M_r is the anhydrous relative molecular mass of the molecule, D is the diffusion coefficient of the molecule, $\bar{v}$ is the partial specific volume of the molecule, ρ is the density of the solvent at 20 °C, R is the molar gas constant, and T is the absolute temperature in K, and the measured values of s and D are corrected to standard conditions of zero concentration of solute in water at 20 °C. Although the relative molecular mass of a molecule may be calculated using equation 5.26, the calculations are, however, complicated by difficulties encountered in the accurate determination of the diffusion coefficient of the particle and for correction in differences in viscosity and temperature. The determination of the relative molecular mass of a macromolecule using sedimentation velocity analysis is therefore less accurate and invariably more time consuming than determination by sedimentation equilibrium.

Sedimentation equilibrium methods are more versatile, and in the majority of cases the most accurate. They can be used to determine relative molecular mass values ranging from a few hundred to several million. This versatility is due to the large range of centrifugal fields available to the ultracentrifuge. The centrifugal field, which varies with the square of the rotor speed, can cover a 7000-fold range at the rotor speeds of 800 to 68 000 rev min^{-1} utilised by the analytical ultracentrifuge.

In the equilibrium method, the ultracentrifuge is operated until a balance is established between sedimentation, under the influence of the centrifugal field, and diffusion of material in the opposite direction, i.e. until there is no net migration of solute throughout the length of the cell. At equilibrium, for a single, ideal solute component, the resulting concentration distribution increases exponentially with the square of the radial position, is invariant with time and is a function of the relative molecular mass of the sedimenting solute. Relative molecular mass can then be calculated from the concentration gradient of the solute that is set up, using the equation

$$M_r = \frac{2RT \ln (c_2/c_1)}{\omega^2 (1 - \bar{v}\rho)(r_2^2 - r_1^2)} \tag{5.27}$$

where c_2 and c_1 are the concentrations of solute at distances r_2 and r_1, respectively, from the centre of rotation.

The relative molecular mass of the molecule to be studied will dictate the rotor velocity to be used. In general, for low speed sedimentation equilibrium a ratio of approximately 4:1 between the ends of the solution column is desirable (i.e. $c_2/c_1 = 4$, in equation 5.27). Therefore it can be calculated, using equation 5.27, that for a molecule with a relative molecular mass of 50 000, a rotor speed of 10 000 rev min^{-1} should be selected. Molecules of higher relative molecular mass require correspondingly lower rotor speeds. However, it is difficult to perform a good low speed sedimentation equilibrium for molecules with a relative molecular mass greater than 5×10^6 owing to the problem of rotor wobble at low centrifuge speeds (e.g. 1000 rev min^{-1}).

A major disadvantage of low speed sedimentation equilibrium used to be the long periods (several days to several weeks) necessary for equilibrium to be achieved. Modern techniques, however, employ analytical cells using short column depths of liquid, usually 1 to 3 mm. Since the time taken to reach equilibrium varies with the square of the depth of solution, a great saving of time is possible. The technique of sedimentation equilibrium, unlike that for sedimentation velocity, does not require a knowledge of the diffusion coefficient (compare equations 5.26 and 5.27), making this method more convenient and hence widely used for the determination of the relative molecular mass of proteins.

High speed equilibrium or meniscus depletion (Yphantis method) methods use short column lengths of liquid (1 to 3 mm), and in principle a technique similar to that of the low speed method. However, the centrifuge is operated at such a high speed that particles move away from the meniscus, resulting in the concentration of the solute at the meniscus becoming essentially zero and producing a concentration gradient due to the solute. The concentrations throughout the cell are then proportional to the difference in refractive index between the meniscus region and any point in the cell. The relative molecular mass is proportional to the slope of a plot of the logarithm of concentration against the square of the distance and can be calculated from

$$M_r = \frac{2RT}{(1 - \bar{v}\rho)\omega^2} \times \frac{\ln \text{concentration}}{(\text{distance})^2} \tag{5.28}$$

Estimates of relative molecular mass, however, are complicated by density heterogeneity in the solution, and possible complex formation in the high concentrations of salts used. The high speed method also suffers from the disadvantage that, for molecules with a relative molecular mass below 10 000, speeds of rotation in excess of 65 000 rev min⁻¹ would be required to ensure zero solute concentration at the meniscus. These excessive speeds can produce cell window distortion even when sapphire windows are used (Section 5.3.6). Nevertheless, this technique is extremely useful for the determination of the relative molecular mass of proteins if the material under study is homogeneous.

5.10.2 Estimation of purity of macromolecules

The analytical ultracentrifuge has been used extensively in the investigation of the purity of DNA preparations, viruses and proteins. Sample purity is of course extremely important if an accurate estimation of the relative molecular mass of the molecule is required. The most widely used methods for the determination of the homogeneity of a preparation include the analysis of the sedimenting boundary using the technique of sedimentation velocity. Several criteria have been devised for assessing the homogeneity of a preparation, although it must be remembered that homogeneity can be presumed only through the absence of detectable heterogeneity. Homogeneity is usually recognised by a single sharp symmetrical sedimenting boundary throughout the duration of the sedimentation velocity experiment. Impurities in the preparation are displayed as additional peaks, shoulders on the main peak, or asymmetry of the main peak. The absence of heterogeneity in sedimentation analysis, however, is no guarantee that all the molecules have the same biological activity or electrical charge. Partial deamidation of a protein sample, for example, while increasing the negative charge on the molecule at neutral pH would have no significant effect on the size, shape or relative molecular mass of the molecule. Such a sample will show no heterogeneity in relative molecular mass or sedimentation coefficient but would show multiple zones in capillary electrophoresis.

5.10.3 Detection of conformational changes in macromolecules

Analytical ultracentrifugation has been applied successfully to the detection of conformational changes in macromolecules. DNA, for example, may exist as single or double strands, each of which may be either linear or circular in nature. If exposed to a variety of agents, for example organic solvents or elevated temperature, the DNA molecules may undergo a number of conformational changes that may or may not be reversible. Changes in conformation may be ascertained by examining differences in the sedimentation velocity of the sample. The more compact the molecule, the lower would be its frictional resistance in the solvent. The more disorganised the molecule becomes, the greater the frictional resistance, and sedimentation occurs more slowly. Changes in conformation may therefore be detected by differences in sedimentation rates of the sample before and after treatment.

In the case of allosteric proteins (e.g. aspartate transcarbamylase) conformational changes may accompany combination of the protein with substrate and/or small ligands (activators or inhibitors). In addition, treatment of the protein with such reagents as urea and 4-chloromercuribenzoate may result in disaggregation of the protein into its subunits (protomers). All of these changes may readily be studied by analytical ultracentrifugation.

5.11 SAFETY ASPECTS IN THE USE OF CENTRIFUGES

Centrifuges can be extremely dangerous instruments if not properly maintained or if incorrectly used. It is therefore essential that all centrifuge users read and understand the operating manual for the particular centrifuge.

The regulations now governing the manufacture of centrifuges have ensured that operators are safeguarded against accidents by the fitting of effective lid locks that prevent access to the rotor chamber while the rotor is still spinning, imbalance detectors, rotor overspeed devices, and the ability of the centrifuge to contain any failure of the rotor. Since zonal rotors are designed for loading and unloading while the rotor is spinning, the normal safety mechanism that prevents activation of the rotor drive while the lid of the centrifuge chamber is still open is overridden, allowing the rotor to be operated at low speeds only. To prevent possible physical injury when zonal rotors are filled and emptied, and in the operation of continuous flow rotors, care must be taken to ensure that the moving rotor is not touched and that long hair and loose clothing (e.g. ties) do not get caught in any rotating part. This is especially important in the use of older centrifuges where the lid can be opened before the rotor has stopped rotating.

To minimise the risk of rotor failure, which is one of the more serious hazards likely to arise, manufacturers' instructions regarding rotor use and care should always be followed (Section 5.4.7). It is important when one is centrifuging hazardous materials (e.g. pathogenic microorganisms, infectious viruses, carcinogenic, corrosive or toxic chemicals, radioactive materials), especially in low speed non-refrigerated centrifuges in which rotor temperature is controlled by air flow through the rotor bowl, that the samples are kept in air-tight, leak-proof containers. This is to prevent aerosol formation arising from accidental spillage of the sample, which would contaminate the rotor, centrifuge and possibly the whole laboratory.

5.12 KEY TERMS

airfuge	equilibrium isodensity	rate zonal centrifugation
analytical cell	equilibrium method	rate zonal technique
analytical centrifugation	fixed-angle rotor	rate zonal separation
analytical ultracentrifuge	frictional coefficient	Rayleigh interference optical system
average radius of rotation	frictional ratio	relative centrifugal field
band sedimentation	fluid cushion	reorienting gradient core
batch flow	high speed equilibrium	Schlieren optical system
bottom loading	isodensity technique	sedimentation coefficient
boundary sedimentation	isokinetic gradients	sedimentation equilibrium
bright-field scanning optical system	isopycnic centrifugation	sedimentation rate
centrepiece	isopycnic technique	sedimentation velocity
centrifugal elutriation	separation	standard core
centrifugal field	isopycnic zonal	standard sedimentation coefficient
centripetal end	$k, k', k*$ factors	step gradient technique
continuous density gradient	linear-log gradients	Stokes equation
continuous flow centrifuge	low speed sedimentation	swinging-bucket rotor
continuous flow rotor	equilibrium	Svedberg equation
counterpoise cell	meniscus depletion	Svedberg unit
density gradient	microfuges	top loading method
density gradient centrifugation	overlay	underlayering method
density gradient maker	overlayering method	upward displacement
differential centrifugation	peripheral edge	vertical tube rotor
discontinuous density gradient	plateau region	Yphantis method
elutriator rotor	preparative centrifugation	zonal rotor
equal density technique	preparative ultracentrifuge	zonal sedimentation

5.13 CALCULATIONS

Question 1   An ultracentrifuge is operated at a speed of 58 000 rev min^{-1}.
Calculate

(i) the angular velocity (ω in radians per second) and the centrifugal field at a point equivalent to 6.2 cm from the centre of rotation.

(ii) How many 'times g' is this equivalent to?

Answer   (i)   The angular velocity may be calculated using the equation

$$\omega = \frac{2\pi \, \text{rev min}^{-1}}{60} = \frac{2 \times 3.14 \times 58\,000}{60} = 6070.7 \text{ radians s}^{-1}$$

The centrifugal field (G) at a point 6.2 cm from the centre of rotation may be calculated using the equation

$$G = \omega^2 r$$

$$G = (6070.7)^2 \times 6.2 = 2.285 \times 10^8 \text{ cm s}^{-2}$$

(ii) How many 'times g' is this equivalent to?

The earth's gravitational field $(g) = 980 \text{ cm s}^{-2}$

$$\text{Relative centrifugal field (RCF)} = \frac{\omega^2 r}{980}$$

and, since $G = \omega^2 r$,

$$\text{RCF} = G/980 = 2.285 \times 10^8/980 = 233\,163 \times g$$

Question 2 Calculate the relative centrifugal field (RCF) exerted at the top and bottom of a centrifuge tube being centrifuged in a fixed-angle rotor, assuming that the rotor dimensions for the minimum radius (r_{min}) at the top of the tube is 4.8 cm and for the maximum radius (r_{max}) at the bottom of the tube is 9 cm, and that the rotor is spinning at a speed of 12 000 rev min^{-1}.

Answer Using the equation

$$\text{RCF} = (1.118 \times 10^{-5})(\text{rev min}^{-1})^2 r$$

$$\text{RCF}_{top} = (1.118 \times 10^{-5})(12\,000)^2 \times 4.8$$
$$= 7728 \times g$$

and $\text{RCF}_{bottom} = (1.118 \times 10^{-5})(12\,000)^2 \times 9$
$$= 14\,489 \times g$$

As can be seen the centrifugal field exerted at the top and bottom of the centrifuge tube differs by nearly two-fold.

Question 3 You are following a method in a research paper that describes a technique for the pelleting of particles, using a particular fixed-angle rotor (rotor A) that has a k factor of 225, in 4 h at its maximum speed.

You wish to save time in the preparation by using a different fixed-angle rotor (rotor B) that has a k factor of 63. Calculate how long you will need to centrifuge, using rotor B at its maximum speed, to pellet the same material.

Answer This may be determined as follows

$$t_1 = t_2(k_1/k_2)$$

where t_1 is the sedimentation time in hours using rotor B, t_2 is the sedimentation time in hours using rotor A, k_1 is the k factor for rotor B at its maximum speed, and k_2 is the k factor for rotor A at its maximum speed.

$$t_1 = 4(63/225) = 1.12\,\text{h} = 1\,\text{h}\,7\,\text{min (approx.)}$$

Question 4 You wish to sediment a preparation of equine encephalitis virus $(s_{20,w} = 300)$. Of the two fixed-angle rotors that are available, rotor A has a $r_{min} = 4$ cm,

$r_{max} = 11.2$ cm, and a maximum speed of 35 000 rev min^{-1}. Rotor B has $r_{min} = 4.2$ cm, $r_{max} = 8.6$ cm, and a maximum speed of 65 000 rev min^{-1}.

(i) Calculate the k factor for each rotor and then estimate the time required to pellet the virus preparation using each rotor, assuming that the rotors are operated at their maximum speed and that the centrifuge tubes are full.

(ii) Which rotor is the most efficient for sedimenting the virus preparation? Give reasons for your answer.

(iii) What is the estimated time required to pellet the virus preparation using each rotor if rotor A is operated at 20 000 rev min^{-1} and rotor B is operated at 40 000 rev min^{-1}?

(iv) What other factors need to be considered in the selection of a suitable rotor for a particular separation?

(v) Sedimentation of the virus preparation was performed using rotor A at its maximum speed but with the centrifuge tubes now only half-filled. Calculate the new r_{min} and the revised k factor and then recalculate the estimated time now required to pellet the virus preparation.

(vi) Will the clearing time be faster or slower using rotor A at its maximum speed and centrifuge tubes only half-filled than when the experiment was performed using rotor A at maximum speed and with the centrifuge tubes completely filled? Give reasons for your answer.

Answer

(i) Calculation of k factor and the estimated time for pelleting the virus preparation.

The k factor may be calculated using the equation

$$k = 2.53 \times 10^{11} \times \frac{[\ln(r_{max}) - \ln(r_{min})]}{(\text{rev min}^{-1})^2_{max}}$$

For Rotor A,

$$k = 2.53 \times 10^{11} \times \frac{[\ln 11.2 - \ln 4]}{(35\,000)^2} = 213$$

For Rotor B,

$$k = 2.53 \times 10^{11} \times \frac{[\ln 8.6 - \ln 4.2]}{(65\,000)^2} = 43$$

Therefore, the time taken for sedimentation with Rotor A will be

$$t = \frac{k}{s_{20,w}} = \frac{213}{300} = 0.71\,\text{h} = 43\,\text{min (approx.)}$$

and with Rotor B

$$t = \frac{k}{s_{20,w}} = \frac{43}{300} = 0.14\,\text{h} = 8.6\,\text{min (approx.)}$$

(ii) Rotor B is more efficient than rotor A. It has a lower k factor, hence less time will be required to sediment the virus preparation.

(iii) The revised k factor may be calculated using the equation

$$k_{revised} = k \times \frac{(\text{rev min}^{-1})^2_{max}}{(\text{rev min}^{-1})^2_{selected}}$$

Operating rotor A at 20 000 rev min^{-1}

$$k_{revised} = 213 \times \frac{(35\,000)^2}{(20\,000)^2} = 652$$

The new clearing time using rotor A will be

$$t = \frac{k}{s_{20,w}} = \frac{652}{300} = 2.17\,h = 2\,h\,10\,min\,(approx.)$$

Operating rotor B at 40 000 rev min^{-1} the revised k factor will be

$$k_{revised} = 43 \times \frac{(65\,000)^2}{(40\,000)^2} = 113$$

The new clearing time using rotor B will be

$$t = \frac{k}{s_{20,w}} = \frac{113}{300} = 0.38\,h = 23\,min\,(approx.)$$

(iv) Other factors that need to be considered include:
  Quantity and sample type.
  The time required for the separation.
  The capacity and resolving power of the rotor.

(v) The tubes are half-filled, therefore the new r_{min} using rotor A will be equal to

$$(r_{max} + r_{min})/2 = (11.2 + 4)/2 = 7.6\,cm$$

The revised k value will be

$$k = 2.53 \times 10^{11} \times \frac{[\ln 11.2 - \ln 7.6]}{(35\,000)^2} = 80$$

and the revised time for sedimentation will be equal to

$$t = \frac{k}{s_{20,w}} = \frac{80}{300} = 0.27\,h = 16\,min\,(approx.)$$

(vi) The clearing time will be faster using centrifuge tubes that are now only half-filled, because the minimum radius has been increased from 4 cm to 7.6 cm. The particles will therefore have a reduced path length to travel and hence start to sediment in a higher 'g' field.

Question 5

A protein was subjected to ultracentrifugal analysis at a rotor speed of 59 780 rev min^{-1} and a temperature of 20 °C. Using the technique of sedimentation velocity, measurements were taken of the radial position of the sedimenting protein boundary as a function of centrifugation time:

Time (min)	Radial position (r in cm)
8	6.089
16	6.179
24	6.270
32	6.362
40	6.454
48	6.549

Unpublished experimental data from D. A. Fell.

(i) From the information provided plot a graph of log r (centimetres) against time (seconds) and hence calculate the sedimentation coefficient of the protein.

(ii) In subsequent analyses, also carried out at 20 °C, the protein was found to have an average diffusion coefficient of 4.0×10^{-11} m^2 s^{-1}, and a partial specific volume of 0.734×10^{-3} m^3 kg^{-1}.

Calculate the relative molecular mass of the protein.

The density of water at 20 °C is 998 kg m^{-3}.

The gradient of the plot of log r (centimetres) against time (seconds) $= s\omega^2/2.3$

where $\omega = \dfrac{2\pi\,\text{rev min}^{-1}}{60}$

$R = 8.314$ J K^{-1} mol^{-1}; 0 °C = 273 K.

| Answer | (i) Calculation of the sedimentation coefficient of the protein: The sedimentation coefficient may be calculated using the equation

$$s = \frac{2.3\,(\text{gradient})}{\omega^2}$$

where $\omega = \dfrac{2\pi\,\text{rev min}^{-1}}{60} = \dfrac{2\pi\,59\,780}{60} = 6260.15$ rads s^{-1}

The gradient of the line is obtained by measuring the radial position of the sedimenting protein boundary (in centimetres) at different times (in seconds) and then plotting log r (centimetres) against time (seconds).

Time (min)	Time (s)	r (cm)	log r (cm)
8	480	6.089	0.7845
16	960	6.179	0.7909
24	1440	6.270	0.7973
32	1920	6.362	0.8036
40	2400	6.454	0.8098
48	2880	6.549	0.8161

From the graph obtained the gradient of the line (log r/time) may be calculated and found to be 1.32×10^{-5}.

Hence

$$s = \frac{2.3 \times 1.32 \times 10^{-5}}{(6260.15)^2} = 7.75 \times 10^{-13}\,\text{s}$$

(ii) Calculation of the relative molecular mass of the protein: The answer may be calculated using the Svedberg equation (p. 302).

Substituting the values given in the question (in SI units) into the equation the answer may be calculated to be

$$M_\mathrm{r} = \frac{RTs}{D(1 - \bar{v}\rho)} = \frac{8.314 \times 293 \times 7.75 \times 10^{-13}}{4 \times 10^{-11}(1 - 0.734 \times 10^{-3} \times 998)} = 176.46\ \text{kg mol}^{-1}$$

Note: The use of SI units in the Svedberg equation gives a value to M_r, technically referred to as the *molar mass*, having units of kg mol^{-1}.

The *relative molecular mass* of a molecule is a relative quantity and is defined as the ratio of the mass of a molecule relative to 1/12 of the mass of the carbon isotope ^{12}C; it is thus dimensionless. The answer obtained from the calculation (i.e. 176.46 kg mol^{-1}) can be converted to a relative molecular mass by dividing by 1 g mol^{-1} (the equivalent of multiplying the answer by 1000 and cancelling units) to give a relative molecular mass of 176 460.

Biochemists have traditionally and continue to think of *molecular mass* expressed in daltons. The molecular mass is the mass of one molecule of a substance expressed in daltons (Da) or atomic mass units (1 dalton = 1 atomic mass unit equals one-twelfth of the mass of one atom of ^{12}C). This may be obtained by multiplying the answer given in the calculation by 1000 to give an answer of 176 460.

5.14 **SUGGESTIONS FOR FURTHER READING**

BIRNIE, G. D. and RICKWOOD, D. (1978). *Centrifugal Separations in Molecular and Cell Biology.* Butterworth, London. (Gives in detail the theory and practice of modern centrifugation techniques in molecular and cell biology.)

FORD, T. C. and GRAHAM, J. M. (1991). *An Introduction to Centrifugation.* Bios Scientific, Oxford. (Intended to provide the novice with an introduction to the basic theory and practical applications of centrifugation, the types of centrifuge, rotors, techniques and density gradient media currently available.)

GRIFFITH, O. M. (1983). *Techniques in Preparative, Zonal and Continuous Flow Ultracentrifugation,* 4th edn. Beckman Instruments Inc., Palo Alto, CA. (Covering preparative and density gradient ultracentrifugation techniques and their application.)

RALSTON, G. (1993). *Introduction to Analytical Ultracentrifugation.* Beckman Instruments Inc., Palo Alto, CA. (Provides an introduction to the sorts of problem that can be solved through the application of analytical ultracentrifugation and describes the different types of experiment that can be performed in an analytical ultracentrifuge and the principles behind them.)

RICKWOOD, D. (ed.) (1984). *Centrifugation,* 2nd edn. Published in the Practical Approaches to Biochemistry Series, IRL Press, Oxford/Washington DC. (Covering the theory and practice of centrifugation, important criteria for optimising centrifugal separations and the protocols of illustrative experiments.)

SHARPE, P. T. (1988). *Laboratory Techniques in Biochemical and Molecular Biology,* vol. 18 *Methods of Cell Separation,* eds. Burden, R. H., and van Knippenberg, P. H. Elsevier, Amsterdam, New York, Oxford. (Chapters 3 and 5 cover the principles and practice of centrifugation and centrifugal elutriation.)

VAN HOLDE, K. E., CURTIS JOHNSON, W. and SHING HO, P. (1998). *Principles of Physical Biochemistry.* Prentice Hall, Upper Saddle River, NJ. (Chapter 5 covers methods and techniques, including sedimentation, used for the separation and characterisation of molecules.)

Chapter 6

Protein structure, purification and characterisation

6.1 IONIC PROPERTIES OF AMINO ACIDS AND PROTEINS

Twenty amino acids varying in size, shape, charge and chemical reactivity are found in proteins and each has at least one codon in the genetic code (Section 2.6.7). Nineteen of the amino acids are α-amino acids (i.e. the amino and carboxyl groups are attached to the carbon atom that is adjacent to the carboxyl group) with the general formula RCH(NH$_2$)COOH, where R is an aliphatic, aromatic or heterocyclic group. The only exception to this general formula is proline, which is an imino acid in which the -NH$_2$ group is incorporated into a five-membered ring. With the exception of the simplest amino acid glycine (R = H), all the amino acids found in proteins contain one asymmetric carbon atom and hence are optically active and have been found to have the L configuration.

For convenience, each amino acid found in proteins is designated by either a three-letter abbreviation, generally based on the first three letters of their name, or a one-letter symbol, some of which are the first letter of the name. Details are given in Table 6.1.

Since they possess both an amino group and a carboxyl group, amino acids are ionised at all pH values, i.e. a neutral species represented by the general formula does not exist in solution irrespective of the pH. This can be seen as follows:

$$
\begin{array}{ccccc}
\text{R} & & \text{R} & & \text{R} \\
| & & | & & | \\
{}^{\alpha}\text{CH}-\overset{+}{\text{N}}\text{H}_3 & \underset{}{\overset{\text{p}K_{a_1}}{\rightleftharpoons}} & {}^{\alpha}\text{CH}-\overset{+}{\text{N}}\text{H}_3 & \underset{}{\overset{\text{p}K_{a_2}}{\rightleftharpoons}} & {}^{\alpha}\text{CH}-\text{NH}_2 \\
| & & | & & | \\
\text{COOH} & & \text{COO}^- & & \text{COO}^- \\
\text{Net positive} & & \text{Zero net} & & \text{Net negative} \\
\text{charge} & & \text{charge} & & \text{charge} \\
& & \text{'zwitterion'} & &
\end{array}
$$

Increasing pH →

Thus, at low pH values an amino acid exists as a cation and at high pH values as an anion. At a particular intermediate pH the amino acid carries no net charge, although it is still ionised, and is called a zwitterion. It has been shown that, in the crystalline state and in solution in water, amino acids exist predominantly as this

Table 6.1 Abbreviations for amino acids		
Amino acid	Three-letter symbol	One-letter symbol
Alanine	Ala	A
Arginine	Arg	R
Asparagine	Asn	N
Aspartic acid	Asp	D
Asparagine or aspartic acid	Asx	B
Cysteine	Cys	C
Glutamine	Gln	Q
Glutamic acid	Glu	E
Glutamine or glutamic acid	Glx	Z
Glycine	Gly	G
Histidine	His	H
Isoleucine	Ile	I
Leucine	Leu	L
Lysine	Lys	K
Methionine	Met	M
Phenylalanine	Phe	F
Proline	Pro	P
Serine	Ser	S
Threonine	Thr	T
Tryptophan	Trp	W
Tyrosine	Tyr	Y
Valine	Val	V

zwitterionic form. This confers upon them physical properties characteristic of ionic compounds, i.e. high melting point and boiling point, water solubility and low solubility in organic solvents such as ether and chloroform. The pH at which the zwitterion predominates in aqueous solution is referred to as the isoionic point, because it is the pH at which the number of negative charges on the molecule produced by ionisation of the carboxyl group is equal to the number of positive charges acquired by proton acceptance by the amino group. In the case of amino acids this is equal to the isoelectric point (pI), since the molecule carries no net charge and is therefore electrophoretically immobile. The numerical value of this pH for a given amino acid is related to its acid strength (pK_a values) by the equation:

$$pI = \frac{pK_{a_1} + pK_{a_2}}{2} \tag{6.1}$$

where pK_{a_1} and pK_{a_2} are equal to the negative logarithm of the acid dissociation constants, K_{a_1} and K_{a_2} (Section 1.4.5).

In the case of glycine, pK_{a_1} and pK_{a_2} are 2,3 and 9.6, respectively, so that the isoionic point is 6.0. At pH values below this, the cation and zwitterion will coexist in equilibrium in a ratio determined by the Henderson–Hasselbalch equation (Section 1.4.5), whereas at higher pH values the zwitterion and anion will coexist in equilibrium.

For acidic amino acids such as aspartic acid, the ionisation pattern is different owing to the presence of a second carboxyl group:

$$
\begin{array}{llll}
\text{COOH} & \text{COOH} & \text{COO}^- & \text{COO}^- \\
| & | & | & | \\
\text{CH}_2 & \text{CH}_2 & \text{CH}_2 & \text{CH}_2 \\
| & | & | & | \\
\overset{+}{\text{CH}}-\text{NH}_3 \underset{2.1}{\overset{\text{p}K_{a_1}}{\rightleftharpoons}} \overset{+}{\text{CH}}-\text{NH}_3 \underset{3.9}{\overset{\text{p}K_{a_2}}{\rightleftharpoons}} \overset{+}{\text{CH}}-\text{NH}_3 \underset{9.8}{\overset{\text{p}K_{a_3}}{\rightleftharpoons}} \text{CH}-\text{NH}_2 \\
| & | & | & | \\
\text{COOH} & \text{COO}^- & \text{COO}^- & \text{COO}^-
\end{array}
$$

| Cation (1 net positive charge) | Zwitterion pH 3.0 (isoionic point) | Anion (1 net negative charge) | Anion (2 net negative charges) |

In this case, the zwitterion will predominate in aqueous solution at a pH determined by $\text{p}K_{a_1}$ and $\text{p}K_{a_2}$, and the isoelectric point is the mean of $\text{p}K_{a_1}$ and $\text{p}K_{a_2}$.

In the case of lysine, which is a basic amino acid, the ionisation pattern is different again and its isoionic point is the mean of $\text{p}K_{a_2}$ and $\text{p}K_{a_3}$:

$$
\begin{array}{llll}
\overset{+}{\text{NH}_3} & \overset{+}{\text{NH}_3} & \overset{+}{\text{NH}_3} & \text{NH}_2 \\
| & | & | & | \\
(\text{CH}_2)_4 & (\text{CH}_2)_4 & (\text{CH}_2)_4 & (\text{CH}_2)_4 \\
| & | & | & | \\
\overset{+}{\text{CH}}-\text{NH}_3 \underset{2.2}{\overset{\text{p}K_{a_1}}{\rightleftharpoons}} \overset{+}{\text{CH}}-\text{NH}_3 \underset{9.0}{\overset{\text{p}K_{a_2}}{\rightleftharpoons}} \text{CH}-\text{NH}_2 \underset{10.5}{\overset{\text{p}K_{a_3}}{\rightleftharpoons}} \text{CH}-\text{NH}_2 \\
| & | & | & | \\
\text{COOH} & \text{COO}^- & \text{COO}^- & \text{COO}^-
\end{array}
$$

| Cation (2 net positive charges) | Cation (1 net positive charge) | Zwitterion pH 3.0 (isoionic point) | Anion (1 net negative charge) |

As an alternative to possessing a second amino or carboxyl group, an amino acid side chain may contain in the R of the general formula a quite different chemical group that is also capable of ionising at a characteristic pH. Such groups include a phenolic group (tyrosine), guanidino group (arginine), imidazolyl group (histidine) and sulphydryl group (cysteine) (Table 6.2). It is clear that the state of ionisation of the main groups of amino acids (acidic, basic, neutral) will be grossly different at a particular pH. Moreover, even within a given group there will be minor differences due to the precise nature of the R group. These differences are exploited in the electrophoretic and ion-exchange chromatographic separation of mixtures of amino acids such as those present in a protein hydrolysate (Section 6.4.2).

Proteins are formed by the condensation of the α-amino group of one amino acid with the α-carboxyl of the adjacent amino acid (Section 6.2). With the exception of the two terminal amino acids, therefore, the α-amino and carboxyl groups are all involved in peptide bonds and are no longer ionisable in the protein. Amino, carboxyl, imidazolyl, guanidino, phenolic and sulphydryl groups in the side chains are, however, free to ionise and of course there may be many of these.

| Table 6.2 | Ionisable groups found in proteins |

Amino acid group	pH-dependent ionisation	Approx. pK_a
N-terminal α-amino	$-NH_3 \rightleftharpoons NH_2 + H^+$	8.0
C-terminal α-carboxyl	$-COOH \rightleftharpoons COO^- + H^+$	3.0
Asp-β-carboxyl	$-CH_2COOH \rightleftharpoons CH_2COO^- + H^+$	3.9
Glu-γ-carboxyl	$-(CH_2)_2COOH \rightleftharpoons (CH_2)_2COO^- + H^+$	4.1
His-imidazolyl		6.0
Cys-sulphydryl	$-CH_2SH \rightleftharpoons -CH_2S^- + H^+$	8.4
Tyr-phenolic		10.1
Lys-ε-amino	$-(CH_2)_4\overset{+}{N}H_3 \rightleftharpoons -(CH_2)_4NH_2 + H^+$	10.3
Arg-guanidino	$-NH-\underset{\overset{\|}{{}^+NH_2}}{C}-NH_2 \rightleftharpoons -NH-\underset{\overset{\|}{NH}}{C}-NH_2 + H^+$	12.5

Proteins fold in such a manner that the majority of these ionisable groups are on the outside of the molecule, where they can interact with the surrounding aqueous medium. Some of these groups are located within the structure and may be involved in electrostatic attractions that help to stabilise the three-dimensional structure of the protein molecule. The relative numbers of positive and negative groups in a protein molecule influence aspects of its physical behaviour, such as solubility and electrophoretic mobility.

The isoionic point of a protein and its isoelectric point, unlike that of an amino acid, are generally not identical. This is because, by definition, the isoionic point is the pH at which the protein molecule possesses an equal number of positive and negative groups formed by the association of basic groups with protons and disso-ciation of acidic groups, respectively. In contrast, the isoelectric point is the pH at which the protein is electrophoretically immobile. In order to determine electro-phoretic mobility experimentally, the protein must be dissolved in a buffered medium containing anions and cations, of low relative molecular mass, that are capable of binding to the multi-ionised protein. Hence the observed balance of charges at the isoelectric point could be due in part to there being more bound mobile anions (or cations) than bound cations (anions) at this pH. This could mask an imbalance of charges on the actual protein.

In practice, protein molecules are always studied in buffered solutions, so it is the isoelectric point that is important. It is the pH at which, for example, the protein has minimum solubility, since it is the point at which there is the greatest opportunity for attraction between oppositely charged groups of neighbouring molecules and consequent aggregation and easy precipitation.

6.2 PROTEIN STRUCTURE

Proteins are formed by condensing the α-amino group of one amino acid or the imino group of proline with the α-carboxyl group of another, with the concomitant loss of a molecule of water and the formation of a peptide bond.

$$\overset{+}{N}H_3-\underset{\underset{R}{|}}{CH}-COO^- + \overset{+}{N}H_3-\underset{\underset{R'}{|}}{CH}-COO^- \xrightarrow{-H_2O} \overset{+}{N}H_3-\underset{\underset{R}{|}}{CH}-\underset{\underset{\underset{\text{Peptide bond}}{\uparrow}}{N}}{CO-NH}-\underset{\underset{R'}{|}}{CH}-COO^-$$

The progressive condensation of many molecules of amino acids gives rise to an unbranched polypeptide chain. By convention, the N-terminal amino acid is taken as the beginning of the chain and the C-terminal amino acid the end of the chain (proteins are biosynthesised in this direction). Polypeptide chains contain between 20 and 2000 amino acids residues and hence have a relative molecular mass ranging between about 2000 and 200 000. Most proteins have a relative molecular mass in the range 20 000 to 100 000. The distinction between a large peptide and a small protein is not clear. Generally peptides contain fewer than 50 amino acids residues and proteins more than 50. Insulin, which is a peptide hormone with 53 amino acid residues, is on the border between the two. Ribonuclease, which is a small protein, has 103 amino acid residues.

The primary structure of a protein defines the sequence of the amino acid residues and is dictated by the base sequence of the corresponding gene(s). Indirectly, the primary structure also defines the amino acid composition (which of the possible 20 amino acids are actually present) and content (the relative proportions of the amino acids present).

The peptide bonds linking the individual amino acid residues in a protein are both rigid and planar, with no opportunity for rotation about the carbon–nitrogen bond, as it has considerable double bond character due to the delocalisation of the lone pair of electrons on the nitrogen atom; this, coupled with the tetrahedral geometry around each α-carbon atom, profoundly influences the three-dimensional arrangement which the polypeptide chain adopts.

Secondary structure defines the localised folding of a polypeptide chain due to hydrogen bonding. It includes structures such as the α-helix and β-pleated sheet. Certain of the 20 amino acids found in proteins, including proline, isoleucine, tryptophan and asparagine, disrupt α-helical structures. Some proteins have up to 70% secondary structure but others have none.

Tertiary structure defines the overall folding of a polypeptide chain. It is stabilised by electrostatic attractions between oppositely charged ionic groups ($-\overset{+}{N}H_3$,

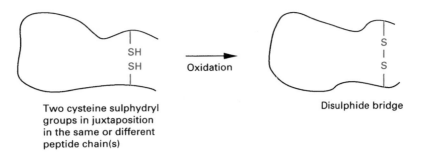

Two cysteine sulphydryl
groups in juxtaposition
in the same or different
peptide chain(s)

Disulphide bridge

Fig. 6.1. The formation of a disulphide bridge.

COO⁻), by weak van der Waals' forces, by hydrogen bonding, hydrophobic interactions and, in some proteins, by disulphide ($-S-S-$) bridges formed by the
oxidation of spatially adjacent sulphydryl groups ($-$SH) of cysteine residues (Fig.
6.1). The three-dimensional folding of polypeptide chains is such that the interior
consists predominantly of non-polar, hydrophobic amino acid residues such as
valine, leucine and phenylalanine. The polar, ionised, hydrophilic residues are
found on the outside of the molecule, where they are compatible with the
aqueous environment. However, some proteins also have hydrophobic residues
on their outside and the presence of these residues is important in the processes
of ammonium sulphate fractionation (Section 6.3.4) and hydrophobic interaction chromatography (Sections 6.3.4 and 13.5.3).

Quaternary structure is restricted to oligomeric proteins, which consist of the
association of two or more polypeptide chains held together by electrostatic
attractions, hydrogen bonding, van der Waals' forces and occasionally disulphide
bridges. Thus, disulphide bridges may exist within a given polypeptide chain
(intra-chain) or linking different chains (inter-chain). An individual polypeptide
chain in an oligomeric protein is referred to as a subunit. The subunits in a protein
may be identical or different: for example, haemoglobin consists of two α- and two
β-chains, and lactate dehydrogenase of four (virtually) identical chains.

Traditionally, proteins are classified into two groups – globular and fibrous. The
former are approximately spherical in shape, are generally water soluble and may
contain a mixture of α-helix, β-pleated sheet and random structures. Globular proteins include the enzymes, transport proteins, hormones and immunoglobulins.
Fibrous proteins are structural proteins, generally insoluble in water, consisting of
long cable-like structures built entirely of either helical or sheet arrangements.
Examples include hair keratin, silk fibroin and collagen. The native state of a
protein is its biologically active form.

The process of protein denaturation results in the loss of biological activity,
decreased aqueous solubility and increased susceptibility to proteolytic degradation. It can be brought about by heat and by treatment with reagents such as acids
and alkalis, detergents, organic solvents and heavy-metal cations such as mercury
and lead. It is associated with the loss of organised (tertiary) three-dimensional

structure and exposure to the aqueous environment of numerous hydrophobic groups previously located within the folded structure.

In enzymes, the specific three-dimensional folding of the polypeptide chain(s) results in the juxtaposition of certain amino acid residues that constitute the active site or catalytic site. Oligomeric enzymes may possess several such sites. Many enzymes also possess one or more regulatory site(s). X-ray crystallographic studies have revealed that the active site is often located in a cleft that is lined with hydrophobic amino acid residues but which contains some polar residues. The binding of the substrate at the catalytic site and the subsequent conversion of substrate to product involves different amino acid residues.

Some oligomeric enzymes exist in multiple forms called isoenzymes or isozymes. Their existence relies on the presence of two genes that give similar but not identical subunits. One of the best-known examples of isoenzymes is lactate dehydrogenase, which reversibly interconverts pyruvate and lactate. It is a tetramer and exists in five forms (LDH1 to 5) corresponding to the five permutations of arranging the two types of subunits (H and M), which differ only in a single amino acid substitution, into a tetramer:

H_4	LDH1
H_3M	LDH2
H_2M_2	LDH3
HM_3	LDH4
M_4	LDH5

Each isoenzyme promotes the same reaction but has different kinetic constants (K_m, V_{max}), thermal stability and electrophoretic mobility. The tissue distribution of isoenzymes within an organism is frequently different, for example, in humans LDH1 is the dominant isoenzyme in heart muscle but LDH5 is the most abundant form in liver and muscle. These differences are exploited in diagnostic enzymology to identify specific organ damage, e.g. following myocardial infarction, and thereby aiding clinical diagnosis and prognosis.

6.3 PROTEIN PURIFICATION

6.3.1 Introduction

At first sight, the purification of *one* protein from a cell and tissue homogenate that will typically contain 10 000–20 000 different proteins, seems a daunting task. However, in practice, on average, only four different fractionation steps are needed to purify a given protein. Indeed, in exceptional circumstances proteins have been purified in a single chromatographic step. Since the reason for purifying a protein is normally to provide material for structural or functional studies, the final degree of purity required depends on the purposes for which the protein will be used, i.e. you may not need a protein sample that is 100% pure for your studies. Indeed, to define what is meant by a 'a pure protein' is not easy. Theoretically, a protein is pure when a sample contains only a single protein species, although in practice it is more or less impossible to achieve 100% purity. Fortunately, many studies on proteins can be carried out on samples that contain as much as 5% to 10% or more contamination with other proteins. This is an important point, since each purification step necessarily involves loss of some of the protein you are trying to purify. An extra (and unnecessary) purification step that increases the purity of your sample from, say, 90% to 98% may mean that you now have a more pure protein, but insufficient protein for your studies. Better to have studied the sample that was 90% pure and have enough to work on!

For example, a 90% pure protein is sufficient for amino acid sequence determination studies as long as the sequence is analysed quantitatively to ensure that the deduced sequence does not arise from a contaminant protein. Similarly, immunisation of a rodent to provide spleen cells for monoclonal antibody production (Section 4.2.3) can be carried out with a sample that is considerably less than 50% pure. As long as your protein of interest raises an immune response it matters not at all that antibodies are also produced against the contaminating proteins. For kinetic studies on an enzyme, a relatively impure sample can be used provided it does not contain any competing activities. On the other hand, if you are raising a monospecific polyclonal antibody in an animal (see Section 4.2.3), it is necessary to have a highly purified protein as antigen, otherwise immunogenic contaminating proteins will give rise to additional antibodies. Equally, proteins that are to have a therapeutic use must be extremely pure to satisfy regulatory (safety) requirements. Clearly, therefore, the degree of purity required depends on the purpose for which the protein is needed.

6.3.2 Protein estimation

The need to determine protein concentration in solution is a routine requirement during protein purification. The only truly accurate method for determining protein concentration is to acid hydrolyse a portion of the sample and then carry out amino acid analysis on the hydrolysate (see Section 6.4.2). However, this is relatively time-consuming, particularly if multiple samples are to be analysed. Fortunately, in practice, one rarely needs decimal place accuracy and other, quicker methods that give a reasonably accurate assessment of protein concentrations of a solution are acceptable. Most of these (see below) are colorimetric methods, where a portion of the protein solution is reacted with a reagent that produces a coloured product. The amount of this coloured product is then measured spectrophotometrically and the amount of colour related to the amount of protein present by appropriate calibration. However, none of these methods is absolute, since, as will be seen below, the development of colour is often at least partly dependent on the amino acid composition of the protein(s). The presence of prosthetic groups (e.g. carbohydrate) also influences colorimetric assays. Many workers prepare a standard calibration curve using bovine serum albumin (BSA), chosen because of its low cost, high purity and ready availability. However, it should be understood that, since the amino acid composition of BSA will differ from the composition of the sample being tested, any concentration values deduced from the calibration graph can only be approximate.

Ultraviolet absorption

The aromatic amino acid residues tyrosine and tryptophan in a protein exhibit an absorption maximum at a wavelength of 280 nm. Since the proportions of these aromatic amino acids in proteins vary, so too do extinction coefficients for individual proteins. However, for most proteins the extinction coefficient lies in the range 0.4 to 1.5; so for a complex mixture of proteins it is a fair approximation to say that a solution with an absorbance at 280 nm (A_{280}) of 1.0, using a 1 cm pathlength, has a protein concentration of approximately 1 mg cm^{-3}. The method is relatively sensitive, being able to measure protein concentrations as low as 10 μg cm^{-3}, and, unlike colorimetric methods, is non-destructive, i.e. having made the measurement, the sample in the cuvette can be recovered and used further. This is particularly useful when one is working with small amounts of protein and cannot afford to waste any. However, the method is subject to interference by the presence of other compounds that absorb at 280 nm. Nucleic acids fall into this category having an absorbance as much as ten times that of protein at this wavelength. Hence the presence of only a small percentage of nucleic acid can greatly influence the absorbance at this wavelength. However, if the absorbance (A) at 280 and 260 nm wavelengths are measured it is possible to apply a correction factor:

Protein (mg cm^{-3}) = 1.55 A_{280} − 0.76 A_{260}

The great advantage of this protein assay is that it is non-destructive and can be measured continuously, for example in chromatographic column effluents.

Even greater sensitivity can be obtained by measuring the absorbance of ultraviolet light by peptide bonds. The peptide bond absorbs strongly in the far ultraviolet, with a maximum at about 190 nm. However, because of the difficulties caused by the absorption by oxygen and the low output of conventional spectrophotometers at this wavelength, measurements are usually made at 205 or 210 nm. Most proteins have an extinction coefficient for a 1 μg cm^{-3} solution of about 30 at 205 nm and about 20 at 210 nm. Clearly therefore measuring at these wavelengths is 20 to 30 times more sensitive than measuring at 280 nm, and protein concentration can be measured to less than 1 μg cm^{-3}. However, one disadvantage of working at these lower wavelengths is that a number of buffers and other buffer components commonly used in protein studies also absorb strongly at this wavelength, so it is not always practical to work at this lower wavelength.

Nowadays all purpose-built column chromatography systems (e.g. fast protein liquid chromatography and high performance liquid chromatography (HPLC)) have in-line variable wavelength ultraviolet light detectors that monitor protein elution from columns.

Lowry (Folin–Ciocalteau) method

In the past this has been the most commonly used method for determining protein concentration, although it is tending to be replaced by the more sensitive methods described below. The Lowry method is reasonably sensitive, detecting down to 10 μg cm^{-3} of protein, and the sensitivity is moderately constant from one protein to another. When the Folin reagent (a mixture of sodium tungstate, molybdate and phosphate), together with a copper sulphate solution, is mixed with a protein solution, a blue-purple colour is produced which can be quantified by its absorbance at 660 nm. As with most colorimetric assays, care must be taken that other compounds that interfere with the assay are not present. For the Lowry method this includes Tris, zwitterionic buffers such as Pipes and Hepes, and EDTA. The method is based on both the Biuret reaction, where the peptide bonds of proteins react with Cu^{2+} under alkaline conditions producing Cu^+, which reacts with the Folin reagent, and the Folin–Ciocalteu reaction, which is poorly understood but essentially involves the reduction of phosphomolybdotungstate to heteropolymolybdenum blue by the copper-catalysed oxidation of aromatic amino acids. The resultant strong blue colour is therefore partly dependent on the tyrosine and tryptophan content of the protein sample.

The bicinchoninic acid method

This method is similar to the Lowry method in that it also depends on the conversion of Cu^{2+} to Cu^+ under alkaline conditions. The Cu^+ is then detected by reaction with bicinchoninic acid (BCA) to give an intense purple colour with an absorbance maximum at 562 nm. The method is more sensitive than the Lowry method, being able to detect down to $0.5\,\mu g$ protein cm^{-3}, but perhaps more importantly it is generally more tolerant of the presence of compounds that interfere with the Lowry assay, hence the increasing popularity of the method.

The Bradford method

This method relies on the binding of the dye Coomassie Brilliant Blue to protein. At low pH the free dye has absorption maxima at 470 and 650 nm, but when bound to protein has an absorption maximum at 595 nm. The practical advantages of the method are that the reagent is simple to prepare and that the colour develops rapidly and is stable. Although it is sensitive down to $20\,\mu g$ protein cm^{-3}, it is only a relative method, as the amount of dye binding appears to vary with the content of the basic amino acids arginine and lysine in the protein. This makes the choice of a standard difficult. In addition, many proteins will not dissolve properly in the acidic reaction medium.

Kjeldahl analysis

This is a general chemical method for determining the nitrogen content of any compound. It is not normally used for the analysis of purified proteins or for monitoring column fractions but is frequently used for analysing complex solid samples and microbiological samples for protein content. The sample is digested by boiling with concentrated sulphuric acid in the presence of sodium sulphate (to raise the boiling point) and a copper and/or selenium catalyst. The digestion converts all the organic nitrogen to ammonia, which is trapped as ammonium sulphate. Completion of the digestion stage is generally recognised by the formation of a clear solution. The ammonia is released by the addition of excess sodium hydroxide and removed by steam distillation in a Markham still. It is collected in boric acid and titrated with standard hydrochloric acid using methyl red–methylene blue as indicator. It is possible to carry out the analysis automatically in an autokjeldahl apparatus. Alternatively, a selective ammonium ion electrode (Section 15.5) may be used to directly determine the content of ammonium ion in the digest. Although Kjeldahl analysis is a precise and reproducible method for the determination of nitrogen, the determination of the protein content of the original sample is complicated by the variation of the nitrogen content of individual proteins and by the presence of nitrogen in contaminants such as DNA. In practice, the nitrogen content of proteins is generally assumed to be 16% by weight.

6.3.3 Cell disruption and production of initial crude extract

The initial step of any purification procedure must, of course, be to disrupt the starting tissue to release proteins from within the cell. The means of disrupting the tissue will depend on the cell type (see Cell disruption, below), but thought must first be given to the composition of the buffer used to extract the proteins.

Extraction buffer

Normally extraction buffers are at an ionic strength (0.1 to 0.2 M) and pH (7.0 to 8.0) that is considered to be compatible with that found inside the cell. Tris or phosphate buffers are most commonly used. However, in addition a range of other reagents may be included in the buffer for specific purposes. These include:

(i) *An anti-oxidant.* Within the cell the protein is in a highly reducing environment, but when released into the buffer it is exposed to a more oxidising environment. Since most proteins contain a number of free sulphydryl groups (from the amino acid cysteine) these can undergo oxidation to give inter- and intramolecular disulphide bridges. To prevent this, reducing agents such as dithiothreitol, β-mercaptoethanol, cysteine or reduced glutathione are often included in the buffer.

(ii) *Enzyme inhibitors.* Once the cell is disrupted the organisational integrity of the cell is lost, and proteolytic enzymes that were carefully packaged and controlled within the intact cells are released, for example from lysosomes. Such enzymes will of course start to degrade proteins in the extract, including the protein of interest. To slow down unwanted proteolysis, all extraction and purification steps are carried out at 4 °C, and in addition a range of protease inhibitors is included in the buffer. Each inhibitor is specific for a particular type of protease, for example serine proteases, thiol proteases, aspartic proteases and metalloproteases. Common examples of inhibitors include: di-isopropylphosphofluoridate (DFP), phenylmethyl sulphonylfluoride (PMSF) and tosylphenylalanyl-chloromethylketone (TPCK) (all serine protease inhibitors); iodoacetate and cystatin (thiol protease inhibitors); pepstatin (aspartic protease inhibitor); EDTA and 1,10-phenanthroline (metalloprotease inhibitors); and amastatin and bestatin (exopeptidase inhibitors).

(iii) *Enzyme substrate and cofactors.* Low levels of substrate are often included in extraction buffers when an enzyme is purified, since binding of substrate to the enzyme active site can stabilise the enzyme during purification processes. Where relevant, cofactors that otherwise might be lost during purification are also included to maintain enzyme activity so that activity can be detected when column fractions, etc. are screened.

(iv) *EDTA.* This can be present to remove divalent metal ions that can react with thiol groups in proteins giving *mercaptids.*

$$R - SH + Me^{2+} \rightarrow R - S - Me^{+} + H^{+}$$

(v) *Polyvinylpyrrolidone (PVP).* This is often added to extraction buffers for plant tissue. Plant tissues contain considerable amounts of phenolic compounds (both monomeric, such as p-hydroxybenzoic acid, and polymeric, such as tannins) that can bind to enzymes and other proteins by non-covalent forces, including hydrophobic, ionic and hydrogen bonds, causing protein precipitation. These phenolic compounds are also easily oxidised, predominantly by endogenous phenol oxidases, to form quinones, which are highly reactive and can combine with reactive groups in proteins causing cross-linking, and further aggregation and precipitation. Insoluble PVP (which mimics the polypeptide backbone) is therefore added to adsorb the phenolic compounds which can then be removed by centrifugation. Thiol compounds (reducing agents) are also added to minimise the activity of phenol oxidases, and thus prevent the formation of quinones.

(vi) *Sodium azide.* For buffers that are going to be stored for long periods of time, antibacterial and/or antifungal agents are sometimes added at low concentrations. Sodium azide is frequently used as a bacteriostatic agent.

Membrane proteins

Membrane-bound proteins (normally glycoproteins) require special conditions for extraction as they are not released by simple cell disruption procedures alone. Two classes of membrane proteins are identified. Extrinsic *(or* peripheral*)* membrane proteins are bound only to the surface of the cell, normally via electrostatic and hydrogen bonds. These proteins are predominantly hydrophilic in nature and are relatively easily extracted by either raising the ionic concentration of the extraction buffer (e.g. to 1 M NaCl) or by changes of pH (e.g. to pH 3 to 5 or pH 9 to 12). Once extracted, they can be purified by conventional chromatographic procedures. Intrinsic membrane proteins are those that are embedded in the membrane (integrated membrane proteins). These invariably have significant regions of hydrophobic amino acids (those regions of the protein that are embedded in the membrane, and associated with lipids, see Section 8.1) and have low solubility in aqueous buffer systems. Hence, once extracted into an aqueous polar environment, appropriate conditions must be used to retain their solubility. Intrinsic proteins are usually extracted with buffer containing detergents. The choice of detergent is mainly one of trial and error but can include ionic detergents such as sodium dodecyl sulphate (SDS), sodium deoxycholate, cetyl trimethylammonium bromide (CTAB) and CHAPS, and non-ionic detergents such as Triton X-100 and Nonidet P-40.

Once extracted, intrinsic membrane proteins can be purified using conventional chromatographic techniques such as gel filtration, ion-exchange chromatography or affinity chromatography (using lectins). However, in each case it is necessary to include detergent in all buffers to maintain protein solubility. The level of detergent used is normally 10- to 100-fold less than that used to extract the protein, in order to minimise any interference of the detergent with the chromatographic process.

Cell disruption

Unless one is isolating proteins from extracellular fluids such as blood, protein purification procedures necessarily start with the disruption of cells or tissue to release the protein content of the cells into an appropriate buffer. This initial extract is therefore the starting point for protein purification. Clearly one chooses, where possible, a starting material that has a high level of the protein of interest. Depending on the protein being isolated one might therefore start with a microbial culture, plant tissue, or mammalian tissue. The last of these has generally been the tissue of choice where possible, owing to the relatively large amounts of starting material available. However, the ability to clone and overexpress genes for proteins from any source, in both bacteria and yeast, means that nowadays more and more protein purification protocols are starting with a microbial lysate. The different methods available for disrupting cells are described below. Which method one uses depends on the nature of the cell wall/membrane being disrupted.

Mammalian cells   Mammalian cells are of the order of 10 μm in diameter and enclosed by a plasma membrane, weakly supported by a cytoskeleton. These cells therefore lack any great rigidity and are easy to disrupt by shear forces.

Plant cells   Plant cells are of the order of 100 μm in diameter and have a fairly rigid cell wall, comprising carbohydrate complexes and lignin or wax that surround the plasma membrane. Although the plasma membrane is protected by this outer layer, the large size of the cell still makes it susceptible to shear forces.

Bacteria   Bacteria have cell diameters of the order of 1 to 4 μm and generally have extremely rigid cell walls. Bacteria can be classified as either Gram positive or Gram negative depending on whether or not they are stained by the Gram stain (crystal violet and iodine). In Gram-positive bacteria (Fig. 6.2) the plasma membrane is surrounded by a thick shell of peptidoglycan (20 to 50 nm), which stains with the Gram stain. In Gram-negative bacteria (e.g. *Escherichia coli*) the plasma membrane is surrounded by a thin (2 to 3 nm) layer of peptidoglycan but this is compensated for by having a second outer membrane of lipopolysaccharide. The negatively charged lipopolysaccharide polymers interact laterally, being linked by divalent cations such as Mg^{2+}. A number of Gram-negative bacteria secrete proteins into the periplasmic space.

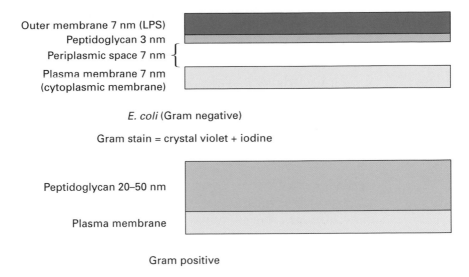

Fig. 6.2. The structure of the cell wall of Gram-positive and of Gram-negative bacteria. LPS, lipopolysaccharide.

Fungi and yeast Filamentous fungi and yeasts have a rigid cell wall that is composed mainly of polysaccharide (80% to 90%). In lower fungi and yeast the polysaccharides are mannan and glucan. In filamentous fungi it is chitin cross-linked with glucans. Yeasts also have a small percentage of glycoprotein in the cell wall, and there is a periplasmic space between the cell wall and cell membrane. If the cell wall is removed the cell content, surrounded by a membrane, is referred to as a spheroplast.

Cell disruption methods

Blenders These are commercially available, although a typical domestic kitchen blender will suffice. This method is ideal for disrupting mammalian or plant tissue by shear force. Tissue is cut into small pieces and blended, in the presence of buffer, for about 1 min to disrupt the tissue, and then centrifuged to remove debris. This method is inappropriate for bacteria and yeast, but a blender can be used for these microorganisms if small glass beads are introduced to produce a bead mill. Cells are trapped between colliding beads and physically disrupted by shear forces.

Grinding with abrasives Grinding in a pestle and mortar, in the presence of sand or alumina and a small amount of buffer, is a useful method for disrupting bacterial or plant cells; cell walls are physically ripped off by the abrasive. However, the method is appropriate for handling only relatively small samples. The Dynomill is a large-scale mechanical version of this approach. The Dynomill comprises a chamber containing glass beads and a number of rotating impeller discs. Cells are ruptured when caught between colliding beads. A 600 cm³ laboratory scale model can process 5 kg of bacteria per hour.

Presses   The use of a press such as a French Press, or the Manton–Gaulin Press, which is a larger-scale version, is an excellent means for disrupting microbial cells. A cell suspension ($\sim$ 50 cm³) is forced by a piston-type pump, under high pressure (10 000 PSI = lbf in.$^{-2} \approx$ 1450 kPa) through a small orifice. Breakage occurs due to shear forces as the cells are forced through the small orifice, and also by the rapid drop in pressure as the cells emerge from the orifice, which allows the previously compressed cells to expand rapidly and effectively burst. Multiple passes are usually needed to lyse all the cells, but under carefully controlled conditions it can be possible to selectively release proteins from the periplasmic space. The X-Press and Hughes Press are variations on this method; the cells are forced through the orifice as a frozen paste, often mixed with an abrasive. Both the ice crystal and abrasive aid in disrupting the cell walls.

Enzymic methods   The enzyme lysozyme, isolated from hen egg whites, cleaves peptidoglycan. The peptidoglycan cell wall can therefore be removed from Gram-positive bacteria (see Fig. 6.2) by treatment with lysozyme, and if carried out in a suitable buffer, once the cell wall has been digested the cell membrane will rupture due to the osmotic effect of the suspending buffer.

Gram-negative bacteria can similarly be disrupted by lysozyme but treatment with EDTA (to remove Ca^{2+}, thus destabilising the outer lipopolysaccharide layer) and the inclusion of a non-ionic detergent to solubilise the cell membrane are also needed. This effectively permeabilises the outer membrane, allowing access of the lysozyme to the peptidoglycan layer. If carried out in an isotonic medium so that the cell membrane is not ruptured, it is possible to selectively release proteins from the periplasmic space.

Yeast can be similarly disrupted using enzymes to degrade the cell wall and either osmotic shock or mild physical force to disrupt the cell membrane. Enzyme digestion alone allows the selective release of proteins from the periplasmic space. The two most commonly used enzyme preparations for yeast are zymolyase or lyticase, both of which have β-1,3-glucanase activity as their major activity, together with a proteolytic activity specific for the yeast cell wall. Chitinase is commonly used to disrupt filamentous fungi. Enzymic methods tend to be used for laboratory-scale work, since for large-scale work their use is limited by cost.

Sonication   This method is ideal for a suspension of cultured cells or microbial cells. A sonicator probe is lowered into the suspension of cells and high frequency sound waves ($>$ 20 kHz) generated for 30 to 60 s. These sound waves cause disruption of cells by shear force and cavitation. Cavitation refers to areas where there is alternate compression and rarefraction, which rapidly interchange. The gas bubbles in the buffer are initially under pressure but, as they decompress, shock waves are released and disrupt the cells. This method is suitable for relatively small volumes (50 to 100 cm³). Since considerable heat is generated by this method, samples must be kept on ice during treatment.

6.3.4 Fractionation methods

Monitoring protein purification

As will be seen below, the purification of a protein invariably involves the application of one or more column chromatographic steps, each of which generates a relatively large number of test tubes (fractions) containing buffer and protein eluted from the column. It is necessary to determine how much protein is present in each tube so that an elution profile (a plot of protein concentration versus tube number) can be produced. Appropriate methods for detecting and quantifying protein in solution are described in Section 6.3.2. A method is also required for determining which tubes contain the protein of interest so that their contents can be pooled and the pooled sample progressed to the next purification step. If one is purifying an enzyme, this is relatively easy as each tube simply has to be assayed for the presence of enzyme activity (Section 7.4).

For proteins that have no easily measured biological activity, other approaches have to be used. If an antibody to the protein of interest is available then samples from each tube can be dried onto nitrocellulose and the antibody used to detect the protein-containing fractions using the dot blot method (Section 4.7.3). Alternatively, an immunoassay such as ELISA or radioimmunoassay (Section 4.7) can be used to detect the protein. If an antibody is not available, then portions from each fraction can be run on a sodium dodecyl sulphate–polyacrylamide gel and the protein-containing fraction identified from the appearance of the protein band of interest on the gel (Section 12.3.1).

An alternative approach that can be used for cloned genes that are expressed in cells is to express the protein as a fusion protein, i.e. one that is linked via a short peptide sequence to a second protein. This can have advantage for protein purification (see Section 6.3.5). However, it can also prove extremely useful for monitoring the purification of a protein that has no easily measurable activity. If the second protein is an enzyme that can be easily assayed (e.g. using a simple colorimetric assay), such as β-galactosidase, then the presence of the protein of interest can be detected by the presence of the linked β-galactosidase activity.

A successful fractionation step is recognised by an increase in the specific activity of the sample, where the specific activity of the enzyme relates its total activity to the total amount of protein present in the preparation:

$$\text{specific activity} = \frac{\text{total units of enzyme in fraction}}{\text{total amount of protein in fraction}}$$

The measurement of units of an enzyme relies on an appreciation of certain basic kinetic concepts and upon the availability of a suitable analytical procedure. These are discussed in Section 7.4.

The amount of enzyme present in a particular fraction is expressed convention-ally not in terms of units of mass or moles but in terms of units based upon the rate of the reaction that the enzyme promotes. The international unit (IU) of an enzyme is defined as the amount of enzyme that will convert 1 μmole of substrate to product in 1 minute under defined conditions (generally 25 or 30 °C at the optimum pH). The SI unit of enzyme activity is defined as the amount of enzyme that will convert 1 mole of substrate to product in 1 second. It has units of katal (kat) such that 1 kat $= 6 \times 10^7$ IU and 1 IU $= 1.7 \times 10^{-8}$ kat. For some enzymes, especially those where the substrate is a macromolecule of unknown relative molecular mass (e.g. amylase, pepsin, RNase, DNase) it is not possible to define either of these units. In such cases arbitrary units are used generally that are based upon some observable change in a chemical or physical property of the substrate.

For a purification step to be successful, therefore, the specific activity of the protein must be greater after the purification step than it was before. This increase is best represented as the fold purification:

$$\text{fold purification} = \frac{\text{specific activity of fraction}}{\text{original specific activity}}$$

A significant increase in specific activity is clearly necessary for a successful pur-ification step. However, another important factor is the yield of the step. It is no use having an increased specific activity if you lose 95% of the protein you are trying to purify. Yield is defined as follows:

$$\text{yield} = \frac{\text{units of enzyme in fraction}}{\text{units of enzyme in original preparation}}$$

A yield of 70% or more in any purification step would normally be considered as acceptable. Table 6.3 shows how yield and specific activity vary during a purifica-tion schedule.

Preliminary purification steps

The initial extract, produced by the disruption of cells and tissue, and referred to at this stage as a homogenate, will invariably contain insoluble matter. For example, for mammalian tissue there will be incompletely homogenised connective and or vascular tissue, and small fragments of non-homogenised tissue. This is most easily removed by filtering through a double layer of cheesecloth or by low speed (5 000 g) centrifugation. Any fat floating on the surface can be removed by coarse filtration through glass wool or cheesecloth. However, the solution will still be cloudy with organelles and membrane fragments that are too small to be conveniently removed by filtration or low speed centrifugation. These may not be much of a problem as they will often be lost in the preliminary stages of protein purification, for example during salt fractionation. However, if necessary they can be removed first by pre-cipitation using materials such as Celite (a diatomaceous earth that provides a large surface area to trap the particles), Cell Debris Remover (CDR) a cellulose-based absorber, or any number of flocculants such as starch, gums, tannins or poly-amines, the resultant precipitate being removed by centrifugation or filtration.

Table 6.3 Example of a protein purification schedule

Fraction	Volume (ml)	Protein concentration (mg ml^{-1})	Total protein (mg)	Activity[a] (U/ml)	Total activity (U)	Specific activity (U mg^{-1})	Purification factor[b]	Overall yield[c] (%)
Homogenate	8500	40	340 000	1.8	15 300	0.045	1	100
45%–70% (NH$_4$)$_2$SO$_4$	530	194	103 000	23.3	12 350	0.12	2.7	81
CM-cellulose	420	19.5	8190	25	10 500	1.28	28.4	69
Affinity chromotography	48	2.2	105.6	198	9500	88.4	1964	62
DEAE-Sepharose	12	2.3	27.6	633	7600	275	6110	50

[a] The unit of enzyme activity (U) is defined as that amount which produces one μmole of product per minute under standard assay conditions.

[b] Defined as: purification factor = (specific activity of fraction/specific activity of homogenate).

[c] Defined as: overall yield = (total activity of fraction/total activity of homogenate).

Reproduced with permission from *Methods in Molecular Biology*, **59**, *Protein Purification Protocols*, ed. S. Doonan (1996), Totowa, NJ, Humana Press Inc.

It is tempting to assume that the cell extract contains only protein, but of course a range of other molecules is present such as DNA, RNA, carbohydrate and lipid as well as any number of small molecular weight metabolites. Small molecules tend to be removed later on during dialysis steps or steps that involve fractionation based on size (e.g. gel filtration) and therefore are of little concern. However, specific attention has to be paid at this stage to macromolecules such as nucleic acids and polysaccharides. This is particularly true for bacterial extracts, which are particularly viscous owing to the presence of chromosomal DNA. Indeed microbial extracts can be extremely difficult to centrifuge to produce a supernatant extract. Some workers include DNAse I in the extraction buffer to reduce viscosity, the small DNA fragments generated being removed at later dialysis/gel filtration steps. Likewise RNA can be removed by treatment with RNase. DNA and RNA can also be removed by precipitation with protamine sulphate. Protamine sulphate is a mixture of small, highly basic (i.e. positively charged) proteins, whose natural role is to bind to DNA in the sperm head. (Protamines are usually extracted from fish organs, which are obtained as a waste product at canning factories.) These positively charged proteins bind to negatively charged phosphate groups on nucleic acids, thus masking the charged groups on the nucleic acids and rendering them insoluble. The addition of a solution of protamine sulphate to the extract therefore precipitates most of the DNA and RNA, which can subsequently be removed by centrifugation. An alternative is to use polyethyleneimine, a synthetic long chain cationic (i.e. positively charged) polymer (molecular mass 24 kDa). This also binds to the phosphate groups in nucleic acids, and is very effective, precipitating DNA and RNA almost instantly. For bacterial extracts, carbohydrate capsular gum can also be a problem as this can interfere with protein precipitation methods. This is best removed by totally precipitating the protein with ammonium sulphate (see below) leaving the gum in solution. The protein can then be recovered by centrifugation and redissolved in buffer. However, if lysozyme (plus detergent) is used to lyse the cells (see Section 6.3.3) capsular gum will not be a problem as it is digested by the lysozyme.

The clarified extract is now ready for protein fractionation steps to be carried out. The concentration of the protein in this initial extract is normally quite low, and in fact the major contaminant at this stage is water! The initial purification step is frequently based on solubility methods. These methods have a high capacity, can therefore be easily applied to large volumes of initial extracts and also have the advantage of concentrating the protein sample. Essentially, proteins that differ considerably in their physical characteristics from the protein of interest are removed at this stage, leaving a more concentrated solution of proteins that have more closely similar physical characteristics. The next stages, therefore, involve higher resolution techniques that can separate proteins with similar characteristics. Invariably these high resolution techniques are chromatographic. Which technique to use, and in which order, is more often than not a matter of trial and error. The final research paper that describes in four pages a three-step, four-day protein purification procedure invariably belies the months of hard work that went into developing the final 'simple' purification protocol!

All purification techniques are based on exploiting those properties by which proteins differ from one another. These different properties, and the techniques that exploit these differences, are as follows.

Stability.   Denaturation fractionation exploits differences in the heat sensitivity of proteins. The three-dimensional (tertiary) structure of proteins is maintained by a number of forces, mainly hydrophobic interactions, hydrogen bonds and sometimes disulphide bridges. When we say that a protein is denatured we mean that these bonds have by some means been disrupted and that the protein chain has unfolded to give the insoluble, 'denatured' protein. One of the easiest ways to denature proteins in solution is to heat them. However, different proteins will denature at different temperatures, depending on their different thermal stabilities; this, in turn, is a measure of the numbers of bonds holding the tertiary structure together. If the protein of interest is particularly heat stable, then heating the extract to a temperature at which the protein is stable yet other proteins denature can be a very useful preliminary step. The temperature at which the protein being purified is denatured is first determined by a small-scale experiment. Once this temperature is known, it is possible to remove more thermolabile contaminating proteins by heating the mixture to a temperature 5 to 10 deg.C below this critical temperature for a period of 15 to 30 min. The denatured, unwanted protein is then removed by centrifugation. The presence of the substrate, product or a competitive inhibitor of an enzyme often stabilises it and allows an even higher heat denaturation temperature to be employed. In a similar way, proteins differ in the ease with which they are denatured by extremes of pH (<3 and >10). The sensitivity of the protein under investigation to extreme pH is determined by a small-scale trial. The whole protein extract is then adjusted to a pH not less than 1 pH unit within that at which the test protein is preciptiated. More sensitive proteins will precipitate and are removed by centrifugation.

Solubility.   Proteins differ in the balance of charged, polar and hydrophobic amino acids that they display on their surfaces. Charged and polar groups on the surface are solvated by water molecules, thus making the protein molecule soluble, whereas hydrophobic residues are masked by water molecules that are necessarily found adjacent to these regions. Since solubility is a consequence of solvation of charged and polar groups on the surfaces of the protein, it follows that, under a particular set of conditions, proteins will differ in their solubilities. In particular, one exploits the fact that proteins precipitate differentially from solution on the addition of species such as neutral salts or organic solvents. It should be stressed here that these methods precipitate native (i.e. active) protein that has become insoluble by aggregation; we have not denatured the protein.

Salt fractionation is frequently carried out using ammonium sulphate. As increasing salt is added to a protein solution, so the salt ions are solvated by water molecules in the solution. As the salt concentration increases, freely available water molecules that can solvate the ions become scarce. At this stage those water molecules that have been forced into contact with hydrophobic groups on the surface of the protein are the next most freely available water molecules (rather than those involved in solvating polar groups on the protein surface, which are bound by electrostatic interactions and are far less easily given up) and these are therefore removed to solvate the salt molecules, thus leaving the hydrophobic patches exposed. As the ammonium sulphate concentration increases, the hydrophobic surfaces on the protein are progressively exposed. Thus revealed, these hydrophobic patches cause proteins to aggregate by hydrophobic interaction, resulting in precipitation. The first proteins to aggregate are therefore those with most hydrophobic residues on the surface, followed by those with less hydrophobic residues. Clearly the aggregates formed are made of mixtures of more than one protein. Individual identical molecules do not seek out each other, but simply bind to another adjacent molecule with an exposed hydrophobic patch. However, many proteins are precipitated from solution over a narrow range of salt concentrations, making this a suitably simple procedure for enriching the proteins of interest.

Organic solvent fractionation is based on differences in the solubility of proteins in aqueous solutions containing water-miscible organic solvents such as ethanol, acetone and butanol. The addition of organic solvent effectively 'dilutes out' the water present (reduces the dielectric constant) and at the same time water molecules are used up in hydrating the organic solvent molecules. Water of solvation is therefore removed from the charged and polar groups on the surface of proteins, thus exposing their charged groups. Aggregation of proteins therefore occurs by charge (ionic) interactions between molecules. Proteins consequently precipitate in decreasing order of the number of charged groups on their surface as the organic solvent concentration is increased.

Organic polymers can also be used for the fractional precipitation of proteins. This method resembles organic solvent fractionation in its mechanism of action but requires lower concentrations to cause protein precipitation and is less likely to cause protein denaturation. The most commonly used polymer is polyethylene glycol (PEG), with a relative molecular mass in the range 6000 to 20 000.

The fractionation of a protein mixture using ammonium sulphate is given here as a practical example of fractional precipitation. As explained above, as increasing amounts of ammonium sulphate are dissolved in a protein solution, certain proteins start to aggregate and precipitate out of solution. Increasing the salt strength results in further, different proteins precipitating out. By carrying out a controlled pilot experiment where the percentage of ammonium sulphate is increased stepwise say from 10% to 20% to 30% etc., the resultant precipitate at each step being recovered by centrifugation, redissolved in buffer and analysed for the protein of interests, it is possible to determine a fractionation procedure that will give a significantly purified sample. In the example shown in Table 6.3, the original homogenate was made 45% in ammonium sulphate and the precipitate recovered and discarded. The supernatant was then made 70% in ammonium sulphate, the precipitate collected, redissolved in buffer, and kept, with the supernatant being discarded. This produced a purification factor of 2.7. As can be seen, a significant amount of protein has been removed at this step (237 000 mg of protein) while 81% of the total enzyme present was recovered, i.e. the yield was good. This step has clearly produced an enrichment of the protein of interest from a large volume of extract and at the same time has concentrated the sample.

Isoelectric precipitation fractionation is based upon the observations that proteins have their minimum solubility at their isoelectric point. At this pH there are equal numbers of positive and negative charges on the protein molecule; intermolecular repulsions are therefore minimised and protein molecules can approach each other. This therefore allows opposite charges on different molecules to interact, resulting in the formation of insoluble aggregates. The principle can be exploited either to remove unwanted protein, by adjusting the pH of the protein extract so as to cause the precipitation of these proteins but not that of the test protein, or to remove the test protein, by adjusting the pH of the extract to its pI. In practice, the former alternative is preferable, since some denaturation of the precipitation protein inevitably occurs.

Finally, an unusual solubility phenomenon can be utilised in some cases for protein purification from *E. coli*. Early workers who were overexpressing heterologous proteins in *E. coli* at high levels were alarmed to discover that, although their protein was expressed in high yield (up to 40% of the total cell protein), the protein aggregated to form insoluble particles that became known as inclusion bodies. Initially this was seen as a major impediment to the production of proteins in *E. coli*, the inclusion bodies effectively being a mixture of monomeric and polymeric denatured proteins formed by partial or incorrect folding, probably due to the reducing environment of the *E. coli* cytoplasm. However, it was soon realised that this phenomenon could be used to advantage in protein purification. The inclusion bodies can be separated from a large proportion of the bacterial cytoplasmic protein by centrifugation, giving an effective purification step. The recovered inclusion bodies must then be solubilised and denatured and subsequently allowed to refold slowly to their active, native configuration. This is normally achieved by heating in 6 M guanidinium hydrochloride (to denature the protein) in the presence of a reducing agent (to disrupt any disulphide bridges). The denatured protein is then either diluted in buffer or dialysed against buffer, at which time the protein slowly refolds. Although the refolding method is not always 100% successful, this approach can often produce protein that is 50% or more pure.

Having carried out an initial fractionation step such as described above, one would then move towards using higher resolution chromatographic methods. Chromatographic techniques for purifying proteins are summarised in Table 6.4, and some of the more commonly used methods are outlined below. The precise practical details of each technique are discussed in Chapter 13.

Charge. Proteins differ from one another in the proportions of the charged amino acids (aspartic and glutamic acids, lysine, arginine and histidine) that they contain. Hence proteins will differ in net charge at a particular pH. This difference is exploited in ion-exchange chromatography (Section 13.7), where the protein of interest is bound onto a solid support material bearing charged groups of the

Table 6.4 Summary of chromatographic techniques commonly used in protein purification

Technique	Property exploited	Capacity	Resolution	Practical points	Further details
Hydrophobic interaction	Hydrophobicity	High	Medium	Can cope with high ionic strength samples, e.g. ammonium sulphate precipitates. Fractions are of varying pH and/or ionic strength. Medium yield. Commonly used in early stages of purification protocol. Unpredictable	Section 13.5.3
Ion-exchange	Charge	High	Medium	Sample ionic strength must be low. Fractions are of varying pH and/or ionic strength. Medium yield. Commonly used in early stages of purification protocol	Section 13.7
Affinity	Biological function	Medium (cost limited)	High	Limited by availability of immobilised ligand. Elution may denature protein. Yield medium–low. Commonly used towards end of purification protocol	Section 13.9
Dye affinity	Structure and hydrophobicity		High	Necessary to carry out initial screening of a wide range of dye-ligand supports	Section 13.9.7
Chromatofocusing	Charge and pI	High–medium	High–medium	Sample ionic strength must be low. Fractions contaminated with ampholytes	Section 13.7.3
Covalent	Thiol groups	Medium–low	High	Specific for thiol-containing proteins. Limited by high cost and long (3 h) regeneration time	Section 13.9.8
Metal chelate	Imidazole, thiol, tryptophan groups	Medium–low	High	Relatively few examples in literature. Expensive	Section 13.9.6
Exclusion	Molecular size	Medium	Low	Commonly used as a final stage of purification. Can give information about protein molecular weight. Good for desalting protein samples	Section 13.8

opposite sign (ion-exchange resin). Proteins with the same charge as the resin pass through the column to waste, after which bound proteins, containing the protein of interest, are selectively released from the column by gradually increasing the strength of salt ions in the buffer passing through the column or by gradually changing the pH of the eluting buffer. These ions compete with the protein for binding to the resin, the more weakly charged protein being eluted at the lower salt strength and the more strongly charged protein being eluted at higher salt strengths.

Another feature of the different charged groups found in proteins is the fact that most proteins will differ in their isoelectric points (Section 4.3.4), i.e. they will differ in the pH value at which they have zero overall charge. This difference in pI can be exploited using chromatofocusing (Section 3.7.3).

Size.   Size differences between proteins can be exploited in molecular exclusion (also known as gel filtration) chromatography. The gel filtration medium consists of a range of beads with slighly differing amounts of cross-linking and therefore slightly different pore sizes. The separation process depends on the different abilities of the various proteins to enter either some, all or none of the beads, which in turn relates to the size of this protein (Section 13.8). The method has limited resolving power, but can be used to obtain a separation between large and small protein molecules and therefore be useful when the protein of interest is either particularly large or particularly small. This method can also be used to determine the relative molecular mass of a protein (Section 13.8.3) and for concentrating or desalting a protein solution (Section 13.8.3).

Affinity.   Certain proteins bind strongly to specific small molecules. One can take advantage of this by developing an affinity chromatography system where the small molecule (ligand) is bound to an insoluble support. When a crude mixture of proteins containing the protein of interest is passed through the column, the ligand binds the protein to the matrix while all other proteins pass through the column. The bound protein can then be eluted from the column by changing the pH, increasing salt strength or passing through a high concentration of unbound free ligand. For example, the protein concanavalin A (con A) binds strongly to glucose. An affinity column using glucose as the ligand can therefore be used to bind con A to the matrix, and the con A can be recovered by passing a high concentration of glucose through the column. Lectins (Section 13.8.4) are particularly useful ligands for purifying glycoproteins by affinity chromatography. Affinity chromatography is covered in detail in Section 13.9.

Hydrophobicity.   Proteins differ in the amount of hydrophobic amino acids that are present on their surface. This difference can be exploited in salt fractionation (see above) but can also be used in a higher resolution method using hydrophobic interaction chromatography (HIC) (Section 13.5.3) A typical column material would be phenyl-Sepharose where phenyl groups are bonded to the insoluble support Sepharose. The protein mixture is loaded on the column in high salt (to ensure hydrophobic patches are exposed where hydrophobic interaction will occur between the phenyl groups on the resin and hydrophobic regions on the proteins. Proteins are then eluted by applying a decreasing salt gradient to the column and should emerge from the column in order of increasing hydrophobicity. However, some highly hydrophobic proteins may not even be eluted in the total absence of salt. In this case it is necessary to add a small amount of water-miscible organic solvent such as propanol or ethylene glycol to the column buffer solution. This will compete with the proteins for binding to the hydrophobic matrix and will elute any remaining proteins.

6.3.5 Engineering proteins for purification

With the ability to clone and overexpress genes for proteins using genetic engineering methodology has also come the ability to aid considerably the purification process by manipulation of the gene of interest prior to expression. These manipulations are carried out either to ensure secretion of the proteins from the cell or to aid protein purification.

Ensuring secretion from the cell

For cloned genes that are being expressed in microbial or eukaryotic cells, there are a number of advantages in manipulating the gene to ensure that the protein product is secreted from the cell:

To facilitate purification. Clearly if the protein is secreted into the growth medium, there will be far less contaminating proteins present than if the cells had to be ruptured to release the protein, when all the other intracellular proteins would also be present.

Prevention of intracellular degradation of the cloned protein. Many cloned proteins are recognised as 'foreign' by the cell in which they are produced and are therefore degraded by intracellular proteases. Secretion of the protein into the culture medium should minimise this degradation.

Reduction of the intracellular concentration of toxic proteins. Some cloned proteins are toxic to the cell in which they are produced and there is therefore a limit to the amount of protein the cell will produce before it dies. Protein secretion should prevent cell death and result in continued production of protein.

To allow post-translational modification of proteins. Most post-translational modifications of proteins occur as part of the secretory pathway, and these modifications, for example glycosylation (see Section 6.4.4), are a necessary process in producing the final protein structure. Since prokaryotic cells do not glycosylate their proteins, this explains why many proteins have to be expressed in eukaryotic cells (e.g. yeast) rather than in bacteria. The entry of a protein into a secretory pathway and its ultimate destination is determined by a short amino acid sequence (signal sequence) that is usually at the N-terminus of the protein. For proteins going to the membrane or outside the cell the route is via the endoplasmic reticulum and Golgi apparatus, the signal sequence being cleaved-off by a protease prior to secretion. For example, human γ-interferon has been secreted from the yeast *Pichia pastoris* using the protein's native signal sequence. Also there are a number of well-characterised yeast signal sequences (e.g. the α-factor signal sequence) that can be used to ensure secretion of proteins cloned into yeast.

Fusion proteins to aid protein purification

This approach requires an additional gene to be joined to the gene of the protein of interest such that the protein is produced as a fusion protein (i.e. linked to this second protein, or tag). As will be seen below, the purpose of this tag is to provide a means whereby the fusion protein can be selectively removed from the cell extract. The fusion protein can then be cleaved to release the protein of interest from the tag protein. Clearly the amino acid sequence of the peptide linkage between tag and protein has to be carefully designed to allow chemical or enzymic cleavage of this sequence. The following are just a few examples of different types of fusion proteins that have been used to aid protein purification.

Flag™.   This is a short hydrophilic amino acid sequence that is attached to the N-terminal end of the protein, and is designed for purification by immunoaffinity chromatography.

   Asp-Tyr-Lys-Asp-Asp-Asp-Asp-Lys-Protein

A monoclonal antibody against this Flag sequence is available on an immobilised support for use in affinity chromatography. The cell extract, which includes the Flag-labelled protein, is passed through the column where the antibody binds to the Flag-labelled protein, allowing all other proteins to pass through. This is carried out in the presence of Ca^{2+} since the binding of the Flag sequence to the monoclonal antibody is Ca^{2+} dependent. Once all unbound protein has been eluted from the column, the Flag-linked protein is released by passing EDTA through the column, which chelates the Ca^{2+}. Finally the Flag sequence is removed by the enzyme enterokinase, which recognises the following amino acid sequence and cleaves C-terminal to the lysine residue

   N-Asp-Asp-Asp-Lys-C

Using this approach, granulocyte–macrophage colony-stimulating factor (GMCSF) was cloned in and secreted from yeast, and purified in a single step. GMCSF was produced in the cell as signal peptide–Flag–gene. The signal sequence used was the signal sequence for the outer membrane protein OmpA. The Flag–gene protein was thus secreted into the periplasm, the fusion protein purified, and finally the Flag sequence removed, as described above.

Glutathione affinity agarose.   In this method the protein of interest is expressed as a fusion protein with the enzyme glutathione *S*-transferase. The cell extract is passed through a column of glutathione-linked agarose beads, where the enzyme binds to the glutathione. Once all unbound protein has been washed through the column, the fusion protein is eluted by passing reduced glutathione through the column. Finally, cleavage of the fusion protein is achieved using human thrombin, which recognises a specific amino acid sequence in the linker region.

Protein A.   As described in Section 4.3.4, protein A binds to the Fc region of the immunoglobulin G (IgG) molecule. The protein of interest is cloned fused to the protein A gene, and the fusion protein purified by affinity chromatography on a column of IgG–Sepharose. The bound fusion protein is then eluted using either high salt or low pH, to disrupt the binding between the IgG molecule and the protein A–protein fusion product. Protein A is then finally removed by treatment with 70% (V/V) formic acid for 2 days, which cleaves an acid-labile Asp-Pro bond in the linker region.

Poly(arginine).   This method requires the addition of a series of arginine residues to the C terminus of the protein to be purified. This makes the protein highly basic (positively charged at neutral pH). The cell extract can therefore be fractionated using cation-exchange chromatography. Bound proteins are sequentially released from the column by applying a salt gradient, with the poly(arg)-containing protein, because of its high overall positive charge, being the last to be eluted. The poly(arg) tail is then removed by incubation with the enzyme carboxypeptidase B. Carboxypeptidase B is an exoprotease that sequentially removes arginine or lysine residues from the C terminus of proteins. The arginine residues are therefore sequentially removed from the C terminus, the removal of amino acid residues stopping when the 'normal' (i.e. non-arginine) C-terminal amino acid residue of the protein is reached.

6.4 PROTEIN STRUCTURE DETERMINATION

6.4.1 Relative molecular mass

There are three methods available for determining protein relative molecular mass, M_r, frequently referred to as molecular weight. The first two described here are quick and easy methods that will give a value to $\pm$ 5% to 10%. For many purposes one simply needs a rough estimate of size and these methods are sufficient. The third method, mass spectrometry, which requires expensive specialist instruments and can give accuracy to $\pm$ 0.001%. This kind of accuracy is invaluable in detecting postsynthetic modification of proteins.

SDS–polyacrylamide gel electrophoresis (SDS–PAGE)

This form of electrophoresis, described in Section 12.3.1, separates proteins on the basis of their shape (size), which in turn relates to their relative molecular masses. A series of proteins of known molecular mass (molecular weight markers) are run on a gel on a track adjacent to the protein of unknown molecular mass. The distance each marker protein moves through the gel is measured and a calibration curve of log M_r versus distance moved is plotted. The distance migrated by the protein of unknown M_r is also measured, and from the graph its log M_r and hence M_r is calculated. The method is suitable for proteins covering a large M_r range (10 000 to 300 000). The method is easy to perform and requires very little material. If silver staining (Section 12.3.8) is used, as little as 1 ng of protein is required. In practice SDS–PAGE is the most commonly used method for determining protein M_r values.

Molecular exclusion (gel filtration) chromatography

The elution volume of a protein from a molecular exclusion chromatography column having an appropriate fractionation range is determined largely by the size of the protein such that there is a logarithmic relationship between protein relative molecular mass and elution volume (Section 13.8.3). By calibrating the column with a range of proteins of known M_r, the M_r of a test protein can be calculated. The method is carried out on HPLC columns ($\sim 1 \times 30$ cm) packed with porous silica beads. Flow rates are about 1 cm^3 min^{-1}, giving a run time of about 12 min, producing sharp, well-resolved peaks. A linear calibration line is obtained by plotting a graph of log M_r versus K_d for the calibrating proteins. K_d is calculated from the following equation:

$$K_d = \frac{(V_e - V_o)}{(V_t - V_o)}$$

where V_o is the volume in which molecules that are wholly excluded from the column material emerge (the excluded volume), V_t is the volume in which small molecules that can enter all the pores emerge (the included volume) and V_e is the volume in which the marker protein elutes. This method gives values that are accurate to $\pm 10\%$.

Mass spectrometry

Using either electrospray ionisation (ESI) or matrix-assisted laser desorption ionisation (MALDI) (see Section 11.6.4) intact molecular ions can be produced for proteins and hence their masses accurately measured by mass spectrometry. ESI produces molecular ions from molecules with molecular masses in excess of 100 kDa, whereas MALDI produces ions from intact proteins in excess of 200 kDa. In either case, only low picomole quantities of protein are needed. The determination of the molecular mass of cytochrome c using ESI is shown in Fig. 11. 22. Note that the observed mass (12 366.20 Da) is in excellent agreement with the molecular mass deduced from the DNA sequence (12 366). In contrast, in another study ESI gave a value of 146 881 for a murine monoclonal antibody that was about 3% higher than that determined from the DNA sequence. This reflected the fact that the IgG molecule contains about 3% carbohydrate, which of course could not be deduced from the DNA sequence. The measured molecular mass was therefore accurate. $\alpha\beta_2$ crystallin protein also gave a molecular mass value (20 200 $\pm$ 0.9), in excellent agreement with the deduced mass of 20 201. However, in addition about 10% of the analysed material produced an ion of mass 20 072.2. This showed that some of the purified protein molecules had lost their N-terminal amino acid (lysine). The deduced mass with the loss of N-terminal lysine was 20 072.8. Clearly mass spectrometry has the ability to provide highly accurate molecular mass measurements for proteins and peptides, which in turn can be used to deduce small changes made to the basic protein structure.

6.4.2 Amino acid analysis

The determination of which of the 20 possible amino acids are present in a particular protein, and in what relative amounts, is achieved by hydrolysing the protein to yield its component amino acids and identifying and quantifying them chromatographically. Hydrolysis is achieved by heating the protein with 6 M hydrochloride acid for 14 h at 110 °C *in vacuo*. Unfortunately, the hydrolysis procedure destroys or chemically modifies the asparagine, glutamine and tryptophan residues. Asparagine and glutamine are converted to their corresponding acids (Asp and Glu) and are quantified with them. Tryptophan is completely destroyed and is best determined spectrophotometrically on the unhydrolysed protein.

The amino acids in the protein hydrolysate may be separated chromatographically and quantified by postcolumn derivatisation with an appropriate reagent. In post-column derivatisation methods, the effluent stream from the chromatography column is mixed, in-line, with a reagent that reacts with the amino groups of amino acids to produce a coloured or fluorescent product. The effluent then continues to pass through an appropriate detector (colorimeter or fluorimeter) and the amount of colour/fluorescence recorded, on a chart recorder, where each amino acid is recorded as a separate peak, the area under the peak being proportional to the amount of that amino acid. The apparatus dedicated to the analysis of amino acids in mixtures by this technique is referred to as an amino acid analyser. In the original procedure, separation was achieved by ion-exchange chromatography on a sulphated polystyrene column and ninhydrin was used as the colour reagent and was sensitive down to about 50 to 100 pmol of the amino acid. Later, *o*-phthalaldehyde (Fig. 6.3) and *fluorescamine*, both of which give fluorescent products, became the reagents of choice, since they enabled as little as 10 pmol of an amino acid to be detected by fluorimetry.

In recent years, precolumn derivatisation of amino acids, followed by separation by reversed-phase HPLC has become attractive and has generally superseded the original ion-exchange method for the quantification of amino acids in a protein hydrolysate. In this approach the amino acid hydrolysate is first treated with a molecule that (i) reacts with amino groups in amino acids, (ii) is hydrophobic, thus allowing separation of derivatised amino acids by reversed-phase HPLC and (iii) is easily detected by its ultraviolet absorbance of fluorescence. Reagents routinely used for precolumn derivatisation include *o*-phthalaldehyde (see Fig. 6.3) and 6-aminoquinolyl-N-hydroxysuccinimidyl carbamate (AQC), which both produce fluorescent derivatives, and phenylisothiocyanate, which produces a phenylthiocarbamyl derivative that is detected by its absorbance at 254 nm. Analysis times can be as little as 20 min, and sensitivity is down to 1 pmole or less of amino acid.

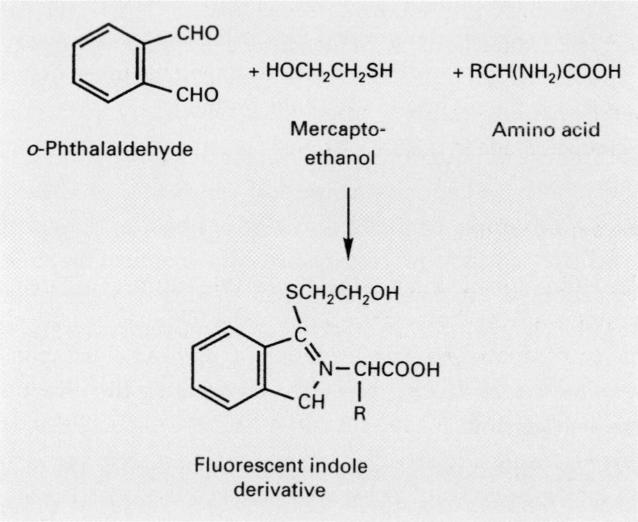

Fig. 6.3. The reaction of an amino acid with *o*-phthalaldehyde for pre- or postcolumn derivatisation.

6.4.3 **Primary structure determination**

For many years the amino acid sequence of a protein was determined from studies made on the purified protein alone. This in turn meant that sequence data available were limited to those proteins that could be purified in sufficiently large amounts. Knowledge of the complete primary structure of the protein was (and still is) a prerequisite for the determination of the three-dimensional structure of the protein, and hence an understanding of how that protein functions. However, nowadays the protein biochemist is normally satisfied with data from just a relatively short length of sequence either from the N terminus of the protein or from an internal sequence, obtained by sequencing peptides produced by cleavage of the native protein. The sequence data will then most likely be used for one of three purposes.

(i)   To search sequence databases to see whether the protein of interest has already been isolated, and hence can therefore be identified. For this type of search extremely short lengths of sequence (three to five residues), known as sequence tags, need to be used. An example of this type of data search is given in Section 12.3.5.

(ii) To search for sequence homology using computerised databases in order to identify the function of the protein. For example, the search may show significant sequence identity with the amino acid sequence of some known protein tyrosine kinases, strongly suggesting that the protein is also a tyrosine kinase. This can then be quickly confirmed by an assay in the laboratory.

(iii) The sequence will be used to design an oligonucleotide probe for selecting appropriate clones from complementary DNA libraries. In this way the DNA coding for the protein can be isolated and the DNA sequence, and hence the protein sequence, determined. Obtaining a protein sequence in this way is far less laborious and time-consuming than having to determine the total protein sequence by analysis of the protein.

A further use of protein sequence data is in quality control in the biopharmaceutical industry. Many pharmaceutical companies produce products that are proteins, for example peptide hormones, antibodies, therapeutic enzymes, etc., and synthetic peptides also require analysis to confirm their identities. Sequence analysis, especially to determine sites and nature of postsynthetic modifications such as glycosylation, is necessary to confirm the structural integrity of these products.

Edman degradation

In 1950, Per Edman published a chemical method for the stepwise removal of amino acid residues from the N terminus of a peptide or protein. This series of reactions has come to be known as the Edman degradation, and the method remains, 50 years after its introduction, the most effective chemical means for removing amino acid residues in a stepwise fashion from a polypeptide chain. The reactions comprise three stages (see Fig. 6.4).

(i) *The coupling reaction.* In this step phenylisothiocyanate (PITC) reacts with the amino group to give the phenylthiocarbamyl (PTC) derivative of the peptide. The reaction is carried out in an inert atmosphere (argon) to avoid oxidation of the sulphur atom in PITC. Following the reaction, the PTC derivative is washed thoroughly with an organic solvent (e.g. benzene) to extract excess PITC and side products, and then dried under vacuum.

(ii) *The cleavage reaction.* In this step, the dried PTC derivative is treated with an anhydrous acid (e.g. heptafluorobutyric acid). This results in the cleavage of the PTC-polypeptide at the peptide bond nearest to the PTC substituent thus releasing the original N-terminal amino acid residue as the 2-anilino-5-thiazolinone derivative, leaving the original polypeptide chain less its N-terminal amino acid residue. Following the cleavage reaction, the anhydrous acid is removed under vacuum and the thiazolinone derivative extracted from the remaining peptide with an organic solvent and recovered by evaporation of the organic solvent.

(iii) *The conversion reaction.* Since the thiazolinone is a derivative of the N-terminal amino acid, it could, in principle, be used for identification of that amino acid. However, in practice this is not done, since thiazolinones are relatively unstable. A more stable derivative is obtained by heating the thiazolinone in 1 M HCl at 80 °C for 10 min to convert it to the more stable, isomeric 3-phenyl-2-thiohydantoin (PTH) derivative. This PTH-amino acid is therefore the end-product of one cycle of the Edman degradation and can be easily identified by reversed-phase (RP) HPLC. Thus, if PTH-alanine is identified, we know that the first amino acid residue in the protein was alanine. The remaining polypeptide chain may now be subjected to further

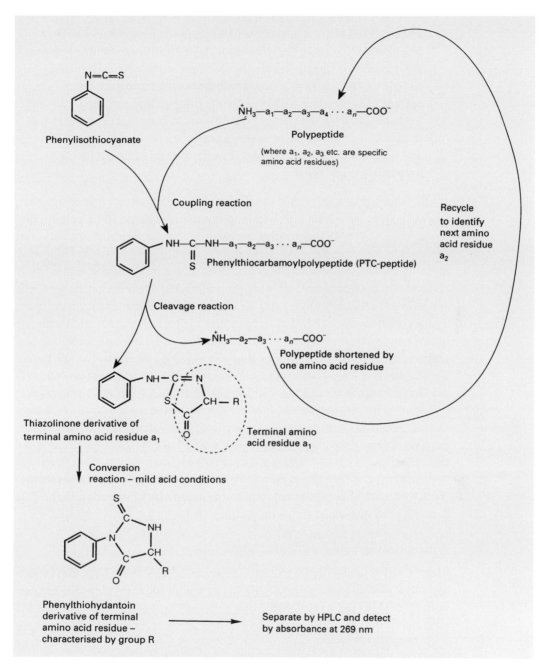

Fig. 6.4. Edman degradation for sequencing of amino acid residues (a, to a_n) in a polypeptide. Each cycle releases the N-terminal amino acid residue as a phenylthiohydantoin derivative, which is then identified chromatographically against reference compounds.

cycles of Edman degradation. At the end of each cycle, a PTH-amino acid is recovered and identified. In this way the amino acid sequence of a polypeptide chain may be determined. Theoretically one should be able to apply a series of Edman degradation reactions to a protein and obtain a complete sequence. In practice this is not possible, since the Edman degradation gives only a 96% to 98% repetitive yield at each step. Thus after a number of cycles, the yield of PTH-amino acid drops and the background level of PTH-amino acids increases. However, sequences of 20 to 40 amino acid residues are not uncommon and are frequently sufficient for the purposes outlined above.

The Edman degradation is invariably carried out in an automated analyser, where all steps, including injection onto the reversed-phase HPLC column and identification of the PTH derivative, are carried out automatically. Analysers can therefore be loaded and run overnight and data obtained first thing the following morning. Protein samples in solution are dried onto a small glass fibre disc that is inserted into the reaction chamber of the machine. This ensures that the protein is spread over a very large surface area (i.e. over every glass thread that goes to make up the glass fibre disc). Therefore, even though the protein is denatured by the rigorous chemical treatments of the Edman degradation, the insoluble protein is precipitated as an extremely thin film, thus allowing high reactivity at each step of the Edman cycle. Even proteins that have been blotted onto membranes from gels can be sequenced in the machine. Following blotting (e.g. from a two-dimensional gel), the protein spot of interest can be cut out and placed in the reaction cartridge. In this case it is necessary to use a particulary resistant form of membrane, poly(vinylidene difluoride) (PVDF), since normal nitrocellular membranes are unstable to many of the reagents involved in the Edman degradation. Nowadays sequence data can be obtained from as little as 10 to 100 ng of protein, the sensitivity of this method being limited only by the sensitivity of detection of the PTH derivatives by ultraviolet absorbance during HPLC.

Protein cleavage and peptide production

Clearly the Edman method determines the amino acid sequence from the N terminus of the protein and requires a free amino group at the N terminus for reaction with PITC. However, it is estimated that 50% to 70% of all proteins have their N terminal amino group blocked (e.g. by a formyl, acetyl or acyl group). For such proteins determining an N-terminal amino acid sequence is not possible, so they have to be cleaved to produce peptides, one or more of which can be purified and sequenced to give details of a region from within the protein. (For the reasons described above for requiring protein sequence data, it is usually immaterial whether the sequence comes from the N terminus or from within the protein.) Peptides can be produced by either chemical or enzymic cleavage of the native protein (see Table 6.5). Chemical methods include the use of cyanogen bromide, which cleaves at methionine residues, and *N*-bromosuccinimide that cleaves at tryptophan residues. Methione is a relatively rare amino acid in proteins, and tryp-

Table 6.5   Specific cleavage of polypeptide

Reagent	Specificity
Enzymic cleavage	
Chymotrypsin	C-terminal side of hydrophobic amino acid residues, e.g. Phe, Try, Tyr, Leu
Endoproteinase Arg-C	C-terminal side of arginine
Endoproteinase Asp-N	Peptide bonds N-terminal to aspartate or cysteine residues
Trypsin	C-terminal side of arginine and lysine residues but Arg-Pro and Lys-Pro poorly cleaved
Endoproteinase Glu-C	C-terminal side of glutamate residues and some aspartate residues
Endoproteinase Lys-C	C-terminal side of lysine
Thermolysin	N-terminal side of hydrophobic amino acid residues excluding Trp
Chemical cleavage	
BNPS skatole	
N-Bromosuccinimide	} C-terminal side of tryptophan residues
o-Iodosobenzoate	
Cyanogen bromide	C-terminal side of methionine residues
Hydroxylamine	Asparagine–glycine bonds
2-Nitro-5-thiocyanobenzoate	N-terminal side of cysteine residues

tophan even rarer, so these methods tend to produce large peptides. Enzymic methods include the use of trypsin, which cleaves C-terminal to arginine and lysine residues, endoproteinase Arg-C, which cleaves C-terminal to arginine only, and endoproteinase Glu-C, which cleaves C-terminal to glutamate and some aspartate residues. Clearly it is useful to have the amino acid composition of the protein (Section 6.4.2) to help to decide which method to use; obviously it is better to cleave at an amino acid that is present at relatively low amounts, thus producing a small number of large peptides rather than a more complex mixture of smaller peptides. The peptide hydrolysate thus produced is then fractionated using RP-HPLC. It may seem a little odd to be separating peptides that invariably contain a large proportion of charged and polar groups using a method based on hydrophobicity. However, the standard conditions used to separate peptides mask the polar groups of peptides and give the peptides an overall hydrophobic characteristic. Peptides are frequently dissolved in 1% (V/V) trifluoroacetic acid prior to RP-HPLC. Under these acid conditions, carboxyl groups ($-COO^-$) in the peptide (from the C terminus and the side-chains of any Asp or Glu residues present) are protonated ($-COOH$) thus masking the charged nature of this group. Any positively charged groups (form the N-terminal amino group and the side-chains of Lys, His and Arg residues), can pair with the trifluoroacetyl group (CF_3COO^-), thus masking the positive charge and indeed now giving these groups hydrophobic character due to the hydrophobic trifluoroacetyl group. The overall appearance of the peptide under these conditions is therefore of a non-charged, hydrophobic molecule, with of course the side-chains of any hydrophobic residues present in the peptide (Leu, Tyr, Phe, etc.) also contributing to the peptide's hydrophobicity. All peptides then bind to a RP-HPLC column and can be sequentially eluted, in order of increasing hydrophobicity, by the application of a linear gradient of acetonitrile (methyl cyanide), which competes for the hydrophobic interaction between the peptide and the column material.

Mass spectrometry

Because of the absolute requirement to produce ions in the gas phase for the analysis of any sample by mass spectrometry (MS), for many years MS analysis was applicable only to small, non-polar molecules (< 500 M_r). However, recent developments in ionisation technology such as the introduction of fast atom bombardment (FAB), ESI and MALDI methods (see Chapter 11), now means that the analysis of large, charged molecules such as proteins and peptides can be achieved. Indeed, the analysis of proteins and peptides by MS is now becoming routine, particularly with the introduction of smaller (and cheaper) bench-top mass spectrometers. Although Edman degradation is still used routinely to obtain sequence data, mass spectrometry is increasingly being used, and in particular has the advantage that postsynthetic modifications (e.g. glycosylation, methylation, phosphorylation, etc.) can be accurately identified, which is not the case with Edman sequencing. Also, of course, proteins with blocked N-terminal residues can be sequenced directly by MS. When peptides are fragmented it is fortunate that the break occurs predominantly at the peptide bond (although it must be noted that other fragmentations, such as interval cleavages, secondary fragmentations, etc. do occur, thus complicating the mass spectrum). This means that the peptide fragments produced each differ sequentially by the mass of one amino acid residue. The amino acid sequence can thus be readily deduced. In particular, if side-chain modifications occur, these can also be observed due to the corresponding increase in mass difference. The use of FAB-MS to sequence a peptide is described more fully in Section 11.6.2. Tandem mass spectrometry (MS/MS or MS^2) is also increasingly being used to obtain sequence data. A digest of the protein (e.g. with trypsin) is separated by MS. The ion corresponding to one peptide is selected in the first analyser and collided with argon gas in a collision cell to generate fragment ions. The fragment ions thus generated are then separated, according to mass, in a second analyser, identified, and the sequence determined as described in Section 11.6.2.

A further method, ladder sequencing, has been developed, and combines the Edman chemistry with mass spectrometry. Edman sequencing is carried out using a mixture of PITC and phenylisocyanate (PIC) (at about 5% of the concentration of PITC). N-terminal amino groups that react with PIC are effectively blocked as they are not cleaved at the acid cleavage step. Consequently at each cycle, approximately 5% of the protein molecules are blocked. Thus, after 20 to 30 cycles of Edman degradation, a nested set of peptides is produced, each differing by the loss of one amino acid. Analysis of the mass of each of these polypeptides using ESI or

MALDI allows the determination of the molecular mass of each polypeptide and the difference in mass between each molecule identifies the lost amino acid residue.

Detection of disulphide linkages

For proteins that contain more than one cysteine residue it is important to determine whether, and if so how many, cysteine residues are joined by disulphide bridges. The most commonly used method involves the use of mass spectrometry. The native protein (i.e. with disulphide bridges intact) is cleaved with a proteolytic enzyme (e.g. trypsin) to produce a number of small peptides. The same experiment is also carried out on proteins treated with dithiothreitol (DTT) which reduces (cleaves) the disulphide bridges. MALDI spectra of the tryptic digest before and after reduction with DTT allows identification of disulphide-linked peptides. Linked peptides from the native protein will disappear from the spectrum of the reduced protein and reappear as *two* peptides of lower mass. Knowledge of the exact mass of each of the two peptides, and knowledge of the cleavage site of the enzyme used, will allow easy identification of the two peptides from the known protein sequence. Thus, if the mass of two disulphide-linked peptides is M, and this is reduced to two separate chains of masses A and B, respectively, then $A + B = M + 2$. The extra two mass units derive from the fact that reduction of the disulphide bond results in an increase of mass of $+ 1$ for both cysteine residues.

$$- S - S - \xrightarrow{2H} - SH + HS -$$

Hydrophobicity profile

Having determined the amino acid sequence of a protein, analysis of the distribution of hydrophobic groups along the linear sequence can be used in a predictive manner. This requires the products of a hydrophobicity profile for the protein, which graphs the average hydrophobicity per residue against the sequence number. Averaging is achieved by evaluating, using a predictive algorithm, the mean hydrophobicity within a moving window that is stepped along the sequence from each residue to the next. In this way, a graph comprising a series of curves is produced and reveals areas of minima and maxima in hydrophobicity along the linear polypeptide chain. For membrane proteins, such profiles allow the identification of potential membrane-spanning segments. For example, an analysis of a thylakoid membrane protein revealed seven general regions of the protein sequence that contained spans of 20 to 28 amino acid residues, each of which contained predominantly hydrophobic residues flanked on either side by hydrophilic residues. These regions represent the seven membrane-spanning helical regions of the protein.

For membrane proteins defining aqueous channels, hydrophilic residues are also present in the transmembrane section. Pores comprise amphipathic α-helices, the polar sides of which line the channel, whereas the hydrophobic sides interact with the membrane lipids. More advanced algorithms are used to detect these sequences, since such helices would not necessarily be revealed by simple hydrophobicity analysis.

6.4.4 Glycoproteins

Glycoproteins result from the covalent attachment of carbohydrate chains (glycans), both linear and branched in structure, to various sites on the polypeptide backbone of a protein. These post-translational modifications are carried out by cytoplasmic enzymes within the endoplasmic reticulum and Golgi apparatus. The amount of polysaccharide attached to a given glycoprotein can vary enormously, from as little as a few per cent to more than 60% by weight. Glycoproteins tend to be found in the serum and in cell membranes. The precise role played by the carbohydrate moiety of glycoproteins includes stabilisation of the protein structure, protection of the protein from degradation by proteases, control of protein half-life in blood, the physical maintenance of tissue structure and integrity, a role in cellular adhesion and cell–cell interaction, and as an important determinant in receptor-ligand binding.

Three major types of protein glycoconjugates exist:

(i)   N-linked;
(ii) O-linked;
(iii) glycosylphosphatidylinositol (GPI)-linked.

N-linked glycans are always linked to an asparagine residue side-chain (Fig. 6.5) at a consensus sequence Asn-X-Ser/Thr where X is any amino acid except proline. O-linked glycosylation occurs where carbohydrate is attached to the hydroxyl group of a serine or threonine residue (Fig. 6.5). However, there is no consensus sequence similar to that found for N-linked oligosaccharides. GPI membrane anchors are a more recently discovered modification of proteins. They are complex glycophospholipids that are covalently attached to a variety of externally expressed plasma membrane proteins. The role of this anchor is to provide a stable association of protein with the membrane lipid bilayer, and will not be discussed further here.

There is considerable interest in the determination of the structure of O- and N-linked oligosaccharides, since glycosylation can affect both the half-life and function of a protein. This is particularly important of course when producing therapeutic glycoproteins by recombinant methods as it is necessary to ensure that the correct carbohydrate structure is produced. It should be noted that prokaryotic cells do not produce glycoproteins, so cloned genes for glycoproteins need to be expressed in eukaryotic cells. The glycosylation of proteins is a complex subject. From one glycoprotein to another there are variations in the sites of glycosylation (e.g. only about 30% of consensus sequences for N-linked attachments are occupied by polysaccharide; the nature of the secondary structure at this position also seems to play a role in deciding whether glycosylation takes place), variations in the type of amino acid–carbohydrate bond, variations in the composition of the sugar chains, and variations in the particular carbohydrate sequences and linkages in each chain. There are eight monosaccharide units commonly found in

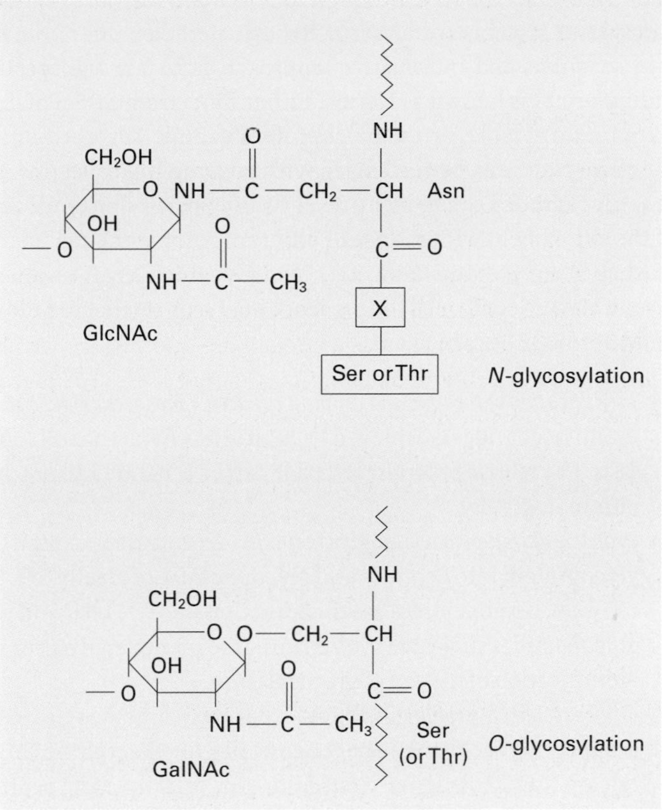

Fig. 6.5. The two types of oligosaccharide linkages found in glycoproteins.

mammalian glycoproteins, although other less common units are also known to occur. These eight are N-acetyl neuraminic acid (NeuNAc), N-glycolyl neuraminic acid (NeuGc), D-galactose (Gal), N-acetyl-D-glucosamine (GlcNac), N-acetyl-D-galactosamine (GalNAc), D-mannose (Man), L-fucose (Fuc) and D-xylose (Xyl). To further complicate the issue within any population of molecules in a purified glycoprotein there can be considerable heterogeneity in the carbohydrate structure (glycoforms). This can include some molecules showing increased branching of sugar side-chains, reduced chain length and further addition of single carbohydrate units to the same polypeptide chain. The complete determination of the glycosylation status of a molecule clearly requires considerable effort. However, the steps involved are fairly straightforward and the following therefore provides a generalised (and idealised) description of the overall procedures used.

The first question to be asked about a purified protein is 'Is it a glycoprotein?' Glycoprotein bands in gels (e.g. on SDS-polyacrylamide gels) can be stained with cationic dyes such as Alcian Blue, which bind to negatively charged glycosaminoglycan side-chains, or by the periodic acid–Schiff reagent (PAS), where carbohydrate is initially oxidised by periodic acid then subsequently stained with

Schiff's reagent. However, although they are both carbohydrate specific (i.e. non-glycosylated proteins are not stained) both methods suffer from low sensitivity. A more sensitive, and informative, approach is to use the specific carbohydrate binding proteins known as lectins. Either blots from SDS–PAGE, dot blots of the glycoprotein sample, or the glycoprotein sample adsorbed onto the walls of a microtitre plates can be challenged with enzyme-linked lectins. Lectins that bind to the glycoprotein can be identified by the associated enzymic activity. By repeating the experiment with a range of different lectins, one can not only confirm the presence of a glycoprotein but also identify which sugar residues are, or are not, present. Having confirmed the presence of glycoprotein the following procedures would normally be carried out.

(i) *Identification of the type and amount of each monosaccharide.* Release of monosaccharides is achieved by hydrolysis in methanolic HCl at 80 °C for 18 h. The released monosaccharide can be separated and quantified by gas chromatography.

(ii) *Protease digestion to release glycopeptide.* A protease is chosen that cleaves the glycoprotein into peptides and glycopeptides of ideally 5 to 15 amino acid residues. Glycopeptides are then fractionated by HPLC and purified glycopeptides subjected to N-terminal sequence analysis to allow identification of the site of glycosylation.

(iii) *Oligosaccharide profiling.* Oligosaccharide chains are released from the polypeptide backbone either chemically, for example by hydrazinolysis to release N-linked oligosaccharide, or enzymically using peptide-*N*-glucosidase F (PNGase F), which cleaves sugars at the asparagine link, or using endo-α-N-acetylgalactosaminidase (*O*-glycanase) which cleaves O-linked glycans. These released oligosaccharides can then be separated either by HPLC or by high performance anion exchange chromatography (HPAEC).

(iv) *Structure analysis of each purified oligosaccharide.* This requires the determination of the composition, sequence and nature of the linkages in each purified oligosaccharide. A detailed description is beyond the scope of this book, but would involve a mixture of complementary approaches including analysis by FAB–MS, gas chromatography–MS, lectin analysis following partial release of sugars and nuclear magnetic resonance (NMR) analysis.

6.4.5 **Tertiary structure**

The most commonly used method for determining protein three-dimensional structure is X-ray crystallography. A detailed description of the theory and methodology is beyond the scope of this book, requiring a detailed mathematical understanding of the process and computer analysis of the extensive data that is generated. The following is therefore a brief and idealised description of the overall process, and ignores the multitude of pitfalls and problems inherent in determining three-dimensional structures.

(i) Clearly the first step must be to produce a crystal of the protein (a crystal should be thought of as a three-dimensional lattice of molecules). Protein crystallisation is attempted using as homogeneous a preparation as possible, such preparations having a greater chance of yielding crystals than material that contains impurities. Because of our inadequate understanding of the physical processes involved in crystallisation, methods for growing protein crystals are generally empirical, but basically all involve varying the physical parameters that affect solubility of the protein – for example pH, ionic strength, temperature, presence of precipitating agents – to produce a state of supersaturation. The process involves extensive trial and error to find a procedure that results in crystals for a particular protein. Initially this involves a systematic screen of methods to identify those conditions that indicate crystallinity, followed by subsequent experiments that involve fine-tuning of these conditions. Basically, nucleation sites of crystal growth are formed by chance collisions of molecules forming molecular aggregates, and the probability that these aggregates will occur will be greater in a saturated solution. Clearly, to produce saturated solutions, tens of milligrams of proteins are required. This used to represent a considerable challenge for other than the most abundant proteins, but nowadays genetic engineering methodology allows the overproduction of most proteins from cloned genes almost on demand. The following are some of the methods that have proved successful.

(a) *Dialysis.* A state of supersaturation is achieved by dialysis of the protein solution against a solution containing a precipitant, or by a gradual change in pH or ionic strength. Because of frequent limitations on the amount of protein available, this approach often uses small volumes ($< 50\ \mu$l) for which a number of microdialysis techniques exist.

(b) *Vapour diffusion.* This process relies on controlled equilibration through the vapour phase to produce supersaturation in the sample. For example, in the hanging-drop method, a microdroplet (2 to 20 μl) of protein is deposited on a glass coverslip; then the coverslip is inverted and placed over a sealed reservoir containing a precipitant solution, with the droplet initially having a precipitant concentration lower than that in the reservoir. Vapour diffusion will then gradually increase the concentration of the protein solution. Because of the small volumes involved this method readily lends itself to screening large numbers of different conditions.

When produced, crystals may not be of sufficient size for analysis. In this case larger crystals can be obtained by using a small crystal to seed a supersaturated protein solution, which will result in a larger crystal.

(ii) Once prepared, the crystal (which is extremely fragile) is mounted inside a quartz or glass capillary tube, with a drop of either mother liquor (the solution from which it was crystallised) or a stabilising solution drawn into one end of the capillary tube to prevent the crystal from drying out. The tube is then sealed and the crystal exposed to a beam of X-rays. Since the

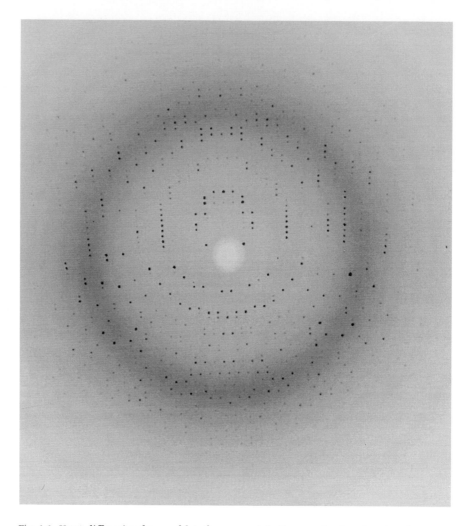

Fig. 6.6. X-ray diffraction frame of data from a crystal of herpes simplex virus type 1 thymidine kinase, complexed with substrate deoxythymidine, at 2 Å resolution. (Picture provided by John N. Champness, Matthew S. Bennett and Mark R. Sanderson of King's College London.)

wavelength of X-rays is comparable to the planar separation of atoms in a crystal lattice, the crystal can be considered to act as a three-dimensional grating. The X-rays are therefore diffracted, interfering both in-phase and out of phase to produce a diffraction pattern as shown in Fig. 6.6. Data collection technology necessary for recording the diffraction pattern is now highly sophisticated. Originally, conventional diffractometers and photographic film were used to detect diffracted X-rays. This involved wet developing of the film and subsequent digital scanning of the negative. Data collection by this method took many weeks. By contrast, modern area-detectors can collect data in under 24 h.

(iii) Unfortunately the diffraction pattern alone is insufficient to determine the crystal structure. Each diffraction maximum has both an amplitude and a phase associated with it, and both need to be determined. Unfortunately the phases are not directly measurable in a diffraction experiment and must be estimated from further experiments. This is usually done by the method of isomorphous replacement (MIR). The MIR method requires at least two further crystals of the protein (derivatives), each being crystallised in the presence of a different heavy-metal ion (e.g. Hg^{2+}, Cu^{2+}, Mn^{2+}). Comparison of the diffraction patterns from the crystalline protein and the crystalline heavy-metal atom derivative allows phases to be estimated. A more recent approach to producing a heavy-metal derivative is to clone the protein of interest into a methionine auxotroph, and then grow this strain in the presence of selenomethionine (a selenium-containing analogue of methionine). Selenomethionine is therefore incorporated into the protein in the place of methionine, and the final purified and crystallised protein has the selenium heavy metal conveniently included in its structure.

(iv) Diffraction data and phase information having been collected, these data are processed by computer to construct an electron density map. The known sequence of the protein is then fitted into the electron density map using computer graphics, to produce a three-dimensional model of the protein (Fig. 6.7.). In the past there had been concern that the three-dimensional structure determined from the rigid molecules found in a crystal may differ from the true, more flexible, structure found in free solution. These concerns have been effectively resolved by, for example, diffusing substrate into an enzyme crystal and showing that the substrate is converted into product by the crystalline enzyme (there is sufficient mother liquor within the crystal to maintain the substrate in solution). In a more recent development, it is now becoming possible to determine the solution structure of protein using NMR. At present the method is capable of determining the structure of a protein up to about 20 000 kDa but will no doubt be developed to study larger proteins. Although the time-consuming step of producing a crystal is obviated, the methodology and data analysis involved are at present no less time-consuming and complex as that for X-ray crystallography.

6.5 KEY TERMS

amino acid analysis	Dynomill	Gram negative
amphipathic α-helices	Edman degradation	Gram positive
bead mill	electron density map	homogenate
bicinchoninic acid method	extrinsic membrane proteins	Hughes Press
Biuret reaction	fibrous proteins	hydrophilic amino acid residues
Bradford method	fold purification	hydrophobic amino acid residues
cavitation	Folin–Ciocalteau reaction	hydrophobic interaction
cell disruption	French Press	hydrophobicity profile
denaturation	globular proteins	inclusion bodies
denaturation fractionation	glycoform	international unit
disulphide bridge	glycosylation	intrinsic membrane protein

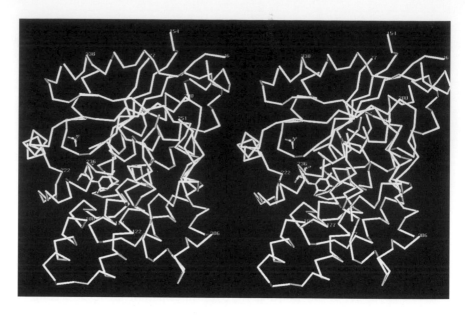

Fig. 6.7. (*Relaxed-eye stereo pair*): A Cα-trace of herpes simplex virus type 1 thymidine kinase from a crystallographic study of a complex of the enzyme with one of its substrates, deoxythymidine. The enzyme is an α–β protein, having a five-stranded parallel β-sheet surrounded by 14 α-helices. The active site, occupied by deoxythymidine, is a volume surrounded by four of the helices, the C-terminal edge of the β-sheet and a short 'flap' segment; a sulphate ion occupies the site of the β-phosphate of the absent co-substrate ATP. (Short missing regions of chain indicate where electron density calculated from the X-ray data could not be interpreted.) (Picture provided by John N. Champness, Matthew S. Bennett and Mark R. Sanderson of King's College London.)

isoelectric point	membrane proteins	secondary structure
isoelectric precipitation	*N*-linked glycosylation	sequence tags
fractionation	*O*-linked glycosylation	SI unit of enzyme activity
isoenzymes	organic solvent fractionation	signal sequence
isoionic point	peptide bond	sonication
isomorphous replacement	peripheral membrane protein	specific activity
isozymes	periplasmic space	tertiary structure
katal	plasma membrane	X-Press
Kjeldahl analysis	post-translational modification	X-ray crystallography
ladder sequencing	primary structure	yield
lipopolysaccharide	protein estimation	zwitterion
Lowry method	quaternary structure	
Manton–Gaulin Press	salt fractionation	

6.6 CALCULATIONS

Question 1 A series of dilutions of bovine serum albumin (BSA) was prepared and 0.1 cm³ of each solution subjected to a Bradford assay. The increase in absorbance at 595 nm relative to an appropriate blank was determined in each case, and the results are shown in the table opposite.

Concentration of BSA

(mg cm^{-3})	A_{595}
1.5	1.40
1.0	0.97
0.8	0.79
0.6	0.59
0.4	0.37
0.2	0.17

Plot a calibration graph of BSA concentration against A_{595}. A sample (0.1 cm^3) of a protein extract from *E. coli* gave an A_{595} of 0.84 in the same assay. Using the graph, determine the concentration of protein in the *E. coli* extract.

Answer   From the graph, the protein concentration of the *E. coli* extracted is 0.85 mg cm^{-3}.

Question 2   Note: In the following example all results are the mean of duplication measurements.
   A tissue homogenate was prepared from pig heart tissue as the first step in the preparation of the enzyme aspartate aminotransferase (AAT). Cell debris was removed by filtration and nucleic acids removed by treatment with polyethyleneimine, leaving a total extract (solution A) of 2 dm^3. A sample of this extract (50 μl) was added to 3 cm^3 of buffer in a 1 cm pathlength cuvette and the absorbance at 280 nm shown to be 1.7.

   (i) Determine the approximate protein concentration in the extract, and hence the total protein content of the extract.
   (ii) One unit of AAT enzyme activity is defined as the amount of enzyme in 3 cm^3 of substrate solution that causes an absorbance change at 260 nm of 0.1 min^{-1}. To determine enzyme activity, 100 μl of extract was added to 3 cm^3 of substrate solution and an absorbance change of 0.08 min^{-1} was recorded. Determine the number of units of AAT actively present per cm^3 of extract A, and hence the total number of enzyme units in the extract.
   (iii) The initial extract (solution A) was then subjected to ammonium sulphate fractionation. The fraction precipitating betweeen 50% and 70% saturation was collected and redissolved in 120 cm^3 of buffer (solution B). Solution B (5 μl (0.005 cm^3)) was added to 3 cm^3 of buffer and the absorbance at 280 nm determined to be 0.89 using a 1 cm pathlength cuvette. Determine the protein concentration, and hence total protein content, of solution B.
   (iv) Solution B 20 μl was used to assay for AAT activities and an absorbance change of 0.21 per min at 260 nm was recorded. Determine the number of AAT units cm^{-3} in solution B and hence the total number of enzyme units in solution B.
   (v) From your answers to (i) to (iv), determine the specific activity of AAT in both solutions A and B.
   (vi) From your answers to question (v), determine the fold purification achieved by the ammonium sulphate fractionation step.
   (vii) Finally, determine the yield of AAT following the ammonium sulphate fractionation step.

Answer

(i) Assuming the approximation that a 1 mg protein cm^{-3} solution has an absorbance of 1.0 at 280 nm using a 1 cm pathlength cell, then we can deduce that the protein concentration *in the cuvette* is approximately 1.7 mg cm^{-3}. Since 50 μl (0.05 cm^3) of the solution A was added to 3.0 cm^3 then the solution A sample had been diluted by a factor of 3.05/0.05 = 61.

Therefore the protein concentration of solution A is 61 × 1.7 mg cm^{-3} =~ 104 mg cm^{-3}. Since there is 2 dm^3 (2000 cm^3) of solution A, the *total* amount of protein in solution A is 2000 × 104 = 208 000 mg or 208 g.

(ii) Since one enzyme unit causes an absorbance change of 0.1 per minute, there was 0.08/0.1 = 0.8 enzyme units in the cuvette. These 0.8 enzyme units came from the 100 μl of solution A that was added to the cuvette.

Therefore in 100 μl of solution A there is 0.8 enzyme units.

Therefore in 1 cm^3 of solution A there is 8.0 enzyme units.

Since we have 2000 cm^3 of solution A there is a total of 2000 × 8.0 = 16 000 enzyme units in solution A.

(iii) Using the same approach as in question 2(i), the protein concentration of solution B is 3.005/0.005 × 0.89 = 601 × 0.89 = 535 mg cm^{-3}.

Therefore the total protein present in solution B = 120 × 535 = 64 200 mg.

(iv) Using the same approach as in question 2(ii), there are 0.21/0.1 = 2.1 units of enzyme activity in the cuvette. These units came from the 20 μl that was added to the cell.

Therefore, 20 μl (0.020 cm^3) of solution B contains 2.1 enzyme units. Thus, 1 cm^3 of solution B contains 1.0/0.02 × 2.1 = 105 units. Therefore, solution B has 105 units cm^{-3}.

Since there are 120 cm^3 of solution B, total units in solution B = 120 × 105 = 12 600.

(v) For solution A, specific activity = 16 000/208 000 = 0.077 units mg^{-1}.
For solution B, specific activity = 12 600/64 200 = 0.197 units mg^{-1}.

(vi) Fold purification = 0.197/0.077 = 2.6 (approx.).

(vii) Yield = (12 600/16 000) × 100% = 79%.

6.7 SUGGESTIONS FOR FURTHER READING

DEUTSCHER, M. (1990). *Guide to Protein Purification.* Academic Press Inc., London and New York. (An extensive volume providing detailed practical procedures for all aspects of protein purification.)

DOONAN, S. (1996). *Protein Purification Protocols.* Human Press, Totowa, NJ. (Detailed theory and practical procedures for a range of protein purification techniques.)

SCOPES, R. K. (1993). *Protein Purification – Principles and Practice* Springer-Verlag, Berlin, Heidelberg, New York. (Extensive theory and some practical detail for the range of protein purification techniques.)

SMITH, B. J. (1997). *Protein Sequencing Protocols.* Humana Press, Totowa, NJ. (Detailed laboratory protocols and relevant theory for all protein sequencing methodologies and related techniques such as amino acid analysis, peptide purification, analysis of disulphide bridges, mass spectrometry methods, etc.)

WILKINS, M. R., WILLIAMS, K. L., APPEL, R. D., and HOCHSTRASSER, D. F. (1997). *Proteome Research: New Frontiers in Functional Genomics.* Spinger-Verlag, Berlin, Heidelberg, New York. (Covers two-dimensional electrophoresis and all associated technologies involved in the characterisation of proteomes.)

Chapter 7

Biomolecular interactions: 1 Enzymes

7.1 RECEPTOR–LIGAND BINDING

The biochemical mechanisms underlying many physiological and pharmacological processes involve the initial binding of one molecule to another molecule. Most commonly, one molecule is a macromolecule such as protein or nucleic acid, generically referred to as the receptor, which possesses a specific site for the binding of the second molecule or ion, generically referred to as the ligand. The binding between the two species involves such non-covalent forces as van der Waals' forces, hydrogen bonds and electrostatic attractions. A characteristic of the binding is the high specificity displayed by the binding site, as a consequence of which only a very small number of structurally related molecules can act as the ligand. Frequently the initial recognition and binding of the ligand by the receptor is followed by a specific response, ranging from the metabolism of the ligand in cases where the receptor is an enzyme to the initiation of a cascade of biochemical reactions that result in such diverse responses as the mobilisation of glycogen as glucose 1-phosphate and the control of gene transcription and translation.

The example of receptor–ligand binding to be considered in this chapter is the binding of substrates and inhibitors to enzymes. The binding of ligands to cell surface receptors and transport proteins is discussed in Chapter 8. In all three cases, the binding of the ligand to the receptor can be quantified by a binding (or affinity or association) constant, K_a, or by the corresponding dissociation constant K_d or K_s, of the resulting receptor–ligand complex. Consideration is given here to the characteristics and importance of these and other constants and to the analytical techniques that may be used to study both the process and the mechanism of binding as well as the initiation of the subsequent response. Some studies with enzymes, receptors and transport proteins can be carried out on unpurified protein preparations, but studies using purified preparations, obtained and characterised using the techniques discussed in Chapter 6, are essential for unambiguous results. Our understanding of the factors that influence the affinity of biomolecular interactions such as those between enzymes, cellular receptors and transport proteins and their ligands is being advanced rapidly by the application of the newer techniques of gene cloning and site-directed mutagenesis, and the impact of the use of these techniques is emphasised in this chapter.

7.2 ENZYMES: CHARACTERISTICS AND NOMENCLATURE

Enzymes are single-chain or multiple-chain proteins that act as biological catalysts with the ability to promote specific chemical reactions under the mild conditions prevailing in most living organisms. Enzymes have three distinctive characteristics.

(i) *High specificity*: the ability to promote a particular chemical reaction on a single or a small number of structurally related substrates. Enzymes commonly exhibit stereospecificity and are able to distinguish between the optical and geometrical isomers of substrates.

(ii) *High reaction rate*: the ability to enhance the reaction rate by factors as high as 10^{12} relative to the non-enzyme-catalysed reaction. Enzymes facilitate the formation of the transition state from substrate to product, thereby lowering the activation energy for the process. They do not alter the position of equilibrium of a reversible reaction but accelerate the establishment of the equilibrium position.

(iii) *High capacity for regulation*: the ability to modify their catalytic activity in response to changing cellular and physiological demands. A range of regulatory mechanisms operate to allow short-, medium- and long-term changes in activity. Examples include feedback inhibition, reversible phosphorylation and gene induction and repression.

Enzymes reversibly bind their substrate at a specific binding site, generally known as the active site, created by the specific three-dimensional structure of the protein molecule. The resulting enzyme–substrate complex undergoes a catalytic reaction, promoted by specific amino acid residues in the active site, resulting in the formation of the product. The enzyme may contain separate regulatory or allosteric sites for the binding of other molecules, commonly distinct from the substrate in their molecular structure, and often key metabolites such as ATP and AMP, which, on binding to the allosteric site, alter the catalytic activity of the enzyme by inducing conformational changes in its active site. These regulatory molecules are termed effectors and may activate or inhibit the enzyme. The allosteric sites may be on either the same or different subunits of the enzyme as is the catalytic site. The catalytic properties of an enzyme are often dependent upon the presence of non-peptide molecules called cofactors or coenzymes which may be tightly bound to the polypeptide chain, in which case they are referred to as a prosthetic group. Examples of coenzymes include NAD^+, $NADP^+$, FMN and FAD, whilst examples of prosthetic groups include haem and oligosaccharides, and simple metal ions such as Mg^{2+}, Fe^{2+} and Zn^{2+}. An enzyme lacking its cofactor is termed the apoenzyme, and the active enzyme with its cofactor is the holo-enzyme.

By international convention, an enzyme is classified into one of six classes on the basis of the chemical reaction which it catalyses. Each class is divided into sub-classes according to the nature of the chemical group and coenzymes involved in the reaction. In accordance with the Enzyme Commission (EC) rules, each enzyme can be assigned a unique four-figure code and an unambiguous systematic name based upon the reaction catalysed. The six classes are:

Group 1: *oxidoreductases*, which transfer hydrogen atoms, oxygen atoms or electrons from one substrate to another.

Group 2: *transferases*, which transfer chemical groups between substrates.

Group 3: *hydrolases*, which catalyse hydrolytic reactions.

Group 4: *lyases*, which cleave substrates by reactions other than hydrolysis.

Group 5: *isomerases*, which interconvert isomers by intramolecular rearrangements.

Group 6: *synthases*, which catalyse covalent bond formation, with the concomitant breakdown of a nucleoside trisphosphate.

As an example, the enzyme alcohol dehydrogenase which catalyses the reaction

$$\text{alcohol} + \text{NAD}^+ \rightleftharpoons \text{aldehyde or ketone} + \text{NADH} + \text{H}^+$$

has the systematic name alcohol:NAD oxidoreductase and the classification number EC 1.1.1.1. The first 1 indicates that it is an oxidoreductase, the second 1 that it acts on a $CH - OH$ donor, the third 1 that NAD^+ or $NADP^+$ is the acceptor and the fourth 1 that it is the first enzyme named in the 1.1.1 subgroup.

The comprehensive study of an enzyme involves the investigation of its

molecular structure:	primary, secondary, tertiary and quaternary (Chapter 6);
protein properties:	pH and temperature stability, isoelectric point, electrophoretic mobility, relative molecular mass, spectroscopic properties;
catalytic activity:	specificity, kinetic constants, thermodynamic constants, catalytic mechanism, regulatory mechanism;
physiological function:	cellular location, integration into a metabolic pathway, metabolic flux.

For such studies, the enzyme generally has to be isolated in pure form and studied *in vitro*. The study of purified enzymes is fundamental to biochemistry because it generates data that allow the biochemist to understand and exploit the cellular situation *in vivo*. This exploitation extends to the design of selective inhibitors that can be used as drugs or biocides, to the industrial use of enzymes to promote specific chemical conversions, and to the use of enzymes in biosensors that are used to assay specific substrates.

7.3 ENZYME STEADY-STATE KINETICS

7.3.1 Measurement of initial rates

When an enzyme is mixed with an excess of substrate there is an initial short period of time (a few hundred microseconds) during which intermediates leading to the formation of the product gradually build up (see Fig. 7.14). This so-called pre-steady state requires special techniques for study and these are discussed in

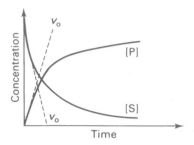

Fig. 7.1. Calculation of initital rate (v_o) from the time-dependent change in the concentration of substrate, [S], and product, [P], of an enzyme-catalysed reaction.

Section 7.6. After this initial state, the reaction rate and the concentration of inter-mediates change relatively slowly with time and so-called steady-state kinetics exist. Measurement of the progress of the reaction during this phase gives the rela-tionships shown in Fig. 7.1. Tangents drawn through the origin to the curves of substrate concentration and product concentration versus time allows the initial rate, v_o, to be calculated.

Measurement of the initial rate of an enzyme-catalysed reaction is fundamental to a complete understanding of the mechanism by which the enzyme works, as well as to the estimation of the activity of an enzyme in a biological sample. Its numerical value is influenced by many factors, including substrate and enzyme concentration, pH, temperature and the presence of activators or inhibitors. Each of these variables is discussed in the following sections.

7.3.2 Monosubstrate–enzyme reactions

For many enzymes, the initial rate, v_o, varies hyperbolically with substrate con-centration, [S], for a fixed concentration of enzyme (Fig. 7.2). At low substrate con-centrations the occupancy of the active sites on the enzyme molecules is low and the reaction rate is related directly to the number of sites occupied. This approxi-mates to first-order kinetics in that the rate is proportional to the substrate con-centration. At high substrate concentrations, effectively all of the active sites are occupied and the reaction becomes independent of the substrate concentration, since no more enzyme–substrate (ES) complex can be formed and zero-order or saturation kinetics are observed. Under these conditions the reaction rate is dependent upon the conversion of the ES complex to products and the diffusion of the products from the enzyme.

The mathematical equation expressing this hyperbolic relationship between initial rate and substrate concentration is known as the Michaelis–Menten equa-tion:

$$v_o = \frac{V_{max}\,[S]}{K_m + [S]} \tag{7.1}$$

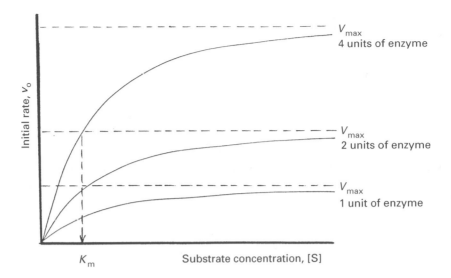

Fig. 7.2. The effect of substrate concentration on the initial rate of a simple enzyme-catalysed reaction in the presence of three different concentrations of enzyme. Doubling the enzyme concentration doubles the maximum initial velocity, V_{max}, but has no effect on K_m.

where V_{max} is the limiting value of the initial rate when all the active sites are occupied, and K_m is the Michaelis constant.

It can be seen from equation 7.1, that when $v_o = 0.5 V_{max}$, $K_m = [S]$. Thus K_m is numerically equal to the substrate concentration at which the initial rate is half of the maximum rate (Fig. 7.2) and has units of molarity. Values of K_m are usually in the range 10^{-2} to 10^{-5} M and are important because they enable the concentration of substrate required to saturate all of the active sites of the enzyme, in an enzyme assay, to be calculated. When $[S] \gg K_m$, equation 7.1 reduces to $v_o \approx V_{max}$, but a simple calculation reveals that when $[S] = 10 V_{max}$, v_o is only 90% V_{max} and that when $[S] = 100 K_m$, $v_o = 99\%$ V_{max}. Appreciation of this relationship is vital in enzyme assays.

As previously stated, enzyme-catalysed reactions proceed via the formation of an ES complex in which the substrate is non-covalently bound to the active site of the enzyme. The formation of this complex for the majority of enzymes is rapid and reversible and is characterised by the dissociation constant, K_s, of the complex:

$$\text{E} + \text{S} \underset{k_{-1}}{\overset{k_{+1}}{\rightleftharpoons}} \text{ES}$$

where k_{+1} and k_{-1} are first-order rate constants for the forward and reverse reactions, respectively.

At equilibrium, the rates of the forward and reverse reactions are equal and the Law of Mass Action can be applied to the reversible process:

$$k_{+1}[E][S] = k_{-1}[ES]$$

Hence, $K_S = \dfrac{[E][S]}{[ES]} = \dfrac{k_{-1}}{k_{+1}}$ (7.2)

It can be seen that when K_S is numerically large, the equilibrium is in favour of unbound E and S, i.e. non-binding, whilst where K_S is numerically small, the equilibrium is in favour of the formation of ES, i.e. binding. Thus K_S is inversely proportional to the affinity of the enzyme for its substrate.

The conversion of ES can be most simply represented by the irreversible equation

$$ES \xrightarrow{k_{+2}} E + P$$

where k_{+2} is the first-order rate constant for the reaction.

In some cases the conversion of ES to E and P may involve several stages and may not necessarily be essentially irreversible. The rate constant k_{+2} is generally smaller than both k_{+1} and k_{-1} and in some cases very much smaller. In general, therefore, the conversion of ES to products is the rate-limiting step such that the concentration of ES is essentially constant but not necessarily the equilibrium concentration. The Michaelis constant, K_m, is defined as

$$K_m = \frac{k_{+2} + k_{-1}}{k_{+1}} = K_S + \frac{k_{+2}}{k_{+1}}$$ (7.3)

It is evident that under these circumstances, K_m must be numerically larger than K_S and only when k_{+2} is very small do K_m and K_S approximately equal each other. The relationship between these two constants is further complicated by the fact that for some enzyme reactions two products are formed sequentially, each controlled by different rate constants:

$$E + S \xrightarrow{k_{+2}} ES \xrightarrow{k_{+3}} EA \longrightarrow E + P_2$$
$$\searrow$$
$$P_1$$

where P_1 and P_2 are products, and A is a metabolic product of S that is further metabolised to P_2.

In such circumstances it can be shown that

$$K_m = K_S \left(\frac{k_{+3}}{k_{+2} + k_{+3}} \right)$$ (7.4)

so that K_m is numerically smaller than K_S. It is obvious therefore that care must be taken in the interpretation of the significance of K_m relative to K_S. Only when the complete reaction mechanism is known can the mathematical relationship between K_m and K_S be fully appreciated and any statement made about the relationship between K_m and the affinity of the enzyme for its substrate.

Whilst the Michaelis–Menten equation can be used to calculate K_m and V_{max}, its use is subject to error owing to the difficulty of experimentally measuring initial

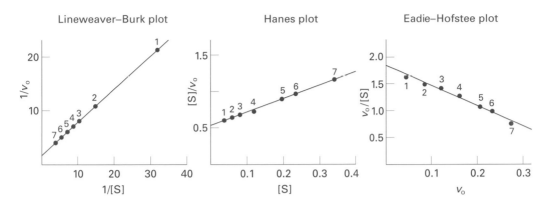

Fig. 7.3. Lineweaver–Burk, Hanes and Eadie–Hofstee linear plots for a set of experimental data of the effect of substrate concentration on the initial rate of an enzyme-catalysed reaction.

rates at high substrate concentrations and hence of extrapolating the hyperbolic curve to give an accurate value of V_{max}. Linear transformations of the Michaelis–Menten equation are therefore preferred. The most popular of these is the Lineweaver–Burk equation obtained by taking the reciprocal of the Michaelis–Menten equation:

$$\frac{1}{v_o} = \frac{K_m}{V_{max}} \times \frac{1}{[S]} + \frac{1}{V_{max}} \tag{7.5}$$

A plot of $1/v_o$ against $1/[S]$ gives a straight line of slope K_m/V_{max}, with an intercept on the $1/v_o$ axis of $1/V_{max}$ and an intercept on the $1/[S]$ axis of $-1/K_m$. Alternative plots are based on the Hanes equation:

$$\frac{[S]}{v_o} = \frac{K_m}{V_{max}} + \frac{[S]}{V_{max}} \tag{7.6}$$

and the Eadie–Hofstee equation:

$$v_o = V_{max} - K_m \times \frac{v_o}{[S]} \tag{7.7}$$

The relative merits of the Lineweaver–Burk, Hanes and Eadie–Hofstee equations for the determination of K_m and V_{max} are illustrated in Fig. 7.3, using the same set of experimental values of v_o for a series of substrate concentrations. It can be seen that the Lineweaver–Burk equation gives an unequal distribution of points and greater emphasis to the points at low substrate concentration that are subject to the greatest experimental error, whilst the Eadie–Hofstee equation and the Hanes equation give a better distribution of points. In the case of the Hanes plot, greater emphasis is placed on the experimental data at higher substrate concentrations and, on balance, it is the statistically preferred plot. It is important to appreciate that whilst K_m is a characteristic of an enzyme for its substrate and is independent of the

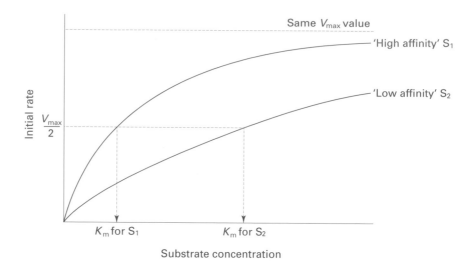

Fig. 7.4. The effect of the Michaelis constant on the kinetic profile of an enzyme acting on two different substrates. At low substrate concentrations the high affinity substrate will be the preferred substrate.

amount of enzyme used for its experimental determination, this is not true of V_{max}. It has no absolute value but varies with the amount of enzyme used. This is illustrated in Fig. 7.2. It is of course possible for two enzymes to have an affinity for the same substrate and, indeed, to have the same V_{max} value at a given enzyme concentration. If the two K_m values differ, however, the Michaelis–Menten plots will be different. This is shown in Fig. 7.4, which illustrates a key concept in the determination of the relative importance of branching in metabolic pathways. The same principle applies to the case where a given enzyme can act on two different substrates with different K_m values but the same or different V_{max} values. The reaction with the numerically smaller K_m value will be preferred at low substrate concentrations.

A valuable catalytic constant in addition to K_m and V_{max} is the turnover number, k_{cat}, defined as:

$$k_{cat} = \frac{V_{max}}{[E_t]} \tag{7.8}$$

where $[E_t]$ is the total concentration of enzyme. The turnover number is the maximum number of moles of substrate that can be converted to product per mole of enzyme in unit time. It has units of reciprocal time in seconds. Its values range from 1 to $10^7 \, s^{-1}$.

Catalase has a turnover number of $4 \times 10^7 \, s^{-1}$ and is one of the most efficient enzymes known. The catalytic potential of turnover numbers can be realised only at high (saturating) substrate concentrations and this is seldom achieved under normal cellular conditions. An alternative constant, termed the specificity constant, defined as being equal to k_{cat}/K_m, is a measure of how efficiently an enzyme converts substrate to product at low substrate concentrations. It has

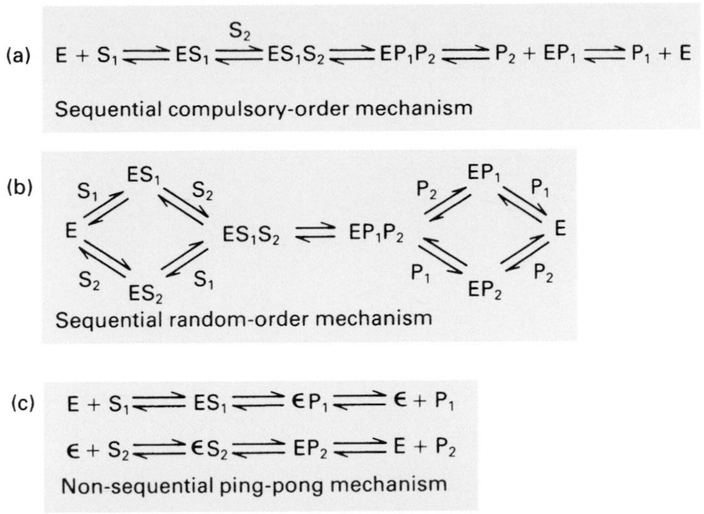

(a) $E + S_1 \rightleftharpoons ES_1 \overset{S_2}{\rightleftharpoons} ES_1S_2 \rightleftharpoons EP_1P_2 \rightleftharpoons P_2 + EP_1 \rightleftharpoons P_1 + E$

Sequential compulsory-order mechanism

(b)

Sequential random-order mechanism

(c) $E + S_1 \rightleftharpoons ES_1 \rightleftharpoons \varepsilon P_1 \rightleftharpoons \varepsilon + P_1$

$\varepsilon + S_2 \rightleftharpoons \varepsilon S_2 \rightleftharpoons EP_2 \rightleftharpoons E + P_2$

Non-sequential ping-pong mechanism

Fig. 7.5. Possible reaction mechanisms for bisubstrate reactions.

units of $M^{-1} s^{-1}$. For a substrate to be converted to product, molecules of the substrate and of the enzyme must first collide by random diffusion and then combine in the correct orientation. Diffusion and collision have a theoretical limiting value of about $10^9 \, M^{-1} s^{-1}$ and yet many enzymes, including acetylcholine esterase, carbonic anhydrase, catalase, β-lactamase and triosephosphate isomerase, have specificity constants approaching this value, indicating that they have evolved to almost maximum kinetic efficiency. Since specificity constants are a ratio of two other constants, enzymes with similar specificity constants can have widely differing K_m values. As an example, catalase has a specificity constant of $4 \times 10^7 \, M^{-1} s^{-1}$, with a K_m of 1.1 M (very high), whilst fumerase has a specificity constant of $3.6 \times 10^7 \, M^{-1} s^{-1}$, with a K_m of 2.5×10^{-5} M (very low). Multienzyme complexes, which are non-covalent associations of a number of enzymes that promote consecutive reactions in a metabolic pathway, overcome some of the diffusion and collision limitations to specificity constants. The product of one reaction is passed directly to the active site of the next enzyme in the pathway as a consequence of its juxtaposition in the complex, thereby eliminating diffusion limitations.

7.3.3 **Bisubstrate–enzyme reactions**

Bisubstrate reactions (Fig. 7.5) such as those catalysed by the transferases, kinases and dehydrogenases, in which two substrates S_1 and S_2 are converted to two products P_1 and P_2 (two-substrate, two-product, bi-bi, reactions), are inherently more complicated than monosubstrate reactions. They may be sequential, in which case both substrates bind at specific regions within the enzyme active site to give a ternary complex before the products are formed. Sequential reactions may be compulsory order, in which case the two substrates bind in a definite sequence, or

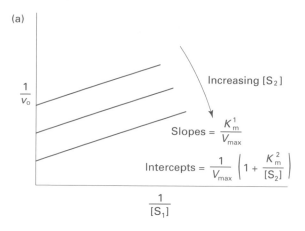

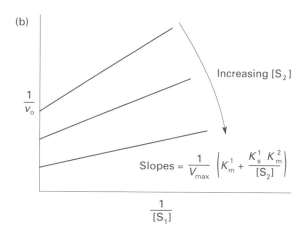

Fig. 7.6. Lineweaver–Burk plots for bisubstrate enzyme-catalysed reactions. (a) For a ping-pong bi-bi mechanism, a series of parallel plots is obtained. (b) For a random or ordered bi-bi mechanism a series of plots that converge to the left of the x-axis is obtained. K_m^1 and K_m^2 are the Michaelis constants for substrates S_1 and S_2, respectively. K_s^1 is the dissociation constant for ES_1.

random order, in which case either substrate can bind first. Alternatively the reaction may be non-sequential, in which case one product is released before the second substrate is bound. One example of this type of mechanism is a ping-pong reaction, which proceeds via a modified form of the enzyme (ϵ) which may take the form of an acylated enzyme. A ping-pong mechanism is indicated, but not confirmed, by a series of parallel lines in Lineweaver–Burk double reciprocal plots when the variation of initial rate with increasing concentrations of one substrate is investigated in the presence of a series of fixed concentrations of the second substrate. Double reciprocal plots give a progressively smaller intercept on the 1/[S] axis as the concentration of second substrate is increased (Fig. 7.6a). A

Table 7.1 **Patterns of product inhibition to distinguish sequential bisubstrate mechanism for the conversion of two substrates S_1 and S_2, to two products, P_1 and P_2**

Mechanism	Product	S_1 variable	S_2 variable
Ordered bi-bi {	P_1	Mixed	Mixed
	P_2	Competitive	Mixed
Random bi-bi {	P_1	Competitive	Competitive
	P_2	Competitive	Competitive

compulsory-order and a random-order ternary complex mechanism both give non-parallel double reciprocal plots with a progressively smaller intercept on the $1/v_0$ axis as the concentration of fixed second substrate is increased (Fig. 7.6b).

In these bisubstrate reactions, V_{max} is defined as the maximum initial rate when both substrates are saturating, and the K_m for a particular substrate as the concentration of that substrate which gives $0.5\,V_{max}$ when the other substrate is saturating. To determine these K_m values, the initial velocity is studied as a function of the concentration of one substrate at a series of fixed second-substrate concentrations. A double reciprocal plot is made for each second-substrate concentration, giving a series of straight lines called primary plots. A secondary plot is then made of the $1/V_0$ intercepts of the primary Lineweaver–Burk plots against the reciprocal of the second (fixed) substrate. This gives a straight line, slope K_m (for the second substrate)/V_{max} and intercept $1/V_{max}$. This study is then repeated reversing the roles of the two substrates. The principle of secondary plots is illustrated in Fig. 7.12.

The elucidation of the reaction mechanism associated with a particular bisubstrate reaction generally involves a study of the variation of the initial rate with the concentration of one substrate at a series of fixed concentrations of the second substrate, in the absence and presence of the two reaction products, and the application of a series of rules formulated by W. Cleland. Two of these rules are:

(i) the intercept on the $1/v_0$ axis of double reciprocal plots is affected only by an inhibitor that binds reversibly to an enzyme form other than that to which the variable substrate binds;

(ii) the slope of double reciprocal plots is affected by an inhibitor that binds to the same enzyme form as the variable substrate or to an enzyme form that is connected by a series of reversible steps to that to which the variable substrate binds.

The consequence of rule (i) is that, if characteristic competitive inhibition (Section 7.3.8) behaviour is observed, the inhibitor and the substrate whose concentration is being varied bind at the same site.

The consequence of rule (ii) is that, if characteristic uncompetitive inhibition (Section 7.3.8) is observed, there must be no reversible link between the inhibitor and the substrate whose concentration is being varied. The pattern for product inhibition for such studies with ordered and random bi-bi reactions is summarised in Table 7.1. Studies applying these rules have revealed, for example, that

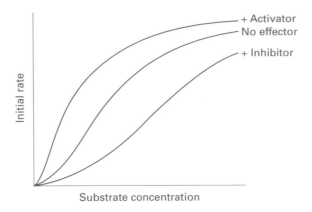

Fig. 7.7. Effect of activators and inhibitors on the sigmoidal kinetics of an enzyme subject to allosteric control.

histamine *N*-methyltransferase operates via a compulsory-order mechanism whereas phosphoglycerate mutase operates via a ping-pong mechanism involving a phosphoryl enzyme intermediate.

7.3.4 **Oligomeric enzyme reactions**

A number of enzymes contain several protein subunits, which may be identical or different, and are said to be oligomeric. They may contain multiple substrate-binding sites and some such enzymes do not display simple Michaelis–Menten kinetics, but give a sigmoidal relationship between initial rate and substrate concentration (Fig. 7.7). Such a curve is indicative of an allosteric enzyme, which is one whose molecular conformation changes as a result of the progressive binding of substrate molecules, a process referred to as a homotropic effect. This conformational change is initiated in one subunit but is transmitted to others. Binding of the substrate to the subunits is therefore said to be cooperative. This cooperativity may result in either increased (positive cooperativity) or decreased (negative cooperativity) activity towards the binding of further substrate molecules. Changes in activity towards the substrate may also be induced by the binding of molecules other than the substrate at distinct allosteric binding sites on one or more subunit. Compounds that induce such changes are referred to as heterotropic effectors. They are commonly key metabolic intermediates such as ATP, ADP, AMP and P_i, which, on binding to the allosteric site, change the conformation of the substrate-binding site. Heterotropic activators increase the reactivity of the enzyme, making the curve less sigmoidal and moving it to the left, whilst heterotropic inhibitors cause a decrease in activity, making the curve more sigmoidal and moving it to the right (Fig. 7.7). The diagnosis of cooperativity by use of the Lineweaver–Burk plot is shown in Fig. 7.11c. The operation of cooperative effects may be confirmed by a Hill plot, which is based on the equation:

$$\log\left(\frac{v_0}{V_{max} - v_0}\right) = h\log[S] + \log K \qquad (7.9)$$

where h is the Hill constant or coefficient, and K is an overall binding constant related to the individual binding constants for n sites by the expression $K = (K_{a1} \times K_{a2} \times \ldots \times K_{an})^{1/n}$.

The Hill constant, which is equal to the slope of the plot, is a measure of the cooperativity between the sites such that: if $h = 1$, binding is non-cooperative and normal Michaelis–Menten kinetics exist; if $h > 1$, binding is positively cooperative; and if $h < 1$, binding is negatively cooperative. At very low substrate concentrations that are insufficient to fill more than one site and at high concentrations at which most of the binding sites are occupied, the slopes of Hill plots tend to a value of 1. The Hill coefficient is therefore taken from the linear central portion of the plot. One of the problems with Hill plots is the difficulty of estimating V_{max} accurately.

It is sometimes argued that h is numerically equal to the number of binding sites, n, for the substrate. This is an oversimplification and very often h is not an integer, indicating incomplete cooperativity between the different binding sites. For example, h for the binding of oxygen to haemoglobin (for which the number of binding sites is known to be 4) is 2.6. In practice, h can be taken to be a minimum estimate of the number of interacting binding sites as well as a measure of the cooperativity.

An example of an enzyme displaying allosteric regulation is phosphofructokinase (PFK), the key regulatory enzyme of glycolysis:

PFK

fructose 6-phosphate + ATP $\rightleftharpoons$ fructose 1,6-bisphosphate + ADP

At low concentrations ATP is a substrate but at higher concentrations it acts as an allosteric inhibitor. The enzyme is also allosterically inhibited by citrate and phosphoenolpyruvate but allosterically activated by ADP, AMP and cyclic AMP. These effects are readily rationalised in terms of cellular energy demands and the associated need for the glycolytic pathway to be activated or inhibited.

The Michaelis constant, K_m, is not used with allosteric enzymes. Instead, the term $[S_{0.5}]$, which is the substrate concentration required to produce 50% saturation of the enzyme, is used. It is important to appreciate that sigmoidal kinetics do not confirm the operation of allosteric effects because sigmoidicity may be the consequence of the enzyme preparation containing more than one enzyme capable of acting on the substrate. It is easy to establish the presence of more than one enzyme as there will be a discrepancy between the amount of substrate consumed and the expected amount of product produced. It is equally important to appreciate that not all enzymes subject to allosteric control display sigmoidal kinetics. Some monomeric enzymes, for example wheat hexokinase, have been shown to be subject to such control but also to display simple Michaelis–Menten kinetics. Several models have been proposed to interpret allosteric regulation. They are all based on the assumption that the allosteric enzyme consists of a number of subunits (protomers), each of which can bind substrate and exist in two

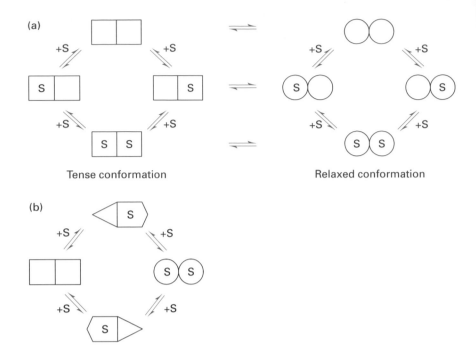

Fig. 7.8. Symmetry and sequential models of allosterism for a dimeric enzyme.
(a) Symmetry model for a dimeric enzyme. The enzyme is assumed to exist in two
conformations T and R, which differ in their affinity for substrate (represented by different
K_d values). Conformational changes within each subunit (protomer) are assumed to be
tightly coupled so that each can exist only in the same conformation. The binding of
substrate disturbs the equilibrium between the T and R states in favour of the R state. Note
that the model cannot explain how binding of a substrate molecule to one protomer
decreases the affinity of the other protomer for substrate (i.e. negative cooperativity).
(b) Sequential model for a dimeric enzyme. Ligand binding to one protomer induces a
change in its conformation and a cooperative interaction with the neighbouring protomer
such that its reactivity towards substrate binding may be either enhanced (positive
cooperativity) or decreased (negative cooperativity). Unlike the symmetry model, the
sequential model does not preserve the symmetry of the enzyme during substrate binding.

conformations referred to as the R (relaxed) and T (tense) states. It is assumed that
the substrate binds more tightly to the R form. One of the most successful models,
due to Jacques Monod, Jeffries Wyman and Jean-Pierre Changeux, is the symmetry
model. It assumes that conformational changes between the R and T states are
highly coupled so that all subunits must exist in the same conformation. Thus
binding of substrate to a T state protomer, causing it to change conformation to
the R state, will automatically switch the other protomers to the R form, thereby
enhancing reactivity (Fig. 7.8). The alternative induced-fit or sequential model of
Daniel Koshland does not assume the tightly coupled concept and hence allows
protomers to exist in different conformations but in such a way that binding to
one protomer enhances the reactivity of others. Conformational changes in a

protein can be studied by spectroscopic and sedimentation techniques but X-ray crystallography gives the most clear-cut evidence. The enzyme aspartate transcarbamylase has been shown by crystallography to display many of the characteristics of the symmetry model.

7.3.5 Effect of enzyme concentration on initial rate

It can be shown that for monosubstrate enzymic reactions that obey simple Michaelis–Menten kinetics

$$v_o = \frac{k_{+2}[E][S]}{k_m + [S]}$$

and hence that

$$v_o = \frac{k_{+2}[E]}{\dfrac{K_m}{[S]} + 1} \qquad (7.10)$$

When the substrate concentration is very large, equation 7.10 reduces to $v_o = k_{+2}[E]$, i.e. the initial rate is directly proportional to the enzyme concentration. This is the basis of the experimental determination of enzyme activity in a particular biological sample (Section 7.4). The importance of the correct measurement of initial rate is illustrated by Fig. 7.13.

7.3.6 Effect of temperature on initial rate and binding constant

The rate of an enzyme reaction varies with temperature according to the Arrhenius equation:

$$\text{rate} = Ae^{-E/RT} \qquad (7.11)$$

where A is a constant known as the pre-exponential factor, which is related to the frequency with which molecules of the enzyme and substrate collide in the correct orientation to produce the ES complex; E is the activation energy (in J mol^{-1}); R is the gas constant (8.2 J mol^{-1} K^{-1}); T is the absolute temperature (K). Thus a plot of the natural logarithm of the initial rate (or better, k_{cat}) against the reciprocal of the absolute temperature allows the value of E to be determined.

Equation 7.11 explains the sensitivity of enzyme reactions to temperature as the relationship between reaction rate and absolute temperature is exponential. The rate of most enzyme reactions approximately doubles for every 10 deg.C rise in temperature (Q_{10} value). At a temperature characteristic of the enzyme, and generally in the region 40 to 70 °C, the enzyme is denatured and enzyme activity is lost. The activity displayed in this temperature range depends partly upon the equilibration time before the reaction is commenced. The so-called optimum temperature, at which the enzyme appears to have maximum activity, is therefore time dependent and for this reason is not normally chosen for the study of enzyme activity. Enzyme assays are carried out routinely at 30 or 37 °C (Section 7.4).

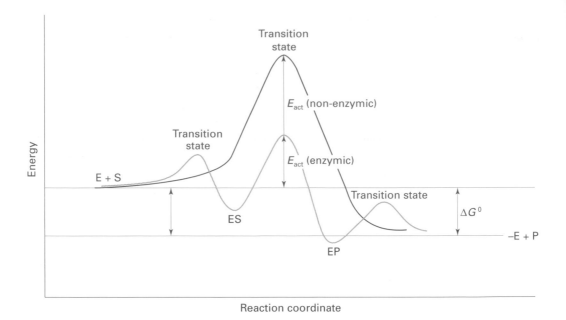

Fig. 7.9. Energy profile for a simple enzyme-catalysed reaction. The formation of ES and EP and subsequent release of E + P proceed via a transition state. The activation energy for the overall reaction is dictated by the initial free energy of E + S and the highest energy transition state (the formation of EP). The non-enzyme-catalysed reaction also proceeds via a transition state but of higher free energy and hence higher activation energy than the enzyme-catalysed reaction.

Enzymes work by facilitating the formation of the transition state and the associated distribution of charges, thereby decreasing the activation energy for the reaction relative to the non-enzyme catalysed reaction (Fig. 7.9). A decrease in the energy barrier of as little as 5.7 kJ mol^{-1}, equivalent in energy terms to a hydrogen bond, will result in a ten-fold increase in reaction rate. The energy barrier is, of course, lowered equally for both the forward and reverse reactions, so that the position of equilibrium is unchanged. As an extreme example of the efficiency of enzyme catalysis, the enzyme catalase decomposes hydrogen peroxide 10^{14} times faster than does the uncatalysed reaction! Figure 7.9 shows a simple energy profile for the conversion of a substrate to products as a function of the reaction coordinate which measures the time-related progress of the reaction. The number of energy barriers in the profile will depend upon the number of kinetically important stages in the reactions. For the majority of enzyme-catalysed reactions the major energy barrier, which dictates the activation energy for the reaction and hence its rate, is the formation of one or more transition states, in which covalent bonds are being made and broken and which, of course, cannot be isolated. An example is shown in Fig. 7.16. However, for a few enzymes, notably ATP synthase, the energy requiring step is the initial binding of the substrate(s) and the subsequent release of the product(s).

Proof that enzymes function by facilitating the creation of the transition state has come from the development of transition state analogues, which mimic the structure of the transition state. For example, the transition state for the esterase hydrolysis of carboxylic acids is a tetrahedral intermediate that is mimicked by a phosphonate ester with similar substituents (Fig. 7.10). If a monoclonal antibody is raised to an antigen consisting of the phosphonate ester as the hapten, one of the antibodies raised will be complementary to the tetrahedral phosphonate ester and will effectively behave as the active site of the esterase (Fig. 7.10). Proof of this ability was confirmed by the ability of the antibody to convert the ester to products in the absence of esterase at an enhanced rate (by factor of up to 10^5) relative to the uncatalysed reaction. The success of these studies lay in using the optimum structures for R and R′. Antibodies with this ability to promote catalysis have been called catalytic antibodies or simply abzymes or mabzymes. Abzyme counterparts of the glycolytic enzyme aldolase, which converts fructose 1,6-bisphosphate to glyceraldehyde 3-phosphate and dihydroxyacetone phosphate, have been produced using a 1,3-diketone hapten. Two abzymes were identified that mimicked aldolase in their display of Michaelis–Menten kinetics and catalytic rates but which had a specificity significantly broader than that of aldolase. This broader specificity has considerable potential in organic synthesis.

The thermodynamic constants ΔG^0, ΔH^0 and ΔS^0 for the binding of substrate to the enzyme can be calculated from a knowledge of the binding constant, K_a ($=1/K_s$). ΔG^0 can be obtained from the equation

$$\Delta G^0 = -RT \ln K_a \tag{7.12}$$

If K_a is measured at two or more temperatures, a plot of $\ln K_a$ versus $1/T$, known as the van't Hoff plot, will give a straight line slope $-\Delta H^0/R$ with intercept on the y-axis of $\Delta S^0/R$, the relevant equation being

$$\ln K_a = \frac{\Delta S^0}{R} - \frac{\Delta H^0}{RT} \tag{7.13}$$

where ΔS^0 and ΔH^0 are the entropy and enthalpy changes, respectively.

7.3.7 **Effect of pH on initial rate**

The state of ionisation of amino acid residues in the active site of an enzyme is pH dependent. Since catalytic activity relies on a specific state of ionisation of these residues, enzyme activity is also pH dependent. As a consequence, a plot of $\log K_m$ and $\log V_{max}$ (or better, k_{cat}) against pH is either bell shaped (indicating two important ionisable amino acid residues in the active site), giving a narrow pH optimum, or it has a plateau (one important ionisable amino acid residue in the active site). In either case, the enzyme is generally studied at a pH at which its activity is maximal. By studying the variation of $\log K_m$ and $\log V_{max}$ with pH, it is possible to identify the pK_a values of key amino acid residues involved in the catalytic process (Section 7.7.3).

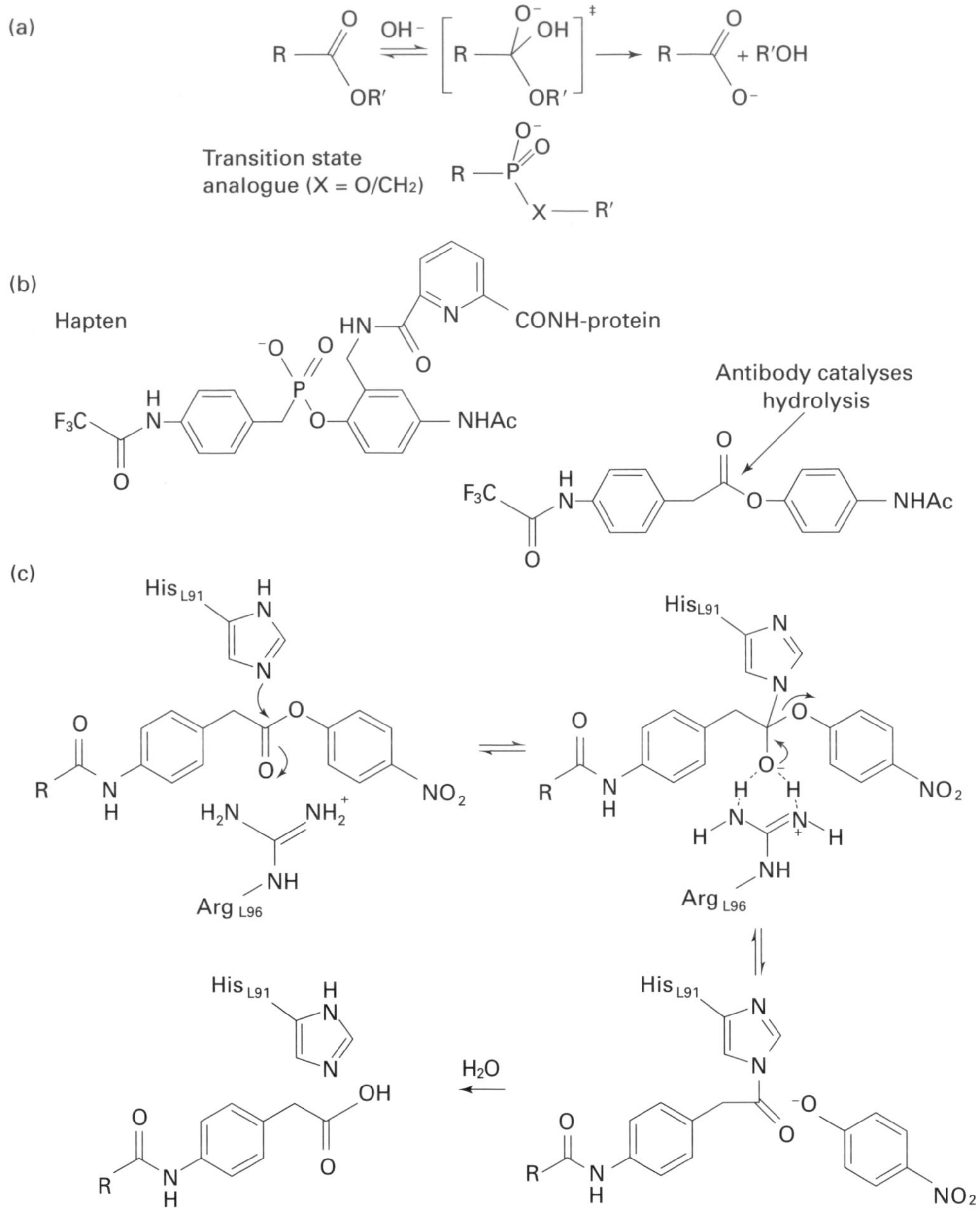

Fig. 7.10. Catalytic antibodies for ester hydrolysis. (a) The catalytic mechanism for ester hydrolysis involves a tetrahedral transition state. (b) The catalytic antibody is based on a hapten containing a tetrahedral organophosphorus compound resembling the ester transition state. The antibody raised against the hapten will contain a structural component complementary to the hapten and hence capable of binding an appropriate ester and facilitating the formation of the transition state. (c) The antibody 43C9 has been shown to promote ester hydrolysis by an acid–base mechanism similar in principle to that of ribonuclease A (Fig. 7.16). (Reproduced by permission of Blackwell Science Limited from Bugg, T. (1997) *An Introduction to Enzyme and Coenzyme Chemistry*, Blackwell Science, Oxford.)

7.3.8 **Enzyme inhibitors**

Enzyme inhibitors act as a ligand and bind specifically with an enzyme in such a way as to reduce its ability to bind substrate and convert it to product. Irreversible inhibitors, such as the organophosphorus and organomercury compounds, cyanide, carbon monoxide and hydrogen sulphide, combine by covalent forces and the extent of their inhibition is dependent upon their reaction rate constant (and hence time) and upon the amount of inhibitor present. The effect of irreversible inhibitors, which cannot be removed by simple physical techniques such as dialysis, is to reduce the amount of enzyme available for reaction. The inhibition involves reactions with a functional group such as hydroxyl or sulphydryl or with a metal atom in the active site or a distinct allosteric site. Thus the organophosphorus compound di-isopropylphosphofluoridate reacts with serine groups in the active site of esterses such as acetylcholinesterase, and the organomercury compound *p*-hydroxymercuribenzoate with cysteine groups, in both cases resulting in covalent bond formation and enzyme inhibition. Such inhibitors are valuable in the study of enzyme active sites (Section 7.7)

Reversible inhibitors combine non-covalently with the enzyme and can therefore be readily removed by dialysis. Competitive reversible inhibitors combine at the same site as the substrate and must therefore be structurally related to the substrate. An example is the inhibition of succinate dehydrogenase by malonate:

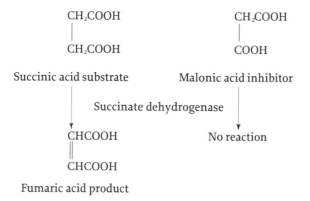

A non-competitive reversible inhibitor combines at a site distinct from that of the substrate but in such a way as to produce a dead-end complex, which cannot convert substrate to product. Uncompetitive reversible inhibitors can bind only to the ES complex and not to the free enzyme, so that inhibitor binding may be at a site created by the binding of the substrate to the active site (i.e. a conformational change occurs on substrate binding) or it may be bound to the substrate molecule. The resulting ternary complex, ESI, is also a dead-end complex. All types of reversible inhibitors are characterised by their dissociation constant K_i, called the inhibitor constant, which may relate to the dissociation of EI (K_{EI}) or of ESI (K_{ESI}).

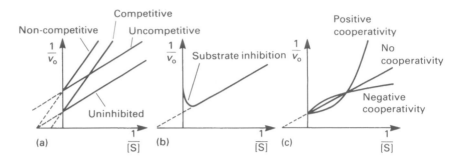

Fig. 7.11. Lineweaver–Burk plots showing (a) the effects of three types of reversible inhibitor, (b) substrate inhibition, and (c) homotropic cooperativity.

For competitive inhibition the following two equations can be written:

$$E + S \rightleftharpoons ES \rightarrow E + P$$
$$E + I \rightleftharpoons EI$$

Since the binding of both substrate and inhibitor involves the same site, the effect of a competitive reversible inhibitor can be overcome by increasing the substrate concentration. The result is that V_{max} is unaltered but the concentration of substrate required to achieve it is increased so that when $v_o = 0.5\, V_{max}$ then

$$[S] = K_m \left(1 + \frac{[I]}{K_i} \right) \tag{7.14}$$

where [I] is the concentration of inhibitor. It can be seen from this that K_i is equal to the concentration of inhibitor that apparently doubles the value of K_m. With this type of inhibition, K_i is equal to K_{EI} whilst K_{ESI} is infinite because no ESI is formed.

In the presence of a competitive inhibitor, the Lineweaver–Burk equation 7.5 becomes:

$$\frac{1}{v_o} = \frac{K_m}{V_{max}} \times \frac{1}{[S]} \left(1 + \frac{[I]}{K_i} \right) + \frac{1}{V_{max}} \tag{7.15}$$

allowing the diagnosis of competitive inhibition (Fig. 7.11a). The numerical value of K_i can be calculated from a Lineweaver–Burk plot for the uninhibited and inhibited reactions. In practice, however, a more accurate value is obtained from a secondary plot (Fig. 7.12). The reaction is carried out in the presence of a series of fixed inhibitor concentrations and a Lineweaver–Burk plot for each inhibitor concentration constructed. Secondary plots of the slope of the primary plot against the inhibitor concentration or of the apparent K_m, K'_m (which is equal to $K_m (1 + [I]/K_i)$ and which can be calculated from the reciprocal of the negative intercept on the I/[S] axis), against inhibitor concentration, will both have intercepts, on the inhibitor concentration axis, of $-K_i$. Sometimes it is possible for two molecules of inhibitor to bind at the active site. In these cases, although all the primary double reciprocal

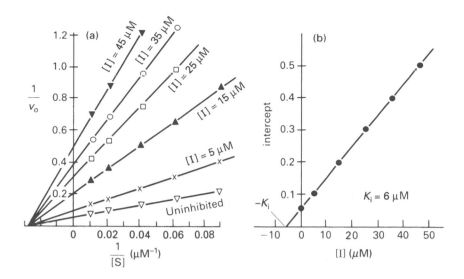

Fig. 7.12. (a) Primary Lineweaver–Burk plots showing the effect of a simple linear non-competitive inhibitor at a series of concentrations and (b) the corresponding secondary plot, which enables the inhibitor constant K_i to be calculated.

plots are linear, the secondary plot is parabolic. This is referred to as parabolic competitive inhibition to distinguish it from normal linear competitive inhibition.

For non-competitive inhibition the inhibitor may also bind to ES:

$$ES + I \rightleftharpoons ESI$$

Since this inhibition involves a site distinct from the active site, the inhibition cannot be overcome by increasing the substrate concentration. The consequence is that V_{max}, but not K_m, is reduced because the inhibitor and substrate do not affect the binding of each other. With this type of inhibition K_{EI} and K_{ESI} are identical and K_i is numerically equal to both of them.

The Lineweaver–Burk equation (7.5) therefore becomes:

$$\frac{1}{v_0} = \frac{K_m}{V_{max}} \times \frac{1}{[S]} + \frac{1}{V_{max}} \left(1 + \frac{[I]}{K_i} \right) \tag{7.16}$$

Once non-competitive inhibition has been diagnosed (Fig. 7.12a), the K_i value is best obtained from a secondary plot of either the slope of the primary plot or of $1/V'_{max}$ (which is equal to the intercept on the $1/v_0$ axis) against inhibitor concentration. Both secondary plots will have an intercept of $-K_i$ on the inhibitor concentration axis (Fig. 7.12).

For uncompetitive inhibition, the inhibitor binds only to ES:

$$E + S \rightleftharpoons ES \longrightarrow E + P$$
$$\quad\quad\quad {-1} \Big\updownarrow {+I}$$
$$\quad\quad\quad ESI$$

As with non-competitive inhibition, the effect cannot be overcome by increasing the substrate concentration, but in this case both K_m and V_{max} are reduced by a factor of $(1 + [I]/K_i)$. An inhibitor concentration equal to K_i will therefore halve the values of both K_m and V_{max}. With this type of inhibitor, K_{EI} is infinite because the inhibitor cannot bind to the free enzyme so K_i is equal to K_{ESI}. The Lineweaver–Burk equation (7.5) therefore becomes:

$$\frac{1}{v_0} = \left(\frac{K_m}{V_{max}} \times \frac{1}{[S]} + \frac{1}{V_{max}} \right) \left(1 + \frac{[I]}{K_i} \right) \tag{7.17}$$

The value of K_i is best obtained from a secondary plot of either $1/V'_{max}$ or $1/K'_m$ (which is equal to the intercept on the $1/[S]$ axis) against inhibitor concentration. Both secondary plots will have an intercept of $-K_i$ on the inhibitor concentration axis.

This classification of enzyme inhibition is not always straightforward or unambiguous. It is possible to observe competitive inhibition in cases where the inhibitor binds to a site other than the active site but in such a way that a conformational change follows the binding of the substrate, thereby preventing binding of the inhibitor. Equally, in some cases of bisubstrate reactions, an inhibitor may competitively inhibit the binding of one substrate and non-competitively inhibit the binding of the second (Section 7.3.3). It is also possible for an ESI complex to have some catalytic activity or for K_{EI} and K_{ESI} to be neither equal nor infinite, in which case so-called mixed inhibition kinetics are obtained. Mixed inhibition is characterised by a linear Lineweaver–Burk plot that does not fit any of the patterns shown in Fig. 7.11a. The plots for the uninhibited and inhibited reactions may intersect either above or below the $1/[S]$ axis. The associated K_i can be obtained from a secondary plot of the slope either of the primary plot or of $1/V_{max}$ for the primary plots against inhibitor concentration. In both cases the intercept on the inhibitor concentration axis is $-K_i$. Non-competitive inhibition may be regarded as a special case of mixed inhibition.

A number of enzymes at high substrate concentration display substrate inhibition, characterised by a decrease in initial rate with increased substrate concentration. The graphical diagnosis of this situation is shown in Fig. 7.12b. It is explicable in terms of the substrate acting as an uncompetitive inhibitor and forming a dead-end complex.

The study of enzyme inhibitors helps our understanding of the mechanisms by which enzymes work. Inhibitors are used widely in the study of metabolic pathways to help in the identification of intermediates. Much of the area of selective toxicity, including the use of antibiotics and insecticides, is based on the exploitation of species differences in susceptibility to enzyme inhibitors.

7.4 ENZYME ASSAYS

7.4.1 General considerations

Enzyme assays may be undertaken for a variety of reasons, but the two most common are, first, to determine the amount (or concentration) of enzyme present in a particular preparation and, secondly, to gain an insight into the kinetic characteristics of the reaction and hence to determine such constants as K_m, V_{max} and k_{cat}. Kinetic studies should be carried out with substrate concentrations ranging from 0.1 to 10 K_m. Enzyme assays should be carried out with excess substrate (at least 10 K_m). All studies should involve an appropriate control that is, in all respects, the same as the test assay but lacking either enzyme or substrate. Changes in the experimental parameter in the control lacking the test enzyme will give an assessment of the extent of the non-enzymic reaction whereas changes in the control lacking added substrate will evaluate any background reaction in the enzyme preparation. All reaction mixtures are incubated at the experimental temperature for at least 2 min before the reaction is started by the addition of either enzyme or substrate. It is worth while assaying the enzyme using different volumes of the test solution to confirm linearity between initial rate and enzyme concentration, thereby confirming the absence of activators or inhibitors in the preparation. Most assays are carried out at 30 °C but some are performed at 37 °C because of the physiological significance of the temperature. Adequate buffering capacity must be used and care should be taken to ensure that all apparatus is scrupulously clean. Analytical methods may be classified as either continuous (kinetic) or discontinuous (fixed time). Continuous methods monitor some property change (e.g. absorbance or gas volume) in the reaction mixture, whereas discontinuous methods require samples to be withdrawn from the reaction mixture and analysed by some convenient technique. The inherent greater accuracy of continuous methods commends them whenever they are available.

For simplicity, initial rates are sometimes determined experimentally on the basis of a single measurement of the amount of substrate consumed or product produced, rather than by the tangent method. This approach is valid over only the short period of time when the reaction is proceeding effectively at a constant rate. This linear section comprises at the most the first 10% of the total possible change and clearly the error is smaller the earlier the rate is measured. In such cases, the initial rate is proportional either to the reciprocal of the time to produce a fixed change (fixed-change assays) or to the amount of substrate reacted in a given time (fixed-time assays). The potential problem with fixed-time assays is illustrated in Fig. 7.13, which represents the effect of enzyme concentration on the progress of the reaction in the presence of a constant initial substrate concentration (Fig. 7.13a). Measurement of the rate of the reaction at time t_0 (by the tangent method) to give the true initial rate or at two fixed times, t_1 and t_2, gives the relationship between initial rate and enzyme concentration shown in Fig. 7.13b. It can be seen that only the tangent method gives the correct linear relationship. Since the correct determination of initial rate means that the observed changes in the concentrations of substrate or product are relatively small, it is inherently more accurate to measure the increase in product concentration because the relative increase in its concentration is significantly larger than the corresponding decrease in substrate concentration. Enzyme units are expressed in either Katals or International Units (Section 6.3.4).

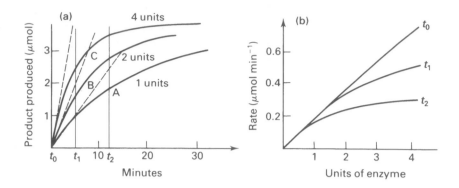

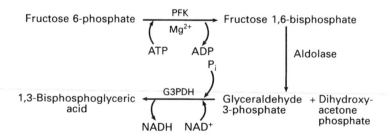

Fig. 7.13. The importance of measuring the initial rate in the assay of an enzyme. (a) Time-dependent variation in the concentration of product in the presence of 1, 2 and 4 units of enzyme; (b) variation of reaction rate with enzyme concentration using true initial rate (t_0) and two fixed times (t_1 and t_2).

7.4.2 **Spectrophotometric methods**

Visible and ultraviolet methods

Many substrates and products absorb light in the visible or ultraviolet region and, provided that the substrate and product do not absorb at the same wavelength and that the Beer–Lambert law (Section 9.4.1) holds, the change in absorbance can be used as the basis of the assays. Studies are best carried out in a double-beam recording instrument with a temperature-controlled cell housing.

A large number of assays are based on the interconversion of NAD^+ and NADH. Both the oxidised and reduced forms of these two nucleotides absorb at 260 nm but only the reduced form at 340 nm. Enzymes that do not directly involve this interconversion may be assayed by using the concept of coupled assays. In such reactions, the enzyme to be assayed is linked to one utilising the NAD^+/NADH system by means of common intermediates. The principle is illustrated by the assay of phosphofructokinase (PFK). It can be linked via aldolase to the glyceraldehyde-3-phosphate dehydrogenase (G3PDH) reaction:

The assay mixture would therefore contain fructose 6-phosphate, ATP, Mg^{2+}, aldolase, G3PDH, NAD^+ and P_i all in excess, so that the rate of NADH production, and hence increase in absorption at 340 nm wavelength, would be determined solely by the concentration of PFK in the known volume of preparation added to the assay mixture. In principle there is no limit to the number of reactions that can be coupled in this way, provided the enzyme under investigation is present in limiting amounts. The number of units of enzyme in the test preparation is calculated as follows:

$$\text{enzyme units (kat cm}^{-3}) = \frac{\Delta E_{340}}{\varepsilon} \times \frac{a}{1000} \times \frac{1000}{x} \tag{7.18}$$

where ΔE_{340} is the control-corrected change in absorption at 340 nm s^{-1}, a is the total volume of reaction mixture (generally about 3 cm^3) in a cuvette of 1 cm light path, x is the volume of test preparation included in the reaction mixture, and ϵ is the molar extinction coefficient for NADH (6.3×10^3 dm^3 mol^{-1} cm^{-1}). A general form of this equation is applicable to all spectrophotometric enzyme assays. In some cases the stoichiometry of the reaction (the number of molecules of compound undergoing the observed change in absorbance) is not unity, in which case a correction for the stoichiometry has to be introduced. The general equation is therefore:

$$\text{enzyme units} = \frac{\Delta E a}{\varepsilon d n} \tag{7.19}$$

where ε is the molar extinction coefficient of the chromophor, n is the stoichiometry, d is the light path in the cuvette (cm), and ΔE is the change in absorbance at experimental wavelength. By dividing equations 7.18 and 7.19 by C_p, the total concentration of protein in the enzyme preparation, the specific activity of the preparation can be calculated.

The scope of visible spectrophotometric enzyme assays can be extended by the use of artificial substrates and by the production of coloured derivatives of the substrate or product. Many enzymes, especially the hydrolases, will act on synthetic analogues of their natural substrate to release a coloured product such as p-nitrophenol and phenolphthalein. An example is the essay of α-glucosidase (maltase):

p-nitrophenyl-α-D-glucopyranoside D-glucose p-nitrophenol (yellow)

An extension of this approach is the use of synthetic dyes for the study of the oxidoreductases. The oxidised and reduced forms of these dyes are different colours. Examples are the tetrazolium dyes, methylene blue, 2,6-dichlorophenol indophenol and methyl and benzyl viologen. Their use, which is discussed fully in Section 15.3.2, depends upon them having an appropriate oxidation–reduction potential relative to that for the substrate.

Substrates or products containing certain functional groups can be converted to a coloured derivative. Examples are the orange dinitrophenylhydroazone derivatives of aldehydes and of ketones. Thus an assay of isocitrate lyase is based on this reaction:

$$
\begin{array}{c}
\underset{\substack{\text{Isocitric}\\\text{acid}}}{\begin{array}{l}\text{CH}_2\text{COOH}\\ |\\ \text{CHCOOH}\\ |\\ \text{HOCHCOOH}\end{array}} \xrightarrow[\text{lyase}]{\text{Isocitrate}} \underset{\substack{\text{Succinic}\\\text{acid}}}{\begin{array}{l}\text{CH}_2\text{COOH}\\ |\\ \text{CH}_2\text{COOH}\end{array}} + \underset{\substack{\text{Glyoxylic}\\\text{acid}}}{\begin{array}{l}\text{COOH}\\ |\\ \text{CHO}\end{array}}
\end{array}
$$

Glyoxylic acid → (Dinitrophenyl hydrazine) → Glyoxylate dinitrophenylhydrazone

Either samples of the reaction mixture are withdrawn periodically and reacted with dinitrophenylhydrazine or, for a fixed-time assay, the whole reaction mixture is reacted with the reagent at a pre-established time. In some cases it is possible to convert the product of an enzyme reaction to a coloured derivative *in situ* without interfering with the enzyme reaction itself. An example is glucose oxidase, whose product, hydrogen peroxide, can be used to oxidise *o*-dianisidine, incorporated into the assay mixture, to a yellow product.

Spectrofluorimetric methods

Although potentially very sensitive, fluorimetric enzyme assays have the practical limitation that trace impurities in the enzyme preparation can quench the emitted radiation (Section 9.5.2). Additionally, many fluorescent compounds are unstable, especially in the presence of ultraviolet light. Nevertheless, the technique is widely applied to enzyme assays. NAD(P)H is fluorescent so that many enzymes can be assayed by coupling to an appropriate reaction, as mentioned above. Equally, synthetic substrates are available that release fluorescent products. Examples include the use of 4-methylumbelliferyl-β-D-glucuronide for the assay of β-glucuronidase (Section 9.5.2).

Luminescence methods

The increasing popularity of bioluminescent reactions (Section 9.8.3), in which the intensity of emitted light is used to study enzyme reactions, is due to the high sensitivity of the technique. One of their problems is occasional lack of reproducibility. Firefly luciferase catalyses the oxidation of luciferin in an ATP-dependent reaction:

$$\text{luciferin} + \text{ATP} + \text{O}_2 \xrightarrow{\text{Luciferase}} \text{oxyluciferin} + \text{AMP} + \text{PP}_1 + \text{CO}_2 + \textit{light}$$

The reaction can be used to assay ATP and appropriate enzymes via coupled reactions. The corresponding bacterial luciferase uses reduced FMN to oxidise long-chain aliphatic aldehydes. The resulting FMN can be coupled to NAD(P)H, thus permitting the assay of many enzymes, e.g. malate dehydrogenase:

$$\text{malic acid} + NAD^+ \xrightarrow{\text{malate dehydrogenase}} \text{oxaloacetic acid} + NADH + H^+$$

$$NADH + H^+ + FMN \xrightarrow{\text{oxidoreductase}} FMNH_2 + NAD^+$$

$$FMNH_2 + RCHO + O_2 \xrightarrow{\text{luciferase}} FMN + RCOOH + H_2O + \textit{light}$$

The luminol/aminophthalic acid system involving microperoxidase can form the basis of the assay of many enzymes, including acetylcholinesterase (ACE) involved in synaptic transmission:

$$\text{acetylcholine} \xrightarrow{\text{ACE}} \text{acetic acid} + \text{choline}$$

$$\text{choline} + O_2 + H_2O \xrightarrow{\text{choline oxidase}} \text{betaine} + 2H_2O_2$$

$$H_2O_2 + \text{luminol} \xrightarrow{\text{microperoxidase}} \text{aminophthalic acid} + N_2 + \textit{light}$$

7.4.3 Radioisotope methods

Although potentially a very sensitive method, the use of radioisotopes (Section 14.6.2) in enzyme assays is restricted to applications where it is possible to separate easily the radiolabelled forms of substrate and product. In those cases where one of the products is a gas, this presents no problem. Thus the assay of glutamate decarboxylase could be based on the evolution of $^{14}CO_2$:

$$\underset{\text{glutamic acid}}{HOOCCH_2CH_2CH(NH_2)^{14}COOH} \xrightarrow{\text{glutamate decarboxylase}} {}^{14}CO_2 + \underset{\gamma\text{-aminobutyric acid}}{HOOCCH_2CH_2CH_2NH_2}$$

The $^{14}CO_2$ evolved could be trapped in alkali and hence the rate of $^{14}CO_2$ evolution measured. In other cases, the substrate and product may be separated by solvent extraction. Thus, in the assay of monoamine oxidase (MAO), samples of the assay mixture could be acidified (thereby converting the monoamine to its salt), the labelled aldehyde removed by ether extraction and the extract added to a sintillation cocktail for counting the radioactivity.

$$\underset{\text{monoamine}}{R^{14}CH_2NH_2} + O_2 + H_2O \xrightarrow{\text{MAO}} \underset{\text{aldehyde}}{R^{14}CHO} + H_2O_2 + NH_3$$

7.4.4 Manometric methods

Enzyme reactions resulting in the net evolution or uptake of a gas such as oxygen and carbon dioxide can be monitored by the Warburg manometer or the Gilson respirometer (Section 1.3.4). Both types of instrument can readily measure small changes in gas volume, provided the temperature is adequately controlled and that corrections are applied for the solubility of the gas in the reaction mixture. The versatility of the method can be extended to examples where one gas is evolved and another taken up, by chemically removing the evolved gas. In the case of CO_2 this would be by absorption in sodium hydroxide solution and in the case of O_2 by absorption by pyrogallol or chromous chloride solution. Enzymes that can be assayed manometrically include glutamate decarboxylase (see above), catalase, malic enzyme and monoamine oxidase (see above):

$$2H_2O_2 \xrightarrow{\text{catalase}} 2H_2O + O_2$$

$$CH_3COCOOH + CO_2 + NADPH + H^+ \xrightarrow[\text{enzyme}]{\text{malic}} HOOCCH(OH)CH_2COOH + NADP^+$$
pyruvic acid   malic acid

7.4.5 Other methods

Ion-selective and oxygen electrodes methods

The development of ion-selective electrodes (Section 15.5), such as those for the ammonium ion, and the oxygen electrode, has afforded attractive methods of enzyme assays. The methods are very sensitive, reproducible and can use very small volumes of reaction mixture.

Immunochemical methods

Polyclonal or monoclonal antibodies (Section 4.2.2) raised to a particular enzyme can be used as the basis for a highly specific ELISA-based assay for the enzyme (Section 4.2.1). Such systems can distinguish between isoenzymes, which, in the context of clinical measurements of enzyme activities, is of considerable diagnostic value. A monoclonal assay is available for serum prostatic acid phosphatase, which is one of the best means of diagnosing carcinoma of the prostate.

Microcalorimetric methods

Most biological reactions are accompanied by a minute change in heat (enthalpy) that gives rise to a temperature change of the order of 10^{-2} to 10^{-4} deg.C. Measurement of such small changes is possible using thermistors, which are temperature-sensitive metal oxides. The technique, which requires stringent insulation of the reaction vessel, may be improved by coupling the primary reaction to a secondary one which generates a larger heat evolution. Reactions releasing protons may be carried out in Tris buffer, which has a large enthalpy change on protonation:

$$\text{glucose} + \text{ATP} \xrightarrow{\text{hexokinase}} \text{glucose 6-phosphate} + \text{ADP} + H^+ \qquad \Delta H^\circ = -28\,\text{kJ mol}^{-1}$$

$$\text{Tris} + H^+ \longrightarrow \text{TrisH} \qquad \Delta H^\circ = -47\,\text{kJ mol}^{-1}$$

7.4.6 **Automated enzyme analysis**

Spectrophotometric methods are the most popular methods for enzyme assays and form the basis of many commercially available reaction rate analysers. These are instruments dedicated to the measurement of enzyme or substrate. Many are automated and based on fixed-change or fixed-time assays. Discrete analysers mix the enzyme and substrate by means of automatic pipettes according to a preprogrammed instruction. Continuous flow analysers pump the substrate continuously through a flow tube and periodically introduce a sample of the enzyme to be analysed into the line, each sample being separated from the next by a bubble. The reactants are mixed in a narrow mixing coil and pumped to the detector. The flow rate ensures that the reactants reach the detector at the correct time. An interesting variant is the fast (centrifugal) analyser. In it the enzyme and substrate are placed in separate wells located near the centre of a horizontal centrifuge plate (rotor) that can accommodate up to 30 separate samples. When the plate is rotated, the reactants are forced centrifugally into a cuvette at the edge of the plate, thus initiating the reaction. The change in absorbance at an appropriate wavelength in each cuvette is continuously recorded, enabling a good estimation to be made of the initial rate.

7.5 **SUBSTRATE ASSAYS**

Enzyme-based assays are very convenient methods for the estimation of the amount of substrates present in a biological sample. In theory, the principle of using excess enzyme and relating the substrate concentration to the observed initial rate could be used but in practice this is not popular because of the difficulty of measuring a rapidly decreasing reaction rate at low substrate concentrations. The procedures employed overcome this problem in a variety of ways but basically they are all variants of the so-called end-point technique. In this approach all of the substrate is converted to product and the total change in parameter (e.g. ultraviolet absorption) recorded. This change is then used to compute the amount of substrate originally present. The technique relies on the use of sufficient enzyme to ensure that the reaction goes to completion in a reasonable time. For reversible reactions it is necessary to adjust the position of equilibrium so that the reaction is effectively complete. This can be achieved by such means as adjusting the pH away from the optimum for the enzyme: in the case of bisubstrate reactions, by using a high concentration of the second substrate, or, in the case of reactions using $NAD(P)^+$, by using an analogue such as acetylpyridine adenine dinucleotide (APAD), which has a more favourable oxidation–reduction potential. Coupled reactions are commonly used in substrate assays. In all cases the substrate concentration should be very much smaller than the K_m and the amount of enzyme used should be adjusted so that that reaction is complete in 2 to 10 min. It can be shown that if the amount of enzyme is such that $V_{max}/K_m \approx 1$, then the reaction will be 99% complete in about 5 min. The detection limits for such assays are determined by the molar extinction coefficient of the compound being monitored. In the case of NAD(P)H, they are of the order of 10^{-2} to 10^{-3} μmol cm^{-3} in a 1 cm cuvette for ultraviolet spectrophotometric assays.

The sensitivity limits for substrate assays can be improved dramatically by the technique of enzymic cycling. The method, which is particularly valuable in those cases where the substrate is present in very low concentrations, involves the regeneration of substrate by means of a coupled reaction. The product accumulated in a given period of time (30 to 60 min) is then measured. A precalibration is necessary, using known amounts of the test substrate and with all the other components in the assay present in excess. The resulting 10^4 to 10^5-fold increase in sensitivity lowers the detection limits for visible and ultraviolet spectrophotometry to 10^{-6} to 10^{-8} μmol cm^{-3}. The method is commonly used for the assay of NAD(P)$^+$ and ATP/ADP. In the latter case, pyruvate kinase and phosphoenolpyruvate are used to regenerate ATP. In the case of NAD$^+$ or NADP$^+$, glutamate dehydrogenase may be used. For example in the assay of NADP$^+$, glucose-6-phosphate dehydrogenase (G6PDH) and glutamate dehydrogenase (GDH) may be coupled:

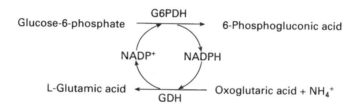

7.6 ENZYME PRE-STEADY-STATE KINETICS

7.6.1 Rapid mixing methods

The experimental techniques so far discussed for steady-state kinetics allow the determination of K_m and V_{max} values, but special techniques must be employed for the determination of the rate constants of the individual steps in the conversion of substrate to product, since the intermediates are transient. Figure 7.14 shows the progress curves in the initial stages of the conversion of substrate to product via ES. The induction period, t, is related to k_{+1}, and k_{+2}.

In the continuous flow method, solutions of the enzyme and substrate are introduced from syringes into a small mixing chamber (typically 100 mm^3 capacity) and then pumped at a preselected speed through a narrow tube to which is attached a light source and a photomultiplier or similar detector. Flow through the tube is fast (typically 10 m s^{-1}) so that it is turbulent, thus ensuring homogeneity of the solution. The precise reaction time, after mixing, at the point of observation can be calculated from the known flow of the two solutions. By varying these rates, the reaction time at the observation point can be varied, allowing the extent of reaction to be studied as a function of time. From these data, rate constants can be calculated. The technique, which requires relatively

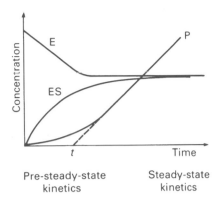

Fig. 7.14. Initial stage progress curve for the reaction $E + S \rightleftharpoons ES \rightarrow E + P$ when $[S] \gg [E]$.

large volumes of reactants, is limited only by the inherent time needed to mix the reactants.

The stopped flow method is a development of the continuous flow method in that, shortly after the reactants emerge from the mixing chamber, the flow is stopped. At this point the recorder is triggered and a continuous recording made of the change in experimental parameter (e.g. absorbance) (Fig. 7.15). The attraction of the method is its conservation of reactants. In both methods, the problem of studying the first few hundred microseconds of the reaction can be partially solved by altering the pH or temperature to slow down the reaction or by using alternative substrates with slower turnover times. The versatility of both the continuous flow and stopped flow techniques is increased by the use of synthetic substrates that either generate a chromophoric leaving group or give a chromophoric acyl or phosphoryl intermediate.

A variant of these rapid flow techniques is the quenching method. In this technique, the reactants from the mixing chamber enter a second chamber where they are mixed with a quenching agent such as trichloroacetic acid, which stops the reaction. The reaction products are then analysed by an appropriate analytical technique. By quenching after a range of reaction times, the progress of the reaction can be followed.

7.6.2 Relaxation methods

The great limitation of the rapid mixing methods is the dead time during which the enzyme and substrate are mixed. In the relaxation method, an equilibrium mixture of the reactants is performed and the position of equilibrium altered by a change in reaction conditions. The most common procedure for achieving this is the temperature jump technique in which the temperature is raised rapidly by 5 to 10 deg.C by the discharge of a capacitor or infrared laser. The rate at which the system adjusts to its new equilibrium (relaxation time τ) is inversely related to the first-order rate constants involved in the reaction sequence. The rate of return to

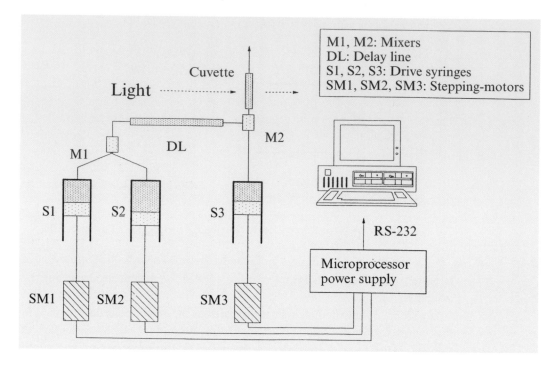

Fig. 7.15. The Bio-Logic stopped-flow apparatus. The reactions (up to three in this apparatus) are each placed in a syringe driven by a microprocessor-controlled stepping motor capable of delivering 0.05 to 6.00 cm^3 s^{-1}, with a minimum injection volume of 20 μl. The reactants from each syringe are premixed before they enter the reaction cuvette, with a deadline of 0.7 ms at 12 cm^3 s^{-1}. The flow can be stopped at any predetermined time, either by stopping the stepping motor or by closing the outlet from the reaction cuvette. The reaction can be studied by visible, ultraviolet, fluorescence or circular dichroism spectroscopy. (Reproduced by permission of BioLogic, France.)

equilibrium is studied by spectrophotometric techniques. It is often advantageous to use more than one such technique, for example ultraviolet absorbance and fluorimetry, since they may yield complementary information. Careful analysis of the total number of relaxation times gives an indication of the number of intermediates involved in the overall process as well as the value of the related rate constants.

Whilst relaxation techniques are best for studying the fastest processess, rapid flow techniques are frequently best for studying the processes involved in the catalytic steps. Rapid kinetic techniques have revealed that enzyme and substrate generally associate very rapidly, with first-order rate constants in the range 10^6 to 10^8 M^{-1} s^{-1}, and dissociate more slowly, with rate constants in the range 10 to 10^4 s^{-1}. The association process is generally slower than that predicted by simple collision theory and indicates the need for specific orientation of the substrate and enzyme, with perhaps conformational changes and the involvement of solvation processes.

7.7 ENZYME ACTIVE SITES AND CATALYTIC MECHANISMS

A complete understanding of the mechanism underlying the binding of a substrate to an enzyme active site and its subsequent catalytic conversion to products must include details of the nature of the binding and catalytic sites and the associated electronic and stereochemical events that result in the formation of the product. A wide range of strategies and analytical techniques has been adopted to gain such an understanding, and brief experimental details and the relative merits of each will now be considered.

7.7.1 X-ray crystallographic studies

This technique is capable of giving, either directly or indirectly, decisive information about the mechanism of enzyme action. It requires the enzyme to be purified and obtained in crystalline form – itself a difficult challenge (Section 6.4.5). X-ray diffraction patterns enable the position of each amino acid residue in the protein to be located and the details of how the substrate binds and undergoes reaction deduced. Such deductions are helped by studying the crystal structure of protein crystals grown in the presence and absence of the substrate, competitive inhibitor and perhaps of effector molecules. The limitation of the technique is that X-ray diffraction provides details of the enzyme in a static, stable state and yet proteins are known to be highly flexible and dynamic in solution. Fortunately, all the evidence to date confirms the validity of the X-ray data. Classic examples of the power of this approach come from studies of lysozyme, ribonuclease, hexokinase, a number of peptidases, phosphorylase and triosephosphate isomerase, all of which have revealed distinct binding clefts or pockets within the protein three-dimensional structure into which the substrate can fit and often induce a structural change or reorientation of specific amino acid residues to create the catalytic site. Such induced changes support the induced-fit theory of active sites rather than the earlier lock and key hypothesis, which visualised the binding site as being a permanent, integral feature of the enzyme. The juxtaposition of specific amino acid residues, within the induced site, to particular covalent bonds in the substrate molecule commonly favours the establishment of hydrogen bonding or electrostatic attractions between the enzyme and the substrate and the formation of the energetically favourable transition state required for reaction. Amino acid residues commonly found in active sites are therefore those with side-chains containing reactive groups, such as aspartic acid, glutamic acid, serine, cysteine, histidine, lysine and arginine.

7.7.2 Irreversible inhibitors and photoaffinity labels

Irreversible inhibitors act by forming a covalent bond with the enzyme (Section 7.3.8). By locating the site of the binding of the inhibitor, information can often be obtained about the identity of specific amino acids in the binding site. Thus cyanide inhibits transition-metal atoms that are important in some enzymes, whilst the organomercury compounds and iodoacetate react with sulphydryl groups of cysteine residues. The organophosphorus compounds, such as di-isopropylphosphofluoridate, are powerful inhibitors of acetylcholinesterase and serine proteases by virtue of the covalent bond they form with a serine hydroxyl group in the active site (Section 7.3.8). This specific labelling of amino acid residues in the active site can be exploited by using an analogue of the natural substrate containing a reactive group that will form a covalent bond with the enzyme. An example is the use of bromohydroxyacetone phosphate to inhibit triosephosphate isomerase.

$$
\begin{array}{c c c}
\mathrm{CH_2O\,PO_3^{2-}} & & \mathrm{CH_2O\,PO_3^{2-}} \\
| & & | \\
\mathrm{CO} & + \mathrm{Enzyme - OH} \rightleftharpoons & \mathrm{CO} \\
| & & | \\
\mathrm{CH_2Br} & & \mathrm{CH_2\text{-}O\text{-}Enz}
\end{array}
$$

3-bromohydroxy-acetone phosphate	triosephosphate isomerase	alkylated enzyme e.g. at a carboxyl group

A development of this approach is the use of photoaffinity labels, which structurally resemble the substrate but contain a functional group, such as azo, which on exposure to bright light is converted to a reactive functional group (e.g. a carbene or nitrene) that forms a covalent bond with a neighbouring functional group in the active site. It is common practice to tag the inhibitor or photoaffinity label with a radioisotope so that its location in the enzyme protein can be easily established experimentally.

$$
\mathrm{RCOCH} = \overset{+}{\mathrm{N}} = \overset{-}{\mathrm{N}} \xrightarrow[\;N_2\;]{\text{Light}} [\mathrm{RCOCH_2:}]^{\ddagger} \longrightarrow \mathrm{RCOCH_2} - \mathrm{Enz}
$$

diazoacetyl compound in which R resembles the natural substrate	carbene-reactive intermediate	inactivated enzyme due to formation of covalent link

7.7.3   Kinetic studies

Kinetic studies, using a range of substrates, carefully selected according to the specificity of the enzyme, and/or competitive inhibitors and the determination of the associated K_m, k_{cat}, and K_i values enables deductions to be made about the structural features of the ligand that facilitate binding and ability to act as a substrate. This in turn allows conclusions to be drawn about the structure of the active site. In the case of bisubstrate reactions, information about the reaction mechanism and substrate binding sequence can be deduced (Section 7.3.2). Further information about the structure of the active site can be gained by studying the influence of pH on the kinetic constants. Specifically, the effect of pH on K_m (i.e. on binding of E to S) and on V_{max} or k_{cat} (i.e. conversion of ES to products) is studied. Plots are then made of the variation of $\log K_m$ with pH and of $\log V_{max}$ or $\log k_{cat}$ with pH. The intersection of tangents drawn to the curves gives an indication of the pK_a values of ionisable groups involved in the active sites. These are then compared with the pK_a values of the ionisable groups known to be in proteins (Section 6.1). For example, pH sensitivity in the range 6 to 8 could reflect the importance of one or more imidazole side-chains of a histidine residue in the active site because of its known pK_a in this range.

7.7.4 Isotope-exchange studies

The replacement of the natural isotope of an atom in the substrate by a different isotope of the same element and the study of the impact of the isotope replacement on the observed rate of enzymic reaction and its associated stereoselectivity often enables deductions to be made about the mechanism of the reaction. Two examples illustrate the principle.

First, alcohol dehydrogenase (ALH), which oxidises ethanol to ethanal using NAD^+:

$$\underset{\text{ethanol}}{CH_3CH_2OH} \underset{NAD^+}{\overset{ALH}{\rightleftharpoons}} \underset{\text{ethanal}}{CH_3CHO} + NADH + H^+$$

The two hydrogen atoms on the methylene (CH_2) group of ethanol are indistinguishable, but if one was replaced by a deuterium or tritium atom they could be identified as either R or S configuration according to the Cahn–Ingold–Prelog rule for defining the stereochemistry of asymmetric centres. Studies have shown that alcohol dehydrogenase exclusively removes the hydrogen atom in the proR configuration, i.e. (R) CH_3CHDOH always loses the D isotope in its conversion to ethanal but (S) CH_3CHDOH retains it. Such a finding can be interpreted only in terms of the specific orientation of the ethanol molecule at the binding site such that the two hydrogens are effectively no longer equivalent.

Secondly, there is the hydrolysis of esters by esterases, which converts the ester to a mixture of acid and alcohol simultaneously incorporating a molecule of water into the products

$$\underset{\text{ester}}{\overset{O}{\overset{\|}{R\,C-O^*R'}}} + H_2O \xrightarrow{\text{esterase}} \underset{\text{acid}}{\overset{O}{\overset{\|}{R\,C-OH}}} + \underset{\text{alcohol}}{R'OH}$$

In this reaction the oxygen atom identified as O^* can be retained either in the acid or in the alcohol, depending on which side of the labelled oxygen atom the bond is broken, with water providing the second oxygen atom in the products. By labelling the oxygen atom in question with O^{18} and studying, by mass spectrometry, its fate after hydrolysis, details about the mechanism of the hydrolysis of the ester by the esterase can be elucidated. In practice, the labelled oxygen is found in the alcohol, which supports the view that the reaction mechanism involves initial attack by water, acting as a nucleophile, on the carbonyl carbon atom and the subsequent elimination of the RO* group.

7.7.5 Spectrophotometric studies

NMR (Section 10.4) and Raman spectroscopy (Section 10.2) have both been used to deduce information about enzyme active sites. In the case of NMR, studies are confined to relatively small enzymes such as ribonuclease A. This single-chain protein contains four histidine residues, two of which were implicated by pH/activity studies (Section 7.7.3) to be involved in enzymic activity, one being protonated and the other unprotonated. NMR studies were possible because the histidine protons give signals quite distinct from those of the mass of the other protons in the enzyme. Changes in NMR signal as a function of pH implicated the two histidine residues in positions 12 and 119. This deduction was confirmed by inhibition studies of ribonuclease A using iodoacetate. Iodoacetate does not normally chemically react with histidine but did react with two histidine residues in ribonuclease A, thereby simultaneously indicating that these two particular histidine residues were more reactive than normal. This was attributed to their being involved in hydrogen bonding within the active site thereby weakening their N — H bond and making it more reactive to the iodoacetate (Fig. 7.16).

7.7.6 Site-directed mutagenesis studies

Advances in molecular biology and particularly in the ability to clone genes and express them in a particular vector (Section 3.3) have opened up the possibility of producing variants of the enzyme in which a partiucular amino acid residue, thought to be involved in substrate binding and catalysis, is replaced by an other amino acid. By studying the impact of the replacement on the catalytic properties of the enzyme, conclusions can be drawn about the role of the amino acid residue that has been replaced. Thus, in the case of ribonuclease A discussed above, replacement of either His12 or His19 would have a deleterious effect on the catalytic properties of the enzyme. In principle it is also possible to produce variants that are more active than the native enzyme. Such studies are, of course, dependent upon the assumption that the impact of the single amino acid replacement is confined to the active site and has not affected other aspects of the enzyme's structure. This needs to be confirmed by complementary structural studies, for example spectroscopic techniques.

7.7.7 Ribonuclease A

RNase A is a small enzyme (molecular mass 13 680 daltons), consisting of only 124 amino acid residues including four histidine residues. It specifically hydrolyses RNA, cleaving a ribose phosphate ester bond attached to the ribose 5'-carbon, with pyrimidine (cytosine or uracil) attached to the ribose in position 1'. The process has been shown to proceed via a 2',3'-phosphate cyclic diester which can be

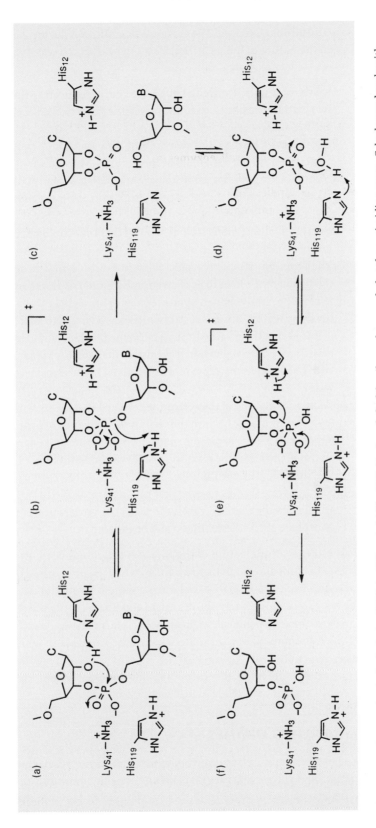

Fig. 7.16. Mechanism for the hydrolysis of RNA by RNase A. (a) The RNA lies in a cleft of the ribonuclease such that the pyrimidine group, C, hydrogen bonds with Thr45. His12, acting as a base, removes a proton from the hydroxyl group, and the oxygen atom, acting as a nucleophile, attacks the phosphate group. (b) The pentavalent phosphorus transition state is attacked by His119, acting as an acid, cleaving the P – O link to the adjacent ribose group to form a cyclic phosphate diester on the first ribose group. (c) The 5'-OH product leaves the site. (d) The cyclic phosphate diester is attacked by a molecule of water which donates a proton to His119, acting as a base. (e) The second pentavelent phosphorus transition state receives a proton from His12, acting as an acid, to give the final 3'-phosphate product shown in (f). (Reproduced by permission of Blackwell Science Limited from T. Bugg (1997) *An Introduction to Enzyme and Coenzyme Chemistry*, Blackwell Science, Oxford.)

isolated and characterised. The evidence that allowed the mechanism of hydrolysis and the nature of the transition states to be deduced was obtained by application of a variety of strategies:

pH-activity studies revealed a bell-shaped curve, indicating the involvement of two histidine residues, one protonated the other not, with pK_a values of 5.4 and 6.4, respectively.

NMR studies gave signals for two protons from two histidine residues displaced from the remainder of the proton NMR signals.

Affinity labelling studies using iodoacetate indicated the involvement of His12 and His119. Similar studies using fluorodinitrobenzene indicated the involvement of Lys41 and possibly Lys7.

Site-directed mutagenesis studies showed that Lys7 could be replaced without loss of activity.

Crystallographic studies revealed a cleft in the molecular structure into which the region of the RNA to be cleaved could bind. The His12 and His119 were in close proximity but on opposite sides of the cleft. Lys7, 41 and 66 were in the same region, as was Asp121, which was adjacent to His119. It was deduced that the positively charged lysine residues would interact with the negatively charged phosphate groups of the RNA backbone and that Asp121, with its negative charge, would be involved in the transfer of a proton from water.

Molecular modelling of the active site revealed that the pyrimidine group (cytosine or uracil) fits into the cleft in such a way as to form two hydrogen bonds with Thr45. Replacement of the pyrimidine by a purine (adenine or guanine) prohibits the formation of these bonds, thereby explaining the specificity for the pyrimidines.

Model substrate studies showed that the enzyme cleaved a $P - O$ ester bond attached to the ribose $5'$-carbon and that the process proceeded via a $2',3'$-phosphate cyclic diester that could be isolated.

This evidence of the nature of the RNase A action has been brought together to deduce the probable catalytic mechanism which is summarised in Fig. 7.16. It is an example of acid–base catalysis, which is common for hydrolase enzymes. Each of the two key histidines act as both an acid and a base during the reaction sequence. Confirmation of a pentavalent phosphoryl intermediate comes from the fact that RNase A is competitively inhibited by uridine vanadate in which the vanadium atom is pentavalent. The lack of a $2'$-hydroxyl group in DNA (containing $2'$-deoxyribose) prevents the formation of the pentavalent intermediates and thereby explains why RNase A does not hydrolyse DNA.

7.8   IMMOBILISED ENZYMES

Studies of immobilised enzymes, in which the enzyme is attached to an insoluble matrix, have shown that they display kinetic behaviour subtly different from that of free enzymes. The reasons for this are complex but involve the perturbation of the three-dimensional structure of the enzyme by the immobilising matrix and changes in the microenvironment of the active site of the immobilised enzyme. Kinetic studies of immobilised enzymes are valuable for our understanding of their action *in vivo*, especially their regulation, since there is evidence that, *in vivo*, enzymes may be less free to diffuse in solution than was originally thought (Section 7.9.3). Immobilised enzymes, however, are also important because of their considerable analytical and industrial potential. Industrially, solutions of enzymes are commonly used to carry out chemical transformations, for example in the synthesis of antibiotics and steroids, and are used increasingly in preference to the techniques of conventional organic chemistry. Enzymes offer the advantages of both chemical specificity and stereospecificity and accordingly give purer products. However, they are frequently unstable and difficult to recover from the reaction mixture. In principle, the ability to immobilise enzymes, pack them into columns and reuse them many times is commercially most attractive.

Enzymes can be immobilised in many ways, and these can be divided into two types, as described below.

7.8.1 Physical immobilisation

Physical immobilisation forms no covalent bonds between the enzyme and the supporting matrix. Adsorption of the enzyme onto animal charcoal or alumina was initially used to achieve immobilisation but current approaches include ionic adsorption onto ion-exchange resins, especially those of the Sephadex (Section 13.8.2) type, and controlled-pore glass. Immobilisation by adsorption has the advantages of simplicity, general applicability, high yield and ability to replace the enzyme when the catalytic activity of the immobilised enzyme has decreased below an acceptable level. A limitation of the technique is the need to control the working conditions for the use of the immobilised enzyme to prevent its desorption. Enzyme entrapment in liposomes (artificially produced concentric spheres of phospholipid bilayers) and in water-insoluble polymers such as polyacrylamide and agarose is also a simple and generally applicable method but the products suffer from poor flow properties, inefficiency and progressive leaching of the enzyme.

A recent advance in physical immobilisation is the production of protein monolayers on a glass surface. The technique involves the production of a protein monolayer in a Langmuir trough and the subsequent transfer of the layer to a glass surface.

7.8.2 Chemical immobilisation

Chemical immobilisation results in at least one covalent bond being formed between the enzyme and the matrix. The chemical procedures used to produce immobilisation are similar to those used in affinity chromatography (Section 13.9). Attachment must not involve amino acid residues in the active site of the enzyme otherwise activity would be lost. The matrix may be polysaccharide, polymers such as nylon, or inorganic carriers such as glass and titanium dioxide.

Immobilised enzymes are finding an increasing number of analytical applications, especially in clinical situations where they offer the potential for fast, sensitive and accurate determinations of analytes such as blood glucose and urea. The most significant development is the combination of immobilised enzymes, with their high specificity, and electroanalytical chemistry with its inherent sensitivity. The so-called enzyme electrode offers the opportunity for accurate analysis without any sample preparation. The principles involved in enzyme electrodes are discussed more fully in Chapter 15.

Another recent development has been the introduction of dry chemistry techniques for quantifying a wide range of enzymes, substrates and other analytes of clinical importance. The techniques involve the impregnation of the reagents, including the enzyme, into an immobile structure, very similar to a photographic film or plate. On adding a drop of the test sample, such as urine, to the slide, the analyte in the sample diffuses to the reagents and initiates an enzyme reaction that results in the production of a coloured product. The intensity of this colour is measured, generally by reflectance spectroscopy, after a predetermined reaction period. The principles of these assays are very similar to those discussed in Section 7.3, but the practice is such that measurements can be made, without access to the usual laboratory facilities, by scientifically unqualified staff. The technique is commonly used in hospitals for quick diagnostic tests for a wide range of analytes including glucose, urea, bilirubin and various diagnostic enzymes such as lactate dehydrogenase.

7.9　CELLULAR CONTROL OF METABOLIC ACTIVITY

7.9.1　Control of metabolic flux

A large proportion of the thousands of enzymes in a cell are involved in the promotion of coordinated chemical pathways such as glycolysis, the citric acid cycle and the biosynthesis of fatty acids and steroids. Each enzyme in a pathway proceeds at a characteristic rate determined by the free energy of activation for the formation of the transition state. Many enzymes in a pathway operate close to equilibrium and are found to operate with relatively small free energy barriers. The consequence is that such enzymes are readily able to accommodate small changes in the concentration of their reactants and/or products. The net rate of flow (flux) of reactants and products along pathways is controlled by a small number, commonly one or two, key regulatory enzymes. For example, in glycolysis only three of the ten enzymes, hexokinase, phosphofructokinase and pyruvate kinase, operate with large negative free energy changes away from equilibrium, and thereby control the overall flux along the pathway. Unlike the other seven enzymes, these three enzymes cannot readily accommodate changes in reactants and/or products since they are essentially saturated and only alteration in their inherent activity can change their rate. As discussed earlier (Section 7.3.4), phosphofructokinase is subject to allosteric control by a number of allosteric effectors that are related to the energy status of the cell. The overall flux through the glycolytic pathway is therefore determined by these rate-determining enzymes and the regulation of their activity.

Enzymes linked in a coordinated pathway are frequently clustered in one of three ways, namely by being located in the same compartment of the cell, or by being physically associated as a multienzyme complex such as that of the fatty acid synthase of *Escherichia coli*, or by being membrane-bound such as the enzymes of the electron transport chain. This clustering facilitates the transport of the product of one enzyme to the next enzyme in the pathway.

The study of these key regulatory enzymes has revealed that they commonly occupy either the first step in a pathway or a branchpoint in a pathway. First enzymes in an unbranched pathway are frequently regulated by end-product inhibition. Here, the final product of the pathway acts as an inhibitor of the first enzyme, thus switching off the whole pathway when the final product begins to accumulate. The inhibition of aspartate transcarbamylase by cytosine triphosphate (CTP) in the CTP biosynthetic pathway is an example of this form of regulation. In branched pathways, product inhibition usually operates on the first enzyme after the branchpoint. Enzymes controlling branchpoints are commonly oligomeric and subject to allosteric control. The greater sensitivity of sigmoidal kinetics, compared with simple Michaelis–Menten hyperbolic kinetics, to changes in substrate or effector concentration offers finer control than could be achieved with a monomeric enzyme.

The biochemical pathways operating in cells contain examples of anabolic and catabolic pathways directly opposing each other. The phosphorylase pathway for the conversion of glycogen to glucose 1-phosphate and the glycogen synthase pathway for the biosynthesis of glucogen from glucose phosphate are examples. The need for the effective control and coordination of pairs of such pathways is obvious. Such control is commonly exerted by the energy charge within the cell, which is defined as the effective mole fraction of ATP in the ATP + ADP + AMP pool. Anabolic and catabolic pathways respond in opposite directions to the prevailing energy charge. Control is greatest when the ATP/ADP ratio is far from equilibrium. Such non-equilibrium ratios can sometimes be established by the operation of substrate cycles. An example is the simultaneous operation of phosphofructokinase and fructose 1,6-bisphosphatase. The former converts fructose 6-phosphate to fructose 1,6-bisphosphate and simultaneously converts ATP to ADP; the latter converts fructose 1,6-bisphosphate to fructose 6-phosphate and inorganic phosphate. The net result is apparently only the hydrolysis of ATP but in fact the resulting displaced energy charge simultaneously stimulates a very large increase in flux through the glycolytic pathway. In the case of muscle, the operation of the cycle enables high activity to be maintained. Superimposed on these various forms of control of enzyme activity may be additional control by hormones, growth factors or neurotransmitters operating via cellular receptors. This is discussed in detail in Chapter 8.

7.9.2 Medium- and long-term control of enzyme activity

The forms of control of enzyme activity discussed so far are essentially short-term control in that they are exerted more or less instantly. The control involves modifications to the enzyme active site by the binding of ligands via weak, non-covalent bonds that are readily made and broken. However, control can also be exerted on a longer time scale. Medium-term control, exerted in minutes or hours, can involve two main mechanisms:

(i) *Irreversible partial proteolysis.* Enzymes subject to such control are synthesised in an inactive form called proenzymes or zymogens. These are activated, when required, by the proteolytic cleavage of peptide fragments by enzymes such as trypsin. Examples include chymotrypsinogen (the precursor of chymotrypsin), prothrombin (the precursor of thrombin), and proelastase (the precursor of elastase).

(ii) *Reversible covalent modification.* This is a more common control mechanism than partial proteolysis for the control of enzyme activity and most frequently involves the phosphorylation of specific threonine, serine and tyrosine residues by a protein kinase. Most significantly, it is reversible by the action of a phosphatase. A large number of protein kinases have been identified and the activity of many of them shown to be subject to control by hormones, growth factors and neurotransmitters operating via cellular receptors. Some enzymes are activated by phosphorylation and deactivated by dephosphorylation whereas other enzymes are deactivated by phosphorylation and activated by dephosphorylation. The phosphate group attached to the threonine, serine and tyrosine residues is a relatively large group carrying negative charges on the oxygen atoms. These negative groups can trigger electrostatic repulsions or attractions with neighbouring ionic groups in the protein and hence induce conformational changes in the active site of the enzyme. The involvement of other enzymes to phosphorylate and dephosphorylate the enzyme explains the medium-term nature of this form of control. A similar form of control can be exerted by the attachment of an adenylyl group to a tyrosine residue. Control by phosphorylation is discussed further in Section 8.4.3. Control can also operate via the binding of calcium ions to calmodulin (Section 8.4.3).

Long-term control, exerted in hours, operates at the level of enzyme synthesis and degradation. Although many enzymes are synthesised at a virtually constant rate and are said to be constitutive enzymes, the synthesis of others is variable and is subject to the operation of control mechanisms at the level of gene transcription and translation. One of the best-studied examples is the induction of β-galactosidase and galactoside permease by lactose in E. coli. The expression of the *lac* operon is subject to control by a repressor protein produced by the repressor gene (the normal state) and an inducer, the presence of which causes the repressor to dissociate from the operator allowing the transcription and subsequent translation of the *lac* genes. The Lac repressor protein binds to the *lac* operator with a K_i of 10^{-13} M and a binding rate constant of 10^7 M^{-1} s^{-1}. This is greater than that possible for a diffusion-controlled process and there is evidence that the DNA facilitates the binding.

The degradation of enzymes resembles the decay of radioisotopes in that it is a first-order process characterised by a half-life. The half-life of enzymes varies from a few hours to many days. Interestingly, enzymes that exert control over pathways have relatively short half-lives. The precise amino acid sequence of an enzyme is thought to influence its susceptibility to proteolytic enzymes. N-terminal leucine, phenylalanine, aspartate, lysine and arginine, for example, appear to predispose the protein to rapid degradation. Proteolytic degradation is believed to involve a small protein (76 amino acid residues), called ubiquitin, which requires ATP and is able to 'tag' proteins for degradation.

7.9.3 Study of enzymology *in vivo*

In the extrapolation of *in vivo* kinetic data to the *in vivo* situation, the assumption is made that intracellular compartments such as the cytosol and the mitochondrial matrix can be regarded as homogeneous bags of enzymes in which the individual enzyme, their substrates and products can freely diffuse. Support for this view has come from cell fractionation studies in which the great proportion of total cell proteins is released when cells are disrupted.

Over the past decade or so, evidence has begun to accumulate that casts doubt on this traditional view of *in vivo* enzymology. For example, studies with high voltage electron microscopy (HVEM) have shown that mammalian cells contain an extensive network of interconnecting strands, termed the microtrabecular lattice (MTL) which appears to connect all the intracellular structures. Critics of the existence of the MTL have argued that such structures are artefacts, but there is increasing acceptance that MTL or closely related structures do represent a good approximation of the structure *in vivo*. The consequence of such a model is that previously regarded freely diffusing enzymes are more likely to be loosely bound to the MTL. Such a view gives rise to the concept of the wide existence of multienzyme complexes, previously regarded as an exception to the norm.

If these revised views of the arrangement of enzymes *in vivo* in a metabolic pathway are correct, then the concept arises of the channelling of products from one enzyme to the next. Channelling could occur by a number of mechanisms including the sequential covalent binding of intermediates to active sites, site-to-site transfer of non-covalently bound intermediates (so-called tight channelling), the transfer of intermediates in an unstirred aqueous layer and the prevention of diffusion of intermediates by electrostatic forces. It has been argued that channelling of metabolic intermediates within an organised enzyme complex could lead to increased flux through the pathway and restriction of flux in competing pathways. Whether or not the loose association of enzymes will result in an influence on their individual kinetic properties is still a matter of debate.

The most successful analytical technique for studying enzymology in individual cells and in whole organisms is NMR (Section 10.4). This non-invasive technique allows the measurement of steady-state metabolite concentrations and of enzyme-catalysed flux using either simple proton NMR, the redistribution of a ^{13}C label among glycolytic intermediates or the use of ^{31}P NMR to measure ATP turnover and flux. Evidence for enzyme–enzyme interaction has been obtained by studying conformational changes in the enzyme protein. This approach requires the protein to be labelled in some appropriate way. One of the most attractive methods is to insert a fluorine atom into the molecule. From an NMR point of view this is an excellent label, since it is a spin half nuclide that is readily studied by NMR. The chemical shift change of the fluorine nucleus is large, making it very sensitive to its local environment in the protein. Moreover, its size is very similar to that of a proton, so that it is unlikely to modify the enzyme's structure. Since fluorine is very rare in biological systems, the NMR signal from the label can be interpreted unambiguously. By studying the relaxation times associated with the fluorine nucleus it should be possible to detect restricted motion of the enzyme in a cell owing to protein–protein aggregation.

A complementary approach to these NMR studies is that of genetic manipulation. Using molecular biological techniques, it is possible to delete, raise or lower the intracellular concentration of selected enzymes and to study the effect on kinetics and flux. The approach requires merely the availability of complementary DNA or a genomic clone for the selected enzyme, coupled with gene disruption and anti-sense RNA methodologies.

7.10 **KEY TERMS**

acid–base catalysis	first-order kinetics	prosthetic group
activation energy	fixed-change assays	protomers
active sites	fixed-time assays	Q_{10} value
affinity constant	flux	rapid mixing methods
allosteric binding	Hanes equation	random order
allosteric enzyme	heterotropic activators	reaction rate analysers
allosteric sites	heterotropic effectors	receptor
apoenzyme	Hill plot	regulatory enzymes
Arrhenius equation	holoenzyme	regulatory sites
association constant	homotropic effect	relaxation methods
bi-bi reaction	immobilised enzymes	relaxed state
binding constant	induced fit	reversible inhibitors
biosubstrate reactions	initial rate	saturation kinetics
catalytic sites	inhibitor constant	secondary plots
chemical immobilisation	irreversible inhibitors	sequential
coenzymes	ligand	sequential model
cofactors	linear competitive inhibition	short-term control
competitive inhibitors	Lineweaver–Burk equation	sigmoidal
compulsory order	Michaelis constant	specificity constant
conformation	Michaelis–Menten equation	steady-state kinetics
constitutive enzymes	mixed inhibition kinetics	stopped flow
continuous flow analyzers	multienzyme complexes	substrate cycles
cooperative	negative cooperativity	substrate inhibition
coupled assays	non-competitive inhibitors	subunits
covalent modification	oligomeric	temperature jump
dead-end complex	optimum temperature	tense state
discrete analysers	parabolic competitive inhibition	ternary complex
dissociation constant	pH optimum	transition state
Eadie–Hofstee equation	photoaffinity labels	transition state analogues
effectors	physical immobilisation	turnover number
end-product inhibition	ping-pong mechanism	uncompetitive
energy barriers	positive cooperativity	van't Hoff plot
enzyme–substrate complex	pre-steady state	zero-order kinetics
enzymic cycling	primary plots	zymogens
fast (centrifugal) analyser	proenzymes	

7.11 CALCULATIONS

Question 1

(i) The enzyme α-glucosidase was studied using the synthetic substrate p-nitro-phenyl-α-D-glucopyranoside (PNPG), which is hydrolysed to release p-nitrophe-nol (which in alkaline solution is yellow) and the absorbance at 400 nm used to study the progress of the reaction (see Section 7.4.2). The Beer–Lambert law for p-nitrophenol was shown to be obeyed under the conditions of the study. A 3 mM solution of PNPG was taken and portions used to study the effect of substrate con-centration on initial rate. The following results were obtained:

PNPG (cm³)	0.1	0.2	0.3	0.4	0.6	0.8	1.2
Initial rate	0.055	0.094	0.130	0.157	0.196	0.230	0.270

The total volume of the assay was 10 cm³. The initial rate was expressed as the absorbance change at 400 nm due to p-nitrophenol release. Calculate the K_m and V_{max} values by means of at least two linear plots.

(ii) The effect of pH on K_m and V_{max} for the reaction was also studied with the follow-ing results:

pH	6.0	6.3	6.5	7.0	7.5	8.0
K_m (mM)	0.120	0.163	0.216	0.250	0.210	0.160
V_{max}	0.430	0.480	0.526	0.530	0.450	0.313

What information can you deduce from these data?

Answer

(i) [PNPG] (mM) = 0.03, 0.06, 0.09, 0.12, 0.18, 0.24, 0.36; K_m (approx.) 0.2 mM; V_{max} 0.4.

(ii) A plot of log K_m versus pH and of log V_{max} versus pH show bell-shaped graphs in-dicating two ionisable groups in the enzyme active site involved in both substrate binding and catalysis. Tangents to the curves indicate pK_a values of 6.2 to 6.4 and 7.2 to 7.3. These can be interpreted as two histidines. [See H. Halvorson & L. Ellias (1958), *Biochim. Biophys. Acta*, **30**, 28–33.]

Question 2

For an enzyme which obeys the mechanism

$$E + S \underset{k_{-1}}{\overset{k_{+1}}{\rightleftharpoons}} ES \overset{k_{+2}}{\longrightarrow} E + P$$

the following values for the rate constants were obtained:

k_{+1}	$10^9\,M^{-1}s^{-1}$
k_{-1}	$10^6\,s^{-1}$
k_{+2}	$10^3\,s^{-1}$
$[E_t]$	1.0 nM

Calculate K_m, K_s, V_{max} and k_{cat}.

Answer

$$
\begin{aligned}
K_m &= k_{-1}/k_{+1} + k_{+2}/k_{+1} = 10^{-3}\,M. \\
K_s &= k_{-1}/k_{+1} = 10^{-3}\,M. \\
V_{max} &= k_2[E_t] = 10^{-6}\,Ms^{-1}. \\
k_{cat} &= V_{max}/[F_t] = 10^3\,s^{-1}.
\end{aligned}
$$

Question 3   If an enzyme has a V_{max} of 150 mmol min^{-1} and gave an initial rate of 50 mmol min^{-1} at a substrate concentration of 1 mM, calculate the K_m of the enzyme assuming that its kinetics obey the Michaelis–Menten equation.

Answer $$V_0 = \frac{V_{max}[S]}{K_m + [S]}$$

$K_m = 2\,\text{mM}$

Question 4   An allosteric enzyme with a V_{max} of 230 mmol min^{-1} gave the following data when the initial rate was investigated as a function of substrate concentration:

[S] (mM)	2	4	6	10	20	40
v_0 (mmol min^{-1})	22	60	110	165	200	215

By means of a Hill plot, determine the value of the Hill coefficient.

Answer   A plot of $\log\left(\dfrac{v_0}{V_{max} - v_0}\right)$ against $\log[S]$ gives a straight line, the slope of which is equal to the Hill coefficient (h) and has a value of approximately 1.9.

7.12 SUGGESTIONS FOR FURTHER READING

BICKERSTAFF, G. F. (ed.) (1997). *Immobilization of Enzymes and Cells.* Methods in Biotechnology, vol. 1. Humana Press, Totowa, NJ. (A good comprehensive coverage of this important topic.)

BUGG, T. (1997). *An Introduction to Enzyme and Coenzyme Chemistry.* Blackwell Science, Oxford. (A good readable text that emphasises the underlying chemistry of the subject.)

EISENTHAL, R. and DANSON, M. J. (1992). *Enzyme Assays: A Practical Approach.* IRL Press, Oxford. (One of a series of 'practical approach' books that gives good advice on the practical details of enzyme assays.)

FELL, D. (1997). *Understanding the Control of Metabolism.* Portland Press, London. (An authoritative coverage of this important topic in which the underlying mathematical concepts are carefully explained.)

PALMER, T. (1995). *Understanding Enzymes,* 4th edn. Prentice Hall, London. (A good general student textbook on enzymology.)

PRICE, N. C. and STEVENS, L. (1989). *Fundamentals of Enzymology,* 2nd edn. Oxford University Press, Oxford. (A general enzymology text, particularly good on mechanisms and control.)

SONNTAG, O. (1993). *Dry Chemistry: Analysis With Carrier Bound Reagents.* Laboratory Techniques in Biochemistry and Molecular Biology, vol. 25. Elsevier, Amsterdam. (An authoritative coverage of this subject.)

TAWFIK, D. S., ESHHAR, A. and GREEN, B. S. (1994). Catalytic antibodies: a critical assessment. *Molecular Biotechnology,* **1**, 87–102. (A review of the principle of catalytic antibodies and how their function supports the principle that enzymes facilitate the formation of the transition state.)

ZUBAY, G. (1993). *Biochemistry,* 3rd edn. William C. Brown, Dubuque, IA. (An excellent general biochemistry textbook with good chapters on enzymology.)

Chapter 8

Biomolecular interactions: II   Cell surface receptors and transporters

8.1 **CELL SURFACE RECEPTOR CLASSIFICATION**

Cells within an organism need to be able to respond to changes in their environment and to be able to communicate with each other in order to ensure their co-ordinated growth and survival. Cells in physical contact with each other can communicate via pores in their membranes but cells that are physically separated need an effective signalling system. This system involves both a molecular signal, which is able to move from its site of synthesis to its target cell, and a molecular detection and transmission system that can stimulate an appropriate cellular response. Cell surface receptors are membrane-bound proteins whose function is to transmit physiological signals originating outside the cell to the internal environment of the cell, which then produces some form of response. The signal takes the form of a ligand, referred to as the first messenger, examples of which include the peptide hormones, neurotransmitters, growth factors and the cytokines. The binding of the ligand to the specific binding site on the receptor is in itself not sufficient to produce a cellular response but the first message has to be transduced into the cell interior either by the 'gating' of ions across the membrane or via the interaction of the intracellular domain of the receptor with enzymes and other proteins in the cell. In the case of many receptors, binding of the first messenger results in the generation, or release from intracellular stores, of one or more of a group of molecules collectively called second messengers. These molecules diffuse to, and react with, various protein targets within the cell, modifying their activity and eventually producing the final cellular response to the binding of the first messenger. One of the biochemical attractions of the first messenger → second messenger cellular transduction pathway is that the series of reactions involved, collectively referred to as a cascade, can result in a large amplification of the final cellular response relative to that which could possibly have been produced by the first messenger acting alone.

Receptor proteins consist of three distinct domains:

Extracellular domain. The external portion of the receptor protein often contains the binding site for the ligand. Recognition of this site by the ligand and its subsequent binding to the site initiates the transduction process.

Transmembrane domain. This region of the protein is inserted into the phospholipid bilayer of the membrane. Many receptors possess several transmembrane regions so that the protein chain loops repeatedly across the membrane. In the case of some receptors, these loops form a channel for the 'gating' of ions, whilst in other receptors they contain the binding site for the ligand.

Intracellular domain. This cytosolic region of the protein has to respond to the extracellular binding of the ligand and, in many cases, interact with intracellular molecules to initiate the cellular response.

It is evident from this three-domain nature, that cell surface receptor proteins must be amphipathic in that they must have a small number of regions of 19 to 24 amino acid residues that are hydrophobic, consisting of non-polar side-chains. They also have other regions that are hydrophilic, consisting of polar and ionised side-chains. The hydrophobic regions, generally in the form of α-helixes, are the transmembrane regions that are inserted into the hydrophobic, long-chain fatty acid portion of the phospholipid bilayer of the membrane. The hydrophilic regions of the receptor are exposed on the outside and inside faces of the membrane, which are in an aqueous, hydrophilic environment. The need for the hydrophobic region to span the membrane is so characteristic of receptors that it is possible to identify the membrane-spanning regions simply by inspecting the amino acid sequence of the protein and associated hydrophobicity profile (Section 6.4.3). Families of receptor proteins can be recognised from the precise number of transmembrane regions each possess (Section 8.3.2).

An important functional feature of receptor proteins is their ability to diffuse laterally within the membrane (Section 8.3.3). This concept of a mobile receptor is essential for the expression of their function and the transduction of the first message into the cell and the production of the final cellular response.

Three main classes of cell surface receptors have been identified on the basis of the type of signal transduction they induce:

The opening of ligand-gated ion channels within the receptor molecule for the movement of ions such as Na^+, K^+ and Cl^-. The opening of these channels and the movement of ions across the membrane initiates a short-term, fast response including the propagation of a membrane electrical potential wave. Examples include the nicotinic acetylcholine receptor and the γ-aminobutyric acid (GABA) receptor type A.

The activation of one of a group of guanine nucleotide binding proteins, collectively known as G-proteins, the modulation of a signal-generating enzyme or effector, and the eventual release of a second messenger such as cyclic AMP, inositol trisphosphate, 1,2-diacylglycerol or calcium ions. Receptors in this class are the most numerous and typically regulate cellular responses occurring on a time scale of minutes. Examples of this type of receptor are the adrenergic, dopamine and histamine receptors.

The phosphorylation of a tyrosine, serine or threonine residue within the C-terminal region of the receptor protein protruding into the cytoplasm. This type of receptor has intrinsic protein kinase enzyme activity, which is essential for production of the final cellular response to the binding of the first messenger. The phosphorylation of other intracellular enzymes by the protein kinase activity of the receptor results in the long-term regulation of the activity of these intracellular enzymes. Examples of this type of receptor are the insulin and epidermal growth factor receptors.

This classification also coincides with classification based on structural characteristics of the receptor proteins. Thus there are three superfamilies of cell surface receptors that have a common structure and transduction mechanism. However, the classification is too exclusive. For example, the receptors for the cytokines do not fall into any of the three classes but their action is similar to that of tyrosine kinase receptors, which are members of the third class. It should be noted that this cell surface receptor categorisation excludes the LDL (low density lipoprotein) receptors located in the cellular membrane, which, although they possess many of the characteristics of other cellular receptors, are linked primarily to the endocytosis of molecules of particles such as the LDL particle and are thus one of a number of transport processes that are considered later in this chapter (Section 8.11.1). It is important to realise, however, that even for the peptide hormone, growth hormone and neurotransmitter receptors, the endocytosis of the receptor–ligand complex is an important component of the various transduction events that govern the overall response of the cell to the initial signal. This process of receptor trafficking is one of the regulatory mechanisms for the control of receptor numbers and hence of the sensitivity of the cell to external first messenger signals.

Much of the early work on the study of cell surface receptor–ligand binding was carried out on isolated tissue preparations and was aimed at the quantification and characterisation of the response as a function of the ligand concentration. The work was driven largely by the search for compounds that could block the binding of the physiological ligand but which did not produce a cellular response in their own right. These so-called ligand blockers had the potential for pharmacological exploitation. In the 1960s it was realised that if such blockers were sufficiently selective in their binding they might be able to distinguish between the various subclasses of the receptor that were believed to exist. The identification of subclasses of receptors could be used to develop blockers as therapeutic agents that would be tissue and response selective and hence more acceptable agents. It was a result of this approach that Sir James Black achieved his pioneering work on β-adrenergic and histamine H_2 receptors, which resulted in the development of the blood pressure-lowering β-blocker, propranolol, and the gastric acid secretion H_2 receptor blocker, cimetidine, used in the treatment of gastric and duodenal ulcers. This approach to receptor classification, coupled with the newer technique of gene cloning, has resulted in the identification of a plethora of receptor subtypes for most receptors.

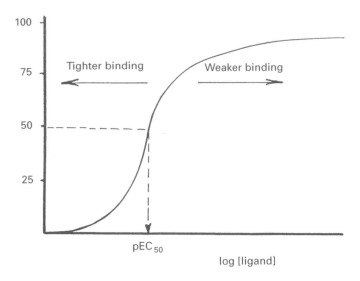

Fig. 8.1. Dose–response curve for the binding of a ligand to its membrane receptor. Agonists differing in their affinity for the receptor move the curve to the left or right as indicated. The y-axis shows percentage response.

8.2 QUANTITATIVE ASPECTS OF RECEPTOR–LIGAND BINDING

8.2.1 Dose–response curves

The graphical relationship between concentration of ligand (dose) and cellular response is hyperbolic, but because such plots often span several hundred-fold variations in ligand concentration, they are best expressed in semi-logarithmic form (Fig. 8.1). These plots, which are sigmoidal, have three components:

(i) an initial threshold below which little or no effect is observed;
(ii) a slope in which response increases rapidly with dose;
(iii) a final maximum response.

The potency of a particular ligand is related to the position of the sigmoidal curve on the log dose axis. It is expressed in a variety of forms including the effective dose or concentration for 50% maximal response (ED_{50} or EC_{50}). On these semilogarithmic plots, the values emerge as pED_{50} or pEC_{50} values (i.e. $-\log ED_{50}$), usually called pD_2 values. Thus a ligand with EC_{50} of 3×10^{-5} M would have a pEC_{50} of 4.5. One of the attractions of semilogarithmic plots is that they are virtually linear within the range 25% to 75% maximal response; hence ED_{50} values can be defined with greater accuracy than by use of hyperbolic plots.

Dose–response studies for a given receptor, using ligands with a wide range of molecular structures, have identified the existence of molecules which can be categorised as:

Agonists: these bind to the receptors and all produce the same maximal cellular response but they differ in their ED_{50} values.

Partial agonists: these bind to the receptors but produce only a partial maximal response even when all the receptors are occupied.

Antagonists: these bind to the receptors but produce no response and can block the binding of agonists including the physiological ligand(s).

Antagonists, like enzyme inhibitors (Section 7.3.8), may be of several types. Competitive reversible antagonists bind reversibly to the receptor at the same site as that to which the agonist binds. Since the binding is reversible, the effect of a competitive antagonist may be overcome by increasing the concentration of agonist. It is characterised by a binding or affinity constant, K_i, which is equal to the concentration of antagonist that would occupy 50% of the receptors at equilibrium if no agonist were present. Its value can be obtained from competitive binding assays, very similar in principle to the determination of K_i for a competitive enzyme inhibitor. The potency of a competitive antagonist is sometimes expressed as a pK_i, pK_B or a pA_2 value. Non-competitive reversible antagonists bind to both the receptor and the receptor–agonist complex. Their effect therefore cannot be overcome by increasing the agonist concentration. They do not change the EC_{50} value for an agonist but they do reduce its maximal response. Irreversible antagonists, like irreversible enzyme inhibitors, form a covalent bond with the receptor. Examples include the α-adrenergic receptor antagonists of the dibenamine type.

The existence of agonists, partial agonists and antagonists emphasises the distinction between the affinity of the ligand for its receptor and its ability to induce a response. The latter property of a ligand is referred to as its intrinsic efficacy. The two-state theory of receptors (Section 8.4.2), put forward to explain the phenomenon, assumes that the resting receptor can exist in two conformations that are in equilibrium with each other, but only one of which on binding the ligand can initiate the response. Ligands are believed to differ in their ability to displace this equilibrium. A second theory, conformational induction, envisages that binding of the ligand deforms the binding site to create the active site and that ligands differ in their ability to induce this conformational change. There are clear similarities between these theories and the symmetry model and the sequential model proposed for the allosteric regulation of enzyme activity discussed previously (Section 7.3.4, Fig. 7.8).

8.2.2 **Receptor–ligand binding parameters**

The general process of ligand binding to a receptor can be represented by the application of the Law of Mass Action as follows:

$$
\underset{\text{receptor}}{R} \; + \; \underset{\text{ligand}}{L} \; \underset{k_{-1}}{\overset{k_{+1}}{\rightleftharpoons}} \; \underset{\substack{\text{receptor–ligand} \\ \text{complex}}}{RL} \tag{8.1}
$$

where k_{+1} is the association first-order rate constant and k_{-1} is the dissociation first-order rate constant.

If, under the conditions of the binding studies, the total concentration of ligand is very much greater than that of receptor, changes in ligand concentration due to receptor binding can be ignored but changes in the free (unbound) receptor concentration cannot. Hence if

[R_t] is the total concentration of receptor that determines the maximum amount of receptor–ligand complex, [RL]$_{max}$ or B_{max} (from binding maximum), that can be formed;

[L] is the ligand concentration;

[RL] is the concentration of receptor–ligand complex at a given ligand concentration, which can be quantified by the amount of ligand bound to the receptor;

[R_t] − [RL] will be the concentration of free receptor.

At equilibrium, the forward and reverse reactions for ligand binding and dissociation (equation 8.1) will be equal:

$$k_{+1}([R_t] - [RL])[L] = k_{-1}[RL]$$

therefore $\dfrac{k_{-1}}{k_{+1}} = K_d = \dfrac{([R_t]) - [RL]\,[L]}{[RL]}$ \hfill (8.2)

where K_d is the dissociation constant for RL.

and $[RL] = \dfrac{[L]\,[R_t]}{K_d + [RL]}$ \hfill (8.3)

The reciprocal of K_d is equal to the affinity constant, K_a, of the receptor for the ligand. Equation 8.3 is of the form of a rectangular hyperbola, which predicts that ligand binding will reach a limiting value as the ligand concentration is increased and therefore that receptor binding is a saturable process. The equation is of precisely the same form as equations 7.1 and 7.2, which define the binding of the substrate to its enzyme in terms of K_m and V_{max}. For the experimental determination of K_d, equation 8.2 is best converted to a linear form. Simple rearrangement of equation 8.2 gives the Scatchard equation:

$$\frac{[RL]}{[L]} = \frac{[R_t]}{K_d} - \frac{[RL]}{K_d}$$ \hfill (8.4)

Hence a plot of bound ligand/free ligand versus bound ligand will be a straight line, of slope $-1/K_d$ with intercept on the x-axis of [R_t]. Sometimes the Scatchard equation is given in the form

$$\frac{[RL]}{[L][R_t]} = \frac{n}{K_d} - \frac{[RL]}{[R_t]K_d}$$ \hfill (8.5)

where n is the number of independent ligand binding sites on the receptor. The expression [RL]/[R_t] is the number of moles of ligand bound to one mole of receptor. If this expression is defined as r, then

$$\frac{r}{[L]} = \frac{n}{K_d} - \frac{r}{K_d}$$ \hfill (8.6)

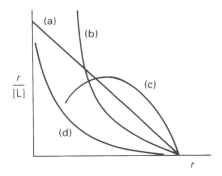

Fig. 8.2. Scatchard plot for (a) a single set of sites with no cooperativity, (b) two sets of sites with no cooperativity, (c) a single set of sites with positive cooperativity, and (d) a single set of sites with negative cooperativity.

In this case, a plot of $r/[L]$ against r will again be linear but the intercept on the x-axis will be equal to the number of ligand binding sites, n, on the receptor (Fig. 8.2). This form of the Scatchard plot can be used only in cases where the molar concentration of the receptor protein in the assay system is known.

Alternative linear plots to the Scatchard plot are

Lineweaver–Burk:

$$\frac{1}{[RL]} = \frac{1}{[R_t]} + \frac{K_d \times 1}{[R_t][L]} \tag{8.7}$$

Hanes:

$$\frac{[L]}{[RL]} = \frac{K_d}{[R_t]} + \frac{[L]}{[R_t]} \tag{8.8}$$

In practice, Scatchard plots are most commonly carried out. It can be seen that when the receptor sites are half saturated, i.e. $[RL] = [R_t]/2$, $[L] = K_d$. This is analogous to $S = K_m$ when $v_o = V_{max}/2$ (Section 7.3.2). Hence K_d will have units of molarity.

The derivation of equations 8.2 and 8.3 is based on the assumption that there is a single set of homogeneous receptors and that there is no cooperativity between them in the binding of the ligand molecules. In practice, two other possibilities arise: first, that there are two or more distinct populations of receptors each with different binding constants and, secondly, that there is cooperativity in binding within a single population. In both cases the Scatchard plot will be curvilinear (Fig. 8.2). If cooperativity is suspected, it should be confirmed by a Hill plot (equation 7.9), which, in its non-kinetic form, is

$$\log\left(\frac{Y}{1-Y}\right) = h\log[L] + \log K_d \tag{8.9}$$

where Y is the fractional saturation of the binding sites (from 0 to 1) and K_d is an overall dissociation constant.

For a receptor with multiple binding sites that function independently, $h = 1$, whereas for a receptor with multiple sites that are interdependent, h is either greater than 1 (positive cooperativity) or less than 1 (negative cooperativity).

Scatchard plots that are biphasic owing to a mixed population of receptors rather than receptor cooperativity are sometimes taken to indicate that the two extreme, and approximately linear, sections of the curvilinear plots represent high affinity (high bound: free ratio at low bound concentration) and low affinity (low bound: free ratio at high bound concentration) sites and that tangents drawn to these two sections of the curve can be used to calculate the associated K_d and $[R_t]$ or n values. This is incorrect, and the correct values can be obtained only from the binding data by means of careful mathematical analysis, generally using computer programes. Discrimination between the two types of receptor is aided by the availability of selective antagonists to one or other site.

8.2.3 Receptor–ligand binding techniques

Preparations of receptors for ligand binding studies may either leave the membrane effectively intact or involve the disruption of the membrane and the release of the receptor with or without membrane fragments. Membrane receptor proteins show no or very little ligand-binding properties in the absence of phospholipid, and purified receptor protein must be introduced into a phospholipid vesicle for binding study purposes.

Common preparations include:

tissue slices, usually 5 to 50 μm thick, cut in a cryostat and adhered to a gelatin-coated glass slide;

isolated whole cells produced by either the mechanical or the enzymic disruption of the whole tissue or by cell culture (Section 1.6);

use of a cloned receptor gene expressed in a specific cell line;

membrane preparations obtained by the use of a variety of methods for cell disruption (Section 6.3.3) coupled with differential centrifugation (Section 5.6.1);

solubilised receptor preparations obtained by the use of detergents as the membrane disruption agents and purified by affinity chromatography using an antagonist as the immobilised ligand (Section 13.9).

Tissue slices are best for the study of receptor distribution and number by autoradiography (Section 14.2.3) or fluorescence spectroscopy (Section 9.5). The kinetics of ligand binding in these preparations are complicated by the existence of diffusion barriers. Receptors on intact isolated cells are used for a wide range of biochemical studies, including receptor post-translational modification, membrane insertion and down regulation, and the study of receptor–response coupling. Binding studies using intact cells have the potential problem that the cells contain metabolic enzymes capable of acting on the physiological ligand, thereby reducing its effective concentration. Ligand-binding data obtained with whole cells are also difficult to interpret, since receptor trafficking and other cellular processes may affect the binding. Care must also be taken to demonstrate the homogeneity of the cell preparation, but the use of receptor gene cloning and expression in a specific cell line effectively overcomes this problem. Whilst cell membrane preparations are an experimentally useful source of receptors, they lack the cytoplasmic components that may affect the regulation of ligand binding. Recombinant receptors are increasingly being used for ligand-binding studies, but care has to be taken to ensure that they have the same functional characteristics as the native receptor. It is particularly important to ensure that post-translational processes have been carried out and that, for example, the receptor protein has been correctly glycosylated. It is equally important to ensure that the cell line used to express the receptor protein also expresses other components, such as G-proteins, to allow a functional assay for the expressed receptor.

Fluorescent-labelled ligands, using, for example, fluorescein or rhodamine, may be used for binding studies but by far the most common technique is to use a radio-labelled ligand. ^{3}H, ^{14}C, ^{32}P, ^{35}S and ^{125}I are the most common radionuclides used. Generally a high specific activity (Section 14.1.6) ligand is used, a large selection of which is available commercially for a wide range of receptors.

Anti-receptor antibodies have been used to study aspects of receptor biochemistry, including cellular location and the location of sites within the receptor for the expression of specific effector functions such as phosphorylation. Anti-receptor antibodies can be raised using cell-bound or membrane-bound receptor protein, purified receptor protein or receptor protein produced by gene cloning. One of the problems associated with the use of anti-receptor antibodies is that they will certainly have more than one epitope, some of which may be located within the membrane or on the intracellular side of the membrane rather than simply on the ligand-binding side of the membrane. Anti-receptor antibodies may therefore bind to sites other than the ligand-binding site and may even trigger receptor aggregation due to their large multivalent nature. The use of monovalent Fab antibody fragments (Section 4.1.1) may help to confirm whether or not the ligand-binding site is being studied.

The direct visualisation of receptor–ligand complexes can be achieved either by the use of electron-dense markers such as ferritin or by the use of colloidal gold particles.

The general experimental approach for studying receptor–ligand binding is to incubate the receptor preparation with the ligand under defined conditions of temperature, pH and ionic concentration for a specific period of time that is sufficient to allow equilibrium to be attained. Using an appropriate analytical procedure, the bound and unbound forms of the ligand are then separated and quantified. The procedure is repeated for a series of ligand concentrations at a fixed receptor concentration and perhaps repeated in the presence of effector molecules. The binding data are then analysed using equations 8.4 to 8.8, often by means of a computer program. Irrespective of the analytical procedure chosen to separate the bound and free ligand, a general problem is the non-specific binding of the ligand to sites other than the specific ligand-binding site(s). Such non-specific binding may involve membrane lipids and other proteins located in the

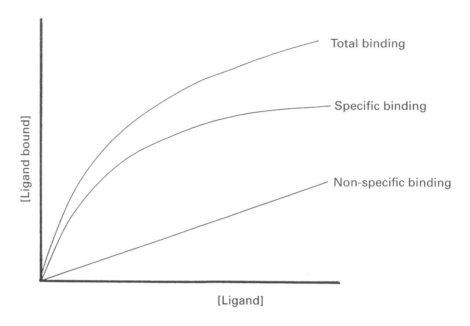

Fig. 8.3. Specific and non-specific binding of a ligand to a membrane receptor. Specific binding is normally hyperbolic and shows saturation. Non-specific binding is linear and is not readily saturated.

membrane. The characteristic of non-specific binding is that it is non-saturable but is approximately linearly related to the total concentration of the ligand. Thus the observed ligand binding is the sum of the saturable (hyperbolic) specific binding to the receptor and the non-saturable (linear) binding to miscellaneous sites. The specific binding component is usually obtained indirectly by carrying out the binding studies in the presence of either excess non-labelled ligand, if a labelled ligand is being used to study binding, or excess unlabelled antagonist (which has a high affinity for the binding site), if labelled antagonist is being used. In both cases the specific binding sites would not be available to the experimental ligand and hence its binding would be confined to non-specific sites (Fig. 8.3).

In practice, a concentration of the competitive ligand of at least 1000 times its K_d would be used and confirmation that under the conditions of the experiment non-specific binding was being studied would be sought by repeating the study using a range of different and structurally dissimilar competitive ligands that should give consistent estimates of the non-specific binding.

Numerous techniques including the ultracentrifugation (Section 5.10), molecular exclusion chromatography (Section 13.8), circular dichroism (Section 9.6) and nuclear magnetic resonance spectroscopy (Section 10.4) have been used to study receptor–ligand binding. In the case of spectrophotometric techniques, information regarding the functional groups in the receptor protein involved in binding the ligand can be obtained in addition to data permitting the calculation of dissociation constants. The principles of these techniques are discussed in the

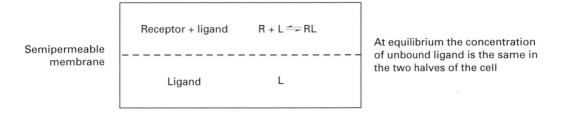

Fig. 8.4. The study of receptor–ligand binding by equilibrium dialysis.

relevant chapters in this book and only details of the two simplest techniques, equilibrium dialysis and ultrafiltration, and the most recent innovation using evanescent wave biosensors, are described here.

Equilibrium dialysis

The receptor and ligand, each in a buffer of the same pH and concentration, are placed in opposite halves of a dialysis cell. The cell, which generally has a total internal volume of about 3 cm^3, is constructed of transparent plastic such as Perspex^R and unscrews into two halves, that are separated by a cellulose acetate or cellulose nitrate semipermeable membrane mounted on an inert mesh support. Many commercial variants of the cell are available, some consisting of banks of up to six cells. The temperature of the cell is thermostatically controlled and the cell is slowly rotated to help the system to reach equilibrium. The ligand molecules, which are small and diffusible, readily cross the membrane until their unbound concentration is the same on both sides (Fig. 8.4). The receptor protein is confined to one half of the cell. At equilibrium, samples are taken from each half of the cell and analysed for ligand. The sample from the receptor half of the cell will give the sum of the bound and unbound ligand concentrations, whereas that in the other half will give merely the unbound ligand concentration, which will be the same as the unbound ligand concentration in the other half of the cell containing the receptor.

For reliable results the binding of both the ligand and protein to the membrane must be minimal and the total ion concentration in each half of the cell equalised to minimise any possibility of a charge inequality on either side of the membrane affecting the distribution of ligand (Donnan effect). The limitations of the technique are the relatively long period of time it takes to establish equilibrium and the fact that it cannot be applied to cases where the ligand is a macromolecule.

Ultrafiltration

The receptor and ligand in a buffered solution are contained in a thermostatically controlled cell (generally 1 to 3 cm^3 capacity) containing a semipermeable membrane on an inert mesh support at its base. Since no diffusion across the membrane is required to establish equilibrium, attainment of equilibrium is rapid (20 min). A small sample (100 mm^3 is then forced across the membrane into a collection cup, either by application of a gas pressure to the mixture side or more simply by placing the cell in a low speed centrifuge and centrifuging at about 3000 g for a few minutes. By analysing the ultrafiltrate (representative of the unbound ligand concentration) and the reaction mixture (bound plus unbound ligand), the influence of ligand concentration on the extent of binding can be studied readily. The attraction of the method is its speed, but binding of the reactants to the membrane must be checked and the volume of the ultrafiltrate kept to a minimum to minimise any possibility that the sampling procedure displaces the equilibrium. As with equilibrium dialysis, the method cannot be used to study macromolecular ligands.

Evanescent wave biosensors

One of the major limitations of many of the techniques commonly used to study receptor–ligand binding is that they can be used to study only the final equilibrium position and are therefore not suitable for studying the rate constants for the formation and dissociation of the receptor–ligand complex. This disadvantage, when coupled with the fact that many of the methods are also slow and not amenable to automation, makes them unattractive for routine, repetitive studies of the kinetics of receptor–ligand binding. Recent developments in gene cloning have opened up the possibility of cloned receptors, including those of unknown physiological function, being available to the pharmaceutical industry as potential targets for new therapeutic agents. This has stimulated the development of automated techniques for the study of biomolecular interactions without the use of fluorescent or radioisotope labels, with the result that a number of dedicated instruments are now available commercially. The theoretical principles underlying the instruments are largely common and based on a phenomenon called surface plasmon resonance.

The receptor under study is immobilised to a sensor surface, such as a hydrogel layer on a glass slide, either via biotin–avidin interactions (Section 12.3.9) or via covalent coupling via amine or thiol reagents (Section 13.9.2). A typical surface concentration of receptor of 1 to 5 ng mm^{-2} is used. An aqueous solution of the ligand is then either allowed to flow over the surface of the immobilised ligand or is stirred over the surface within a small cell. The binding of the receptor to the ligand is monitored continuously, exploiting changes in refractive index caused by the molecules on the interacting surface. The measurement is based on the principle of total internal reflection of light. The interacting ligand–receptor surface is monitored by a light beam angled to the surface to cause total internal reflection, which is possible because glass and the surface on which the ligand is immobilised have different refractive indices. When light is totally internally reflected at the interface, an electromagnetic component, called an evanescent wave, is formed and propagated into the lower refractive index medium (the receptor-containing liquid) where it rapidly decays. The characteristics of this wave are dependent upon the refractive index of the medium it is penetrating. If the refractive index changes, owing to receptor–ligand interactions, the profile of the evanescent wave changes. This is measured indirectly by exploiting the fact that if a thin layer of gold is also placed at the glass–ligand layer interface its electron cloud can be made to resonate by interaction with the incident light beam. This surface plasmon resonance absorbs energy, reducing the intensity of the reflected light. The angle at which this resonance occurs depends on several factors, one of which is the refractive index into which the evanescent wave is propagated (Fig. 8.5). The reflectance angle needed to cause resonance varies linearly with surface receptor–ligand interaction, hence allowing, by appropriate calibration, binding constants and rate constants to be calculated.

8.2.4 Receptor–ligand binding data

Receptor occupancy

The K_d values generally observed for receptor binding to their physiological ligand are in the range 10^{-6} to 10^{-10} M, which is indicative of a higher affinity than is typical of enzymes for their substrates. It is relatively easy to calculate from binding data the number of receptors on cell membranes. The number is in the range 10^{-3} to 10^{-6}. Although this may appear large, it represents only a small fraction of the total membrane protein, which partly explains why receptor proteins are sometimes difficult to purify. From a knowledge of receptor numbers and the associated K_d values, it is possible to calculate the occupancy of these receptors under normal physiological concentrations of the ligand. In turn it is possible to calculate how the occupancy and the associated physiological response will respond to changes in the circulating concentration of the ligand. The percentage response change will be greater the lower the normal occupancy of the receptors. This is seen from the shape of the dose–response curve within the physiological range of change of the ligand concentration. It is clear that if the normal occupancy is high, the response to change in ligand concentration is small. Under such conditions, the response is likely to be larger if the receptor–ligand binding is a positively cooperative process.

Binding studies have revealed that some agonists can stimulate the maximal response from the receptors preparation without all the receptors being occupied. This has given rise to the concept of spare receptors that are indistinguishable from the occupied receptors. It is believed that spare receptors maximise the sensitivity of the cell to the available ligand. However, binding studies have shown that the number of receptors in a membrane varies with time. The number is subject to up regulation or down regulation depending upon the needs of the cell. Control of receptor numbers is exerted at a number of levels, ranging from transcription and translation to endocytic internalisation and subsequent degradation by lysosomal enzymes. Some receptors can be shown by labelling studies to be recycled back into the membrane following endocytosis, the whole cycling time taking as little as a few minutes (see Section 8.11.2). The half-life of the insulin receptor is 9 h. Prolonged exposure of receptors to their ligand has been shown to result in desensitisation in some cases. The mechanism of this process is discussed later (Section 8.4.4).

(a)

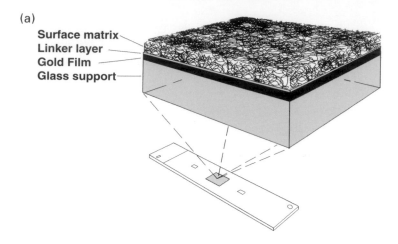

Surface matrix
Linker layer
Gold Film
Glass support

(b)

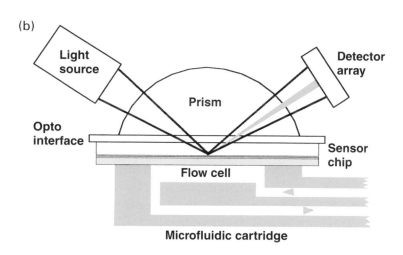

Light source

Detector array

Prism

Opto interface

Sensor chip

Flow cell

Microfluidic cartridge

Fig. 8.5. The Biacore surface plasmon resonance (SPR) instrument for studying ligand–receptor interactions in real time. (a) The surface of the sensor chip consists of four layers: glass, a thin gold film and an inert linker layer bonding a surface matrix. Gold is chosen because of its chemical inertness and good SPR response. The surface matrix, to which the receptor is immobilised, provides a hydrophilic environment for ligand interaction. (b) The optical system and flow cell. A solution of the ligand is passed through the flow cell where it interacts with the immobilised receptor on the sensor chip, the surface of which is exposed to the circulating ligand by means of a tight seal. As the interaction proceeds, the concentration of the ligand in the surface layer increases, giving an SPR response that can be monitored by a fixed array of light-sensitive diodes covering the whole wedge of reflected light. By using a wedge of incident light and a fixed array of detectors, the response angle (see the text) can be monitored continuously. (Reproduced by permission of Biacore AB, Sweden.)

Receptor subclasses

Binding studies using both agonists and antagonists have revealed the heterogeneity of many membrane receptors. Classification of receptor subclasses based on such studies is not without ambiguity and indeed controversy, and clearly identifies the need for such classification studies to be paralleled by those based on a gene cloning approach. This dual approach has confirmed the existence of over a dozen types of 5-hydroxy tryptamine (5-HT, serotonin) receptor. An interesting feature of receptor subclasses is that not only do they have different binding characteristics, but they may also trigger contrasting cellular responses. As an example, β-adrenergic receptors are activated by adrenaline and noradrenaline, but there are three subclasses, β_1, β_2 and β_3, with different amino acid composition, affinities for agonists and physiological responses. Thus β_1-adrenergic receptors mediate cardiac responses, β_2-adrenergic receptors are involved in skeletal and smooth muscle function, and β_3-adrenergic receptors are involved in metabolic responses. Synthetic agonists, such as salbutamol, readily discriminate between the three subtypes.

8.3 RECEPTOR STRUCTURES

8.3.1 Binding domains

The experimental strategies adopted for the study of receptor proteins are very similar to those used so successfully for the study of enzymes (Fig. 8.6). Purification of the protein by affinity chromatography (Section 13.9), lectin affinity chromatography (Section 13.9.4) or hydrophobic interaction chromatography (Section 13.5.3) has been particularly successful. Affinity labelling (Section 7.7.2) has also been adopted with success. In the case of the insulin receptor, 4-azido-2-nitrophenyl-[^{125}I]insulin was used as a photoaffinity label. Once the label was bound to the insulin receptor, the receptor–label complex was exposed to ultraviolet light, which converted the azido group to a nitrene, which covalently attached itself to the binding site. An alternative approach for binding site studies is the use of cross-linking agents. In the case of the insulin receptor, [^{125}I]insulin was bound to the receptor and the resulting receptor–insulin complex cross-linked by the use of disuccinimidyl suberate (Fig. 8.7), which reacts with free amino group on both the insulin- and the receptor-binding site. The rationale for the use of the cross-linking agents is that only the cross-linked products (generally only one), containing the [^{125}I]insulin will give information about the receptor. The products are studied by polyacrylamide gel electrophoresis (Section 12.3) in the presence of detergent. In the case of the insulin receptor the cross-linking reagent was found to be linked to an α-subunit. The insulin receptor consists of two α-subunits (molecular mass 84 000 daltons) and two β-subunits (molecular mass 70 000 daltons) linked as a tetramer by disulphide bridges. Hydrophobicity studies revealed that only the two β-subunits span the membrane and protrude into the intracellular region. The two α-subunits are entirely on the outside of the membrane and contain the insulin-binding sites. The N-terminal region of each

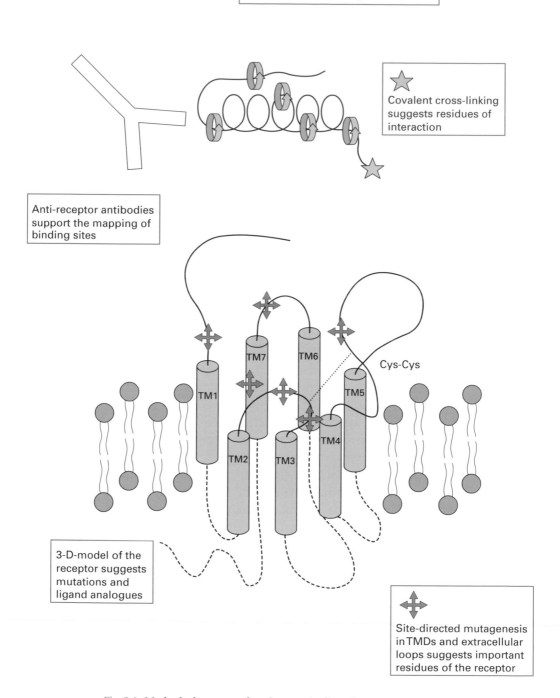

Replacement of certain residues gives information on relevant positions of the ligand

Covalent cross-linking suggests residues of interaction

Anti-receptor antibodies support the mapping of binding sites

TM1
TM2
TM3
TM4
TM5
TM6
TM7

Cys-Cys

3-D-model of the receptor suggests mutations and ligand analogues

Site-directed mutagenesis in TMDs and extracellular loops suggests important residues of the receptor

Fig. 8.6. Methods that are used to characterise ligand–receptor interactions. TMDs, transmembrane domains; 3-D, three-dimensional. (Reproduced by permission of Elsevier Science from A. G. Beck-Sickinger (1996), *Drug Development Today*, **1** (12), 511.)

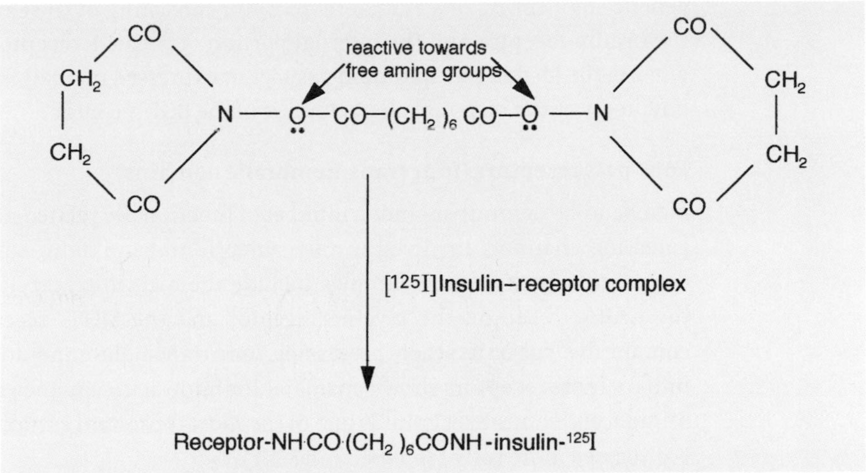

Fig. 8.7. Cross-linking of the insulin receptor with disuccinimidyl suberate.

α-subunit is cysteine rich and contains a binding domain that has similarities to the binding site identified for the epidermal growth factor receptor.

8.3.2 Receptor superfamilies

The general strategies for the investigation of receptor structure have led to the identification of receptor superfamilies that are groups of receptors having similar structures and mechanisms for the transduction of the cellular response. Their classification is based on the number of transmembrane domains the receptor possesses.

Single-pass receptors (one transmembrane domain)

Members of this group include the epidermal growth factor (EGF) receptor, the platelet-derived growth factor (PGDF) receptor and the insulin receptor, which works like a dimer of the EGF or the PGDF receptor, each of which have intrinsic tyrosine kinase activity (Section 8.4.3; see Fig. 8.10). The EGF receptor is a single-chain protein in which the EGF-binding site is near the N-terminal end (see Fig. 8.11). The intracellular C-terminal region contains a region of 250 residues with tyrosine kinase activity that is similar in sequence to that of pp60[v-src], a tyrosine kinase encoded by the Rous sarcoma virus. It also contains a tyrosine residue that is autophosphorylated by the tyrosine kinase domain in response to EGF binding. The insulin receptor, as discussed in the previous section, contains two α and two β subunits but only the β-subunits span the membrane, so that it looks like a dimer of the EGF receptor (see Fig. 8.11). The intracellular β-subunit regions, like that of the EGF receptor, possess tyrosine kinase activity and a tyrosine residue that is autophosphorylated in response to insulin binding. The EGF and insulin receptors are able to cross-phosphorylate each other, confirming their similarity. Further proof of the similarity between these two receptors comes from the genetic engineering of a chimaeric receptor consisting of the external portion of the insulin receptor and the internal portion of the EGF receptor. The chimaera, when embedded in phospholipid vesicles or expressed in a cell line, binds insulin but produces the response characteristic of the EGF receptor.

Four-pass receptors (four transmembrane domains)

Members of this group include a number of functionally related neurotransmitter-gated ion channels involved in fast synaptic transmission, particularly in the central nervous system. Examples include the nicotinic acetylcholine receptor, the $GABA_A$ receptor, the glycine receptor and the $5-HT_3$ receptor. They each contain five subunits, each possessing four transmembrane domains. The subunits of these receptors show considerable amino acid sequence identity. The nicotinic acetylcholine receptor is one of the most thoroughly studied receptors and is discussed more fully later (Section 8.4.1).

Seven-pass receptors (seven transmembrane domains)

Members of this family include the receptors for adrenaline, noradrenaline, dopamine and serotonin, and also rhodopsin, a visual pigment. As the family name implies, the proteins all have seven transmembrane regions within a single protein chain. Affinity and photoaffinity labelling studies have revealed that part of the transmembrane regions forms part of the receptor-binding site for relatively small lipophilic ligands such as adrenaline, but not for peptide ligands such as lutropin. A common feature of these receptors is the glycosylation of asparagine residues near the extracellular N-terminal end.

8.3.3 Receptor mobility

The ability of receptors to interact with other membrane-associated molecules, essential for the process of signal transduction, requires the receptor to diffuse freely within the two-dimensional lipid bilayer. This receptor mobility can be studied by the technique of fluorescence recovery after photobleaching (FRAP), which requires the receptor to be labelled by a fluorescent molecule such as a labelled antibody, lectin or photoaffinity label. Labelled receptors within a small circular region of the membrane (1 to 10 μm^2) are then exposed to an intense attenuated laser beam that irreversibly bleaches the fluorescent receptors within the beam. The subsequent time-dependent increase in fluorescence within this bleached area, due to diffusion into the area of non-bleached fluorescent receptor molecules, is then monitored, allowing the rate of diffusion of the receptors to be calculated. Such studies have revealed that a given receptor can traverse the whole surface of a cell in times ranging from 4 min to 7 h.

8.4 MECHANISMS OF SIGNAL TRANSDUCTION

As previously indicated, cellular receptors have been classified according to the mechanism for the transduction of the original signal initiated by the binding of the first messenger. The three classes – ligand-gated ion channels, activators of G-proteins, and receptors with intrinsic protein kinase enzyme activity – are discussed in turn below.

8.4.1 Ligand-gated ion channels

The characteristic of this class of receptors is that the binding of the first messenger directly triggers the opening (gating) of a cation or anion channel that is part of the total structure of the receptor. Since this mechanism of transduction is independent of any other membrane component or intracellular molecule, the cellular response is virtually spontaneous. This class includes numerous receptors that are involved in signal transmission between neurones, between glia and neurones, and between neurones and muscles.

One of the most thoroughly studied examples of these ion channels is the nicotinic acetylcholine receptor found in large amounts in the eel and electric ray where receptors act cooperatively to produce electric shocks. The receptors are also present at the mammalian skeletal neuromuscular junction where they are located on the membrane of the postsynaptic cell adjacent to the synaptic neurone and are involved in muscle contraction. Nicotinic acetylcholine receptors cause an excitatory response on binding acetylcholine. The snake venom toxin, α-bungarotoxin, binds irreversibly to the receptors, to block the action of acetylcholine. The torpedo or eel receptor consists of five subunits of four types, α, β, γ and δ, with a stoichiometry of $\alpha_2\beta\gamma\delta$, whilst in adult mammalian muscle the γ-subunit is replaced by a homologous ϵ-subunit, giving a stoichiometry of $\alpha_2\beta\epsilon\delta$. Each receptor can bind two molecules of acetylcholine, one on each α-subunit, in a positively cooperative fashion with a Hill coefficient (see Section 7.3.4) of nearly 2, or two molecules of α-bungarotoxin at the acetylcholine-binding sites. Each of the five subunits spans the membrane four times, mainly with α-helical structure, but with some β-structure. The α-helical regions have been designated M1 to M4 and the experimental evidence from photoaffinity labelling studies and the production of point mutations support the view that each of the M2 regions of the five subunits lines the ion channel, with the M1 and M3 regions forming a scaffold to support the channel. Genes encoding the subunits have been cloned and expressed in eggs of *Xenopus laevis*; these cells do not normally express acetylcholine receptors. Hybrid clones have confirmed the importance of all five types of subunit but appear to indicate a central role for the δ-subunit.

Electron microscopy of *Torpedo* electric organ postsynaptic membrane has given an indication of the three-dimensional structure of the receptor. The channel is funnel shaped, with a large proportion of the receptor outside the membrane, protruding into the postsynaptic cleft. The channel is 25 to 30 Å wide at the entrance and only 6.4 Å wide at its narrowest point. Three rings of negatively charged amino acid residues, all on the M2 helices, line the narrow part of the channel and appear to determine its ion selectivity. The importance of these amino acid residues has been confirmed by mutagenesis studies. The distance between the acetylcholine binding site, shown by photoaffinity labelling to be on

(a)

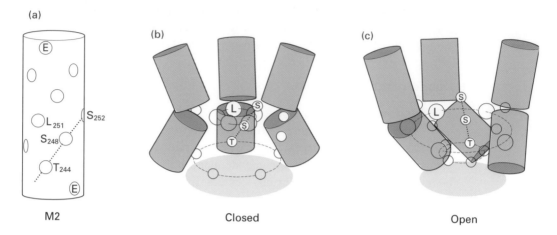

M2   Closed   Open

Fig. 8.8. Proposed mechanism for the opening of the acetylcholine ion channel. The channel is formed by the M2 regions of the five constituent subunits (see the text). (a) The channel-facing part of the M2 region of the α-subunit. Key amino acid residues are two glutamates (E), two serines (S), a threonine (T) and a leucine (L). In the closed state (b), the M2 segments are kinked, with the leucine residues in equivalent positions at the narrow kink-point of the channel. Ligand binding induces a movement of the M2 regions such that the leucine residues move backwards, widening the channel so that its narrowest part (9 to 10 Å) is now created by the serine and threonine residues (c). (Reproduced by permission of Macmillan Magazines Limited from N. Unwin, *Nature* (1995), **373**, 42.)

the N-terminal region of the α-subunits, and the narrowest part of the channel is 50 Å. Details of the mechanism by which acetylcholine binding induces channel opening are not fully known but a model has been proposed (Fig. 8.8).

Patch clamp studies (Section 8.10.2) have enabled the kinetics of channel opening to be evaluated. The whole process may be represented as follows:

$$\text{ACh} + \text{RR}' \rightleftharpoons \text{R AChR}' \rightleftharpoons \text{R AChR}'\text{ACh} \rightleftharpoons (\text{RAChR}' \text{ACh})^*$$
closed   closed   closed   open

where R and R' are the two binding sites, one on each α-subunit, each for one molecule of acetylcholine (ACh).

Measurement of the rate constants for these three reversible processes revealed that the final conformational change from closed to open channel is energetically favoured. Since binding of the acetylcholine molecules is positively cooperative, it follows that, in the presence of high acetylcholine concentrations, which occur on its release from the nerve terminal, the receptor channel should be open. On opening, ions flow through the channel down their electrochemical gradient, leading to a change in membrane potential. The channel remains open until either the acetylcholine is depleted from the synaptic cleft or desensitisation occurs, probably as a consequence of phosphorylation.

All five subunits contain potential sites for phosphorylation between the M3 and M4 regions and phosphorylation of the receptor has been shown to occur at two serine residues on each of the γ- and δ-subunits. Each phosphate group introduces two negatively charged oxygen atoms, which could induce important conformational changes in the receptor structure. Mutagenesis studies of these serine residues have shown that their replacement by non-polar amino acids minimises the susceptibility of the receptor to acetylcholine-induced desensitisation. In contrast, replacement of the serine residues by glutamic acid residues, which contain negatively charged groups, permanently desensitises the receptor. This phosphorylation-induced modulation of receptor function is found in many other types of channel protein, indicating a common mechanism. Thus the nicotinic acetylcholine receptor may be a model for many of these ligand or voltage-gated ion channels, conformational changes in their ion channel being induced either by ligand binding or by changes in membrane potential.

8.4.2 Second messengers – the role of G-proteins

Receptor–ligand binding studies have shown that many receptors, especially those of the seven-pass superfamily (Section 8.3.2), are linked to second messengers by a family of membrane-associated proteins that can bind GTP and GDP and are known collectively as G-proteins. The essential components of this transduction pathway are a receptor, a G-protein and an ion channel or an enzyme (effector) that generates a second messenger such as cyclic AMP, inositol trisphosphate or diacylglycerol. It has been estimated that approximately 3% to 4% of all the genes encoded by the human genome are devoted to receptors linked to G-proteins.

G-proteins are heterotrimeric, consisting of one each of the α-, β- and γ-subunits, which are loosely attached to the inner surface of the cellular membrane. In the normal resting state, the G-protein consists of the trimer, with a molecule of GDP bound to the α-subunit. When the receptor–ligand complex interacts by diffusion translocation and binds to the G-protein it induces the dissociation of GDP to form a transient 'empty state'. This then binds GTP and, in the presence of Mg^{2+}, triggers a conformational change in the α-subunit, which dissociates into a free GTP-linked α-subunit (GTPα) leaving the $\beta\gamma$-subunits as a dimer. In the case of a receptor using the cyclic AMP second messenger system, for example the β-adrenergic receptor, the GTPα subunit binds to inactive adenylyl cyclase, resulting in its activation and the conversion of ATP to cyclic AMP (Fig. 8.9). The GTPα subunit also possesses intrinsic GTPase activity that is activated by receptor binding. Hydrolysis of GTP to GDP terminates the activation of adenylyl cyclase and facilitates the reassociation of the α-subunit with the $\beta\gamma$ dimer.

The response of the binding of an agonist, partial agonist and antagonist to the receptor can be rationalised by this need to form a ternary complex with a G-protein and by application of the two-state model of receptors. Thus, if the receptor existed as an equilibrium mixture of an inactive or resting state (R_r), which could not interact with a G-protein to form a ternary complex, and an active state (R_a), which could form a ternary complex, then agonists would bind to the R_a conformation, disturbing the equilibrium between R_r and R_a states, which is

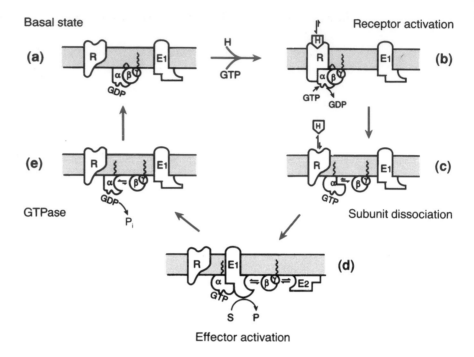

Fig. 8.9. G-protein-mediated transmembrane signal transduction. (a) The basal state consists of GDP tightly bound to the α-subunit of the heterotrimer. The receptor (R) is unoccupied and the effector (E_1), e.g. adenylyl cyclase, is inactive. (b) Ligand binding induces a conformational change, resulting in the replacement of GDP by GTP. (c) GTP binding causes the G-protein to dissociate from the receptor and the α-subunit–GTP complex (GTPα) to dissociate from the βγ-subunits. (d) The GTPα complex binds to, and activates, the effector. The βγ-subunit complex may activate a second effector (E_2) (e) The GTPase activity of the α-subunit causes the hydrolysis of the GTP to GDP and the deactivation of, and dissociation from, the effector. The GDPα reassociates with the βγ-complex, returning the system to its basal state. Examples of effectors E, and E_2 include adenylyl cyclase and phospholipase C. (Reproduced by permission of Elsevier Science, from J.R. Hepler and A.G. Gilman (1992), *Trends in Biochemical Sciences*, **17**, 383.)

normally in favour of R_r, in favour of the R_a state. Competitive antagonists would bind to both the R_r and R_a conformations, stabilising them both equally, and have little effect on the equilibrium. Partial agonist binding would result in only a small, but detectable and characteristic, displacement of the equilibrium in favour of the R_a state. Importantly, the normal equilibrium between R_r and R_a contains a small number of the active R_a receptors, which are responsible for the basal, low level of signal produced in the absence of ligand. The model envisages the existence of a fourth category of ligand, termed an inverse agonist, which would displace the equilibrium below its resting state, thereby reducing the basal level of signal.

A variety of methods have been used to study G-proteins and their interaction with receptors. Examples include the following.

The use of analogues of GTP that are poorly hydrolysed, for example [^{35}S]GTPγS.

The use of toxins that act by virtue of the fact that they are ADP ribosyl transferases and stimulate the transfer of the ADP-ribose moiety of NAD$^+$ to G-proteins, thereby 'fixing' them in either the active or inactive state. In practice ^{32}P-labelled NAD$^+$ is used.

The use of *N*-ethylmaleimide as a reversible inhibitor of α-subunits, which it selectively alkylates.

The use of photoaffinity labelling using analogues of GTP such as GTP-azidoanilide, which is converted to a nitrene by light and covalently labels the α-subunit (see Section 7.7.2).

The use of antibodies raised to each subunit.

The use of gene cloning and site-directed mutagenesis techniques and expression of the clones in appropriate cell lines.

The production of chimaeras.

The synthesis and use of a range of ligand analogues to identify the structural and kinetic features of receptor–ligand binding. The advent of combinatorial chemistry, which allows the simultaneous synthesis of a very large number of structurally related compounds, has increased the importance of this approach.

Studies have revealed a very complex picture of the G-proteins. Twenty different α-subunits, 6 β-subunits and 12 γ-subunits have been identified. The potential number of different Gαβγ functional trimers is therefore very large. Eight families of G-proteins have been classified on the basis of their action. The G$_s$ subgroup stimulates adenylyl cyclase whilst the G$_i$ subgroup inhibits the enzyme, the G$_q$ subgroup couples receptors to phospholipase C and the C$_o$ subgroup couples receptors to Ca^{2+} channels. Contrary to the indication of early studies on G-proteins, the Gβγ dimer may, like Gα, have a direct receptor binding and regulation role including the activation of some forms of adenylyl cyclase and phospholipase C. A given G-protein may be activated by a large number of different receptors, whilst a given receptor may interact with different G-proteins and/or produce more than one response. Thus adrenergic receptors can stimulate two second messenger pathways, by the activation of G$_s$α in the case of β-adrenoceptors, or G$_q$α in the case of α-adrenoceptors. Equally, different agonists binding to a given receptor subtype can activate different pathways via G-proteins. Whilst at first sight this may appear surprising, there are possible mechanisms to rationalise this phenomenon. The rationale lies in the fact that agonist binding induces conformational changes in both the receptor protein and the G-protein effector. Subtle differences in these conformational changes could be highly significant to the subsequent activation process. Since agonists differ in their intrinsic activity for the receptor, it is possible to visualise strong (high affinity) agonists that could induce conformational changes recognised by several G-protein subtypes, whilst weak agonists could stimulate only a single pathway. It is known from point mutation studies, for example, that the α$_2$-adrenergic receptor couples to G$_i$ protein via the second intracellular loop whilst coupling to G_s protein is via the third intracellular loop. The ability of a given receptor–ligand complex to initiate more than one response is referred to as agonist trafficking, since it appears to be a function of the agonist rather than the receptor per se. The crystal structures of $G\alpha\beta\gamma$ and $G\beta\gamma$ have been determined. The β-subunit within $G\beta\gamma$ has a 'propeller' structure consisting of four antiparallel β-strands that can interact with the γ-unit and, in principle, more than one type of α-subunit. The N-terminal end of the α-subunit is involved in binding to $G\beta\gamma$ whilst the C-terminal end binds to the receptor. The GTPase domain consists of five α-helical and six β-sheet structures.

G-proteins are involved in the production of second messengers in addition to cyclic AMP. The activated G-protein G_q activates the effector enzyme phospholipase C, which cleaves phosphatidylinositol 4,5-bisphosphate, a component of the cell membrane, to give the two second messengers inositol 1,4,5-trisphosphate and diacylglycerol. Inositol 1,4,5-trisphosphate stimulates the release of Ca^{2+} from the endoplasmic reticulum which in turn activates a very large number of enzymes via the action of the calcium-binding protein calmodulin. Diacylglycerol, which remains attached to the membrane, activates protein kinase C, which is also membrane-bound and responsible for the modulation of the activities of several enzymes. Among the enzymes controlled by these two second messengers is a group of phosphoinositide kinases that have key roles in a wide range of biochemical processes ranging from lysosomal targeting to membrane trafficking and the mediation of the effects of growth factors.

In addition to the stimulation of second messenger release, G-proteins can also regulate ion channels. The muscarinic acetylcholine receptor can control the opening of K^+ channels in the heart via a G_K protein, although it itself contains no intrinsic ion channel, in contrast to the nicotinic acetylcholine receptor.

The heterogeneity of G-proteins and the diversity of the responses they may induce via the transduction pathways, offer two main biochemical advantages, namely amplification and control. Each $G\alpha$–GTP complex on binding, for example to adenylyl cyclase, may result in the synthesis or release of many molecules of second messenger, each of which may induce multiple responses (amplification) from the other components of the cascade system to which they are linked (Section 8.5). Control is exerted at the level of the receptor by virtue of the fact that binding of the $G\alpha$–GTP complex to the receptor results in a decreased affinity for the ligand (increased K_d), thus encouraging the release of the ligand, whilst hydrolysis of GTP to GDP reverses the affinity change. Overall, G-protein-mediated signal transduction allows cross-talk between different transduction pathways to reflect changes in cellular priorities.

8.4.3 Receptors with intrinsic protein kinase activity

An important group of cellular receptors, including those that have the common feature of binding growth factors as the first messenger, has the important property of possessing intrinsic tyrosine kinase activity. This activity is switched on by ligand binding, resulting in both the autophosphorylation of a tyrosine residue

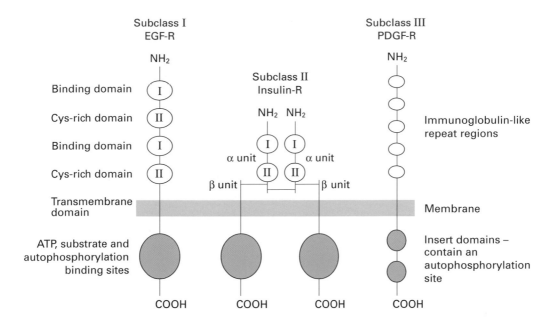

Fig. 8.10. Diagrammatic representation of receptor tyrosine kinase subclasses. The EGF subclass contains two ligand-binding domains that are located in juxtaposition so that the ligand binds in the cleft between the two domains. The two cysteine-rich domains are both located near the membrane surface. On ligand binding, both the EGF and the PDGF subclass receptors dimerise so that the intracellular tyrosine kinase domains possess elevated activity and enhanced ligand binding affinity relative to the monomeric forms. The insulin subclass receptors are effectively dimeric, but, as with the subclasses I and III, there is allosteric interaction between the two $\alpha\beta$ halves of each receptor on ligand binding. The tyrosine kinase domains of the three subclasses show the greatest degree of homology between the subclasses.

within the intracellular region of the receptor protein and in the activation of the tyrosine kinase activity of the intracellular domain towards intracellular proteins. Three subgroups of the receptors are known (Fig. 8.10), characterised by the EGF receptor (Fig. 8.11), the insulin receptor and the PDGF receptor. They each have a large, glycosylated, extracellular domain that binds the ligand monovalently, an intracellular region that contains a tyrosine residue that can be auto-phosphorylated, and a tyrosine-kinase-binding domain that binds and phosphorylates other intracellular proteins. These intracellular proteins possess a similar binding domain for the autophosphorylated receptor tyrosine kinase, referred to as SH2 domains, which are homologous to a non-catalytic region of the C-*src* protooncogene. Proteins activated by this route include phosphatidylinositol 3-kinase and phospholipase C; the activity of the latter enzyme may also be controlled via a G-protein (Section 8.3.2). Once activated, these enzymes initiate a cascade of events resulting in the final cellular response. The autophosphorylation of the EGF receptor, which appears to release an intrinsic binding constraint for these SH2 domains, requires the initial dimerisation of the receptor, which

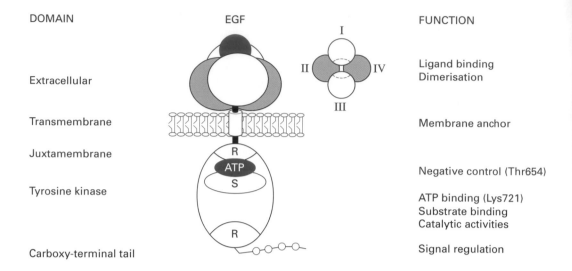

Fig. 8.11. The proposed structure–function topology of the EGF receptor. The cleft between domains II and III determines the EGF binding affinity. Domains II and IV are cysteine rich. S and R refer to sites for substrate and regulatory factors. (Reproduced by permission of Cell Press from A. Ullrich and J. Schlessinger (1990), *Cell*, **61**, 205.)

explains why the EGF and insulin receptors can activate each other by cross-phos-phorylation. Autophosphorylation increases the V_{max} values but does not alter the K_m for these intracellular proteins. The importance of this autophosphorylation to the expression of the tyrosine kinase activity has led to receptor tyrosine kinases being called membrane-associated allosteric enzymes. One of the characteristic features of receptor tyrosine kinases is their rapid internalisation by endocytosis after their autophosphorylation. The importance of this endocytic process to the control of receptor activity is discussed in Section 8.11.

Complementary to the tyrosine kinase group of receptors is a second group of protein kinase receptors characterised by their ability to autophosphorylate serine and threonine residues in the intracellular domain of the receptor. These protein serine/threonine kinase receptors are specific for members of the transforming growth factor (TGF) β superfamily, which regulates growth, differentiation, migration and cell adhesion. They are classified into a number of subgroups on the basis of their structure, particularly their serine/threonine kinase domain. They are all single transmembrane receptors, which on binding of their ligand form heterooligomeric complexes between subgroup types. This stimulates autophosphorylation and activation of the serine/threonine kinase activity towards other cytosolic proteins that are components of the transduction pathway.

Recently a histidine protein kinase receptor has been identified as a component of the chemotactic signalling system. Receptors for the cytokines, which include the interferons, monokines, chemokines and lymphokines, lack inherent autoprotein kinase activity, but binding of the cytokine to the receptors stimulates dimerisation of the receptor with tyrosine kinase receptors, resulting in the phosphorylation of tyrosine residues on the cytokine receptor intracellular domain and the activation of tyrosine kinase activity towards other components of the transduction pathway.

Like the G-proteins, receptor protein kinases stimulate numerous transduction pathways by means of phosphorylation. The downstream members of these transduction pathways include the phospholipases and phosphoinositide kinases, which are also involved in the G-protein transduction pathways. Among a number of effectors unique to the protein kinases is Ras, a membrane-bound guanosine-binding protein with intrinsic GTPase activity, involved in cell growth and development in all eukaryotes. Crucial to the control of transduction by the protein kinases is the existence of a group of protein phosphatases that can either deactivate or activate pathways by dephosphorylation. Phosphatases specific for tyrosine and others that act on serine and threonine as well as tyrosine have been identified. Some are purely cytoplasmic whilst others are receptor-like with a transmembrane domain. Most have two phosphatase domains for reasons that are not yet clear, but their specificity may be linked to interaction between the two sites. The activity of the phosphatases appears to be linked to their own phosphorylation and a significant number have an SH2 domain for the receptor tyrosine kinases.

The role of Ca^{2+} in transduction pathways involving both G-proteins and protein kinases is very important. Many cellular responses to first messengers are linked to changes in cellular Ca^{2+} concentrations. Calmodulin is one of a number of molecules that sense changes in Ca^{2+} concentration and transduce the information to other effectors. Cells have two sources of Ca^{2+}: extracellular and organellar. Ca^{2+} levels are 10 000-fold higher outside the cell than inside, hence there is a large electrochemical gradient favouring entry. Influx is regulated by various forms of channel include voltage and receptor-mediated forms. Ca^{2+} excretion from cells is mediated by a number of different pumps, including the P-type Ca^{2+}-ATPase discussed in Section 8.10.3. These opposing influx–eflux mechanisms result in pulses of Ca^{2+} and there is a possibility that Ca^{2+} signalling may be linked to the frequency of these pulses rather than to their absolute value.

8.4.4 **Receptor desensitisation**

Prolonged exposure of a receptor to its ligand commonly results in its desensitisation, characterised by a reduction or termination of the cellular response despite the continued presence of the ligand. There appears to be a number of mechanisms responsible for this loss of activity. A common one is the phosphorylation of the receptor in the case of the ligand-induced ion channels and G-protein linked receptors. Phosphorylation introduces a polar phosphate group, which induces conformational changes that are deleterious to the normal functioning of the receptor. Thus, in the case of the β-adrenergic receptor, its phosphorylation uncouples it from its G-protein. Phosphorylation of the receptor may also trigger its internalisation by endocytosis, a process that is linked directly to the control of receptor numbers. Desensitisation and down regulation of receptors may also be linked to the generation of cyclic AMP and cyclic AMP-dependent changes in mRNA levels for the receptor protein. Cyclic AMP is known to regulate the transcription of some genes via a DNA element called the cyclic AMP response element.

8.5 SIGNAL AMPLIFICATION

It was pointed out above (Section 8.4.2) that one of the biochemical advantages of linking receptor occupancy to cellular response via second messengers, such as cyclic AMP, is that it affords the opportunity for amplification of the signal produced by the first messenger. The mobilisation of glycogen as glucose 1-phosphate provides a good illustration of this principle. The components of the biochemical cascade are the receptor, the ligand, a G_s protein, adenylyl cyclase and cyclic AMP, protein kinase, phosphorylase kinase, phosphorylase and glycogen. Cyclic AMP released from adenylyl cyclase activates cyclic AMP-dependent protein kinase, which in its inactive form is a tetramer consisting of two regulatory (R) and two catalytic (C) subunits. Two cyclic AMP (cAMP) molecules bind to each of the R subunits in a positively cooperative manner, causing them to dissociate:

$$R_2C_2 \quad + 4cAMP \rightleftharpoons 2(R - cAMP) + 2C$$
inactive   active

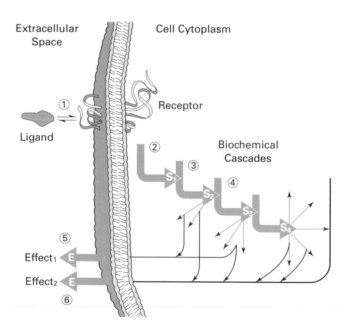

Fig. 8.12. A schematic representation of cytosolic biochemical cascades linking drug–receptor interaction at the cell surface membrane to cellular response. The final cellular response may be intracellular or extracellular. E, effect; S, substrates. (Reproduced by permission of Blackwell Science from T. Kenakin (1997), *Molecular Pharmacology: A Short Course*, p. 126.)

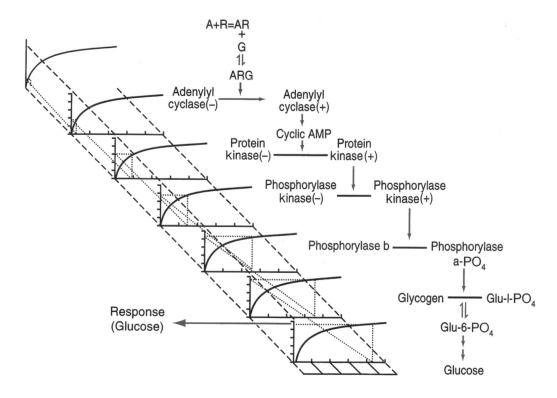

Fig. 8.13. A typical biochemical cascade showing the stages from the initial binding of the first messenger (A) to its cell-surface receptor (R), the resultant activation of a G-protein (G) by the AR complex, through the activation of adenylyl cyclase and the release of cyclic AMP to the final cellular response, namely the release of glucose. Each step in the cascade is represented as a hyperbolic function. The initial low receptor occupancy triggers a sequence of progressively amplified responses so that the final release of glucose is a nearly maximal response. (Reproduced by permission of Blackwell Science from T. Kenakin (1997), *Molecular Pharmacology: A Short Course*, p. 122.)

The active units act as a kinase and in the presence of ATP phosphorylate and thereby activate glycogen phosphorylase kinase:

$$\text{phosphorylase kinase} + \text{ATP} \xrightleftharpoons[\text{}]{\text{C unit}} \text{phosphorylated phosphorylase kinase} + \text{ADP}$$
$$\text{inactive} \qquad\qquad\qquad\qquad\qquad \text{active}$$

The activated glycogen phosphorylase kinase activates phosphorylase b by phosphorylation to give phosphorylase a and it in turn degrades glycogen to glucose 1-phosphate. Phosphorylase b can also metabolise glycogen but it requires high concentration of cyclic AMP as an allosteric effector. The phosphorylated phosphorylase a is far less dependent on cyclic AMP and has a decreased K_m for inorganic phosphate. Both phosphorylases a and b are believed to exist in two conformations, T and R, such that in phosphorylase b the T/R ratio is 3000 whilst in phosphorylase a it is reduced to 10. Hence phosphorylation enhances the formation of the catalytically favourable R state. At each step in the phosphorylase cascade there is at least 100-fold amplification, moving the associated dose–response curve nearer the maximum (Figs. 8.12 and 8.13). Thus occupation of only a very small percentage of the membrane receptors is needed to produce a response approaching the maximum. It is evident that the larger the number of components in the cascade, the greater the potential amplification.

The mobilisation of glycogen is reversed by glycogen synthetase, which is inactivated by phosphorylation and activated by a phosphatase that simultaneously inactivates glycogen phosphorylase kinase and glycogen phosphorylase a. The process of controlling the activity of proteins by phosphorylation and dephosphorylation is extremely common. Phosphorylation can be studied by the use of $[32_P]$ATP followed by the separation of the phosphorylated products by isoelectric focusing (Section 12.3.4). Control of enzyme activity by the kinase/phosphatase principle is found in a broad range of organisms, indicating its early evolution. It operates with the net consumption of ATP, but with considerable gain in sensitivity, amplification and flexibility, which more than compensates for the ATP consumed.

8.6 KEY TERMS

agonist	photobleaching	non-specific binding
agonist trafficking	G-protein	partial agonist
amphipathic	intrinsic efficacy	PDGF receptor
amplification	insulin receptor	receptor occupancy
antagonist	intrinsic protein kinase enzyme	receptor superfamilies
cascades	activity	receptor trafficking
chimaeric receptor	inverse agonist	Scatchard equation
competitive reversible antagonists	ion channel	Scatchard plot
conformational induction	irreversible antagonists	second messenger
control	K_d	seven-pass receptors
down regulation	ligand	single-pass receptors
desensitisation	ligand blockers	signal transduction
ED_{50}, EC_{50}	ligand-gated channel	spare receptors
EGF receptor	membrane-associated allosteric	surface plasmon resonance
endocytosis	enzymes	transduced
equilibrium dialysis	mobile receptor	transduction
evanescent wave	nicotinic acetylcholine receptor	two-state theory of receptors
first messenger	non-competitive reversible	up regulation
fluorescence recovery after	antagonists	ultrafiltration

8.7 MEMBRANE TRANSPORT PROCESSES

Cellular and organellar membranes act to preserve the internal environment of the cytoplasm and the organelle, respectively. Large differences in ion and nutrient concentration that exist across membranes are essential for effective cellular function and it is the dual function of membranes to maintain such gradients whilst permitting selecting transport to meet cellular needs. Membranes contain small aqueous pores that allow the passage of water and other small molecules such as urea. Transport of larger molecules across a membrane must occur via either the phospholipid bilayer or the proteins that are inserted into it. Kinetic studies of these two options have characterised three types of transport process for small to medium-size ions and molecules:

(i) *Physical diffusion*: molecules cross the phospholipid bilayer from a high concentration to a low concentration until equilibrium of concentration is achieved.

(ii) *Facilitated transport*: molecules associate with a specific carrier protein and are transported across the membrane from high concentration to low concentration so as to equilibrate their concentration.

(iii) *Active transport*: molecules or ions associate with a specific carrier protein and are transported against a concentration gradient (i.e. from low to high concentration) which, since it is an endergonic process, requires the expenditure of energy via a coupled reaction.

For large molecules, such as proteins and structures such as low density lipoprotein, viruses and bacteria, totally different transport strategies are needed. The processes of receptor-mediated endocytosis involves a small region of the membrane engulfing the molecule or particle, bound to a specific receptor, to form a vesicle (endosome) which, when internalised, commonly fuses with a lysosome, resulting in either the degradation of the molecule or particle. Exocytosis is the reverse of endocytosis and is important in, for example, the secretion of proteins from the Golgi complex out of a cell. Transport processes are commonly studied by the use of radiolabelled solutes and isolated membrane preparations or artificial membranes. Plasma membrane preparations may be obtained either by disrupting the cell by gentle homogenisation in a hypotonic medium or by nitrogen cavitation, in which nitrogen gas is forced into the cell under pressure and the pressure then released causing the cell to disrupt. The membrane fragment of choice is isolated by isopycnic centrifugation (Section 5.6.2). Organellar membranes are obtained from the isolated organelle in a similar way. Nuclei and mitochondria have a double membrane structure that may be separated by the use of detergents. One of the problems to be considered in membrane isolation is the potential for the isolation process to cause the membrane to be 'inside out', i.e. its orientation is the reverse of that in the intact cell.

8.8 **PHYSICAL DIFFUSION**

Physical diffusion, also called passive diffusion, involves the molecule partitioning from its aqueous environment into the lipid bilayer and crossing the membrane to a region of lower concentration. The process is driven by the concentration gradient and will continue until it is zero. Clearly the process does not involve any form of ligand binding and hence does not fit within the broad theme of this chapter. However, its main characteristics are discussed as it is of biochemical importance.

The rate of physical diffusion of a molecule across a membrane is described by Fick's law, which states simply that the rate of diffusion is proportional to the concentration gradient of the molecule across the membrane:

$$\text{rate of physical diffusion} = P(C_{\text{out}} - C_{\text{in}}) \tag{8.10}$$

where P is the permeability (or diffusion) coefficient of the molecule, C_{in} is the concentration of molecule on the inside of the membrane, and C_{out} is the concentration of molecule on the outside of the membrane.

It can be seen that when C_{out} is equal to C_{in}, i.e. when the concentration gradient is zero, physical diffusion will cease. The diffusion coefficient is a measure of the ability of the molecule to pass across each unit area of the membrane from the aqueous external environment to the non-polar (hydrophobic) region of the membrane and back into the internal aqueous environment. Its value for a given molecule should therefore be related to its partition coefficient between oil and water. In practice, partition coefficients are commonly measured between octanol and water and expressed as a logarithm in order to convert the value to a small number (positive or negative).

Experimental studies have revealed that small, non-polar molecules that are lipophilic readily cross membranes by physical diffusion. The rate is related directly to the concentration of the molecule (a first-order process) and is non-saturable. Moreover, several molecules crossing the membrane by physical diffusion can do so independently of each other, i.e. the process is non-competitive. If the diffusing molecule is a weak acid or weak base it will exist as an equilibrium mixture of ionised and unionised forms defined by the Henderson–Hasselbalch equation (equation 1.27, Section 1.4.5). Thus a weak acid will exist as -COOH and -COO$^-$ and a weak base as -NH$_2$ and -$\overset{+}{\text{N}}$H$_3$. The ionised forms will less lipophilic and hence not be expected to diffuse physically across the membrane. This is the basis of the pH hypothesis of physical diffusion of weak electrolytes, which states that the pK_a (or pK_b) of the electrolyte and the prevailing pH will determine physical diffusion in addition to its partition coefficient. Physical diffusion of the unionised species will continue until its concentration (as opposed to the sum of ionised and unionised species) is the same on both sides of the membrane. Of course, some of the transported unionised species will revert to the ionised form in order to establish the correct balance between ionised and unionised in accordance with the Henderson–Hassalbalch equation and the prevailing pH. Thus,

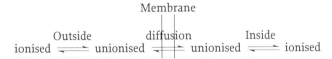

If there is a significant difference in pH on the two sides, the phenomenon of ion trapping can cause a significant imbalance of total concentration of the molecule on the two sides.

Distribution coefficients (D) are similar to partition coefficients but take into account the proportion of the unionised species at the prevailing pH. Log D values are measured for convenience in order to obtain a small number.

Physical diffusion is very important for the passage of drugs across membranes. This includes the processes for their absorption from the gastrointestinal tract, distribution to body tissues and excretion via the kidneys. Lipophilic drugs are generally well absorbed from the gut and retained by the kidneys, and require the process of metabolism to polar metabolites to intervene to facilitate their excretion from the body. Most drugs are organic molecules with relative molecular masses in the region 200 to 400 and in general the pH hypothesis does explain their transport characteristics. However, some drugs that are ionised at physiological pH have been shown to cross membranes, with all the characteristics of physical diffusion. One such drug is proxicromil, an anti-asthma compound, with a pK_a of 1.93. At pH 7, therefore, it exists entirely as the anion but is readily absorbed and distributed. Radiolabel studies have revealed that it crosses membranes as an ion-pair with a counter cation, with a stoichiometry of 1, 2 or 3 with mono-, di- and tri-valent cations, respectively. This process of ion-pairing identifies the importance of an electrical potential gradient as well as a concentration gradient in the diffusion process. Studies of the physical diffusion of lipophilic drugs with a very broad range of molecular structures have revealed a sigmoidal rather than linear relationship between the rate of diffusion and diffusion coefficient. This indicates that the model of physical diffusion, which requires the partitioning of the molecule from an aqueous environment into a lipid environment, is perhaps too simple and ignores both the presence of an unstirred water layer at the surface of the membrane and local variations of pH within this water layer.

8.9 **FACILITATED TRANSPORT**

Some non-polar molecules cross membranes at a rate that is considerably greater than that predicted by Fick's law for physical diffusion. One example is glucose. Its transport across erythrocyte membranes has been shown to obey a hyperbolic relationship with glucose concentration and to display saturation kinetics. This is characteristic of facilitated transport in which a membrane-bound carrier protein, variously termed a transporter, carrier or translocase, is involved. It has a specific binding site exposed on the external side of the membrane to which the molecule to be transported first binds. This binding can be characterised by a K_m or K_d value, exactly analogous to that for enzymes and membrane receptors, and a V_{max} or J_{max} (maximum flux) value, which is the observed flux when all the binding sites on the transporter are occupied. K_m and K_d are numerically equal to the concentration of substrate when the observed transport rate is half the maximum rate. Hence

$$\text{transport rate, } V = \frac{J_{max}[S]}{K_m + [S]} \tag{8.11}$$

where [S] is the substrate concentration on the external side of the membrane.

Typically for this type of system, the transporter displays both specificity and competition. For the transport of D-glucose across the erythrocyte membrane, the K_d is 1.5 mM whilst the L-glucose is it 3000 mM. The transporter will convey other D configured monosaccharides such as galactose and mannose, structurally related

(a) Carrier ionophore   (b) Channel-forming ionophore

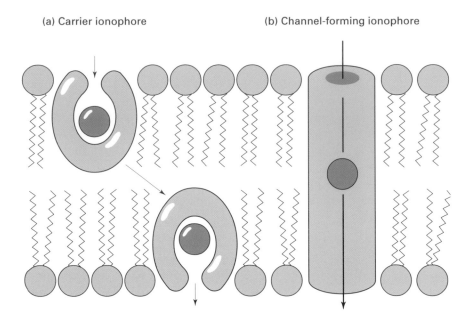

Fig. 8.14. The diagrammatic representation of the modes of ion transport by ionophores. (a) Carrier ionophores such as valinomycin coordinate the ion, diffuse through the lipid bilayer and release the ion. (b) Channel-forming ionophores such as gramicidin span the membrane with a channel through which the ions diffuse. (Reproduced by permission of John Wiley and Sons Inc. from D. Voet and J. G. Voet (1990), *Biochemistry*.)

to D-glucose. When two such sugars are exposed simultaneously to the glucose transporter, they will display classical competitive inhibition towards each other (Section 7.3.8), confirming the availability of a limited number of transport sites.

Facilitated transport operates along a concentration gradient and, like physical diffusion, cannot go against one. In the case of glucose transport in erythrocytes and liver, once inside the cell, the glucose is phosphorylated to glucose 6-phosphate, thereby helping to maintain the concentration gradient for glucose. By analogy with ion trapping discussed earlier, this process is referred to a metabolic trapping. The glucose transporter has been purified and five forms identified. All have approximately 500 amino acid residues and possess a high degree of sequence identity. Each is a glycoprotein with 12 α-helical membrane-spanning regions that are thought to constitute a hydrophilic channel through which the glucose passes. The precise transport mechanism is an example of a gated pore. Studies of the glucose transporter, in which glucose derivatives with substituents on the free hydroxyl groups were used as the substrate, have revealed that the C1 hydroxyl must be free for binding on the external side of the transporter, whilst the C6 hydroxyl is required for binding on the internal side. Such studies lead to the conclusion that binding of the glucose via the C1 hydroxyl triggers a conformational change in the structure of the channel (gate), closing it on the outside and simultaneously opening it on the inside. The glucose molecule then dissoci-

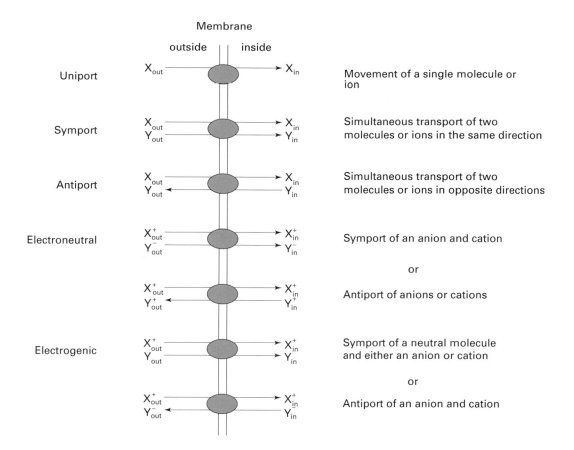

Fig. 8.15. Possible profiles of facilitated transport of molecules or ions.

ates from the binding site, triggering conformational changes that re-expose the external binding site. The sensitivity of glucose uptake to insulin is believed to be due to the ability of the insulin to release glucose transporters from storage vesicles. Thus, in the presence of insulin, the K_d for glucose is unchanged but the maximal uptake rate is increased 10-fold.

A number of antibiotics such as valinomycin and gramicidin facilitate the transport of ions across membranes by a mechanism that resembles facilitated transport. The two antibiotics are examples of ionophores, which are substances that enhance the permeability of membranes to specific ions. Valinomycin is a cyclic compound based on the three repeated units of L-Val-D-hydroxyisovaleric acid-D-Val-L-lactic acid. The six valine residues coordinate a K^+ with octahedral geometry and the resulting ionophore $-K^+$ complex diffuses across the membrane and releases the K^+ on the other side. The uncomplexed ionophore then diffuses back to the extracellular side of the membrane and repeats the K^+ transfer process (Fig. 8.14). In contrast, gramicidin, which is a 15-residue polypeptide, dimerises to form a transmembrane channel through which K^+ can diffuse selectively. The two mechanisms by which the ionophores operate can be easily distinguished experimentally owing to the relative insensitivity of the channel formers to reduced temperature.

Mediated transport, including active facilitated transport, can be classified in two main ways (Fig. 8.15):

(i) Based on the stoichiometry and direction of the transported species:
    Uniport: movement of a single molecular species at a time.
    Symport: simultaneous movement of two molecular or ionic species in the same direction.
    Antiport: simultaneous movement of two molecular or ionic species in opposite directions.
(ii) Based on the electrical consequences of the transport process:
    Electrogenic: results in a net movement of charge and an increase in electrical potential across the membrane.
    Electroneutral: no net change in charge as a consequence of the transport. Thus either symport results in the transport of an anion and cation or antiport of similarly charged ions.

8.10 ACTIVE TRANSPORT AND ION CHANNELS

8.10.1 Energetic considerations

The transport processes discussed so far all operate down a concentration gradient, resulting in a positive entropy change and a negative free energy change. In contrast, some other transport mechanisms can operate against a concentration gradient, provided a suitable compensatory free energy source is available. This coupling of endergonic and exergonic processes is the characteristic of active transport. It is generally associated with a carrier system. Active transport very commonly involves the transmembrane movement of ions and hence is associated with the prevailing membrane potential, $\Delta \Psi$. The free energy change associated with ion transport depends on both the relative concentration of ions $[X^+]$ on the inside and outside of the membrane and the prevailing membrane potential (Section 1.2.5):

$$\Delta G^0 = {}^-nF\Delta\Psi - RT\ln\left(\frac{[X^+]_{out}}{[X^+]_{in}}\right) \tag{8.12}$$

where n is the charge on the transported species and F is the Faraday constant $(0.0965\,\mathrm{kmol^{-1}\,_mV^{-1}})$.

Whether or not the free energy change will be negative (exergonic reaction) will depend upon the relative size of the two expressions in the equation. If ΔG^0 is positive (endergonic reaction) the reaction could only proceed if it were coupled to a free-energy-releasing process (ΔG^0 negative) such as the hydrolysis of ATP. Such coupled transport mechanisms are referred to as active transport and are dependent upon the coupling of the transport to cell metabolism. They are therefore sensitive to metabolic poisons that block the synthesis of ATP. Some of the active transport systems are said to be primary in that the transport process is directly coupled to an energy-releasing process such as the hydrolysis of ATP. In secondary active transport systems the energy required to transport against a concentration gradient is coupled to the movement of a second molecule or ion down a concentration gradient. In this case the negative free energy change associated with the movement of the second species down a concentration gradient is used to drive the transport of the first species with a positive free energy change. For both primary and secondary active transport the precise molecular mechanisms of transport must explain how the 'downhill' transport of the first species is physically prevented by the coupled reaction. The explanation must lie in terms of gated channels and free energy barriers. In the case of the Na^+, K^+-ATPase system to be considered later, the explanation lies partly in the relative affinities of the binding sites on the carrier for the transported species.

8.10.2 **Patch clamp studies**

Although cells contain an equal number of anions and cations and are electrically neutral, the concentration of individual ions is often grossly different within the cell relative to the external environment. This is true of organic anions and a number of cations such as K^+, Na^+, Ca^{2+}, and Mg^{2+}. As an example, the approximate basal concentration of K^+ and Na^+ in mammalian cells is 140 mM and 10 mM, respectively, whilst the corresponding extracellular concentrations are 5 mM and 150 mM. These large ion gradients are maintained by active transport systems.

Owing to differences in the permeability of the membrane to different ions, most cells possess a membrane potential such that the inside of the cell is negative relative to the outside. The membrane potential in resting cells is in the range -10 to -560 mV. Its precise value is dictated by the Nernst equation (Section 1.2.5). When this potential is related to the thickness of the cell membrane (approximately 4 nm), the potential gradient is as high as $20\,000$ V cm^{-1} which is a large driving force for the movement of ions across the membrane, complementary to the drive by concentration gradients. The transmembrane transport of ions and the presence of the associated electrical activity form the basis of two experimental techniques for the study of ion transport in addition to those already discussed based on the study of the associated protein and its conformational changes:

(i) *Ion fluxes*: the study of the rate of concurrent movement of ions across a unit area of membrane. The technique most commonly involves the use of radioactive isotope forms of the ions being studied and the time-related changes in intra- and extracellular ion concentrations. Studies have revealed that with the Na^+, K^+-ATPase antiport transport system three Na^+ are exchanged for two K^+.

(ii) *Patch clamp study of ion channels*: a more detailed way of measuring ion fluxes across the membrane was developed by Bert Sakmann and Erwin Neher in the late 1970s. The technique involves a glass micropipette with a tip diameter in the order of micrometres, which is brought into contact with the

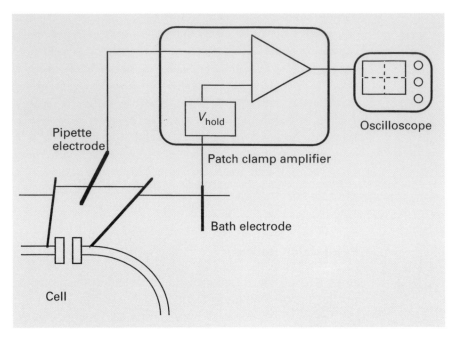

Fig. 8.16. Diagram of a patch clamp set-up in voltage mode. The potential between a bath electrode and a pipette electrode is compared with a reference potential V_{hold}. Current is injected via a feedback circuit until the two potentials are equal. Ion flow across the patch membrane is therefore represented by the required current injected to maintain V_{hold} across the two electrodes. (Reproduced by permission of E. Molleman, University of Hertfordshire.)

membrane of a cell. The glass will form a very high resistance seal with the membrane, thus electrically isolating the patch of membrane covered by the pipette tip. The salt solution in the electrode is connected through an Ag/AgCl junction to a device that allows simultaneous recording of current and control of potential ('voltage clamp'), or vice versa ('current clamp') over the patch of membrane (Fig. 8.16). The former is used far more than the latter, because the activity of many ion channels is dependent on the potential across the membrane. If the patch contains one or only a few ion channels, ionic currents through individual channels can be recorded. The magnitude of these currents is in the order of a few picoamperes (10^{-12} A). Single-channel traces show the characteristic instantaneous jumps representing transitions between the open and closed states of the ion channel. The great power of the technique is that many configurations are possible (Fig. 8.17), depending on the researcher's wish to manipulate the intra- or extracellular medium during the experiment, or to record single-channel activity or whole-cell (macro)currents. Our present knowledge of the physiology of ion channels, both voltage dependent and ligand gated, and their modulation is owed almost entirely to patch clamp work. In recent years, the restriction that the technique could be applied only to isolated cells has been overcome,

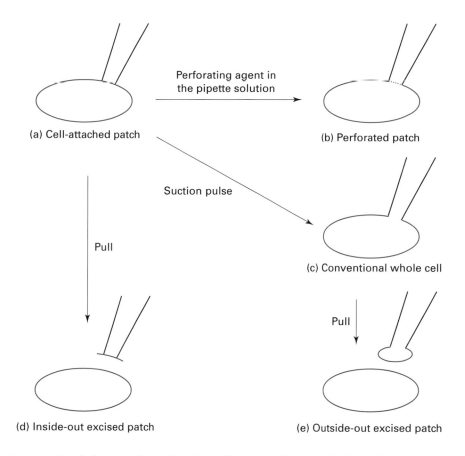

Fig. 8.17. Patch clamp configurations. In configurations (b), (c) and (e) the medium on the extracellular side of the membrane under study can be changed during a recording. In configuration (d) the intracellular side can be manipulated. Configurations (a) and (b) leave the cytoplasm relatively intact. (Reproduced by permission of E. Molleman, University of Hertfordshire.)

at least in neuroscience, by the development of patch clamping in brain slices. This has opened the way to studies of intercellular communication, for example, interactions between neurones *in situ*.

8.10.3 **ATP-driven active transport**

A large number of different carrier-mediated and ion channel transport systems have been identified and shown to operate via a variety of mechanisms in which the stimulus for a conformational change in the protein and the concomitant transport of the ion comes from processes such as:

changes in Ca^{2+} concentration;
binding of cyclic AMP released by the activation of adenylyl cyclase by a $G\alpha$ subunit;

binding of cyclic GMP produced by the activation of guanylyl cyclase by a
   neurotransmitter binding to its receptor or by the binding of nitric oxide to
   the haem group of guanylyl cyclase;
binding of a $G\alpha$ or $G\beta\gamma$ subunit released from a G-protein as a result of receptor
   binding by a neurotransmitter;
changes in membrane potential (voltage-gated channels);
phosphorylation by diacylglycerol-sensitive protein kinase C;
phosphorylation by ATP;
phosphorylation by phosphoenolpyruvate.

The Danish Nobel Laureate Jen Skou has led the discovery and study of the ATP-
driven antiporter for Na^+ and K^+. It is a dimeric transmembrane protein consisting of an α-subunit, which contains the cation-binding sites, and β-subunit, which
is a glycoprotein with no catalytic function presumed to be involved in the maintenance of the structure of the functional transporter. The $\alpha\beta$ complex has a relative molecular mass of 160 000 and contains ten transmembrane domains. There
are two distinct binding sites, that for ATP is located in loop 4 and is accessible only
from the cytoplasmic site of the membrane, whilst the location of the ionophore
site, to which the Na^+ and K^+ bind in turn, is not clear. Kinetic studies indicate that
the transporter functions as a dimer, i.e. $(\alpha\beta)_2$. The complete functional cycle of
the protein results in the hydrolysis of ATP and the transport of three Na^+ to the
outside of the cell and two K^+ into the cell, both against an electrochemical gradient. The protein is therefore referred to as a Na^+, K^+-ATPase or simply the Na^+, K^+
pump.

Skou's key discovery was that the ATP phosphorylates an aspartate residue in
the presence of Na^+ and that the phosphorylated enzyme transports Na^+. The
release of the Na^+ on the outside of the cell enables K^+ to bind. The subsequent
hydrolysis of the phosphate group on the outside of the membrane triggers the
transport of the K^+ into the cell. This process identifies many interesting features:

The high affinity Na^+ binding sites are on the inside of the membrane
   (K_m 0.2 mM) and when occupied enable ATP to bind to give the ternary
   complex enzyme–$3Na^+$–ATP. The cardiac glycoside ouabain blocks Na^+
   binding.
The ternary complex in the presence of Mg^{21} (a normal cofactor for the
   majority of kinases) reacts to produce the phosphorylated aspartate residue,
   which is a 'high energy' acylphosphate group. This triggers a conformational
   change and the translocation of Na^+ through the protein molecule to the
   outside of the cell.
On the outside of the membrane the acylphosphate group 'relaxes' to a low
   energy conformation, which can be isolated and characterised, and causes
   the protein to release Na^+.
The cation-binding sites are then occupied by two K^+ (K_m 50 mM) and the
   phosphate group is hydrolysed, triggering a second conformational change
   and the translocation of K^+ to the inside of the membrane where they are
   released (Fig. 8.18).

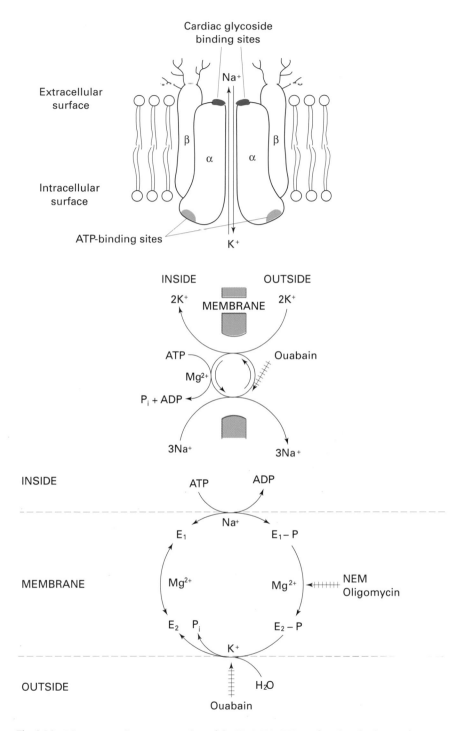

Fig. 8.18. Diagrammatic representation of the Na$^+$, K$^+$-ATPase showing the ion- and ATP-binding sites, stoichiometry and sensitivity to ouabain, oligomycin and *N*-ethylmaleimide (NEM) (Reproduced by permission of M. Davis, University of Hertfordshire.)

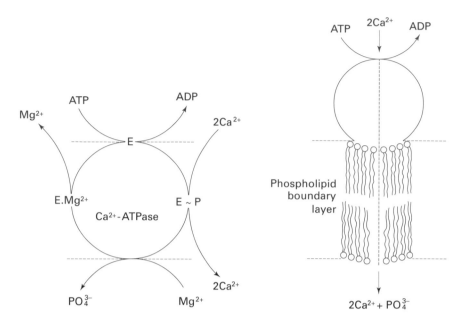

Fig. 8.19. Schematic representation of the Ca^{2+}-ATPase. E, non-phosphorylated enzyme; $E \sim P$, phosphorylated (energy-rich) enzyme. (Reproduced by permission of M. Davis, University of Hertfordshire.)

The transport of Na^+ and K^+ occurs in a compulsory sequence of events driven by the net hydrolysis of ATP which, energetically, enables the ion transport to proceed against a concentration gradient. The free energy change for the binding of the Na^+ is large and negative and occurs at a low Na^+ concentration. In contrast, the release of Na^+ at a higher concentration results in a free energy change that must be less negative. Energy is therefore needed to reduce the binding affinity for Na^+ and this is supplied by ATP, although there is no direct contact between the ATP molecule or the Asp phosphorylation site and the binding of the Na^+.

The discovery of the Na^+, K^+-ATPase has been followed by the identification of similar pumps, including ones for the transport of Ca^{2+} in muscle cells and for proton transport in the stomach. The Ca^{2+}-ATPase is responsible for the transport of Ca^{2+} across the plasma membrane, the inner mitochondrial membrane and the endoplasmic reticulum. It is asymmetrically located in the membrane and, like the Na^+, K^+-ATPase, has 10 transmembrane domains, the major loops being located within the cytoplasm. For each molecule of ATP used to phosphorylate the protein, two Ca^{2+} are transported out of the cytoplasm by a mechanism very similar to that for the Na^+, K^+-ATPase (Fig. 8.19). The ionophone-binding site has been identified as a number of carboxyl groups, which are good ligands for Ca^{2+}, in transmembrane regions IV to VIII. The unusual feature of the Ca^{2+}-ATPase is that its activity is controlled by Ca^{2+} via calmodulin. At low Ca^{2+} concentrations the activity is low, but at concentrations greater than $1\,mM$ the Ca^{2+}–calmodulin complex forms, resulting in activation of the Ca^{2+}-ATPase and the excretion of Ca^{2+}, the activation being characterised by a decreased K_m for Ca^{2+}.

The H^+, K^+-ATPase of gastric mucosa has many similarities with the Na^+, K^+- and Ca^{2+}-ATPase pumps. These three types of ATPase are referred to as P-type, indicating that the transport mechanism involves the phosphorylation of the protein. Three other classes of ATPases have been characterised on the basis of their sensitivity to various inhibitors. None of them are phosphorylated by ATP:

(i) *F-type*. This is found in mitochondrial, chloroplast and bacterial membranes and are sensitive to azide ions. They translocate ions, normally protons and consist of F_1 and F_o (the 'o' subscript refers to oligomycin sensitivity) portions, each consisting of multiple subunits. The F_1 portion contains the ATPase activity and the F_o an ion channel. Such ATPases are more commonly known as ATP synthases.

(ii) *V-type*. This is found in endoplasmic reticulum, Golgi apparatus, endosomes and lysosomes (V, vacuolar). Pumps translocate protons and are sensitive to *N*-ethylmaleimide but are not separable into F_1 and F_o portions.

(iii) *A-type*. This is found in bacterial cells and translocates anions.

The P-type consist of single-chain proteins, whilst the others have at least eight subunits. The four types differ in their sensitivity to various inhibitors that have been valuable in the elucidation of the mechanism of action of the pumps. They are all reversible in their action and can transfer ions down a concentration gradient and in the process synthesise ATP. Under normal physiological conditions, however, and with the exception of the F-type, they all work in one direction using the free energy of hydrolysis of ATP to create an electrochemical potential gradient. The F-types, better known as ATP synthases, synthesise ATP by chemiosmotic coupling. The P-type transporters include the cystic fibrosis transmembrane regulator (CFTR) and many drug-resistance transporters in bacteria, and accordingly are the targets for the development of new drugs.

There are some secondary transport proteins that use an existing potential gradient, for example that created by the Na^+, K^+-ATPase, to drive a transport process. An example is the Na^+-glucose symport system found in the brush border cells of the intestine and the epithelial cells that line the kidney tubule. It uses a Na^+ gradient to drive the absorption of glucose. The transmembrane protein has distinct binding sites for Na^+ and glucose, which can bind in a random order to form a ternary complex that undergoes a conformational change to release both the Na^+ and glucose within the cell. The glucose subsequently leaves the cell to enter the bloodstream via the glucose transporter discussed in Section 8.9.

8.11 RECEPTOR-MEDIATED ENDOCYTOSIS

8.11.1 LDL receptor

The transmembrane transport systems so far discussed are not suitable for the selective uptake of large molecules such as proteins or macromolecular structures such as low density lipoprotein (LDL), the carrier of cholesterol. Receptor-mediated endocytosis is the solution to this particular transport process. It involves specific membrane receptors that bind the particle or macromolecule with characteristics of affinity and selectivity typical of the receptors for the growth factors, peptide hormones and neurotransmitters previously discussed.

Research by Joseph Goldstein and Michael Brown on the LDL receptor and its link to the development of atherosclerosis resulted not only in the award of the Nobel Prize for Medicine, but also in a considerable understanding of both the molecular nature of the receptor and the endocytosis process in general. LDL is a spherical particle, 20–25 nm in diameter, consisting of an outer phospholipid monolayer containing inserted proteins and cholesterol, and an internal core of triglyceride and cholesterol ester. It is the main vehicle for the transport of cholesterol around the body and elevated levels are linked to the premature development of atherosclerosis and coronary heart disease. The main transmembrane protein in the monolayer is apoprotein B100 (apoB100), part of which is the ligand for the LDL receptor. Unusually, therefore, both the receptor and its ligand are membrane-bound proteins. Several apoB100 molecules are in the membrane of each LDL particle. The LDL receptor is a dimer of two identical single chain proteins. Each has a transmembrane domain of 22 amino acid residues near the C-terminal end, which protrudes into the cytoplasm. A region of 48 amino acid residues on the immediate extracellular face of the membrane is rich in serine and threonine and is glycosylated. The N-terminal end is cysteine-rich, containing an eight-fold repeating sequence of 40 amino acid residues and is believed to be the binding site for apoB100 and apoE. The latter is found in high density lipoprotein (HDL) and is a particle smaller than LDL but also involved in cholesterol transport. Interestingly, a region of 350 amino acid residues located between the glycosylation and binding sites possesses considerable sequence similarity to the EGF-precursor receptor. Labelling studies have revealed that there are between 15 000 and 70 000 LDL receptors per cell membrane that are not evenly distributed, but located mainly in coated pits, regions in the membrane in which a protein called clathrin is located on the cytoplasmic side of the membrane. Clathrin consists of three heavy and three light chains that can polymerise to form a cage-like structure or lattice which attaches to the C-terminal end of the LDL receptor. Clathrin plays an important role in the endocytosis process.

The K_d for binding apoB100 to the LDL receptor is 1×10^{-10} M, which implies that, given the normal circulatory concentration of LDL, the receptors are permanently saturated. The occupied LDL receptors in the coated pit are endocytosed (engulfed) to create a coated vesicle or endosome. This endocytotic process is promoted by clathrin, which forms a polyhedral polymeric network on the cytoplasmic side of the membrane thereby triggering 'budding' and coating the outside of the endosome. The polymerisation of clathrin into the network involves the phosphorylation of the light chains at several sites possibly involving different kinases. This phosphorylation is energy dependent and drives the whole endocytosis process. Ca^{2+} are involved in both the stabilisation of the clathrin network and its subsequent breakdown. Within the cell, the clathrin coat is depolymerised, probably by the heat shock protein hsp70, with the concomitant hydrolysis of ATP. The decoated vesicle eventually fuses with a lysosome. This fusion is subject to control by a number of factors, possibly including phosphatidylinositol 3-kinase, the activity of which is subject to control by phosphorylation (Section 8.4.3).

As a result of a prevailing pH of 5.0 within the fused endosome–lysosome, the LDL particle dissociates from its receptor and is degraded by lysosomal hydrolytic enzymes. The majority of the receptors escape degradation and are recycled, whilst the internalised cholesterol controls both *de novo* synthesis of further cholesterol and the synthesis of new LDL receptors. The lack of functional LDL receptors, crucially therefore, has implications for total cellular cholesterol levels and ultimately for the development of atherosclerosis.

Goldstein and Brown worked with cultured fibroblast cells, which are a good source of LDL receptors, grown in a medium of high and low cholesterol concentrations. They linked radiolabelled LDL to ferritin via a monoclonal antibody to the LDL receptor protein, to enable them to study the fate of the LDL simultaneously by electron microscopy and radiolabel uptake. They were able to show that endocytosis is fast and that receptors are recycled in 10 to 12 min. From a clinical point of view they also demonstrated that individuals with genetically linked elevated plasma cholesterol levels suffered from a total lack of LDL receptors, dysfunctional receptors or a reduced number of functional receptors.

8.11.2 Cell surface receptor trafficking

The endocytotic cycle described for LDL uptake also operates for the uptake of transferrin, bacterial toxins and some viruses. It is now established that cellular receptors of the G-protein-linked and protein kinase classes also undergo the same endocytotic trafficking cycle that constitutes a vital part of the control mechanism for receptor numbers and hence for the sensitivity of the cell to external signals. There are, however, some fundamental differences in the details of the endocytosis of LDL, and related structures and molecules, and that for the trafficking of receptors for hormones, growth factors and neurotransmitters. LDL and transferrin receptors are located in coated pits, whether free or ligand-bound. In contrast, receptors for hormones and growth factors are distributed evenly over the membrane and only accumulate in coated-pits after ligand binding. This accumulation is triggered by interaction between the intracellular domain of the receptor and a protein adaptor molecule complex, AP2, associated with the clathrin. The phosphorylation of the intracellular domain of the receptor, also triggered by ligand binding, may be important in the endocytotic process. In the case of the insulin and EGF receptors, the endocytosed receptors continue to exert their tyrosine kinase activity, as the receptor cytoplasmic domain remains exposed to the cytoplasm (Fig. 8.20). The factors that influence endosomal sorting, which directs the endocytosed receptor either to degradation or to recycling, have not been totally established but are clearly fundamental to the regulation of cellular receptor numbers. One important determinant appears to be the ease with which the ligand dissociates from the receptor within the endosome,

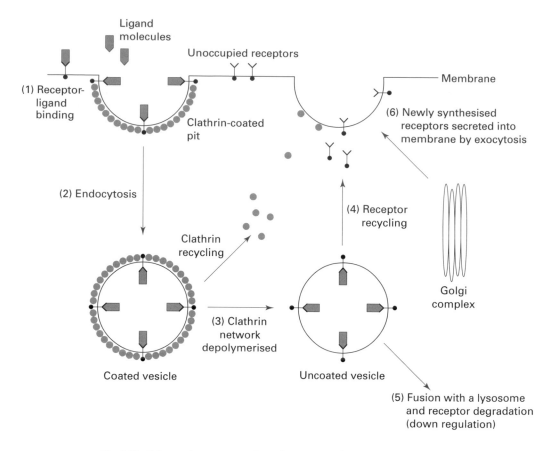

Fig. 8.20. Schematic representation of receptor endocytosis and recycling. (1) The ligand binds either to a receptor located in a coated pit or elsewhere in the surface of the membrane, in which case the ligand–receptor complex then migrates to a coated pit facilitated by an adaptor molecule complex (not shown) attached to the clathrin. (2) The coated pit 'buds' into the cell cytoplasm aided by clathrin, which forms a network around the vesicle to give a 'coated vesicle' (endosome). Note that the cytoplasmic domain of the receptor remains exposed to the cytoplasm following endocytosis. (3) The clathrin network is depolymerised to give an uncoated endosome and the clathrin redirected to the inner membrane surface. (4 and 5) The ligands dissociate from their receptors, which are either recycled to the outer membrane surface or degraded following fusion of the endosome with a lysosome. (6) The Golgi complex secretes newly synthesised receptor molecules to the outer membrane surface by a process called exocytosis, which is the reverse of endocytosis. The balance between receptor recycling, receptor degradation and receptor synthesis determines the number of functionally active receptors on the membrane surface at any time.

triggered by the progressive acidification of the endosome owing to its electrogenic proton-pumping ATpase. EGF is resistant to dissociation from its receptor, which is predominantly degraded. The same is true for the PDGF receptor but not for the insulin receptor. A second factor appears to be the presence of lysosomal sorting signals present in the exposed C-terminal tail of the receptor molecule in the endosome. These signals are recognised by lysosomes and result in the eventual degradation of the receptor. The absence of such signals would encourage the recycling of the receptor molecules.

The temporal variation in the number of cell surface receptors available for ligand binding is the net result of receptor trafficking (recycling and degradation) and of new receptor synthesis, which takes place in the rough endoplasmic reticulum. A leader sequence in the protein results in its recognition and transport to the Golgi complex, where it is glycosylated, packaged into coated vesicles and inserted into the membrane by exocytosis, which is essentially the reverse of endocytosis and in which the protein clathrin plays a vital part. The fusion of the coated vesicle with the membrane ensures that the receptor proteins are inserted into the membrane with the correct orientation (Fig. 8.20).

8.12 **KEY TERMS**

active transport	exocytosis	partition coefficient
antiporter	facilitated transport	patch clamp study of ion
adaptor molecule complex	Fick's law	channels
carrier	gated pore	patch clamping
clathrin	ion flux	permeability coefficient
coated pits	ionophore	physical diffusion
coated vesicle	ion-pairing	receptor-mediated endocytosis
diffusion coefficient	ion trapping	symport
distribution coefficients	LDL receptor	translocator
effector	membrane potential	transporter
electrogenic	metabolic trapping	uniport
electroneutral	Na^+, K^+-ATPase	voltage-gated channels
endosome	Na^+, K^+-pump	

8.13 **CALCULATIONS**

Question 1   Amphetamine is a weakly basic drug with a pK_a of 9.5. Given that the pH of the stomach is 1.0, that of the small intestine is 7.3, and that of the plasma 7.4, by use of the Henderson–Hasselbalch equation, calculate the ratio of the conjugate acid to free base of amphetamine in the stomach, intestine and plasma and hence by applying the principles of physical diffusion and of ion-trapping, show that amphetamine should not be absorbed from the stomach by physical diffusion but that it should be absorbed from the small intestine. Show by similar calculations that you would expect more amphetamine to be excreted by the kidneys with an acid urine (pH 4.5) than with an alkaline urine (pH 8.5).

Answer   Since amphetamine is a weak base, we can calculate the relative amount of the free base (unionised) and conjugate acid (ionised) from the Henderson–Hasselbalch equation:

$$pH = pK_a + \log\left(\frac{[base]}{[conjugate\ acid]}\right)$$

Thus, at pH 1 (stomach),

$$1 = 9.5 + \log\left(\frac{[\text{base}]}{[\text{conjugate acid}]}\right)$$

if $x = [\%\text{ base}]$, then $100 - x = [\%\text{ conjugate acid}]$.
Therefore

$$-8.5 = \log\left(\frac{x}{100 - x}\right)$$

$$3.2 \times 10^{-9} = \frac{x}{100 - x}$$

$$3.2 \times 10^{-7} - 3.2 \times 10^{-9}x = x$$

The $3.2 \times 10^{-9}x$ can be ignored.

Hence $3.2 \times 10^{-7}\%$ (i.e. virtually none) of the amphetamine will exist as the conjugate base, which is unionised and able to physically diffuse across membranes, but virtually all the drug will exist as the ionised conjugate acid which cannot physically diffuse from the stomach to plasma. Thus the drug will not be absorbed from the stomach.

For the drug in the intestine, the comparable equations become:

$$7.3 = 9.5 + \log\left(\frac{x}{100 - x}\right)$$

$$-2.2 = \log\left(\frac{x}{100 - x}\right)$$

$$6.3 \times 10^{-3} = \frac{x}{100 - x}$$

Therefore,

$$0.63 - 6.3 \times 10^{-3}x = x$$

$$0.63 = 1.0063x$$

$$x = 0.63$$

i.e. 0.63% of the amphetamine in the intestine will exist as the unionised free base and hence 99.37% will exist as the ionised conjugate acid. Although the proportion of the unionised form is still small, it is sufficient to diffuse across the intestinal barrier into the plasma. In the plasma it will be predominantly protonated to the conjugate acid thereby displacing the equilibrium, which favours the further absorption of amphetamine. Thus we have:

This is an example of the amphetamine becoming ion-trapped in the plasma, thereby favouring absorption from the intestine. The natural circulation of the plasma will further displace the equilibrium and favour absorption. In the kidneys, with an acid urine, similar calculations show that the majority of the amphetamine will be present as the conjugate acid, which will be glomerularly filtered into the primary urine and hence not able to be reabsorbed by physical diffusion during passage through the loop of Henle. In an alkaline urine, in contrast, a greater proportion of the amphetamine will exist as the free base which will be able to physically diffuse back into the plasma and hence be retained in the body. You may wish to extend these principles by considering what would happen in the stomach, the intestine, the plasma and the kidneys if the drug in question was a weak acid (e.g. a barbiturate) with a pK_a of 5.0.

Question 2

The study of the binding of a ligand to its membrane receptor gave the following data when studied by equilibrium dialysis:

Bound ligand per mole receptor protein (mM)	5.9	3.3	1.98	1.18	0.29
Free ligand (mM)	1.0	1.5	2.0	2.5	3.5

By means of a Scatchard plot, determine the value of the binding constant, K_a, and the number of binding sites on the receptor.

Answer

A Scatchard plot of bound/free versus bound has a slope of $-K_a$ of $-2\ mM^{-1}$ therefore $K_a = 2\ mM^{-1}$. The intercept on the x-axis is equal to $n = 4$.

8.14 SUGGESTIONS FOR FURTHER READING

Membrane Receptors

CHALLIS, R. A. J. (ed.) (1997). *Receptor Signal Transduction Protocols.* Methods in Molecular Biology series, **83**. Humana Press: Totowa, NJ. (Provides a diverse range of protocols for the study of receptor–ligand interactions.)

HARDIE, D. G. (1991). *Biochemical Messengers: Hormones, Neurotransmitters and Growth Factors.* Chapman and Hall: London. (An excellent and readable text of membrane receptors and cell–cell signalling.)

HULME, E.C. (1992). *Receptor–Ligand Interactions: A Practical Approach.* IRL Press, Oxford. (A good coverage of the practical aspects of this subject.)

JANS, D.A. (1997). *The Mobile Receptor Hypothesis: The Role of Membrane Receptor Lateral Movement in Signal Transduction.* Springer-Verlag, Berlin Heidelberg, New York. [A comprehensive review of the central importance of receptor diffusion to signal transduction.]

KENAKIN, T. (1997). *Molecular Pharmacology: A Short Course.* Blackwell Scientific, Cambridge, MA. (An excellecent and authoritative text that covers the characterisation and measurement of receptor activity and their use in the development of new drugs.)

LAUFFENBURGER, D.A. and LINDERMAN, J. J. (1993). *Receptors: Models for Binding Trafficking and Signaling.* Oxford University Press, New York. (Presents a lucid, but thorough, introduction to the mathematical and physical basis for the quantitative analysis of receptor-mediated events.)

MILLIGAN, G. (ed.) (1992). *Signal Transduction: A Practical Approach*, IRL Press, Oxford. (A good coverage of the practical aspects of this topic.)

NICOLA, N. A. (ed.) (1994). *Guidebook to Cytokines and their Receptors*. Oxford University Press, Oxford. (A comprehensive coverage of this important group of receptors.)

WINZOR, D. J. and SAWYER, W. H. (1995). *Quantitative Characterization of Ligand Binding*. Wiley-Liss, New York. (A good coverage of the methodologies of receptor–ligand studies and of the mathematical interpretation of the binding data.)

Transport processes

AIDLEY, D. J. and STANFIELD, P. R. (1996). *Ion Channels: Molecules in Action.* Cambridge University Press: Cambridge. (An excellent, readable and authoritative coverage of this important aspect of ion transport.)

BOULTON, A. A., BAKER, G. B. and WALZ, W. (ed.) (1995). *Patch Clamp Applications and Protocols. Human Press*, Totowa, NJ. (A practical guide to this important experimental technique.)

BROWN, M.S. and GOLDSTEIN, J. L. (1986). A receptor-mediated pathway for cholesterol homeostasis. *Science*, **232** 34–47. (A personal account of their discovery of the LDL receptor and its endocytosis.)

LEFF, P. (1995). 2 State model of receptor activation. *Trends in Pharmacological Sciences*, **16**, 89–97. (An authoritative discussion of this important mode of receptor activation.)

General reading

MINGARRO, I., VON HEIJNE, G. and WHITLEY, P. (1997). Membrane protein engineering. *Trends in Biotechnology*, **15**, 432–7.

Chapter 9

Spectroscopic techniques: I   Atomic and molecular electronic spectroscopy

9.1 INTRODUCTION

9.1.1 Properties of electromagnetic radiation

The interaction of electromagnetic radiation with matter is essentially a quantum phenomenon and is dependent both upon the properties of the radiation and the appropriate structural parts of the material involved. This is not surprising, as the origin of the radiation is due to energy changes within the matter itself. An understanding of the properties of electromagnetic radiation and its interaction with matter leads to a recognition of the variety of types of spectra and consequently spectroscopic techniques and their application to the solution of biological problems. Also the transitions which occur within matter (see e.g. Section 9.1.2) are quantum phenomena and the spectra which arise from such transitions are, at least in principle, predictable. Table 9.1 shows the various interactions, with parts of matter, of the electromagnetic spectrum and corresponding wavelengths. The various parts of matter both give rise to and are affected by the radiation in the corresponding region of the spectrum.

Electromagnetic radiation (Fig. 9.1) is composed of both an electric vector and magnetic vector (which gives rise to the name), which oscillate in planes at right angles (normal) to each other and mutually at right angles to the direction of propagation.

9.1.2 Interaction with matter

Electromagnetic phenomena exhibit energy, frequency, wavelength and intensity. All these are interrelated and can be explained either in terms of waveforms or particles termed photons or quanta. These phenomena are best exemplified by considering electronic spectra. Electrons in either atoms or molecules may be distributed between several energy levels but principally reside in the lowest levels or ground state. In order for an electron to be promoted to a higher level (or excited state), energy must be put into the system and this gives rise to an absorption spectrum if the energy is derived from electromagnetic radiation. Only the exact amount of energy equivalent to the difference in energy level, in accordance with the rules of quantum mechanics, will be absorbed. This is termed one quantum of

Table 9.1 Interaction of electromagnetic radiation and the various parts or 'structures' of matter

Phenomenon	Region of spectrum	Wavelength
Nuclear	Gamma	0.1 nm
Inner electrons	X-rays	0.1–1.0 nm
Ionisation	Ultraviolet	0–200 nm
Valency electrons	Near ultraviolet and visible	200–800 nm
Molecular vibrations	Near infrared and infrared	0.8–25 μm
Rotation and electron spin orientation in magnetic fields	Microwaves	400 μm–30 cm
Nuclear spin orientation in magnetic fields	Radiowaves #	100 cm and above

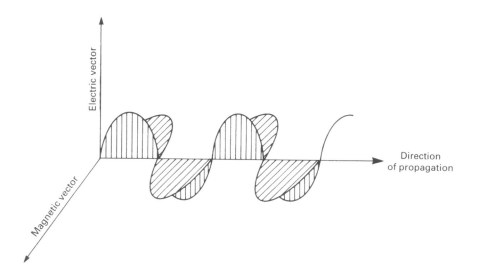

Fig. 9.1. The electric and magnetic vectors or 'oscillations' of electromagnetic radiation and the direction of propagation.

energy for a single-electron transition, and the absolute magnitude of each quantum will differ according to the difference in energy levels involved. When an electron falls from a higher to lower level, then exactly one quantum of energy is emitted from the system, giving rise to an emission spectrum. Energy in other forms may be put into the system; for example, the heating of metals achieves the promotion of electrons to higher energy levels and, if sufficient energy has been input, when they return to lower levels visible light is emitted. This gives rise to the effect of the glowing of heated metals.

Figure 9.2a is a diagrammatic representation of electron transitions in the sodium atom. These transitions in most atoms give rise to relatively simple line spectra. The situation in molecules is somewhat more complicated, although the

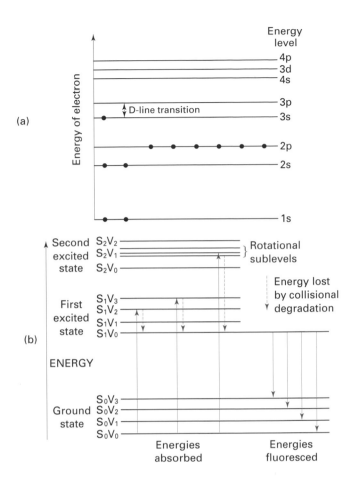

Fig. 9.2. Energy levels and transitions of electrons: (a) in the sodium atom and (b) in a fluorescent organic molecule. Note: for clarity, rotational sublevels have been indicated only for vibrational sublevel S_2V_1.

same basic principles apply, because more different kinds of energy level exist. Moreover the atoms in molecules may vibrate and rotate about a bond axis, which gives rise to vibrational and rotational sublevels. This situation is shown diagrammatically in Fig. 9.2b but, owing to the subdivision of energy levels in molecules, molecular spectra are usually observed as band spectra.

The energy change for an electron transition is defined in quantum terms by the following simple relation;

$$\Delta E = E_1 - E_2 = h\upsilon \tag{9.1}$$

where ΔE is the change in energy state of the electron or the energy of electromagnetic radiation absorbed or emitted by an atom or molecule, E_1 is energy of electron in original state, E_2 is the energy of electron in the final state, h is the Planck constant $(= 6.63 \times 10^{-34}\,\text{J s})$, υ is the frequency of the electromagnetic radiation in hertz (c/λ) where c is speed of electromagnetic radiation $(3 \times 10^8\,\text{m s}^{-1})$, and λ is

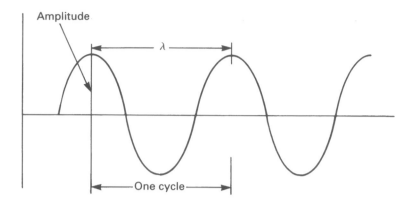

Fig. 9.3. Representation of terms in a single sinusoidal waveform. (The number of cycles occurring in unit time (second) is the frequency measured in hertz.)

the wavelength of electromagnetic radiation ($1/\bar{v}$ or $c\bar{v}$, where $\bar{v}$ is the wave number of electromagnetic radiation in waves cm^{-1} (kaysers)). Despite the simplicity of the relation, it is of fundamental importance. Figure 9.3 shows some of the interrelationships. It should be noted that wavelength should be expressed in submultiples of the metre, i.e. nanometre (nm), micrometre (μm), centimetre (cm) etc. (not ångströms (Å) or mμ or μ) and frequency expressed in hertz (not cycles s^{-1}).

In Fig. 9.2a,b, electron transitions in atoms or molecules give rise to the electronic spectra generally observed as absorption, emission or fluorescence phenomena (Section 9.5) in the ultraviolet and visible regions of the electromagnetic spectrum. The basic quantum relationships hold for other regions also. Of course, different energy transitions occur in these other regions and these will be indicated as each appropriate part of the system is dealt with.

In the following subsections each region of the electromagnetic spectrum is treated in terms of the interaction involved, instrumentation used and application to appropriate biological problems. The treatment is unequal, however, and some sections are presented in considerably more detail to reflect usage.

9.2 γ-RAY SPECTROSCOPY AND γ-RAY RESONANCE SPECTROSCOPY

9.2.1 Principles

γ-Rays are of nuclear origin, but they are also part of the electromagnetic spectrum and so, in principle, it is possible to develop spectroscopic methods involving them. Owing to their considerable penetrating power, the main applications in a biological context are in imaging but also in radiotherapy. The rays arise from energy transitions occurring within the nucleus, the mechanisms of which are not described here. For further details, see the literature cited in Section 9.13.

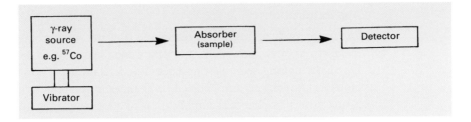

Fig. 9.4. Layout of a simple Mössbauer spectrometer.

An important application of the use of γ-ray emission spectroscopy is the use of the element technicium, Tc, which does not occur naturally but is a product of the nuclear industry. This element may be used for medical studies, because, if it is complexed to a compound that is preferentially concentrated in specific biological tissues, particularly bone, liver or brain, its location can be determined by its emission spectrum. The emitted radiation is detected using a device known as a γ-camera, enabling the shape and structure of the tissue under study to be investigated. Despite the name given to the instrument, in this type of application the technique is essentially spectroscopic.

Nuclear γ-resonance, the so-called Mössbauer effect, was discovered in 1957. Many isotopes exhibit the effect but the main emphasis appears to have centred around the ^{57}Fe isotope. Although the applications have been somewhat limited, there is considerable potential for the study of biologically important metal-containing complexes.

9.2.2 Mössbauer spectroscopy

Principles

The γ-ray energy from a radioactive nucleus may be modulated by giving a Doppler velocity to the source. The Doppler effect (observed in all waveforms, sound and electromagnetic) is recognised as the apparent change in frequency that occurs when the source is moving relative to the detector (observer). The change in frequency is proportional to the source velocity and any velocity may be chosen to give the required frequency. γ-Rays of discrete energy can be absorbed resonantly by appropriate nuclei. The source used is usually ^{57}Co; this emits a range of γ-rays with different energies, an appropriate one of which may be selected. The selected ray is then modulated by the imposed Doppler phenomenon.

Instrumentation

Figure 9.4 shows a very simplified diagram of the arrangement required to perform Mössbauer spectroscopy. Usually, because of the energies and wavelengths involved, the Doppler velocity can be imposed by rapidly vibrating the ^{57}Co source.

Applications

The major applications of this technique is in the study of the coordination of metal atoms by ligands of an appropriate complexing agent. Model compounds have been investigated, enabling a better understanding of how certain metals of biological importance are affected by changes in the binding properties of the ligand either by chemical modification or local environment differences. An example is sickle cell anaemia, where, compared with normal haemoglobin, the iron atom is distorted out of the plane of the haem moiety.

9.3 X-RAY SPECTROSCOPY

9.3.1 Principles

Whereas γ-rays are of nuclear origin, X-rays arise from displacement of inner, extranuclear electrons. The electrons, with principle quantum numbers 1, 2 and 3, in an atom can be imagined to occupy shells – K, L and M, respectively. Should a bombarding electron from an external source have sufficient energy to displace a K shell (innermost) electron in a target atom, then this vacancy is filled within a time span of 10^{-4} s by an L shell electron and an X-ray of appropriate wavelength is emitted. The energy transition from L to K is, of course, governed by quantum rules and $E = h\nu$ must be satisfied; hence the frequency and wavelength of the emitted X-ray are determined.

X-rays can be absorbed by matter and this gives rise to X-ray absorption spectra. The rules applying to the relationship between an incident beam of monochromatic X-radiation (I_0) and the transmitted portion I, are similar to the Beer–Lambert case described in Section 9.4.1. If μ is the linear absorption coefficient of the absorbing material then

$$I = I_0 e^{-\mu x} \tag{9.2}$$

where x is the thickness of the absorber.

If X-rays have wavelength shorter than the so-called K absorption edge of an atom, then it is possible for the incident radiation to dislodge K electrons. This then results in the emission of X-rays (because of K electron displacement) of a frequency different from that of the incident ray. The phenomenon is called X-ray fluorescence and gives rise to X-ray fluorescence analysis (XRFA). The general principles of fluorescence are considered in Section 9.5.

9.3.2 Instrumentation and applications

A suitable X-ray source is required that can be focused into the specimen chamber where the substance under test is excited by the incident beam. A monochromator is required also to disperse the fluorescent (emitted) radiation and finally a suitable detector and data-processing facilities are needed. Figure 9.5 is a simple representation of the required layout.

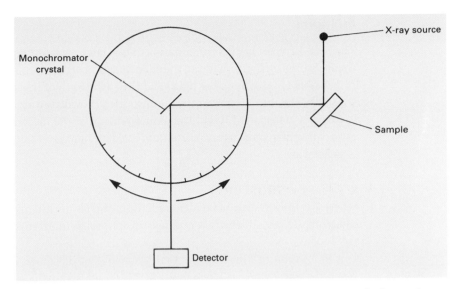

Fig. 9.5. X-ray fluorescence analysis. Dispersion of fluorescent X-rays may be detected at various angles.

The technique has wide applications in forensic science and environmental pollution studies, because it enables many elements to be detected and concentrations measured. Of course the analysis is essentially concerned with elements but can be a useful adjunct to, for example, the detection and measurement of trace elements in fertilisers. Such elements may well find their way into the food chain, with possible toxic consequences if they potentially interfere with normal metabolism. An example of such an application would be the study of the uptake of lead in plants at various distances from, say, a heavily used thoroughfare.

Absorption and emission spectra are obtained in ways similar to those described below for the ultraviolet/visible region of the electromagnetic spectrum (Section 9.4). A clinical application for performing bone densitometry measurements involves either single-photon or dual energy X-ray absorptiometry (DEXA). These studies are useful for monitoring hormone replacement therapy (HRT) in female patients. X-ray spectrometers obviously require a more rigorous approach to the incorporation of safety features, but the essential requirements of source, monochromator and detector are the same.

9.4 ULTRAVIOLET AND VISIBLE LIGHT SPECTROSCOPY

These regions of the electromagnetic spectrum and their associated techniques are probably the most widely used, both for routine analytical work and research into biological problems. The energy transitions that occur here are exactly those described in Section 9.1.2. It is convenient, however, to deal here with the appropriate laws related to the absorption of 'light', that region of the electromagnetic spectrum for which these laws were developed.

9.4.1 Principles

The Beer–Lambert law is a combination of two laws, each dealing separately with the absorption of light, related to the concentration of the absorber (the substance responsible for absorbing the light) and the pathlength or thickness of the layer (related to the absolute amount of the absorber). Provided an absorbing substance is partially transparent it will transmit a portion of the incident radiation. The ratio of the intensities of transmitted and incident light gives the transmittance, T, expressed as:

$$T = I/I_0 \tag{9.3}$$

where I_0 is the intensity of incident radiation, and I is the intensity of transmitted radiation. (Note: intensity = number of photons interacting in unit time (seconds).)

A 100% value of T represents a totally transparent substance, with no radiation being absorbed, whereas a zero value of T represents a totally opaque substance, which, in effect, represents complete absorption. For intermediate values we can define the absorbance (A) or extinction (E), which is given by the logarithm (base 10) of the reciprocal of the transmittance:

$$A = E = \log(1/T) = \log(I_0/I) \tag{9.4}$$

Absorbance used to be called optical density (OD) but continued use of this term should be discouraged. Also, as absorbance is a logarithm it is by definition unitless and has a range of values from 0 ($\equiv 100\% \, T$) to ∞ ($\equiv 0\% \, T$).

It is now possible to define the Beer–Lambert law, which, as described above, states that the absorbance is proportional to both the concentration of absorber and thickness of the layer, as

$$A = \epsilon_\lambda cl \tag{9.5}$$

where ϵ_λ is the molar absorbance coefficient (or molar extinction coefficient) for the absorber at wavelength λ, c is the concentration of absorbing solution, and l is the pathlength through the solution (or thickness).

In the strictest use of SI units the concentration should be expressed as mol m^{-3} (which is not molar) and the pathlength in metres. As A is unitless this would give units for ϵ_λ as mol^{-1} m^2 (derived from 1/(mol m^{-3} m), if equation 9.5 is rearranged to give $\epsilon_\lambda = A/(cl)$). This is to be expected, as the value of the absorbance is also dependent upon the area of illumination by the incident radiation. As this area is identical for both sample and reference it can be ignored in any calculations. It may also be instructive for the reader to show for himself or herself that mol m^{-3} is equivalent to mmol dm^{-3}. Hence, sometimes a millimolar absorbance coefficient is quoted and this does not contravene strict SI rules. However, more practical units for ϵ_λ are dm^3 mol^{-1} cm^{-1}, which conform to the definition of molarity (despite being incoherent in SI terms) and the common use of 1 cm pathlength cuvettes. Sometimes molar absorbance coefficients are extremely large and in such cases a more convenient way of expressing values is to quote the absorbance of a 1 cm thick sample of a 1% solution of the absorbant. This is distinguished by writing the coefficient as $A_{1cm}^{1\%}$.

9.4.2 Instrumentation

The material used in the optical parts of the instrument depends on the wavelength used. In the ultraviolet region it is necessary to use prisms, gratings, reflectors and cuvettes made of silica. Above 350 nm wavelength, borosilicate glass may be used but also there are now some plastic materials (e.g. disposable cuvettes) available that are transparent over virtually the whole of the visible region and into the near ultraviolet.

Wavelength selection is obviously of crucial importance. In the visible region where the analyte may not absorb, but can be readily modified chemically to produce a coloured product, coloured filters may be used which absorb all but a certain limited range of wavelengths. This limited range is known as the bandwidth of the filter. The methods that use filter selectors and depend on the production of a coloured compound are the basis of colorimetry; such methods give moderate accuracy, as even the best filters (interference types) do not have particularly narrow bandwidths. The usual procedure is to use two optically matched cuvettes, one containing a blank in which all the materials are mixed except the sample under test, an equivalent volume of solvent being added to this mixture, and the other containing the coloured material to be measured. It is necessary to standardise or zero the instrument using the blank, change cuvettes and read the absorbance. The best analytical procedure requires the zero to be reset between each measurement as colorimeters, and some filters, are influenced by temperature changes. It is also good practice to work from the most dilute (least colour) to the most concentrated because even if the cuvette is rinsed between each measurement the possibility of carryover should be minimised. Table 9.2 shows a number of commonly used colorimetric assays.

If the wavelength is selected using prisms or gratings, the technique is called spectrophotometry. In both colorimetry and spectrophotometry, the usual procedure is to prepare a set of standards and produce a concentration versus absorbance calibration curve, which is linear because it is a Beer–Lambert plot. Absorbances of unknowns are then measured and the concentration interpolated from the linear region of the plot. Interpolation is critical because:

(i) one should never extrapolate beyond the region for which any instrument has been calibrated, and
(ii) particularly in colorimetry, a phenomenon known as the Job effect (see below) occurs.

If we continue to take measurements beyond the colour reagent limit, it is observed that the linearity of the Beer–Lambert calibration does not continue indefinitely but forms a plateau, at a point which indicates that there is insufficient reagent to produce any more colour. This phenomenon is known as the Job effect. To extrapolate beyond the linear portion of the curve, therefore, would

Table 9.2 Common colorimetric assays

Substance	Reagent	Wavelength (nm)
Inorganic phosphate	Ammonium molybdate; H_2SO_4; 1,2,4-aminonaphthol; $NaHSO_3$, Na_2SO_3	600
Amino acids	(a) Ninhydrin	570 (proline 420)
	(b) Cupric salts	620
Peptide bonds	Biuret (alkaline tartrate buffer, cupric salt)	540
Phenols, tyrosine	Folin (phosphomolybdate, phosphotungstate, cupric salt)	660 or 750 (750 more sensitive)
Protein	(a) Folin	660
	(b) Biuret	540
	(c) BCA reagent (bicinchoninic acid)	562
	(d) Coomassie Brilliant Blue	595
Carbohydrate	(a) Phenol, H_2SO_4	Varies, e.g. glucose 490, xylose 480
	(b) Anthrone (anthrone, H_2SO_4)	620 or 625
Reducing sugars	Dinitrosalicylate, alkaline tartrate buffer	540
Pentoses	(a) Bial (orcinol, ethanol, $FeCl_3$, HCl)	665
	(b) Cysteine, H_2SO_4	380–415
Hexoses	(a) Carbazole, ethanol, H_2SO_4	540 or 440
	(b) Cysteine H_2SO_4	380–415
	(c) Arsenomolybdate	Usually 500–570
Glucose	Glucose oxidase, peroxidase, o-dianisidine, phosphate buffer	420
Ketohexose	(a) Resorcinol, thiourea, ethanoic acid, HCl	520
	(b) Carbazole, ethanol, cysteine, H_2SO_4	560
	(c) Diphenylamine, ethanol, ethanoic acid, HCl	635
Hexosamines	Ehrlich (dimethylaminobenzaldehyde, ethanol, HCl)	530
DNA	Diphenylamine	595
RNA	Bial (orcinol, ethanol, $FeCl_3$, HCl)	665
α-Oxo acids	Dinitrophenylhydrazine, Na_2CO_3, ethyl acetate	435
Sterols	Liebermann–Burchardt reagent (acetic anhydride, H_2SO_4, chloroform)	625
Steroid hormones	Liebermann–Burchardt reagent	425
Cholesterol	Cholesterol oxidase, peroxidase, 4-aminoantipyrine, phenol	500

potentially introduce enormous errors. Furthermore, if a particular sample gives a very high absorbance reading, it is incorrect procedure merely to dilute that sample. This achieves nothing as all the materials in the sample are diluted to the same extent. The correct procedure is to return to the original material and dilute that appropriately and then perform all the steps required to produce colour.

If high precision is not required and the absorbances of the test and standard are close in value, the Beer–Lambert linear relation may be assumed for this experiment and an approximate concentration obtained from the simple relationship

$$\text{concentration} = \frac{\text{test absorbance}}{\text{standard absorbance}} \tag{9.6}$$

Of course, such an assumption for individual experiments is valid only if the Beer–Lambert relationship has been established for that particular reaction on a previous occasion.

It is important to note that when plotting calibration curves, despite the fact that the Beer–Lambert relationship implies that there is zero absorbance at zero concentration, and that the instrument is physically zeroed, it is wrong to force the drawn line through zero. This would be to give greater credence to this point than any other and assume an unjustified level of precision. The best straight line should be drawn through the points, either by eye or by regression methods.

A further point to note is that the accuracy of the instrument is not uniform throughout the transmission range. The final measurement is an electrical one involving a galvanometer. The maximum accuracy can be shown to occur at 36.8% transmission, and between 20% and 80% the relative error is about $\pm 2\%$. Owing to the nature of galvanometric measurements, the errors at low and high absorbance can be large. This indicates that the analysis should be designed to give absorbance readings in the middle of the range of the transmission scale.

In a colorimeter, the bandwidth of the wavelengths is determined by the filter. A filter that appears red to the human eye is transmitting red light and absorbing almost everything else. This kind of filter would be used to examine blue solutions as they would absorb red light. In general the filter should be of a colour complementary to that of the solution under test.

The arrangement in such an instrument can be very simple, consisting merely of a light source (lamp), filter, cuvette and photosensitive detector to collect the transmitted light. Another detector is required to measure the incident light, or a single detector is used to measure incident and transmitted light alternately. This latter design is both cheaper and analytically better as it eliminates variation between detectors.

The spectrophotometer is a much more sophisticated instrument. A photometer is a device for measuring 'light' and 'spectro' implies the whole range of continuous wavelengths that the light source is capable of producing. The detector in the photometer is generally a photocell in which a sensitive surface receives photons and a current is generated that is proportional to the intensity of the light beam reaching the surface. In instruments for measuring ultraviolet/visible light, two lamps are usually required: one, a tungsten filament lamp, produces wavelengths in the visible regions; the second, a hydrogen or deuterium lamp, is suitable for the ultraviolet. There is a switchover point, usually 350 nm, although often both lamps are lit all the time that an instrument is in use if both ultraviolet and visible are to be used. The 'switch' in the latter case is then just a mechanical means of directing the appropriate beam along the optical axis, using mirrors or lenses.

(a)

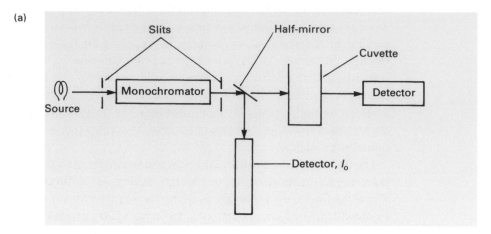

(b)

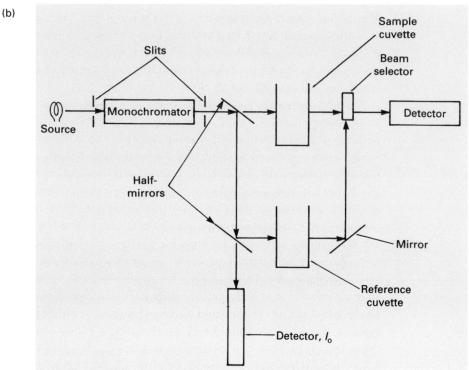

Fig. 9.6. Optical arrangements in (a) a simple single-beam spectrophotometer and (b) a double-beam spectrophotometer.

Mirrors are more frequently used, owing to cheapness and the fact that less light is lost, due to chromatic aberration, in a reflectance than a refraction system. The arrangement may be very simple, as in a colorimeter, but this really defeats the object of the instrument. Figure 9.6a shows the optical arrangement in a single-beam instrument. Here, first the blank and then the sample must be moved into the beam, adjustments made and readings taken. Figure 9.6b illustrates the double-beam device. In this arrangement the beam is split into two parts, one passing through the blank, or reference, at the same time as the other part passes through the sample. This approach obviates any problems of variation in light intensity, as both reference and sample would be affected equally. The resultant measured absorbance is the difference between the two transmitted beams of light recorded by the matched detectors. Multibeam instruments are available that allow the simultaneous recording of absorbance changes at two or more predetermined wavelengths.

The light or radiation emittted from the source lamps covers the whole range of wavelengths that the lamp is capable of producing. In colorimeters, as described above, the filter is used to obtain an appropriate range of wavelengths within the bandwidth it is capable of selecting. In spectrophotometers the bandwidth is selected by the monochromator, which is the optical system used in these devices. Theoretically, these systems select a single wavelength of monochromatic radiation, the emergent light being a parallel beam. The bandwidth here is defined as twice the half-intensity bandwidth, which is the range of wavelengths for which the transmitted intensity is greater than half the intensity of the chosen wavelength and it is a function of the slit width.

The optical systems used are usually either prisms, which split the multiwavelength source radiation into its component parts by the phenomenon known as refraction (an analogy is the natural water-droplet prisms that produce a rainbow), or gratings, which achieve the same thing by diffraction. Refraction occurs because radiation of different wavelengths travels along different paths in the denser medium of the prism material. In order that velocity conservation is maintained overall, a potentially slower moving wavepacket must travel a shorter distance in a dense medium than does a faster one. Diffraction occurs by reflectance at a surface upon which is engraved a series of fine lines. The distance apart of the lines has to be of the same order of magnitude as the wavelength of the radiation being diffracted. The resolution of wavelengths is greater from gratings than from prisms and, originally, gratings were only available in the most expensive research instruments because they were hand engraved. With the advent of photoreproduction in the semiconductor industry, gratings of high quality can be reproduced in large numbers and hence are now relatively cheap.

The optical slit width affects the bandwidth, and the narrower the slit width the more reproducible are measured absorbance values. In contrast, sensitivity becomes less as the slit narrows, because less radiation travels through to the detector. In the most sophisticated instruments, a high level of control is available to the operator, usually via a computer.

The cuvettes used in either spectrophotometry or colorimetry are an integral part of the system. They should be optically matched for the most precise and accurate work, the optical faces parallel and the pathlengths identical. In flow cells, used in continuous flow systems, the parallelism of the optical faces and the pathlength are less critical because the reference (baseline) solution and the sample both occupy the same cell successively in time. Microcells are available for

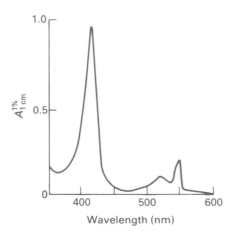

Fig. 9.7. Absolute absoption spectrum of reduced cytochrome *c*.

limited specimens and the extreme of this is the microscale spectophotometer, where a very narrow parallel beam of monochromatic radiation passes through the microcell and then enters a microscope optical system.

The major advantage of the spectrophotometer, however, is the facility to scan the wavelength range over both ultraviolet and visible and obtain absorption spectra. These are plots of absorbance versus wavelength and a typical example is shown in Fig. 9.7. This shows the extent of absorbance (absorption peaks) at various wavelengths for reduced cytochrome *c*. Absorption spectra in the ultraviolet (200 to 400) and visible (400 to 700) nm ranges arise owing to the kinds of electron transitions described above (Section 9.1.2), usually the delocalised π-bonding electrons of carbon–carbon double bonds and the lone pairs of nitrogen and oxygen. The wavelengths of light absorbed are determined by the actual electronic transitions occurring and hence specific absorption peaks may be related to known molecular substructures. The term chromophore relates to a specific part of the molecule that independently gives rise to distinct parts of an absorption spectrum. Conjugation of double bonds lowers the energy (lower frequency) required for electronic transitions and hence causes an increase in the wavelength at which a chromophore absorbs. This phenomenon is termed a bathochromic shift. Conversely a decrease in conjugation (e.g. protonation of an aromatic ring nitrogen) causes a hypsochromic shift to lower wavelength. Changes in peak maxima (increase or decrease in absorbance) can also occur. A hyperchromic shift describes an increase and a hypochromic shift a decrease in absorption maximum.

There are a number of specialised types of spectrophotometer available other than those already mentioned above. Recording spectrophotometers are usually capable of both scanning a predetermined spectrum (the prism or grating angle is changed by a motor-driven system, thereby emitting a continuously changing bandwidth along the optical axis), or monitoring changes at a predetermined wavelength. Although data are commonly recorded on a chart as hard copy, the more sophisticated devices capture and store data in computer systems and in some cases computer control is an option. Variable chart and scanning speeds and absorbance scale expansion are available. It is also possible to incorporate automatic cell changers and measurement at predetermined time intervals for time-dependent changes (e.g. kinetic studies, see Section 7.4.4). Measurement at the temperature of liquid nitrogen (-196 °C) increases the resolution, owing to the reduced thermal motion of the molecules. The absorbance generally increases also as the apparent pathlength is increased, because of internal reflections occurring in the frozen sample. Reflectance instruments measure the radiation absorbed when a light beam is reflected by the sample, for example pastes and suspensions of microorganisms that are too opaque to transmit the radiation. In such cases, internal reflection and refraction is occurring and hence the true pathlength is unknown; the strict Beer–Lambert law is therefore inapplicable, making quantification difficult. A reference reflecting surface is required and magnesium oxide is frequently used.

9.4.3 **Applications**

Qualitative analysis may be performed in the ultraviolet/visible regions to identify certain classes of compound both in the pure state and in biological mixtures, for example proteins, nucleic acids, cytochromes and chlorophylls. The technique may also be used to indicate chemical structures and intermediates occurring in a system. The most precise analysis, however, is obtained by infrared methods.

Quantitative analysis may be performed by making use of the fact that certain chromophores, for example the aromatic amino acids in proteins and the heterocyclic bases in nucleic acids, absorb at specific wavelengths. Proteins may be measured at 280 nm and nucleic acids at 260 nm, although corrections are usually necessary to account for interfering substances. Such corrections commonly require the measurement of the absorbance, by the interfering substance, at a wavelength remote from that for the compound under test, plus a knowledge of the absorbance at the test wavelength. If the ratio of the absorbances of the interfering substance is known for the remote and test wavelengths then the correction is simple, for example (Section 6.3.2) the $A_{280/260}$ ratio for proteins in the presence of nucleic acid. More sophisticated algebraic techniques are available for the more complicated cases, for example R. A. Morton's and D. W. Stubbs' correction for the amount of vitamin A in saponified oils.

The amounts of substances with overlapping spectra, such as chlorophylls a and b in diethylether may be estimated if their extinction coefficients are known at two different wavelengths. For n components absorbance data are required at n wavelengths.

A phenomenon known as Rayleigh light scattering (Section 9.7) occurs with moderate concentrations of some biological macromolecules (e.g. large DNA fragments) measured at 260 nm. This introduces an interference leading to error but may be accounted for by measuring the scattering in a region of the spectrum where DNA does not absorb, for example at 330 to 430 nm.

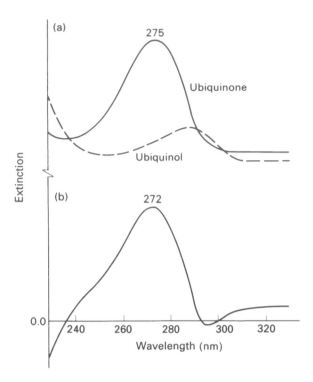

Fig. 9.8. (a) Absolute and (b) difference spectra of ubiquinone and ubiquinol.

A difference spectrum is the difference between two absorption spectra. There are essentially two ways in which difference spectra may be obtained: first, indirectly, by subtraction of one absolute spectrum from another (Fig. 9.8a); secondly, directly, by placing one compound in the reference cell and the other in the test cuvette (Fig. 9.8b). Figure 9.8a shows the two absolute spectra of ubiquinone and ubiquinol and differences in absorbance may be calculated at wavelength points with suitable regular intervals between them. The resultant absorbance values may then be plotted at the same wavelength points. Figure 9.8b shows this difference spectrum, which is obviously the same, although obtained in a different manner. Difference spectrophotometry has the advantage of enabling the detection of small absorbance changes in a system with a high background absorbance. An example of this kind of investigation is the measurement of changes in the oxidation state of components of the respiratory chain in intact mitochondria and chloroplasts.

The following important observations should be made:

(i) Difference spectra may contain negative absorbance values.
(ii) Both absorption maxima and minima may be displaced and extinction coefficients are different from those of absolute absorption peaks.
(iii) There are points of zero absorbance in the difference spectrum, equivalent to those wavelengths where both the reduced and oxidised forms of the

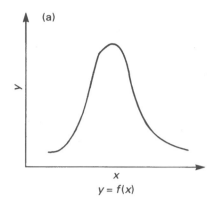

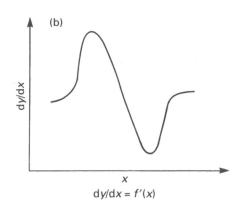

Fig. 9.9. First-differential spectra.

compound exhibit identical absorbances (isobestic points) and which may be used for checking for the presence of interfering substances.

A more complex example is that of the cytochrome a_3–CO complex minus cytochrome a_3, the difference spectrum being obtained by using anaerobic bacteria in the reference cuvette and the same system complexed with CO in the sample or test cuvette. Cytochrome a_3 is the terminal electron carrier and is the only component in the system that reacts with carbon monoxide.

Frequently the term difference spectrum refers specifically to the absolute reduced spectrum minus the absolute oxidised spectrum, for example the difference spectrum of cytochrome c corresponds to the cytochrome c_{red} minus cytochrome c_{ox} difference spectrum. A similar difference spectrum may be obtained for a suspension of mitochondria using the so-called reversal technique. This involves measuring the change in absorbance at each wavelength when the preparation passes from the aerobic to the anaerobic state. The resultant spectrum obtained is a combined difference spectrum, for the cytochromes a, a_3, b, c, c_1 and NAD^+ and flavoprotein. Shoulders on peaks observed in difference spectra obtained at room temperature may be resolved into distinct peaks at $-196\,°C$ by measuring low temperature difference spectra.

An alternative to low temperature studies of unresolved absorption spectra (difference or absolute) is a purely mathematical one and is termed differential spectroscopy. If the algebraic relationship that governs the shape of a symmetrical peak is known then it may be differentiated and the differential plotted against the original variable. An ideal example is shown in Fig. 9.9a and b.

Almost always the algebraic relationship is unknown. However the results may be readily obtained by digital computer techniques by sampling the curve at small intervals of the x-axis (wavelength). This process gives $\Delta y/\Delta x$ or $\Delta abs/\Delta\lambda$. If the $\Delta\lambda$ intervals were infinitesimally small, the limiting value would be dy/dx. Furthermore, higher order differential spectra may be obtained by feeding the data back to the processor chip as many times as are required. The value of higher-order calculations is in many cases dubious but second-order differential spectra (d^2y/dx^2) solve a number of otherwise intractable problems and instruments are commercially available, with the facility for making the calculations. The binding of a monoclonal antibody to its antigen may be monitored using second-order differential spectroscopy.

Binding spectra or substrate binding spectra may be used to study the extent of interaction between an enzyme and its substrate. The binding of a substrate to a haem group containing a ferric ion in the high spin state perturbs the spectrum by displacing the ligand water from the sixth position of the ferric ion, causing it to change to the low spin state. The process may be followed spectrophotometrically. An example of this is the binding of a drug (substrate) to liver microsomal mono-oxygenase (mixed function oxidase), which causes a blue shift of the cytochrome P450 component of the enzyme from 420 nm to 390 nm (a hypsochromic shift).

Valuable structural studies may be performed on some particular biological macromolecules such as proteins and nucleic acids. In proteins, the spectrum of a chromophore depends largely on the polarity of the microenvironment. A change in the polarity of a solvent in which the protein is dissolved changes the spectrum of a particular amino acid chromophore without changing the conformation of the protein. This phenomenon is known as solvent perturbation and obviously, to be accessible to the solvent, the amino acid residue must be on the surface of the protein. Solvents or solutions miscible with water must be used and examples are dimethylsulphoxide, dioxane, glycerol, mannitol, sucrose and polyethylene glycol.

The aromatic amino acids are powerful chromophores in the ultraviolet. Processes such as denaturation (unfolding) of a polypeptide chain by pH, temperature and ionic strength can be monitored as more of these residues become exposed to the incident radiation.

Many other processes may be followed, particularly if the amino acid residue tyrosine is involved, for example protein–protein binding, protein–metal or protein–small molecule interactions. The range may be extended by the use of reporter group techniques in which an artificial chromophore is attached to the appropriate region of the protein.

In nucleic acid studies, solvent perturbation may be used to estimate the number of unpaired bases in RNA. If normal water is replaced by 50% ^2H_2O as solvent the ^2H_2O only changes the spectral components due to unpaired nucleotides. Also the denaturation of the helical structure of DNA in solution may be investigated when the double-stranded DNA is heated through its transition temperature (Section 2.3.1). The extinction at 260 nm increases (hyperchromic shift) on denaturation and decreases again (hypochromic shift) on renaturation, which occurs on cooling. Effects on the secondary structure of DNA by pH and ionic strength may be studied in a similar way.

In certain situations an action spectrum may be shown as a plot of a physiological (non-extinction) parameter against wavelength. In many complex biological systems such a spectrum often corresponds to the absorption spectrum of a single key compound. An example is the plotting of the rate of oxygen evolution by green plant tissue against the wavelength of light used to irradiate the system. This results in a graph similar to the spectrum of the chlorophylls.

9.5 **SPECTROFLUORIMETRY**

9.5.1 **Principles**

Fluorescence is an emission phenomenon, the energy transition from a higher to lower state within the molecule concerned being measured by the detection of this emitted radiation rather than the absorption. In order for the transition from higher to lower states to occur, an earlier excitation event, for example caused by absorption of electromagnetic radiation, must have taken place. The wavelength(s) of absorbed radiation must be at lower values (higher energy) than the emitted (fluoresced) wavelength. The difference between these two wavelengths is known as the Stokes shift and in general the best results are obtained from compounds involving large shifts. It is possible for a compound to absorb (be excited) in the ultraviolet region and emit or fluoresce in the visible.

In Fig. 9.2b an example of the various permissible energy levels is shown. Most electrons will occupy the ground state S_0V_0 at room temperature. Elevation to a higher energy level, S_1, S_2, etc., may be achieved by absorption of electromagnetic energy (photons) in less than 10^{-15} s. Energy may be lost very rapidly (as heat) by collision degradation, resulting in minimal vibrational energy in the lowest excited state, S_1V_0. Electrons in this state return to the ground state in less than 10^{-8} s, the emitted energy being manifested as fluorescence. Many organic molecules absorb in the ultraviolet/visible regions but do not fluoresce. Fortunately, of those that do, many are of biological interest. Also, although a knowledge of the structure of an organic molecule may allow predictions about its absorption spectrum, this is not true with fluorescence. Aliphatic molecules, which are usually flexible, tend to photodissociate rather than fluoresce, whereas aromatic compounds with delocalised π-electrons sometimes fluoresce.

The emitted radiation appears as band spectra because there are many closely related values (for the wavelengths) dependent upon the final vibrational and rotational energy levels attained. These band spectra are usually independent of the wavelength of the exciting radiation and have a mirror image relationship with the absorption peak with the greatest wavelength.

An associated phenomenon is phosphorescence, but this emission has long decay times and usually persists when the exciting energy is no longer applied. Phosphorescence arises as a result of intersystem crossing to the lowest triplet state. This light emission usually occurs at longer wavelengths than does fluorescence.

Fluorescence spectra give information about events that occur in less than 10^{-8} s. The ratio

$$Q = \frac{\text{quanta fluoresced}}{\text{quanta absorbed}} \tag{9.7}$$

gives Q as the quantum efficiency and is usually independent of the exciting wavelength. At low concentrations, the intensity of fluorescence (I_f) is related to the intensity of the incident radiation (I_0) by

$$I_f = 2.3 I_0 \epsilon_\lambda \, cdQ, \qquad \text{i.e. } I_f \alpha c \tag{9.8}$$

where c is the concentration of the fluorescing solution (molar), d is the light path in fluorescing solution (cm), and ϵ_λ is the molar extinction coefficient for the absorbing material at wavelength λ (dm^{3}mol^{-1}cm^{-1}).

The technique of spectrofluorimetry is most accurate at very low concentrations, whereas absorption spectrophotometry is least accurate at these concentrations. For example, 100 pg of catecholamines or NADH may be measured fluorimetrically, whereas absorption spectrophotometry requires 100 μg each of the catecholamines serotonin and adrenaline. This is due to increased sensitivity, which is easily adjustible over a large range by amplification of the detector signal. The technique allows great spectral selectivity because, owing to the Stokes shift, two monochromators may be used, one for the exciting wavelength and the other for the emitted fluorescence. Although no reference cuvette is required, a calibration curve must be obtained.

Susceptibility to pH, temperature, solvent polarity and the inability to predict whether a particular compound will fluoresce, are disadvantages but the major one is the phenomenon of quenching. This occurs because energy that might have been emitted as fluorescence is lost to other molecules by collisional interaction. This partly explains the increased sensitivity and accuracy in low concentrations because there are fewer molecules, and hence collisions, although the effects of solvent must not be neglected. Many materials such as detergents, stopcock grease, filter paper and some tissues may cause interference by the release of fluorescing agents.

9.5.2 Instrumentation

The direct relationship between fluorescence intensity and concentration, allows relatively simple electronics and optics to be used. Two monochromators may be employed, the first (M_1) for selecting the excitation wavelength. Fluorescence emission occurs in all possible directions and one direction (90°) is chosen and the second monochromator (M_2) is used for determination of the fluorescence spectrum. The radiation source is generally either a mercury lamp or a xenon arc, excitation wavelengths frequently being selected in the ultraviolet region and the emission wavelengths in the visible region. The detector is usually a sensitive photocell, for example a red-sensitive photomultiplier for wavelengths greater than 500 nm. Temperature control is required for accurate work as the intensity of fluorescence may vary between 10% and 50% for a 10 deg.C change at approximately 25 °C.

Two approaches are possible for the illumination of the sample: the simplest is the basic 90° illumination (Fig. 9.10), the alternative approach being front-face illumination (FFI; Fig. 9.11) which obviates pre- and postfilter effects. These latter

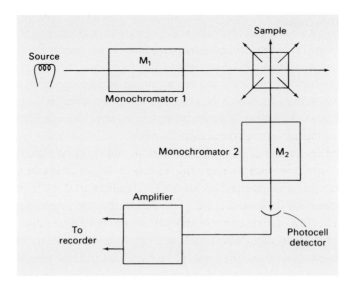

Fig. 9.10. The basic component of a spectrofluorimeter set up for 90° illumination.

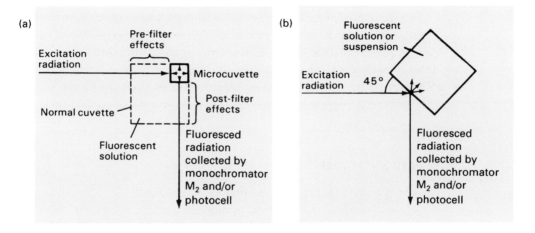

Fig. 9.11. Reduction of filter effects using (a) microcuvettes and (b) front-face illumination.

effects arise owing to the absorption of radiation prior to it reaching the fluorescent molecules (prefilter absorption) and the reduction in the amount of emitted radiation escaping from the cuvette (postfilter effects). Such effects are more evident in concentrated solutions, and the use of microcuvettes (containing less material) can be of value (Fig. 9.11a). FFI is essential for examining suspensions, and cuvettes with only one optical face are required. Excitation and emission occur at the same face but generally the technique is somewhat less sensitive than 90° illumination.

9.5.3 **Applications**

Applications of the technique are many and varied, despite the fact that relatively few compounds exhibit the phenomenon. A compound may have its fluorescence and absorption spectra compared as an aid to identification; the effects of pH, solvent composition and the polarisation of fluorescence may all contribute to structural elucidation. The measurement of phosphorescence and phosphorescence lifetimes can also be of value in compound identification.

The detection of non-fluorescent compounds may be achieved by coupling a fluorescent probe (or fluor) in a similar way to the use of reporter groups in absorption spectrophotometry (Section 9.4.3). This is termed extrinsic fluorescence as distinct from intrinsic fluorescence, where the native compound exhibits the property. The use of such probes is valuable in both qualitative and quantitative analysis. For instance amino acids and peptides separated by chromatography or electrophoresis may be identified by coupling to their primary amino groups either dansyl chloride or o-phthalaldehyde (Section 13.2.6). The latter conjugates fluoresce intensely blue and the total oligopeptide fingerprint may be determined on only 10^{-5} g of protein. If the separation methods are used in column form, then quantification is possible by forming derivatives postcolumn. Acridine orange is an extrinsic fluor that can be used to determine the strandedness of polynucleotides as the Stokes shifts differ between conjugates of single- and double-stranded polynucleotides, which fluoresce red and green, respectively. The fluor should be tightly bound at a specific site, its fluorescence should be sensitive to environmental changes and it should not have adverse effects on the system being studied. Some structures of fluorescent probes are shown in Fig. 9.12.

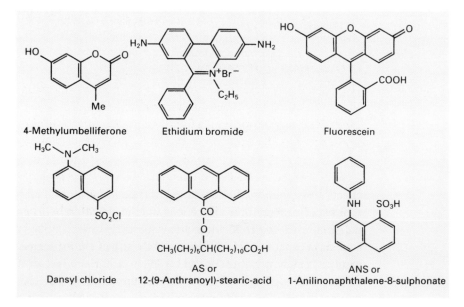

Fig. 9.12. Structure of some fluorescent probes.

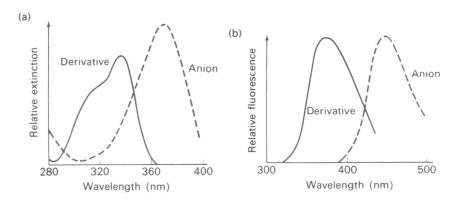

Fig. 9.13. Spectra of the methylumbelliferone anion and derivatives of 4-methylumbelliferone at pH 10: (a) absorption spectra; (b) fluorescence spectra.

The major use of fluorimetry in biochemistry is in quantitative determination of materials present in concentrations too low for absorption spectrophotometry. Assays of vitamin B_1 in foodstuffs, NADH, hormones, drugs, pesticides, carcinogens, chlorophyll, cholesterol, porphyrins and some metal ions indicate the range. Self- and contaminant quenching can be determined by adding a known quantity of a standard to an unknown quantity of a pure compound and measuring the fluorescence before and after the addition.

Ca^{2+} may be measured in the cytoplasm by the chelating agent Quin-2, which preferentially binds the metal. The fluorescence increases about five-fold on binding. More sensitive probes for this analysis are Fura-2 and Indo-1. Quin-1 is a chelating agent that may be used as a fluorescent probe to monitor intracellular pH changes in the range 5 to 9. Over this range, there is a 30-fold increase in fluorescence.

Enzyme assays and kinetic analysis

The general principles of enzyme assays, which are discussed in Section 7.4.1, often rely on the use of spectrofluorimetric assays. An example is the anion of 4-methylumbelliferone, which fluoresces at 450 nm. Its rate of appearance may be monitored when it is produced as a result of enzymic action on an ether or ester derivative of the fluor. The enzymes used are group-specific hydrolases and their kinetics may be studied by fluorescence measurement; Fig. 9.13a and b shows typical absorption and fluorescence spectra. Irradiation is usually at 350 to 400 nm wavelength and virtually all the fluorescence measured between 450 and 500 nm is due to the anion product. It is claimed that one molecule of β-galactosidase may be detected when it acts on fluorescein bis(β-D-galactopyranoside) as substrate because the sensitivity of the method is so great. Hence actual numbers of molecules in a single bacterial cell may be determined, as may the synthesis of the enzyme in individual cells in a population.

Spectrofluorimetry can be applied widely in metabolic studies where NAD forms are involved as cofactors. This arises because NADH and NADPH fluoresce, whereas the oxidised equivalents do not. Therefore redox processses may be followed kinetically *in vitro* at concentrations similar to those encountered *in vivo*, and also followed in intact cells or organelles (e.g. mitochondria).

Protein structure

The presence of tryptophan and FAD as cofactors allows fluorescence to be measured in proteins. The binding and release of cofactors, inhibitors, substrates etc., at sites close to the fluor, cause changes in the associated fluorescence spectra. Information about conformational changes, denaturation and aggregation may be gleaned. The absence of an intrinsic fluor can be overcome by coupling a suitable extrinsic fluor such as anilino-napthalene-8-sulphonate (ANS), dansyl chloride and derivatives of fluorescein or rhodamine.

Membrane structure

The fluorescent properties of a molecule are affected by its mobility and environment, particularly the polarity of the latter. These effects in the vicinity of a fluorescent probe may be monitored by measuring changes in fluorescence. Various probes having charged and hydrophobic regions (ANS and *N*-methyl-2-anilino-6-naphthalene sulphonate (MNS)) and hence able to orient themselves across lipid/aqueous interfaces may be used to study membrane structure and gain information about the properties of such interfaces. Incorporation of phospholipids containing 12-(9-anthroanoyl)-stearic acid and 2-(9-anthroanoyl)-palmitic acid into membranes yields information about the regions 0.5 nm and 1.5 nm, respectively, from the phosphate head groups of the lipid bilayer. The basic membrane structure and also the effects of temperature and certain biological phenomena may be studied. Changes in mitochondrial membranes during energy transduction have also been monitored using an ANS probe.

Fluorescence bleaching recovery

If a fluor is exposed to a pulse of high intensity radiation it may be irreversibly bleached, i.e. permanently lose its ability to fluoresce. Fluorescently labelled phospholipids incorporated into a biological membrane may be subjected to this treatment and then the motion of such entities (in the membrane) can be studied by monitoring (with low intensity radiation) the re-emergence of fluorescence as the bleached and unbleached molecules interdiffuse. Applications include the lateral motion of extrinsically labelled rhodopsin in the photoreceptor membrane, the study of polymerisation of proteins such as actin and the diffusion of fluorescently labelled proteins microinjected into cells (see also Section 8.3.3).

Energy transfer studies

In a number of cases energy may be transferred, by resonance energy transfer, from a donor to an acceptor fluor, provided there is overlap between the donor fluorescence spectrum and the acceptor absorption spectrum. The fluors must also be closely situated and transfer efficiency is related to spatial separation. This efficiency may be measured either as quenching of the donor fluorescence by acceptor or as the intensities of fluorescence of acceptor when the latter is irradiated both in the presence and in the absence of the donor.

Intrinsic fluors such as tryptophan or extrinsic ones attached to amino acids, -SH groups, sugars or fluorescent analogues of substrates, inhibitors, cofactors or phospholipids may be employed in energy transfer experiments to deduce distances within protein molecules. Accuracy is limited to about ± 0.5 nm and determinations include the localisation of metals in metalloproteins, the measurement of the extent of conformational changes in enzymes when substrate binding occurs, the distances between various pairs of proteins in the ribosome and the three-dimensional structure of transfer RNAs.

Fluorescence depolarisation

The excitation wavelengths used may be polarised by introducing a suitable polariser between the first monochromator (M_1) and the sample. The emitted radiation may be totally unpolarised or partially polarised and may be detected by using a second polariser between the emission monochromator (M_2) and the detector.

Molecular rotations affect fluorescence depolarisation: for instance, the rotation of an absorber chromophore and energy transfer between chromophores increase the depolarisation effect. High concentrations of chromophore and high viscosity of the solvent result in the measurement of mainly energy transfer. At low concentrations and low viscosity the effects of molecular motion predominate.

The mobility of whole molecules, or parts thereof, may be investigated using this technique. The lifetimes of intrinsic fluors of proteins and nucleic acids are usually too short, as these biological macromolecules move relatively slowly. Hence extrinsic fluors are frequently used in these studies. Examples of such studies include the binding of fluorescent substrates, the binding of inhibitors and cofactors to enzymes, reduction of mobility (increase of overall mass and hence inertia); and the antigen/antibody complexation reaction. The association and dissociation of multisubunit proteins, such as lactate dehydrogenase and chymotrypsin, and the viscosity of living cells may also be measured.

An interesting historical aside involves the use of highly viscous glycerol to slow down the rotation and translation of large molecules in depolarisation experiments. It was knowledge of this totally unconnected fact that gave the clue to the use of glycerol as a matrix in fast atom bombardment mass spectrometry (Section 11.6.2).

Microspectrofluorimetry

In this technique a microscope is combined with a spectrofluorimeter equipped with fibre optics to enable the examination of single bacterial cells binding fluorescent antibodies and also the fluorescent intensity of subcellular structures. The extra amount of nucleic acid that tends to be present in malignant cells will take up more of the fluorescent probe acridine orange than do normal cells. This observation may be used to detect malignant cells in biopsy tissue.

The fluorescence-activated cell sorter

This system, described in Section 4.8.5 makes use of the light emitted by cells carrying a fluorescently labelled antibody to trigger their physical separation from unlabelled cells as they flow through a fine capillary.

Fluorescence immunoassay

These methods are dealt with extensively in Section 4.7.6 but are worthy of a brief mention here.

Several immunoassays have been developed using fluorescent probes to label either antigen or antibody. The binding of a labelled hapten by an antibody may alter the intensity of fluorescence, thus enabling the complex formation to be monitored. Changes in polarisation methods applied to immunoassay have been mentioned above. A major disadvantage of either of these approaches is the high background fluorescence which often accompanies the process and interferes with the measurement. The most promising development in this area is time-resolved fluorescence immunoassay. Two approaches have been combined to reduce the effects of background fluorescence and hence increase the sensitivity. First, europium chelates are usually used as the fluor, as they have large Stokes shifts and long-lived fluorescence. Secondly, a fluorimeter has been designed that delays the measurement of the emitted light by 400 μs, during which time the non-specific background fluorescence has almost completely decayed. Such an approach has led to the development of dissociation-enhanced lanthanide fluoro-immunoassay (DELFIA).

Multicomponent analysis by synchronous luminescence spectrometry

Despite its name this is really a fluorescence technique and allows the simultaneous analysis of multicomponent mixtures without the need to resort to the use of rather complicated algorithms and sophisticated computer techniques. For this reason it is included in this section.

In conventional luminescence spectrometry an emission spectrum is monitored by scanning the emission wavelength λ_{em} while the luminescent (fluorescent) compound is excited at a fixed excitation wavelength λ_{exc}. Conversely an excitation spectrum is obtained by scanning λ_{exc} while the emission is monitored at a fixed λ_{em}.

A combined method involves scanning both λ_{em} and λ_{exc} together, i.e. varying both simultaneously or synchronously. This is feasible despite the loss of constant excitation energy employed in the conventional method.

The luminescence intensity, I_s, is obtained from equation 9.9, the right-hand side of which is derived from the Beer-Lambert law:

$$I_s = KcdE_X(\lambda - \Delta\lambda)E_M(\lambda) \tag{9.9}$$

where K is an aggregate constant; c is concentration of analyte; d is the optical pathlength; λ is the emission wavelength; $E_M(\lambda)$ is the emission spectrum; $E_X(\lambda - \Delta\lambda)$ is related to the experimentally determined exitation spectrum, which involves excitation at a wavelength λ'. It is a specific requirement of this technique that the difference between excitation and emission wavelengths remains fixed, i.e. $\Delta\lambda = \lambda - \lambda'$. Hence $\lambda' = \lambda - \Delta\lambda$ in the expression above. It is often convenient in practice to choose $\Delta\lambda$ to be the same as the Stokes shift.

A number of advantages of the method are that complex spectra may be reduced to a single peak, spectral bands are generally narrowed, a spectral range is produced (this is of particular advantage to the analytical scientist as against the requirements of the purist spectroscopist); and spectra of multicomponent systems may be simplified. In addition, multiplicity of scan rates for both monochromators allows for considerable variability in the operation of the technique.

Amongst the applications of the technique is the measurement of the fluorescence associated with benzo(a)pyrene (BP) molecules covalently attached to nucleic acids, both DNA and RNA, isolated from the epidermis of BP-treated mice. The measurements were made at 77 K in frozen aqueous solutions by use of a photon-counting fluorimeter operating in synchronous scanning mode. A $\Delta\lambda$ of 28 nm was chosen, which corresponds to the Stokes shift for the fluorescence of bound BP. Other applications have involved the measurement of the carcinogenic polycyclic hydrocarbon dibenz(a,h)anthracene in extracts of cigarette smoke, resolution of tyrosine and tryptophan in proteins and polypeptides, and quantitative determination of hallucinogens (e.g. LSD). Derivative spectra may also be obtained, enabling the resolution of phenylalanine, tyrosine and tryptotphan in admixture, protein mixtures, and catecholamines. The method offers potential for applications in clinical analysis.

9.6 CIRCULAR DICHROISM SPECTROSCOPY

9.6.1 Principles

It has been known for some time that optical isomers (isomers whose mirror images are non-superimposable) possess the property of allowing the rotation of plane-polarised light. Electromagnetic radiation oscillates in all possible directions and it is possible to select preferentially waves oscillating in a single plane. This is achieved using a polarising material such as Polaroid or a nicol prism. The technique of polarimetry essentially measures the angle through which the plane of polarisation is changed after such light is passed through a solution containing a chiral (optically active) substance. Optical rotary dispersion (ORD) spectroscopy is a technique for measuring this ability to rotate the plane of polarisation, as a function of the wavelength. However, such chiral substances may also absorb the plane-polarised radiation at certain wavelengths. In such cases the chromophore is termed an optically active chromophore or chiral centre, as it may only be part of a complex molecule. The technique of ORD has been largely supplanted by circular dichroism (CD) spectroscopy, which gives rather better information about the three-dimensional structure of macromolecules containing chiral centres. In CD, circularly polarised light is used and this is obtained by superimposing two plane-polarised light waves of the same wavelengths and amplitudes but differing in phase by one quarter of a wavelength and in their planes of polarisation by 90°.

Just as plane-polarised light may be left (L) or right (R) handed, so can circularly polarised light. Whether R or L circularly polarised light is produced depends on the relative positions of the peaks of the two plane-polarised waves.

The asymmetry inherent in the structure of chiral molecules or centres interact differently with polarised light. Not only are the R and L waves of plane-polarised light differentially absorbed and refracted, resulting in a beam in a different plane (the basis of polarimetry), but in the case of circularly polarised light a similar differential interaction occurs. In the latter case, the resultant beam, after having passed through the sample, is a recombination of the R and L components to give an emergent beam of elliptically polarised light. In polarimetry the specific rotation $[\alpha]_\lambda$ would be measured, whereas in CD spectroscopy it is the ellipticity, θ, which is measured:

$$\theta = 2.303\,\Delta A$$
$$\quad = 33\,\Delta A\ \text{degrees} \tag{9.10}$$

where ΔA is the difference in absorption between R and L components.

A CD spectrum is usually a plot of ellipticity versus wavelength and information regarding the structure of certain entities may be gleaned from it.

9.6.2 Instrumentation

The basic layout of a CD spectrometer is shown in Fig. 9.14. Both L and R circularly polarised light may be produced alternately, from a single monochromator, by the passage of plane-polarised light through an electrooptic modulator. This modulator is a crystal that, when subjected to alternating currents, transmits either the R or the L component, depending on the polarity of the electric field to which it is exposed. The photomultiplier detector produces a voltage proportional to the ellipticity of the resultant beam emerging from the sample container.

9.6.3 Applications

The major application of CD is the study of conformation of biological macromolecules and complements data generated from nuclear magnetic resonance experiments (Chapter 10).

Proteins

Information can be gained about the relative proportions of secondary structure, α-helical, β-sheet and random coil, in solution. The application of CD to tertiary structure is limited, owing to inadequate theoretical understanding of the influences of different parts of these molecules at this level of structure. The CD spectra of poly-L-amino acids have been obtained and are used as standards for calculating the percentage of each form of secondary structure in proteins. Curve-fitting procedures using computer processing have been used to apply the method to unknown proteins.

One of the most important benefits to be gained from CD spectroscopy is the

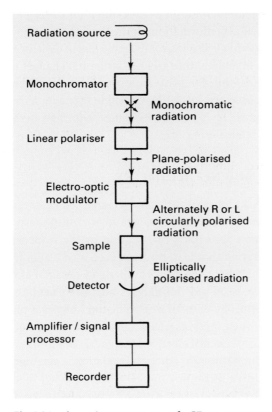

Fig. 9.14. The main components of a CD spectrometer.

study of conformational changes during, or because of, interactions with other entities. Examples are the determination of binding constants of substrates, cofactors, inhibitors or activators of virtually any enzyme. The binding of the inhibitor 3-cytidilic acid to the active site of pancreatic ribonuclease changes the CD spectrum of a remotely situated tyrosine residue. The binding of this inhibitor must therefore cause a conformational change in a distant part of the enzyme. CD spectroscopy is very sensitive and may be used to monitor the conversion of α- and β-structures to random coil (a major event of the denaturation process).

Nucleic acids

It is possible to calculate the CD spectrum of a single strand of DNA from the known nearest-neighbour frequency. Experimentally determined deviations from this calculated spectrum are indicative of a variation in structure, for example double strandedness. The CD spectrum of double-stranded DNA appears to be independent of the base composition in the range of wavelengths usually used.

A large increase in the CD spectrum of mononucleotides is observed when they link to form even short oligonucleotide chains. This observation provides evidence that hydrophobic interactions between stacked bases are important in stabilising the double-stranded structure of DNA.

All nucleotides exhibit chiral properties, and their CD is greatly increased on the adoption of a helical conformation. Hence the technique may be used to study structural changes in nucleic acids, for example loss of helicity of single-stranded DNA as a function of temperature and pH, structural changes on the binding of cations and proteins, transfer RNA–amino acid binding, transitions between single- and double-stranded DNA, DNA histone interactions in chromatin, the structure of ribosomal RNA in the ribosomes, and the interaction of double-stranded DNA and intercalating drugs.

9.7 TURBIDIMETRY AND NEPHELOMETRY

The two similar techniques of turbidimetry and nephelometry are both associated with the estimation of the concentrations of dilute suspensions. In turbidimetry, the apparent absorption of radiation by the suspension is measured. The apparent absorption should be measured at a wavelength where *true* absorption is not occurring; hence the Beer–Lambert law does not apply in turbidimetry. When radiation is passed through a transparent medium, for example a solution in a cuvette, one or both of two distinct physical phenomena might occur. In the case of extinction, true absorption of energy occurs and allows changes in the energy states of electrons, magnetic conditions, molecular vibrations, etc. The medium through which the radiation is passing and in which the absorption is occurring, is termed optically empty, when this is the only phenomenon occurring. However, in the case of a suspension, a quite distinct radiative phenomenon may occur in which the light is scattered by the suspended particles. This scattering is due to reflection and refraction and gives rise to the Tyndall effect; it occurs in all directions and is an example of the more general Rayleigh scattering.

In turbidimetry the incident and transmitted radiation may be measured in an ordinary colorimeter or spectrophotometer, but the contribution of true absorption, if any, is small and the Beer–Lambert law is not strictly applicable as it holds only for very thin layers or very dilute suspensions.

The scattered light or Tyndall light may also be measured, usually at right angles (normal) to the incident radiation. This gives the Tyndall ratio, which is the ratio of the Tyndall intensity to that of the incident radiation. If this ratio is measured directly, a Tyndall meter would be used. If, however, the Tyndall intensity is compared with that of a standard suspension of known concentration, then the instrument is known as a nephelometer (measures cloudiness). The concentrations of suspensions of microorganisms may be obtained using nephelometry and those of proteins and some other biological macromolecules by turbidimetry.

These techniques are difficult to use but in experienced hands can be of value. The relationship between energy input (incident radiation) and measured output (transmitted or scattered), however, is complicated and non-linear. It should be noted that these techniques are not strictly spectroscopic but are included here for completeness.

9.8 **LUMINOMETRY**

9.8.1 **Principles**

The emission and radiative techniques discussed above all depend on some physical phenomenon within the molecules concerned. The phenomenon also depends on the prior input of energy, frequently obtained from electromagnetic radiation. The radiative phenomenon luminescence arises in a different way. Although it is essentially the emission of electromagnetic radiation in the visible region (i.e. light), it arises as the result of a chemical reaction. Luminometry is the technique used to measure this luminescence, and, although not a spectrophotometric technique, it is included for completeness as it is an important method in biological science.

Chemiluminescence occurs as a result of excited electrons relaxing to the ground state (see Fig. 9.2b). The prior excitation arises as a result of a chemical reaction that yields a fluorescent product, and the chemiluminescent spectrum of a reaction such as luminol with oxygen to produce 3-aminophthalate is the same as the fluorescent spectrum of the product. A similar phenomenon is bioluminescence, so-called because the light emission arises from an enzyme-catalysed reaction (Section 7.4.2) usually involving luciferase. The colour of the light emitted in the latter case depends on the source of the enzyme and varies between 560 nm (greenish yellow) and 620 nm (red) wavelengths. This method has the distinct advantage of high sensitivity, as a result of the reaction having a high quantum yield – 100% under favourable conditions.

9.8.2 **Instrumentation**

It is not electromagnetic radiation that is the source of the excitation energy, hence no monochromator is required. Luminometry can therefore be performed with relatively simple photometers. Two minor complications are the need to amplify the output signal prior to recording and the need to maintain fairly strict temperature control. This control is necessary owing to the sensitivity of reactions to temperature, particularly in the case of enzyme-catalysed reactions.

Figure 9.15 shows the layout of the main components. The reactants are introduced into a suitable light-protected reaction vessel in which adequate mixing takes place. The emitted light is collected by a photomultiplier tube, which is connected to a direct current amplifier with a wide range of sensitivity and linear response.

9.8.3 **Applications**

The firefly luciferase system

Details for the firefly luciferase system are given in Section 7.4.2. ATP concentration may be measured in an assay that is rapid to carry out and whose accuracy is comparable to spectrophotometric and fluorimetric assays. The sensitivity is,

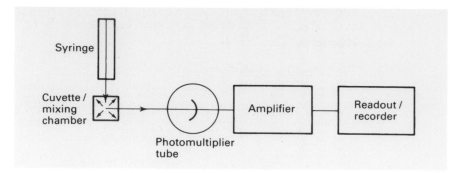

Fig. 9.15. Diagram of the main components of a simple luminometer.

however, vastly increased, having a limit of detection of 10^{-15} M and a linear range of 10^{-12} to 10^{-6} M ATP. The concentrations of ADP, AMP and cyclic AMP may also be determined using appropriate enzymes, for example pyruvate kinase for ADP $\rightarrow$ ATP, adenylate kinase for AMP $\rightarrow$ ADP, and phosphodiesterase for cyclic AMP $\rightarrow$ AMP. In principle, all the enzymes and metabolites involved in ATP inter-conversion reactions may be assayed by this method. Examples are the enzymes creatine kinase, hexokinase and ATP sulphurase, and the substrates creatine phosphate, glucose, GTP, phosphoenolpyruvate and 1,3-diphosphoglycerate.

The bacterial luciferase system

Details of the bacterial luciferase system also are given in Section 7.4.2. The determination of nicotinamide adenine dinucleotides (and phosphates) and flavin mononucleotides, in their reduced states (i.e. NADH, NADPH and $FMNH_2$) may be made in assays which use this system. A concentration range of 10^{-9} to 10^{-12} M is achievable, which is much more sensitive than the corresponding spectrophotometric and fluorimetric assays, although the NADPH assay is less sensitive than the NADH assay by a factor of about 20. The method can be applied to a whole range of coupled enzyme reaction systems of the redox type that involve these nucleotides as coenzymes.

The aequorin system

Despite the development of calcium-specific electrodes, the calcium ion concentration may be determined with high sensitivity, intracellularly, using the phosphoprotein aequorin. The protein is isolated from luminescent medusae (jellyfish) and is practically non-fluorescent. In the presence of Ca^{2+}, however, it is converted from its natural yellow reflective colour to the blue fluorescent protein (BFP). The bioluminescent spectrum of the reaction is identical with the fluorescent spectrum of BFP:$2Ca^{2+}$ but different from BFP:Ca^{2+}.

Ease of use, high sensitivity to, and relative specificity for, calcium and the non-toxicity of aequorin to living cells are advantages. The disadvantages are the scarcity of the protein, its large molecular size, consumption during the reaction and the non-linearity of the light emission relative to calcium concentration. Also the reaction is sensitive to its chemical environment and the limited speed in which it can respond to rapid changes in calcium concentration, for example influx and efflux in certain cell types.

Chemiluminescence

Luminol and its derivatives can undergo chemiluminescent reactions with high efficiency. For instance, enzymically generated H_2O_2 may be detected by the emission of light at 430 nm wavelength in the presence of luminol and microperoxidase (Section 7.4.2).

Competitive binding assays may be used to determine low concentrations of hormones, drugs and metabolites in biological fluids. Such assays depend on the ability of proteins such as antibodies and cell receptors to bind specific ligands with high affinity (Section 7.4.2). Competition between labelled and unlabelled ligand for appropriate sites on the binding compound occurs. If the concentration of the binding compound is known, i.e. the number of available sites is known and a limited but known concentration of labelled ligand is introduced, then under saturation conditions all sites are occupied and the concentration of unlabelled ligand can be determined. Use of labelled ligand allows the concentration of only binding compound (the number of sites) to be determined. A variety of labels, including radioisotopes, is in common use, enabling the fractions in the bound and free states to be distinguished. Labelling with a luminol derivative, completing the binding reaction, separating bound and free fractions allows the protein to be assayed by its chemiluminescence. The system must be calibrated using standards and, under the most favourable conditions, 10^{-12} M of a compound may be determined.

Whilst polymorphonuclear leukocytes are phagocytosing, singlet molecular oxygen is produced that exhibits chemiluminescence. The effects of pharmocological and toxicological agents on these and other phagocytic cells can be studied by monitoring this luminescence.

9.9 ATOMIC SPECTROSCOPY

All of the methods described above, with the exception of nuclear phenomena in the γ- and X-ray regions, have dealt essentially with molecular spectroscopy. The general theory of electron transitions was discussed in Section 9.1.2 and for simplicity the phenomena were described mainly in atomic terms, although the extension to molecules is not too difficult. It was indicated above (Section 9.1.2) that, in general, molecules give rise to band spectra and atoms to clearly defined line spectra. These lines can be observed by eye either as light, associated with a particular wavelength, which are atomic emission spectra or black lines against a bright background, which are atomic absorption spectra. Some elements, particularly metals, have an important role to play in biological systems, whether as simple cofactors in enzymes, the central atom in biological macromolecules such as iron in haemoglobin or magnesium in chlorophyll, or as toxic substances that affect metabolism. Use of atomic spectroscopy will enable data to be obtained that are important in understanding the biological roles of these elements.

In a spectrum of an element, the wavelengths at which absorption or emission are observed are associated with transitions where the minimal energy change occurs. For example, in Fig. 9.2a is shown the $3s$–$3p$, or D-line transition in the sodium atom that gives rise to the emission of orange light. When electron transitions occur in an atom they are limited by the availability of an empty orbital or level. An orbital or level could not be overfilled without contravening the Pauli exclusion principle (Section 9.1.2). In order for energy changes to be minimal, transitions tend to occur between levels close together in energy terms. These limitations mean that emission and absorption lines are absolutely characteristic of the element concerned. At least for simple atoms it is theoretically possible to deduce their electronic structure from their line spectra. The wavelengths emitted from excited atoms may be identified using a spectroscope, spectrograph or a direct reading spectrophotometer that use as detectors the human eye, a photographic plate or a photoelectric cell, respectively.

In general, and in contrast to molecular spectroscopy, atom concentrations are not measured directly in solution. The atoms have to be volatilised either in a flame or electrothermally in an oven. In this state the elements will readily emit or absorb monochromatic radiation at the appropriate wavelength. Usually nebulisers (atomisers) will be used to spray the standard or test solution into the flame through which the light is passed. Alternatively the light beam is passed, in an oven, through a cavity containing the vaporised material.

9.9.1 **Principles of atomic flame spectrometry**

This technique takes advantage of the properties described above to determine the amounts of a specific element that may be present. The emission of light is measured by emission flame spectrophotometry and absorption by atomic absorption flame spectrophotometry.

The energy absorbed or emitted is proportional to the number of atoms in the optical path. In the case of emission it is strictly the number of excited atoms, but under reproducible standard conditions this will be the same as that for a calibrating standard. Flame instability, variation in temperature and composition of the flame make standard conditions difficult to achieve. Sodium gives high backgrounds and hence should be measured first and then a similar amount added to all other standards. Excess hydrochloric is usually added as chloride compounds are often the most volatile salts. Calcium and magnesium emission is enhanced by the addition of alkali metals and suppressed by addition of phosphate, silicate and aluminate (by the formation of non-dissociable salts). This suppression effect may be relieved by the addition of lanthanum and strontium salts. Cyclic analysis may be performed that involves the estimation of each interfering substance in a mixture and then the standards for each component in the mixture are 'doped' with each interfering substance. The process is repeated (usually only two to three cycles are necessary) with refined estimates of interfering substance, until self-consistent values are obtained for each component; this implies minimal interference effects resulting from the concentrations approaching those in the unknown sample.

Flame instability requires that assays are carried out in triplicate and it is advantageous to bracket a determination of an unknown with measurements of the same standard to achieve the greatest accuracy. The use of lithium as an internal standard improves the technique. Polythene bottles should be used for storage if possible, as metal ions are both absorbed and released by glass.

Biological samples are usually converted to ash prior to the determination of metals. This can be done dry if sublimation losses are prevented. Wet ashing (in solution) is often used; this employs an oxidative digestion similar to the Kjeldahl method (see Section 6.3.2).

9.9.2 Instrumentation

Atomic emission spectrophotometry

The nebulisers used are usually of the type that involves passing a stream of air over a capillary tube whose other end dips into the solution under test. Larger droplets tend not to remain in the hottest part of the flame long enough, in direct injection systems, for their constituents to be volatilised and hence are allowed to settle out in a cloud chamber. Combustion of air and natural gas gives a temperature of 1500 °C, which is adequate for sodium determination. Calcium is better assayed at 2000 to 2500 °C and magnesium and iron require 2500 °C, obtained from an air/acetylene gas mixture. Bandwidth selection using a filter device may be used for routine analyses of moderate accuracy. More accurate measurements require a monochromator. The best accuracy achieves a resolution of 0.1 to 0.2 nm over the range 200 to 1000 nm. Table 9.3 lists the wavelengths used for a number of metals, together with their detection limits. Detectors are often of the photocell type but flame instability limits their value as their potential accuracy is not realised. Multichannel polychromators allow the emission of up to six elements at one time to be measured. The basic layout of an atomic (flame) emission spectrophotometer is shown in Fig. 9.16.

Atomic absorption spectrophotometry

In these instruments either a double monochromator with a source of white light or a hollow cathode discharge lamp is used to produce radiation in a very narrow bandwidth. Discharge lamps emit radiation at a wavelength specific for the element being assayed. This specificity can be obtained only from a pure sample of the element that is excited electrically to produce an arc spectrum of that element, and electrodeless discharge lamps are now available. Nebulisers and burners are similar to the emission devices but 10 cm flames are often used to obtain an increased optical length. Both single and double beam instruments are available, the latter often incorporating a chopper to give intermittent pulses and prevent stray light from the flame reaching the detector. The most useful wavelength range is 190 to 850 nm.

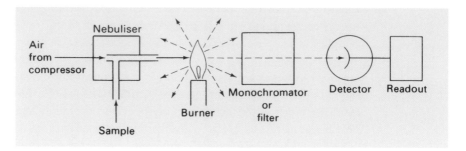

Fig. 9.16. The main components of an atomic emission (flame) spectrophotometer.

Flameless instruments

A flameless atomic absorption spectrophotometer incorporates a graphite tube as an oven, which may be heated electrothermally to 3000 °C. Monochromatic light specific to the element being assayed is produced either by a hollow cathode discharge lamp or an electrodeless discharge lamp. The graphite tube forms an optical cavity, in which the sample resides and through which the monochromatic radiation is passed. Absorption is measured continuously as the temperature is raised and computer methods allow the superimposition of absorption and temperature profiles, with time, to be produced. This approach allows optimum conditions to be determined for future analyses. The flameless technique is 100 times more sensitive than flame methods and has the distinct advantage of being able to be automated as the inherent dangers of using combustible gases have been eliminated.

9.9.3 Applications

Sodium and potassium may be assayed at concentrations of a few parts per million (< 5) using simple filter photometers. The more sophisticated emission flame spectrophotometers may be used to assay some 20 elements in biological samples, the most common being calcium, magnesium and manganese. Absorption flame spectrophotometers are usually more sensitive than emission types and can usually detect < 1 p.p.m. of each of more than 20 elements. Exceptions to this are the alkali metals. Relative precision is about 1% in a working range of 20 to 200 times the detection limit (Table 9.3).

The techniques are widely used in clinical laboratories, for the determination of metals in body fluids. These determinations aid diagnosis and are valuable in the monitoring of many therapeutic regimes. In physiological and pharmacological research, sodium, potassium, calcium, magnesium, cadmium and zinc may be measured directly, but copper, lead, iron and mercury require prior extraction from the biological source. The methods are also widely used in element determination in soil and plant materials and, after suitable ashing procedures, may be used for metals in macromolecules, organelles, cells and tissues.

Table 9.3 The detection limits for various elements in emission and absorption flame spectrophotometry, flameless absorption spectrophotometry, and ion-selective electrodes

Element	Emission		Absorption				Ion-selective electrode: detection limit (p.p.m.)
	Detection limit (p.p.m.)	Wavelength (nm)	Detection limit (p.p.m.)			Wavelength (nm)	
			Flame	Flameless			
Calcium	0.005	442.7	0.1	0.00007		442.7	0.02
Copper	0.1	324.8	0.1	0.0001		324.8	0.0006
Iron	0.5	372.0	0.2	0.0001		248.3	
Lead			0.5	0.0002		283.3	0.21
Lithium	0.001	670.7	0.03	0.0001		670.7	
Magnesium	0.1	285.2	0.01	0.00001		285.2	
Manganese	0.02	403.3	0.05	0.00004		279.5	
Mercury			10.0	0.018		253.8	
Potassium	0.001	766.5	0.03	0.00003		766.5	0.04
Sodium	0.0001	589.0	0.03	0.00001		589.0	0.02
Strontium	0.01	460.7	0.06	0.0001		460.9	

9.9.4 **Atomic fluorescence spectrophotometry**

Prior excitation of atoms by electromagnetic radiation rather than by thermal energy is required (cf. molecular fluorescence, Section 9.8.1). Atoms are again required to be in the vapour state: the phenomenon is not observed in solution as it is with molecules. The source beam must be intense but less spectrally pure than that required for atomic absorption spectrophotometry, as only the resonant wavelengths will be absorbed and lead to fluorescence. Direct emission from the flame being recorded by the detector must be avoided and this may be achieved by modulation of the detector amplifier to the same frequency as that of the primary source. Although limited to only a few metals, the extreme sensitivity achievable in appropriate cases make it better than comparable methods. For example, zinc and cadmium may be detected at levels as low as 1 and 2 parts per 10^{10}, respectively.

9.10 **LASERS**

Laser is an acronym for *l*ight *a*mplification by *s*timulated *e*mission of *r*adiation. A detailed explanation of how laser light is generated is not possible here. A simple view is that electromagnetic radiation used as the excitation agent can be considered as the input of photons to an absorbing material. This results in elevation of an electron to a higher energy level as described above (Section 9.1.2). If, while the electron is in an excited state, another photon of precisely the correct energy arrives, then, instead of the electron being promoted to an even higher energy level, it returns to its original ground state. This return is accompanied by the emission of two coherent photons. These photons have associated wavelengths which are exactly in phase, hence the term coherent. A laser-producing material has to be pumped and this is often achieved by surrounding the material with a rapidly flashing high intensity flash tube that gives an ample supply of suitable photons.

The emitted, coherent light has considerable advantages, but in particular it can be produced with zero bandwidth, i.e. unique invariant wavelengths can be selected to excite molecules or atoms in a very precise way. It is also possible to generate, from appropriate sources, groups of selected wavelengths should this be required. Various applications are under development in spectroscopic and spectrophotometric methods that take advantage of the spectral purity of laser light.

An important application is the laser reflectance method for determining complementary DNA (cDNA) in nucleic acid studies. The use of reverse transcriptase and DNA polymerase (see Section 2.13.2) allows the nucleotide sequence corresponding to the primary sequence of a peptide fragment or protein to be synthesised. Chain growth occurs at the 3' end from a primer section, and chain termination occurs when a dideoxynucleotide is incorporated into the growing complementary strand (Chapter 2). Four 'channels' are required, each containing primer, all four deoxynucleoside triphosphates and one of each of the four dideoxy compounds. In each of the four channels, chain termination occurs at different points. Also, at the 5′-end of the primers a different fluorescent label is attached that has no influence on the subsequent reactions but can be used to identify uniquely components of the resulting mixtures in each channel. Mixtures are separated by gel electrophoresis (see Section 12.2.2) in which distance travelled in the gel is effectively inversely proportional to the mass of the fragment. The gel is illuminated with a narrow beam of laser light and fluorescent emission from each label is measured (a different wavelength is emitted from each label). The band on the gel can be identified by including, to interrupt the emitted beam, a rotating filter disc that contains four sectors, each of which allows only one fluorescent wavelength to pass. By design, which fluor relates to which dideoxy terminator is known and mobility, position and amount are determined. The system can be automated and avoids the use of radioisotopes. It is reliable and precise, and data interpretation can be done by computer.

9.11 **KEY TERMS**

absorbance	emission flame spectrophotometry	phosphorescence lifetimes
absorber	emission spectrum	photocell
absorption	energy	photons
absorption edge	excited state	polarisation
absorption spectrum	extinction	prism
action spectrum	extrinsic fluorescence	quanta
atomic absorption flame	fluor	quantum
spectrophotometry	fluorescence	quantum efficiency
atomic absorption spectra	fluorescent probe	quenching
atomic emission spectra	frequency	Rayleigh scattering
band spectra	grating	reflectance
bandwidth	ground state	refraction
bathochromic shift	hyperchromic shift	reporter group
Beer–Lambert law	hypochromic shift	rotational sublevel
binding spectra	hypsochromic shift	shells
bioluminescence	intensity	single photon X-ray
calibration curve	intrinsic fluorescence	absorptiometry
chemiluminescence	isobestic point	solvent perturbation
chromophore	Job effect	spectrofluorimetry
circular dischroism spectroscopy	laser	spectrophotometry
colorimetry	line spectra	Stokes shift
difference spectrum	luminescence	substrate binding spectra
differential spectroscopy	luminescence spectrometry	time-resolved fluorescence
diffraction	magnetic vector	immunoassay
dissocation-enhanced lanthanide	molar absorbance coefficient	turbidimetry
fluoroimmunoassay	monochromator	Tyndall effect
Doppler effect	Mössbauer effect	vibrational sublevel
dual energy X-ray absorptiometry	nephelometry	waveforms
electric vector	optical rotatory dispersion	wavelength
electromagnetic spectrum	spectroscopy	X-ray fluorescence
ellipticity	particles	X-ray fluorescence analysis
emission	phosphorescence	

9.12 CALCULATIONS

Question 1

An aliquot of a solution containing a light-absorbing substance at a concentration of 5 g dm^{-3}, was placed in a 2 cm light path cuvette. The cuvette was placed in a spectrophotometer and a beam of light of wavelength λ was passed through the cuvette containing the solution. A transmission value of 80% was recorded.

Find (i) the absorbance of the solution, and (ii) the molar extinction coefficient if the molecular mass of the substance is known to be 410.

Answer

(i) As the concentration is given in terms of absolute mass per unit volume, it is necessary to find a 'specific extinction coefficient', ϵ_s.

The transmission, T, is expressed as the percentage $100 \times I_t$, of the incident light I_0;

$$T = 80\% = 100 \times \frac{I_t}{I_0}$$

If $I_0 \equiv 100\%$ of the light, then

$$I_t \equiv 80\%$$

$$\frac{I_t}{I_0} = \frac{80}{100} = 0.8$$

Absorbance $= A = \log(1/T) = \log(1/0.8) = \log(1.25) = 0.0969$

$$A = \epsilon_s \times c \times \ell = \epsilon_s \times 5 \times 2$$

Therefore,

$$\epsilon_s = \frac{0.0969}{10} = 9.69 \times 10^{-3} \text{ g}^{-1} \text{dm}^3 \text{cm}^{-1}$$

(ii) As the specific extinction coefficient relates to 'per gram', the molar extinction coefficient is obtained simply by multiplying by the relative molecular mass.
Hence,

$$\epsilon_s \times 410 = \epsilon_m$$

$$9.69 \times 10^{-3} \times 410 = 3.973 \text{ mol}^{-1} \text{dm}^3 \text{cm}^{-1}$$

Question 2

If a solution containing ATP is found to have an absorbance of 0.17 in a 1 cm cuvette and the molar extinction coefficient is $1.54 \times 10^4 \text{ mol}^{-1} \text{dm}^3 \text{cm}^{-1}$, find

(i) the concentration of ATP solution,
(ii) the transmission of the solution in a 1 cm cuvette
and (iii) the absorbance of a $2.5 \times 10^{-2} \text{ mM}$ solution of ATP in a 4 cm cuvette.

Answer

(i) The concentration is found by the direct application of the Beer–Lambert Law.

$$A = \log\left(\frac{I_0}{I_t}\right) = \epsilon_\lambda c\ell$$

$$0.17 = 1.54 \times 10^4 \times c \times 1$$

Therefore,

$$c = [\text{ATP}] = \frac{0.17}{1.54 \times 10^4 \times 1} = 1.104 \times 10^{-5}\,\text{mol dm}^{-3}$$

(ii) $A = \log\left(\dfrac{I_0}{I_t}\right) = \log\left(\dfrac{1}{T}\right)$

Therefore,

$$0.17 = \log\left(\frac{1}{T}\right)$$

$$\frac{1}{T} = \text{antilog}\,(0.17) = 1.4791$$

and $T = 0.676$ or 67.6%

(iii) As we have a value of the molar extinction coefficient we must convert the given concentration to mol dm^{-3} (M).

Hence $2.5 \times 10^{-2}\,\text{mM} = 2.5 \times 10^{-5}\,\text{M}$

Then   absorbance $= A = \epsilon_m \times c \times \ell$

or $A = 1.54 \times 10^4 \times 2.5 \times 10^{-5} \times 4 = 1.54$

As an aside, it is worth recalling that absorbance (because it is a logarithm) is unitless by definition. This is clearly demonstrated by performing 'quantity algebra' on the units of each term.

e.g. $\epsilon_m\,\text{mol}^{-1}\,\text{dm}^3\,\text{cm}^{-1}$

$c\,\text{mol dm}^{-3}$

$\ell\,\text{cm}$

Hence,

$\epsilon_m \times c \times \ell \equiv \text{mol}^{-1}\,\text{dm}^3\,\text{cm}^{-1} \times \text{mol dm}^{-3} \times \text{cm}$

and all units cancel.

Question 3 In biochemical redox systems many enzyme-catalysed processes may be monitored by the interconversion of NAD$^+$ (NADP$^+$) and NADH (NADPH). This may be done by taking measurements of absorbance at two wavelengths: 260 nm, where both oxidised and reduced forms both absorb; and 340 nm, where only the reduced forms absorb.

Find the concentrations of NAD$^+$ and NADH in a mixed solution from the following data obtained in a 1 cm cuvette.

Molar extinction coefficients, ϵ_m (mol^{-1} dm^3 cm^{-1}), at 260 nm are 1.5×10^4 for NADH and 1.84×10^4 for NAD$^+$.
At 340 nm only NADH absorbs with an ϵ_m of 6.22×10^3 mol^{-1} dm^3 cm^{-1}.
The mixed solution gave absorbances of 1.362 and 0.382 at 260 nm and 340 nm, respectively.

Answer   At 340 nm, all the absorbance in the mixture arises from the reduced component, NADH. Hence the concentration may be found from:

$$A_{NADH} = \epsilon_m \times c \times \ell$$

$$0.382 = 6.22 \times 10^3 \times c \times 1$$

Therefore,

$$c = [NADH] = \frac{0.382}{6.22 \times 10^3 \times 1} = 6.141 \times 10^{-5}\, mol\, dm^{-3}$$

Clearly, the concentration of NADH is the same at 260 nm (where NAD^+ also absorbs). The absorbance owing to NADH at 260 nm is given by

$$A_{NADH} = 1.5 \times 10^4 \times 6.141 \times 10^{-5} \times 1$$
$$= 0.9212$$

The total absorbance (for NAD^+ and NADH) = A_t = 1.362.
Hence,

$$A_{NAD^+} = A_t - A_{NADH}\, (at\, 260\, nm)$$
$$= 1.362 - 0.9212$$
$$= 0.4408$$

Now the concentration of the oxidised form may be calculated by the application of the Beer–Lambert Law again, with the appropriate parameters for this wavelength.
Hence,

$$A_{NAD^+} = \epsilon_m \times c \times \ell$$

$$0.4408 = 1.84 \times 10^4 \times c \times 1$$

and $c = [NAD^+] = \dfrac{0.4408}{1.84 \times 10^4 \times 1} = 2.396 \times 10^{-5}\, mol\, dm^{-3}$

Quoting results to an acceptable level of precision;

$$[NAD^+] = 2.40 \times 10^{-5}\, mol\, dm^{-3}$$

and $[NADH] = 6.14 \times 10^{-5}\, mol\, dm^{-3}$

Question 4   The concentrations of two components X1 and X2 may also be found if they both absorb at two wavelengths, provided the standard parameters are known.

Measurements were made in an 0.01 m cuvette at wavelengths of 340 nm and 380 nm. The total absorbance values obtained at each wavelength were 0.42 and 0.284, respectively. The absorptivities of X1 and X2 are 1.6×10^7 and $8.2 \times 10^6\, mol^{-1}\, m^2$, respectively, at 340 nm and 3.65×10^6 and $6.2 \times 10^6\, mol^{-1}\, m^2$, respectively, at 380 nm.
Find the concentrations of X1 and X2.

Answer   Where two components both absorb at two different wavelengths it is necessary to establish simultaneous equations. Also values are given in absorptivities, in this example, so concentrations, for calculation purposes, will be in $mol\, m^{-3}$. Using [ ] to represent concentration:

$$A_{340} = \{\epsilon_{m340[X1]} \times [X1] \times 0.01\} + \{\epsilon_{m340[X2]} \times [X2] \times 0.01\}$$

$$0.42 = 0.01\{(1.67 \times 10^7 \times [X1]) + (8.2 \times 10^6 \times [X2])\} \tag{1}$$

and

$$A_{380} - \{\epsilon_{m380[X1]} \times [X1] \times 0.01\} + \{\epsilon_{m380[X2]} \times [X2] \times 0.01\}$$

$$0.284 = 0.01\{(3.65 \times 10^6 \times [X1]) + (6.2 \times 10^6 \times [X2])\} \tag{2}$$

From equation (1), [X1] may be expressed in terms of [X2], as follows:

$$1.67 \times 10^7 \times [X1] = \frac{0.42}{0.01} - (8.2 \times 10^6 \times [X2])$$

or

$$[X1] = \frac{1}{1.67 \times 10^7} \left\{ \frac{0.42}{0.01} - (8.2 \times 10^6 \times [X2]) \right\}$$

$$= 2.515 \times 10^{-6} - (0.491 \times [X2]) \tag{3}$$

This value for [X1] may now be substituted into equation (2), as follows:

$$0.284 = 0.01\{(3.65 \times 10^6 \times (2.515 \times 10^{-6} - (0.491 \times [X2]))) + (6.2 \times 10^6 \times [X2])\}$$

This can now be solved for [X2], the only unknown variable in this equation.

$$\frac{0.284}{0.01} = 9.7197 - (1.792 \times 10^6 \times [X2]) + (6.2 \times 10^6 \times [X2])$$

$$= 9.1797 + (4.4078 \times 10^6 \times [X2])$$

Hence, $$[X2] = \frac{28.4 - 9.1797}{4.4078 \times 10^6} = 4.3605 \times 10^{-6} \, \text{mol m}^{-3}$$

This value may now be substituted into equation (3) above and the concentration of X1 found.

So, $$[X1] = 2.515 \times 10^{-6} - (0.491 \times 4.3605 \times 10^{-6})$$

$$= 2.515 \times 10^{-6} - 2.141 \times 10^{-6}$$

$$= 3.7399 \times 10^{-7} \, \text{mol m}^{-3}$$

To convert to more familiar units remember that $\text{mol m}^{-3} \equiv \text{mmol dm}^{-3}$. Hence,

$$[X1] = 3.7399 \times 10^{-7} \, \text{mmol dm}^{-3}$$

$$= 3.74 \times 10^{-1} \, \text{nmol dm}^{-3}$$

and

$$[X2] = 4.36 \times 10^{-6} \, \text{mmol dm}^{-3}$$

$$= 4.36 \, \text{nmol dm}^{-3}$$

both above values being rounded off to an acceptable level of precision.

For n components and measurements at n wavelengths it is necessary to resort to the methods of matrix algebra to deconvolute the data.

Question 5   The enzyme glucose-6-phosphate dehydrogenase (in the presence of Mg^{2+} and $NADP^+$) catalyses the conversion of glucose-6-phosphate to 6-phosphogluconic acid δ-lactone. If an excess of NADP$^+$ is used the equilibrium is displaced to the right and the reaction essentially goes to completion.

A 1.0 cm^3 portion of a solution containing glucose 6-phosphate was taken and to it was added 1.0 cm^3 of a solution containing excess NADP$^+$ and MgCl$_2$. The change in absorbance with time was monitored in a 1 cm cuvette, at 340 nm, and reached a maximum (plateau) value of 0.61 on complete consumption of the glucose 6-phosphate. Calculate the original concentration of glucose 6-phosphate, given that the molar extinction coefficient of NADPH is 6.22×10^3 mol^{-1} dm^3 cm^{-1} at 340 nm.

Answer   By ensuring that excess oxidised coenzyme is present the reaction will essentially go to completion. The maximum absorbance measured enables the determination of the final concentration of NADPH (initial concentration zero). This is the only component which absorbs at 340 nm and its production is stoichiometrically related to the consumption of glucose 6-phosphate.

Applying the Beer–Lambert Law,

$$A = \epsilon_m \times c \times \ell$$

$$0.61 = 6.22 \times 10^3 \times c \times 1$$

Therefore

$$c = \frac{0.61}{6.22 \times 10^3 \times 1} = 9.807 \times 10^{-5} \, \text{mol dm}^{-3}$$

However, the original solution was diluted 1:1 when the reagents were added so the concentration above must be doubled to take account of the dilution factor.

Hence,

$$c_{\text{orig}} = 1.96 \times 10^{-4} \, \text{mol dm}^{-3}$$

Question 6   A metabolite M was isolated from cerebrospinal fluid (CSF). After excitation at $\lambda_1 = 280$ nm the material fluoresced at $\lambda_2 = 360$ nm.

Using a standard spectrofluorimeter:

(i)   the instrument scale was set to zero with solvent (e.g. buffer) and the 100% mark using a pure sample of M as standard (conc. 100 ng/100 cm^{-3}),

(ii) a blank was measured on a solution containing all the components except M and gave a reading of 11.2%,

(iii) an extract including M gave a total fluorescence measurement of 67%,

(iv) an overall fluorescence reading of 92% was observed when the extract above had an amount of pure M added, as internal standard, to give an equivalent concentration of 1 µg dm^{-3}. (Note this concentration is equivalent to 100 ng 100 cm^{-3}.)

Calculate the concentration of M in the sample of CSF in µg dm^{-3} and the proportion of quenching, if any. Also state the Stokes shift for the assay.

Answer   The best way to proceed is to define the individual intensities.

Let I_s be the 100% value due to the standard.
Let I_b be the 11.2% value due to the blank.

Let I_t be the 67% value due to the total fluorescence.

Let I_f be the 92% value due to the overall fluorescence when sample is 'spiked' with internal standard.

Let I_u be the 55.8% value due to the blank correction $I_t - I_b$ (67 − 11.2).

Let I_{as} be the 25% value due to the 'quenched' internal standard $I_f - I_t$ (92 −67).

Then

$$\frac{\text{assay fluorescence of unknown}}{\text{assay fluorescence of int. std}} = \frac{\text{amount of unknown}}{\text{amount of int. std}}$$

$$\frac{I_u}{I_{as}} = \frac{\text{amount of unknown}}{1 \, \mu\text{g dm}^{-3}}$$

$$\text{amount of unknown} = \frac{I_u \times 1 \, \mu\text{g dm}^{-3}}{I_{as}} = \frac{55.8}{25} = 2.2 \, \mu\text{g dm}^{-3}$$

The degree of quenching is found as follows:

pure standard gives $I_s = 100\%$
equivalent amount of standard in assay $I_{as} = 25\%$

Hence, quenching,

$$Q = 100 \times \left(\frac{100 - 25}{100} \right) = 75\%$$

The value of the Stokes shift is the difference between the emission and excitation wavelengths,

$$\Delta\lambda = \lambda_2 - \lambda_1 = 360 - 280 = 80 \, \text{nm}$$

9.13 SUGGESTIONS FOR FURTHER READING

Note: Some of the suggestions listed at the end of Chapter 10 are also appropriate for this chapter.

BANCROFT, G. M. (1975). *Mössbauer Spectroscopy*. McGraw-Hill, New York. (Early chapters contain details of the instrumentation and theory.)

BROWN, S. B. (1980). *An Introduction to Spectroscopy for Biochemists*. Academic Press, London. (Contains comprehensive sections on the principles, instrumentation and chemical applications of many of the techniques considered in this chapter.)

DELUCA, M. A. (ed.) (1978). *Methods in Enzymology*, vol. 57 *Bioluminescence and Chemiluminescence*. Academic Press, London. (Contains a comprehensive coverage of basic luminescence methods)

GILBERT, B. (1984). *Investigation of Molecular Structure: Spectroscopy and Diffraction Methods*, 2nd edn. Bell and Hyman, London. (A basic introduction to classical spectroscopy techniques.)

HESTER, R. E. and GIRLING, R. B. (eds.) (1991). *Spectroscopy of Biological Molecules*. Royal Society of Chemistry Special Publication, Cambridge. (Comprehensive account of applications.)

LAKOWICZ, J. R. (1983). *Principles of Fluorescence Spectroscopy*. Plenum Press, New York. (Starts with basic principles but contains topics of further interest.)

ROST, F. N. D. (1992, 1994). *Fluorescence Microscopy*, vols. 1 and 2, Cambridge University Press. (A definitive text with a large and comprehensive appendix on fluorochromes.)

WHISTON, C. (1987). *X-ray Methods*. ACOL Series. John Wiley and Sons, London. (An open learning text for those needing a deeper understanding of the principles.)

Chapter 10

Spectroscopic techniques: II   Vibrational spectroscopy and electron and nuclear spin orientation in magnetic fields

10.1 INTRODUCTION

In Chapter 9 it was established that the electromagnetic spectrum was a continuum of frequencies from the high energy γ-rays of nuclear origin to the long wavelength region of the radiofrequencies. The energy associated with the spectrum decreases as it is traversed from the high to low frequency regions, according to the rules of quantum theory. There is therefore no obvious logical dividing point where this overall spectrum may be split. The split presented in this text is one of convenience. The justification is purely pragmatic and is based on 'common practice'. The biologist or biomedical scientist, having isolated a 'new' material (compound), is faced, initially, with the requirement to identify this isolate. Amongst the spectroscopic and spectrometric techniques available, assuming sufficient pure material has been obtained, the first analytical procedures to be used would, in practice, involve the methods described in this chapter. There are two important reasons for this approach: first, a considerable amount of information is obtained from a 'single' analysis and, secondly, the techniques are non-destructive. In view of the latter reason, replicate analyses may be performed in many cases, to improve signal-to-noise ratios, and precious samples can be recovered that may then be subjected to other analytical investigations.

In Chapter 11 the mass spectrometric techniques are encountered. These techniques give information different from and complementary to the spectroscopic ones. They have the distinct advantage of being considerably more sensitive and hence the investigator, often faced with having too small a sample to make use of the spectroscopic techniques, is forced to use mass spectrometry. However, it is essential to recognise that the spectroscopic techniques give information that is not available from mass spectrometry alone. Also, a disadvantage with mass spectrometry is that the technique is destructive and some of the sample is lost during the analytical procedure, although, with the most sensitive systems now available, the loss is probably insignificant. In many situations the amount of sample destroyed during analysis is less than losses arising from sample transfer!

10.2 INFRARED AND RAMAN SPECTROSCOPY

With reference to the introductory statement of Section 10.1, the region of the electromagnetic spectrum, ranging from γ-rays to the near ultraviolet/visible

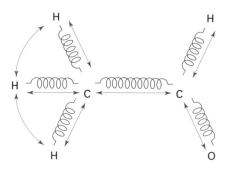

Fig. 10.1. Possible vibrations in acetaldehyde.

(0.1 nm to 800 nm), contains frequencies that are sufficiently energetic to cause electron transitions, and the highest energy γ-rays are associated with nuclear transitions. From the near infrared region onwards there is insufficient energy to effect transitions of the kind alluded to above. Over the portion of the electromagnetic spectrum encompassing the range 0.8 μm to 25 μm the phenomena involve 'bond vibrations'. The term must be interpreted in a rather wider sense than just uniform oscillations and taken to include bending deformations as well.

10.2.1 **Principles**

These two spectroscopic methods are complementary, giving similar information, but the criteria for the phenomena to occur are different for each type. It is also true that, for asymmetric molecules, absorptions will give rise to both types and virtually the same information could be gained from either. However, for symmetrical molecules having a centre of symmetry, the fundamental frequencies that appear in the Raman do not appear in the infrared and vice versa. The two methods are then truly complementary.

The reasons are the two different mechanisms on which the two types depend. Both are indicated in Fig. 10.1 for a simple molecule, acetaldehyde. For the purposes of this discussion the bonds between atoms can be considered as flexible springs so that the atoms are in constant vibrational motion, i.e. the molecule is not fixed and rigid.

Bonds can either stretch or deform (bend) and theory predicts that if a molecule contains n atoms there will be $3n - 6$ fundamental vibrations in total. Of these, $2n - 5$ cause bond deformations and $n - 1$ cause bond stretching. In Table 10.1 are listed the most important fundamental frequencies observed in acetaldehyde molecules.

The region of the electromagnetic spectrum ranges from the red end of the visible to the microwave lengths. Energy is input by irradiating in the appropriate region with electromagnetic radiation. The criterion for an infrared spectrum is that there is a change in dipole moment, i.e. a change in charge displacement. Conversely, if there is a change in the polarisability of the molecule, a portion of

Table 10.1 Some fundamental frequencies associated with vibrations in acetaldehyde

Functional group	Vibration type	Frequency (cm^{-1})
$- CH_3$	Bending	1460
		1365
$- C - C -$	Stretching	1165
$- C = O$	Stretching	1730
$- C - H$ (in CH_3)	Stretching	2960
		2870
$- C - H$ (in CHO)	Stretching	2720

the scattered radiation will have a frequency different from that of the incident radiation. These different frequencies constitute Raman spectra. It should be noted that more information can be gained about oscillations in molecules by proceeding even further into the microwave region and using microwave spectroscopy.

The fundamental frequencies observed are characteristic of the functional groups concerned and are absolutely specific. This gives rise to the term fingerprint for the infrared pattern obtained. As the number of functional groups increases in more complex molecules, the absorption bands in the infra-red patterns become more difficult to assign. However, group frequencies arise that help to simplify interpretation. These groups of certain bands regularly appear near the same wavelength and may be assigned to specific molecular groupings, just as particular chromophores absorb in the ultraviolet and visible regions. Such group frequencies are extremely valuable in structural diagnosis. It should be noted that, in infrared spectra, which are vibrational spectra, it is usual to work in frequency units, hertz (Hz), rather than wavelength.

The frequency associated with a particular group varies slightly, owing to the influence of the molecular environment. This is extremely useful in structural biochemistry studies as it is possible to distinguish between $C - H$ vibrations in methylene ($-CH_2$) and methyl groups ($-CH_3$). Decrease in wavelength also occurs when double bonds are formed as the stretching frequency increases.

10.2.2 Instrumentation

The most common source is a Nichrome alloy coil heated to incandescence. This region of the electromagnetic spectrum contains the heat waves. Samples of solids are either prepared in mulls such as nujol and held as layers between salt planes such as NaCl or pressed into KBr discs. Non-covalent materials must be used for sample containment and also in the optics, as these materials are transparent to infrared.

Detectors are of the heat recognition type. The Golay cell contains gas or liquid whose expansion is registered when the energy is absorbed. Thermal detectors such as thermocouples can also be employed. Analysis using a Michelson interferometer allows Fourier transform infrared spectroscopy (FT–IR) to be performed. This instrument involves fixed and rotating mirrors that split the incident beam into two. The beams are recombined after passage through the sample but as the two pathlengths are different, interference patterns arise that may be analysed by Fourier transform methods (see Section 10.4.1 for consideration of FT methods). The Beer–Lambert law applies in all cases except complex mixtures, where more complicated mathematical procedures are required.

10.2.3 Applications

The use of infrared and Raman spectroscopy is mainly in biochemical research for intermediate-sized molecules such as drugs, metabolic intermediates and substrates. Examples are the identification of substances such as penicillin and its derivatives, small peptides and environmental pollutants. It is an ideal and rapid method for measuring certain contaminants in foodstuffs and can be coupled to a gas–liquid chromatograph (GC–IR) when it is also frequently used for the analysis of drug metabolites. Figure 10.2 shows the major bands of an FT-IR spectrum of the drug phenacetin. Gas analysis is rapid, particularly for measuring different concentrations of gases such as CO_2, CO and $CH = CH$ (acetylene) in biological samples. Use in the study of photosynthesis and respiration in plants is valuable, particularly for CO_2 metabolism.

10.3 ELECTRON SPIN RESONANCE SPECTROSCOPY

10.3.1 Magnetic phenomena

Prior to any detailed discussion of electron spin resonance (ESR) and nuclear magnetic resonance (NMR) (Section 10.4) methods it is worth while considering the more general phenomena applicable to both.

An important consideration is magnetism and how it arises. All substances are magnetic, and magnetism arises from the motion of charged particles. This motion is controlled by internal forces in a system and, for the purposes of this discussion, the major contribution to magnetism in molecules is due to the spin of the charged particle.

Consider the situation in the chemical bonds of a molecule where electrons (negatively charged) have the property of spin controlled by strict quantum rules. The simplest view of the chemical bond is that of paired electrons with opposite spins. It is true that in many chemical systems the electrons may become delocalised, ie. lose their association with a particular atom, but the essential argument still applies in that for pairs of electrons in molecular orbitals the spins must be opposite (no two electrons can have all the quantum numbers identical: the Pauli principle). Each of these spinning electronic charges generates a magnetic effect, but in electron pairs the effect is almost self-cancelling. The mathematical considerations do not in general apply exactly in molecules but in atoms a value for

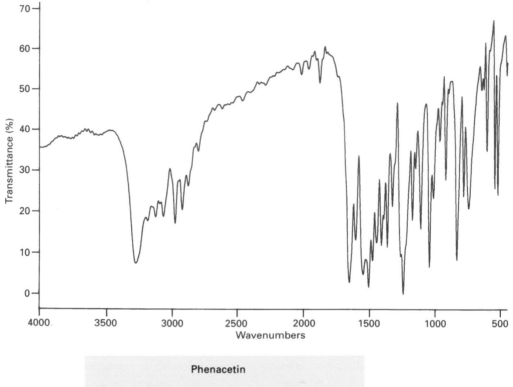

Fig. 10.2. FT-IR spectrum of phenacetin. Bands at the appropriate frequencies (cm^{-1}) are shown, indicating the bonds with which they are associated and the type (s, stretching; b, bending or deformation).

magnetic susceptibility may be calculated and is of the order of $-10^{-6}\,g^{-1}$. This is diamagnetism possessed by all substances because all substances contain the miniscule magnets, i.e. electrons. Diamagnetism is temperature independent.

If an electron is unpaired there is no counterbalancing opposing spin and the magnetic susceptibility is of the order of $+10^{-3}$ to $+10^{-4}\,g^{-1}$. In cases where this possibility arises, the underlying diamagnetism is so small by comparison that it is irrelevant and the free electron case gives rise to paramagnetism. Free electrons can arise in a number of examples, the most notable of which is in the structure of certain metals such as iron, cobalt and nickel. These metals exhibit an extreme case of paramagnetism that is termed ferromagnetism and are the materials from which permanent magnets, with which everyone is familiar, can be made. Some crystal structures allow free electrons to exist but free radicals (free electron entities) are probably the most important systems in biological investigations.

The way in which a substance behaves in an externally applied magnetic field allows us to distinguish between diamagnetism and paramagnetism. A paramagnetic material is attracted by an external magnetic field and a diamagnetic substance is rejected. This principle is employed in the GUOY balance, which allows the quantification of the magnetic effects. A balance pan is suspended between the poles of a suitable electromagnet (to supply the external field). The substance under test is weighed in air with the current switched off. The same sample is then reweighed with the current on, the result being that a paramagnetic substance apparently weighs more and a diamagnetic substance apparently less.

Exactly similar arguments can be made regarding atomic nuclei. Of course, it is not now the extranuclear electrons but the subnuclear particles that are the spinning charged particles. Strictly speaking (because of interchangeability) it is the number of nucleons (protons plus neutrons) that determine whether a species will exhibit nuclear paramagnetism. It is beyond the scope of this discussion to explore why neutrons (which are neutral and uncharged; Section 14.1.1) are involved. It is sufficient to note that the hydrogen atoms in a molecule exhibit residual nuclear magnetism and, if some or all are replaced by deuterium, then there is no magnetism from the dueterium. Hydrogen contains a single proton, whereas deuterium contains one proton and one neutron (two nucleons, an even number). Carbon-12 (^{12}C) contains six protons plus six neutrons – an even number, no residual magnetism. ^{13}C contains six protons (because it is carbon) but seven neutrons, an odd number of nucleons; hence it exhibits residual nuclear magnetism.

10.3.2 **The resonance condition**

In both ESR and NMR techniques (Section 10.4) two possible energy states exist for either electronic or nuclear magnetism in the presence of an external magnetic field;

(i) Low energy state E_1: the field generated by the spinning charged particle lies with, or is parallel to, the external field
(ii) High energy state E_2: the field generated by the spinning charged particle lies against, or is antiparallel to, the external field.

The resonance condition is satisfied when the transition from the low to high energy states occurs and equation 10.1 is satisfied. Energy must be absorbed for these transitions to occur: one quantum or $h\upsilon$ (where h is the Planck constant). In the appropriate external magnetic fields it is shown that the frequency of applied radiation, υ, occurs in the microwave region for ESR (sometimes called electron paramagnetic resonance (EPR)) and the radiofrequency region for NMR (sometimes called nuclear paramagnetic resonance). In both techniques, two possibilities exist for determining the absorption of electromagnetic energy (at the resonance point):

(i) either a constant frequency is employed and the external magnetic field swept, or
(ii) a constant external magnetic field is used and the appropriate region of the spectrum swept.

For technical reasons the more commonly employed option is (i), but the same results would be obtained if either option were chosen.

10.3.3 Principles

The quantum of energy required to cause the resonance condition to be satisfied, and transition between energy states in an ESR experiment, may be quantified as

$$h\upsilon = g\beta H \tag{10.1}$$

where g is the spectroscopic splitting factor (a constant), β is magnetic moment of the electron (termed the Bohr magneton), and H is the strength of the applied external field.

The frequency of the absorbed microwave radiation is a function of the paramagnetic species, β and the applied magnetic field strength H (equation 10.1). This indicates that either may be varied to the same effect. The absorption of the energy is recorded as a peak in the ESR spectrum and is indicative of the presence of a paramagnetic species. The area under the peak is proportional to the concentration of that species, strictly the number of unpaired electron spins. Calibration of the instrument with known standards allows the concentration to be calculated. The standard, containing a known number of spins, must have the same line shape as the unknown for a reliable comparison to be made. Examples of standards are solutions of peroxylamine disulphonate or the solid 1,1-diphenyl-2′-picryl-hydrazyl (DPHH). The solid standard contains 1.53×10^{21} unpaired spins per gram in the pure state and may be diluted by admixture with carbon black in order to give lower concentrations.

For a delocalised electron (some free radicals), $g = 2.0023$ but for localised electrons, for example in transition metal atoms, g varies and its precise value gives information about the nature of the bonding in the environment of the unpaired electron within the molecule. When resonance occurs, the absorption peak is broadened owing to spin–lattice interactions, i.e. the interaction of the unpaired electron with the rest of the molecule. This gives further information about the structure of the molecule.

High resolution ESR may be performed by examining the hyperfine splitting of the absorption peak, which is caused by interaction of the unpaired electron with adjacent nuclei. This yields information about the spatial location of atoms in the molecule. Proton (^{1}H) hyperfine splitting for free radicals occurs in the region of

0 to 3×10^{-3} tesla (1 tesla $= 10^4$ gauss and is a measure of the magnetic induction, which is linearly related to the magnetic field strength) and yields data analogous to those obtained in high resolution NMR. In fact a considerable improvement in the effective resolution of an ESR spectrum may be achieved by using the electron nuclear double resonance (ENDOR) technique. In this approach the sample is irradiated simultaneously with microwaves for ESR and RF (radiofreqeuncy) for NMR. The RF signal is swept for a fixed point of the ESR spectrum. The output display is the ESR signal height versus swept nuclear RF. The approach is particularly useful when there is a large variety of nuclear levels that broaden the normal electron resonance line. A similar but different technique is electron double resonance (ELDOR), in which the sample is irradiated with two microwave frequencies. One is used for observation of the ESR signal at some point in the spectrum, whilst the other is used to sweep other parts of the spectrum. This is used to display the ESR signal as a function of the difference of the two microwave frequencies. ELDOR finds use in the separation of overlapping multiradical spectra and to study relaxation phenomena, for example chemical spin exchange.

10.3.4 Instrumentation

Figure 10.3 is a diagram of the main components of an ESR instrument. The field strengths generated by the electromagnets are of the order of 50 to 500 millitesla, and variations of less than 1 in 10^6 are required for highest accuracy. The monochromatic microwave radiation is produced in the Klystron oscillator, the wavelength being of the order of 3×10^{-2} m (9000 MHz).

The samples are required to be in the solid state; hence biological samples are usually frozen in liquid nitrogen. The first-order differential (dA/dH) is usually plotted against H, not A versus H (cf. Section 9.4.3). Hence a plot similar to that in Fig. 9.9 is obtained and this shape is called a 'line' in ESR spectroscopy. Generally there are relatively few unpaired electrons in a molecule, resulting in fewer than 10 lines, which are not closely spaced.

10.3.5 Applications

ESR spectroscopy is one of the main methods used to study metalloproteins, particularly those containing molybdenum (xanthine oxidase), copper (cytochrome oxidase and copper blue enzymes) and iron (cytochrome, ferredoxin). Both copper and non-haem iron, which do not absorb in the ultraviolet/visible regions, possess ESR absorption peaks in one of their oxidation states. The appearance and disappearance of their ESR signals are used to monitor their activity in the multienzyme systems of intact mitochondria and chloroplasts, as well as in isolated enzymes. In metalloproteins there exists a specific stereochemical structure whereby a characteristic number of ligands (frequently amino acid residues of the protein) are coordinated to the metal. ESR studies show that the structural geometry is frequently distorted from that of model systems and the distortion may be related to biological function.

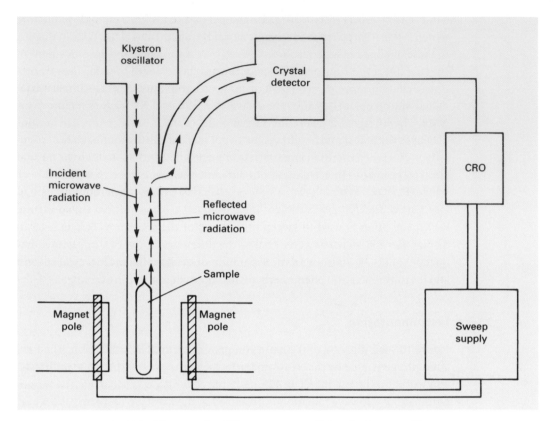

Fig. 10.3.   Diagram of an ESR spectrometer. CRO, cathode ray oscilloscope.

Spin labels are stable and unreactive free radicals used as reporter groups or probes. The procedure of spin labelling is the attachment of these probes to biological molecules that lack unpaired electrons. The label can be attached to either a substrate or a ligand. Often the spin label contains the nitric oxide moiety. These labels enable the study of events that occur with a frequency of 10^7 to 10^{11} s^{-1}. If the motion is restricted in some directions, only anisotropic motion may be studied, for example in membrane–rigid spin label in bilayers. Here the label is attached so that the NO group lies parallel to the long axis of the lipid.

Intramolecular motions and lateral diffusion of lipid through the membrane may be observed and measured. This study is achieved by either (i) concentrating the spin-labelled lipids into one region of the bilayer, or (ii) randomly incorporating, usually into model membranes. The diffusion of the spin labels allows them to come into contact with each other and causes line broadening in the spectrum. Another label used to study lipid motion in bilayers is 2,2,6,6-tetramethylpiperidine-1-oxyl (TEMPOL). Labelling of glycerophosphatides with this compound allows measurement of the flip rate between inner and outer surfaces as well as lateral diffusion.

Spin trapping is a process whereby an unstable free radical has stability conferred upon it by reacting it with a compound such as 5,5-dimethylpyrroline-1-oxide (DMPO). Hyperfine splittings are observed that depend upon the nature of the radical R·.

Molecules in the triplet (phosphorescent) state (Section 9.5.1) may also be studied by ESR. This gives data complementary to that obtained in the ultraviolet/visible region of the spectrum. For instance, free radicals due to the triplet state of tryptophan have been observed in cataractous lenses.

Free radicals are found in many metabolic pathways and as degradation products of drugs and toxins. Electron transfer mechanisms in mitochondria and chloroplasts involve paramagnetic species, for example the Fe − S centres. Other redox processes involving the flavin derivatives FAD, FMN and semiquinones lend themselves readily to exploration by this approach. The $g = 2.003$ signal is associated mainly with mitochondria, but different cell lines show different intensities. This phenomenon is also dependent on metabolic state. Factors that increase metabolic activity also lead to an increase in organic radical signal. Many studies have involved the free radical polymer melanin and the ascorbyl radical. The latter has been used to study the effects of certain drugs on sperm maturation.

Carcinogenesis is an area where free radicals have been implicated and where their study has been of value. There is, in general, a lower concentration of free radicals in tumours than in normal tissues. Also a concentration gradient is observed, being higher in the peripheral non-necrotic surface layers than in the inner regions of the tumour. The free radicals may, of course, initiate the neoplasia. The development of implanted tumours in mice has also been studied. Chemical carcinogens are in many cases associated with generation of free radicals. An example is the prediction of carcinogenicity of certain polycyclic hydrocarbons. Polycyclic hydrocarbons arise by the successive linking of benzene rings along ring edges. Examples of such compounds are naphthalene (two rings), and anthracene and phenanthrene (three rings). As more rings are added the structures become increasingly complicated. As these compounds possess 'aromatic' character it becomes increasingly possible for the free electron of the radical to be accommodated, i.e. these kinds of radicals become more stable and therefore possibly more long lived. The fact that they may survive for extended periods of time allows more damage to be done. Many of the precursors of these radicals exist in natural sources such as coal tar, tobacco smoke and other products of combustion, hence the environmental risk.

Many metabolic studies have made use of ESR. Examples are the metabolism of drugs, processes occurring in the microsomes of the liver, peroxidation mechanisms and the free radical products of oxygen. Superoxide dismutases scavenge oxygen-related (dioxygenyl) free radicals $O_2^{\pm}$ (that have been associated, for example, with inflammation and ageing). Nitric oxide, NO, as an independent entity, operates as a physiological messenger regulating the nervous, immune and cardiovascular systems. It has been implicated in septic (toxic) shock, hypertension, stroke and neurodegenerative diseases. Although NO is involved in normal synaptic transmission, excess levels are neurotoxic. Superoxide dismutase attenuates the neurotoxicity by removal of $O_2^{\pm}$, hence limiting its availability for reaction with NO to produce peroxynitrite.

Another source of free radicals is the irradiation, for example with γ-rays, of biological material. For instance -S — S- cross-linkages in proteins may be identified by irradiating the protein, and the free radical produced has the free electron localised in the -S — S- region. Another major application in this area is examining irradiated foodstuffs for residual free radicals. The technique can be used to establish whether the packed foodstuff has been irradiated or not. A similar biomedical/ environmental application involves the study of hard biological materials such as bone or teeth. When such materials are exposed to ionising radiation, energy is stored in them and this energy may give rise to the production of free radicals. Clearly ESR may be used to detect these radicals and is used in 'dose assessment' in nuclear radiation accidents.

10.4 NUCLEAR MAGNETIC RESONANCE SPECTROSCOPY

The essential background theory of the phenomena that allow nuclear magnetic resonance (NMR) to occur has been dealt with in Section 10.3.1. The miniscule magnets involved here are nucleons (in effect protons) rather than electrons. The specific principles, instrumentation and applications are treated below.

10.4.1 Principles

Again there is considerable similarity with ESR. Most studies involve the use of ^{1}H (hence the term proton magnetic resonance (PMR) but ^{13}C, ^{15}N and ^{31}P isotopes are used in biochemical studies.

The resonance condition in NMR is satisfied in an external magnetic field of several hundred millitesla, with absorptions occurring in the region of radiowave 40 MHz frequency for resonance of the ^{1}H nucleus. The actual field scanned is small compared with the total field applied and the radio frequencies absorbed are specifically stated on such spectra.

The molecular environment of a proton governs the value of the applied external field at which the nucleus resonates. This is recorded as the chemical shift (τ) and is measured relative to an internal standard, frequently tetramethylsilane (TMS), whose structure $(CH_3)_4Si$ contains 12 identical protons. The chemical shift arises from the applied field inducing secondary fields (15×10^{-4} to 20×10^{-4} tesla) at the proton by interacting with the adjacent bonding electrons. If the induced field opposes the applied field, the latter will have to be at a slightly higher value for resonance to occur. Alternatively if the induced and applied fields are aligned the latter is required to be at a lower value for resonance. In the opposing field case, the nucleus is said to be shielded, the magnitude of the shielding being proportional to the electron-withdrawing power of proximal substituents. In the aligned field case, the nucleus is said to be deshielded. The field axis may be calibrated in units on a scale from 0 to 10, with TMS at the maximum value. The type of proton may thus be identified by the absorption peak position, i.e. its chemical shift and the area under each peak being proportional to the number of such protons in a particular group. Figure 10.4 is a simplified diagram of an ethyl

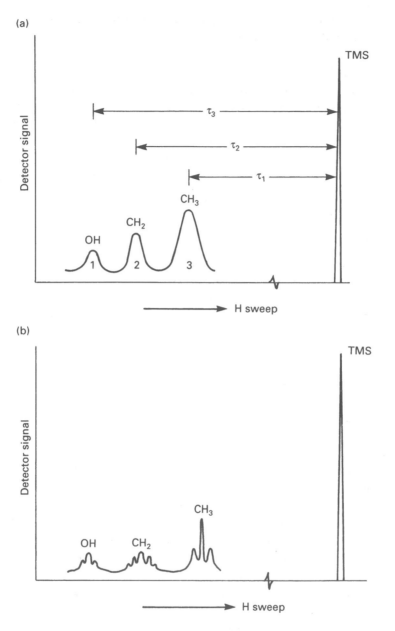

Fig. 10.4. NMR spectrum of ethyl alcohol (a) at low resolution and (b) at high resolution. The latter resolved only in very pure samples. TMS, trimethylsilane.

alcohol spectrum in which there are three methyl, two methylene (methene) and one alcohol group protons. The peaks appear in the area proportions 3:2:1.

High resolution NMR yields further structural information derived from the observation of hyperfine splitting. This arises owing to spin-spin splitting or coupling, owing to the interaction of bonding electrons with like or different spins, and may extend to nuclei four or five bonds apart. It is shown as fine-structure splitting of peaks already separated by chemical shifts. NMR spectra are of great value in elucidating chemical structures. Both qualitative and quantitative information may be obtained, and hyperfine splitting yields information about the near-neighbour environment of a nucleus. The advances in computing power have made possible many of the more advanced NMR techniques. Weak signals may be enhanced by running many scans and accumulating the data; baseline noise, which is random, then tends to cancel out whereas the real signal increases. This approach significantly improves the signal-to-noise ratio and the method is known as computer averaging of transients or CAT scanning. On combining CAT scanning with the very rapid acquisition and data processing of pulse-acquire/Fourier transform methods, very powerful tools become available. In addition the facile manipulation of data postacquisition and the generation of difference spectra has dramatically improved the usefulness and applicability of the basic technique.

Despite the value and continued use of what might be termed 'conventional' proton NMR, much more structural information may be obtained by resorting to pulsed input, of the radiofrequency energy, and subjecting the resulting output to computer analysis by Fourier transform. This approach has given rise to a wide variety of procedures that allow the production of multidimensional spectra (four dimensional in the most sophisticated experiments), ^{13}C and other odd-isotope NMR spectra and the determination of multiplicities and scan images.

In common with all of the spectroscopic techniques already discussed, the energy is input in the form of electromagnetic radiation and 'entities' are promoted from lower to higher states. The 'entities' are electrons in the ultraviolet/visible techniques, bond oscillations and deformations in the infrared, Raman and microwave techniques and magnetic spin orientations in ESR and NMR. All these processes follow the strict quantum rules already described. Clearly (after a certain, albeit short, time span) the entities that were previously promoted to the higher states may return to the original condition. The general term for this process is relaxation. A very simple example is observable in the ultraviolet/visible region, where an absorption spectrum arises when the energy is input and absorbed and an emission spectrum when the system relaxes.

Pulse-acquire and Fourier transform methods

A number of approaches to the method used for the production of spectra exists but mainly one of two options are used. In 'conventional' spectroscopy the electromagnetic energy is supplied, from the source, as a continuously changing frequency over a preselected spectral range. The response is detected by an appropriate device and whether the scan is from shorter to longer wavelength (higher to lower frequency), or the reverse, is irrelevant. The essential point is that the change is smooth and regular between fixed limits. The alternative is to put all the energy, i.e. all the resonant frequencies between the fixed limits, in at the same time. This is achieved by irradiating the sample with a broadband pulse of all these frequencies at one go. The output is, of course, also measured simultaneously and the observed result is, in general, a very complicated interference pattern. Fortunately these patterns are amenable to analysis by Fourier transform methods, which, although being quite complicated mathematical procedures, can be performed readily using modern computer facilities and appear transparent to the user.

The approaches differ with the spectroscopic technique. As indicated in Section 10.2.2, FT–IR involves the method of interferometry and the interferograph that results arises from observation of the frequencies which pass through the sample and are not absorbed. What is detected in FT–NMR is known as the free induction decay (FID). This is akin to the emission spectrum referred to in ultraviolet/visible methods in that the FID arises from the excited species re-emitting the absorbed frequencies. The discussion so far has, for the sake of simplicity, attempted to describe the observed phenomena in terms of single entities, i.e. single nuclei. In a real sample of material in which bulk magnetism may be observed, this arises from the accumulation of all the miniscule nuclear magnets. It may be demonstrated using Boltzmann statistics that, when the sample is placed in an external magnetic field, at thermal equilibrium there will be a slight excess of spins, the so-called α-spins, aligned or parallel with this field. Note that this is the normal low energy condition, the high energy state being that of the antiparallel β-spins. This gives rise to the bulk magnetisation vector, M, and, by agreed convention, it is taken to lie along the z-axis of a three-dimensional Cartesian coordinate system, the z-axis being parallel to the direction of the external magnetic field. The magnetic induction of the external field is designated B_0. Now consider the input of a pulse of the appropriate radio frequency radiation. Recall that this is electromagnetic radiation comprising an electric and a magnetic vector. The magnetic vector of the RF radiation has an associated magnetic field whose magnetic induction may be designated B_1. If the transmitter coils supplying the pulse of RF radiation are arranged so that B_1 is perpendicular to the z-axis along which the bulk magnetisation vector, M, lies, then M will be rotated through an angle θ towards the x–y plane. The value of θ depends upon the magnitude of the B_1 field and the duration of the pulse. Figure 10.5a, b is a diagrammatic representation of this process, with $\theta = \pi/2$ for simplicity (see multidimensional NMR, below, for further explanation). The cumulative spins comprising M are no longer parallel to the external magnetic field, i.e. M no longer lies along the z-axis. In the absence of a further pulse of RF radiation the system will relax, M returning to lie along the z-axis. It is this return or relaxation, which is first-order exponential, that gives rise to the free induction decay alluded to above and data are acquired during the decay period. As described, this would be known as a simple pulse-acquire experiment. Multipulse RF input, possibly at different angles, gives rise to a large array of different experiments, resulting in the production of extremely valuable data. Two relaxation processes are important in NMR and associated techniques. The first-order exponential decay observed in FID arises from energy dissipation by spin–lattice or longitudinal relaxation. In this situation the energy is lost to the matrix (surroundings). The time span for this process is designated T_1. An alternative process is spin–spin or transverse relaxation with time span T_2, where energy

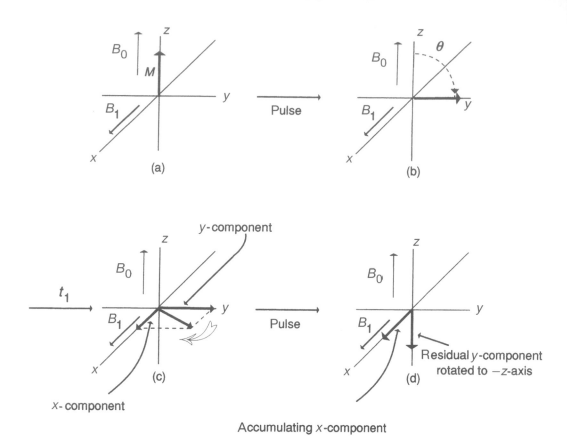

Fig. 10.5. Rotation of magnetism during radiofrequency pulses.

is dissipated between spins rather than the environment. T_1 is always greater than or equal to T_2 and for small organic molecules they are equal.

It is beyond the scope of this text to examine the specific details of the Fourier transform method. It is sufficient to recognise that the mathematical procedure effects the translation of a signal in the time domain to a corresponding 'peak' in the frequency domain. For a sine wave of single frequency, v Hz (cycles per second), 1 cycle is mapped in $1/v$ seconds. The ordinary sine wave is normally shown in the time domain as a portion of an infinite cycle of oscillations of constant amplitude. The frequency appears as a single peak in the frequency domain, also of fixed amplitude. Figure 10.6a shows the effect of the translation between domains for a single sine wave and Fig. 10.6b that for the single FID pattern. All complicated interference patterns may be separated into their constituent sine and cosine waves by Fourier analysis and transformed between domains. Figure 10.7 shows the transform of a waveform comprising three sine waves of different frequency and amplitude.

The time domain oscillograph representing the FID from a real NMR experiment would of course be much more complicated, as it would comprise many

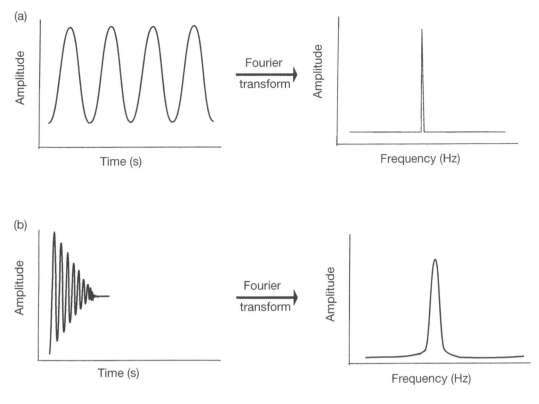

Fig. 10.6. Diagrammatic representation of the Fourier transformation of a single frequency sine wave and single FID. (a) Sine wave, (b) single free induction decay.

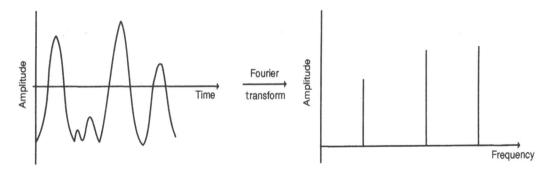

Fig. 10.7. FT of a three-sine-wave combination.

more contributory sine and cosine waves. These would be extracted, transformed to the frequency domain and presented as peaks in a spectrum.

In Section 10.3.2 it was indicated that spins or spinning nuclei generate magnetic fields that may extend their influence through space. Proximal neighbours are subject to this influence, directly, and the general term for this phenomenon is dipolar interaction. If the signal intensity of a resonance is observed to change when the state of a near neighbour is perturbed from the equilibrium, then what is being seen is an example of the nuclear Overhauser effect (NOE). This effect is of profound importance in the elucidation of the three-dimensional stereochemistry of the molecular species under investigation. The magnetic influences encountered in the dipolar interaction are transmitted through space over a limited distance and for the NOE to be observed the distance between nuclei must be of the order of about 0.4 nm or less. Clearly this spatial constraint enables information to be gained about the three-dimensional geometry of the molecule being examined when considered together with scalar coupling (spin–spin coupling) information, this being the influence whose effects occur through bonds.

It is possible to saturate spins in a given population (the perturbation) with a selective 90° irradiation giving ample time for the acquisition of proton spectra involving ^{1}H–^{1}H interactions giving rise to NOE enhancements. By performing a second irradiation at a point in the RF spectrum that is remote from any resonant frequencies, off-resonance irradiation, a control spectrum (no NOEs produced) is generated that may be subtracted from the previously acquired one, resulting in the cancelling out of any signals that are not NOE enhancements. The results obtained are referred to as steady-state NOEs and the method is termed the NOE difference experiment.

One of the main advantages to be gained from the use of pulse-acquire/Fourier transform methods coupled to signal averaging, together with the development of high field magnets, is the ability to obtain ^{13}C NMR spectra. This isotope of carbon exists in low abundance, 1.108% (see Section 11.3.2) and compared to the essentially 100% abundance of ^{1}H it may be recognised that, in general, signal intensities are likely to be low. Despite the advances described above, about ten times the amount of sample, in most cases, is required for ^{13}C NMR spectra compared with that for ^{1}H spectra.

Owing to the low abundance of the ^{13}C nucleus, the chance of finding two such species next to each other in a molecule is very small. This is considered in more detail in Chapter 11. In consequence of this, ^{13}C–^{13}C interactions (homonuclear couplings) do not arise. It is true that ^{1}H–^{13}C interaction (heteronuclear coupling) is possible but, for technical reasons such as band overlap, it is usual to generate decoupled spectra. The result is that, in general, ^{13}C spectra are very much simpler and cleaner and have improved signal-to-noise ratios (albeit with higher sample loadings) compared with their proton resonance counterparts. There are clear advantages in this approach but at least one considerable disadvantage. The ability to observe multiplicities has been lost, i.e. whether a particular ^{13}C is associated with a methyl (CH_3), methene (CH_2) or methyne (CH) group. Some of this information may be regained by performing the decoupling using off-resonance irradiation as in the NOE difference experiments described above. However, a method that has become routine is distortionless enhancement by polarisation transfer (DEPT). This method requires a multipulse excitation sequence at different angles, frequently 45°, 90° or 135°. Although interactions have been decoupled, in this situation the resonances exhibit positive or negative signal intensities, or signal phases, which are dependent on the number of protons directly attached to the carbon nucleus. For example, in a DEPT-135 experiment: CH and CH_3 are both positive; CH_2 is negative. Clearly a single DEPT-135 experiment would suffice if no methyl groups are present. DEPT signals for the above primary, secondary or tertiary carbons, from irradiations at 45° and 90°, are either positive or zero.

Multidimensional NMR

Consider further the processes described in Fig. 10.5a–d. The magnetisation vector M is originally aligned along the z-axis parallel to the vector direction of the external field, B_0. A pulse B_1 is applied, at right angles, i.e. parallel to the x-axis and M is rotated to the y-axis through 90°, provided the pulse is of sufficient magnitude and lasts for a sufficient time (Fig. 10.5a,b). Apart from the decay process this vector will precess (rotate) in the x–y plane, towards the x-axis (Fig. 10.5c) with a characteristic frequency, the Larmor frequency during a period of time t_1. This is quite distinct from the decay process, FID, which overlaps it. At any point between the x- and y-axes the vector M may be resolved into components along these two axes. If, during t_1, a second B_1 pulse is applied then the component along the y-axis will again be rotated, in this instance towards the $-z$-axis. The component along the x-axis is unaffected because it is parallel to B_1. If the time t_1 is zero, i.e. there are immediately consecutive B_1 pulses, then M rotates from the z- to the y-axis with the first pulse and then immediately to the $-z$-axis with the second pulse. For $t_1 = 0$ there will be no x component as there has been no time available for it to be established. For values of $t_1 > 0$ a component of M along the x-axis will be established whose magnitude depends on the length of t_1. The longer t_1 the greater will be the magnitude of the x component because M will have moved nearer to this axis. By applying successive B_1 pulses with increasing lengths of t_1, an accumulated x component of magnetisation is produced and a series of FIDs may be measured and stored separately in the computer. The y- and $-z$-components are not measurable. This accumulation of FIDs gives rise to a second dimension in the time domain and each may be transformed by Fourier methods.

Two-dimensional frequency diagrams are produced as contour maps. Values on the diagonal correspond to chemical shifts, etc. that would have been shown in a one-dimensional experiment. It is the asymmetrical, off-diagonal information that is new. These data arise from the correlation of coupling interactions between nuclei, the main advantage being that the information is all gathered in one experiment, an achievement entirely dependent on the use of multipulse excitation. Proton–proton correlation gives rise to homonuclear correlation spectroscopy (COSY). Proton–carbon correlation gives rise to heteronuclear chemical shift correlation spectroscopy (hetero-COSY or HETCOR).

The achieved and potential sophistication of NMR experiments is quite phenomenal, allowing more useful two-dimensional and extension into three- and four-dimensional spectra. Considering again Fig. 10.5a–d (the COSY pulse sequence), the second 90° pulse rotates the magnetisation vector along the $-z$-axis. Various transverse components are removed by electronic control and the vector in the $-z$ direction accumulates (cf. the process described above for the COSY case). A third 90° pulse is then applied and produces magnetisation, which can be measured. Repeat of the pulse sequence for varying (increasing) values of t_1 give rise to changes that are observable during the final 90° pulse. The outcome is a two-dimensional experiment that allows the detection of NOEs and is known as nuclear Overhauser effect spectroscopy (NOESY). This can be improved upon yet further by studying phenomena in the rotating frame coordinate system rather than fixed Cartesian coordinates. Such an experiment involves rotating frame nuclear Overhauser effect spectroscopy (ROESY). A significant problem is that, for ^{1}H NOESY NMR to be of value, all the NOEs should be resolved. In the study of biological macromolecules this becomes less likely with the increase in molecular mass. The use of triple pulse sequences (three time variables) in conjunction with a COSY or NOESY sequence generates a three-dimensional spectrum. This, in effect, is a cube and is akin to stacking two-dimensional spectra one on top of the other. Note that this is a near analogy and not a simple stacking procedure. In order to achieve this it is necessary to incorporate into the molecule under investigation an isotopically labelled nuclide such as ^{13}C or ^{15}N. A whole new range of interactions between ^{1}H, ^{13}C and/or ^{15}N is now possible and adds extensively to the analytical procedure. To obtain the resolution advantages of the four-dimensional spectrum, both ^{13}C and ^{15}N must be incorporated, the heavy isotope of carbon being deliberately introduced at particular points in the carbon chain in order to be associated with specific aliphatic hydrogens. Essentially, three separate two-dimensional experiments are combined, the different interactions being ^{1}H–^{1}H, ^{1}H–^{13}C and ^{1}H–^{15}N. It is interesting to note that, in the four-dimensional case, the manipulation of the generated data by powerful computer techniques results in substantially improved resolution without a corresponding increase in complexity.

10.4.2 Instrumentation

The essential details of an NMR instrument are shown diagrammatically in Fig. 10.8. It will be seen yet again that the layout is almost identical to that of ESR, except that instead of a Klystron oscillator being present to generate microwave radiation, two sets of coils, a transmitter and a receiver, are used for generation and reception, respectively, of the appropriate RF. Samples in solution are contained in sealed tubes, which are rotated rapidly in the cavity to eliminate irregularities and imperfections; in this way an average and uniform signal is reflected to the receiver to be processed and recorded. Solid state and high field NMR are more recent and rapidly advancing techniques enable hitherto difficult or impossible investigations. The latest developments allow multidimensional NMR to be performed, permitting even more sophisticated structural analyses to be carried out. Many of these developments in instrumentation differ from the simple design shown in Fig. 10.8 in terms of the geometric layout of the coils, for the multipulse methods described above, sophisticated electronics and advanced computer facilities.

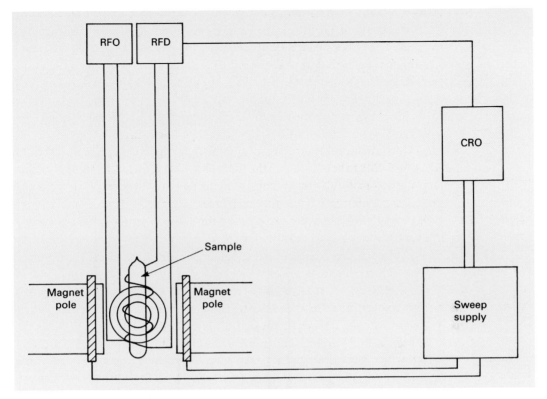

Fig. 10.8. Diagram of an NMR spectrometer. CRO, cathode ray oscilloscope; RFO, radio frequency oscillator; RFD, radio frequency detector.

10.4.3 **Applications**

The study of molecular structure, conformational changes and certain types of kinetic investigation is the main use of NMR in the biological field. Most work is done in solution, and in order to eliminate solvent effects the equivalent deuterated solvent (for proton NMR) would be used. The use of the technique in drug metabolism studies is of increasing importance, particularly when coupled with infrared and X-ray diffraction data, which can then be used in molecular modelling methods using sophisticated computer techniques to try to elucidate drug action. Figure 10.9 shows a high resolution proton resonance spectrum of phenacetin and, together with the FT-IR spectrum shown in Fig. 10.2, yields substantial structural information. For comparative purposes, the two-dimensional COSY spectrum of phenacetin is shown in Fig. 10.10, where contours along the diagonal give information equivalent to that shown in Fig. 10.9. The off-diagonal contours represent additional information; for explanation, see the legend.

An examination of the scientific literature in the field shows a plethora of results for biological macromolecules using the whole battery of techniques described above. For peptide and protein structural studies the species tend to be

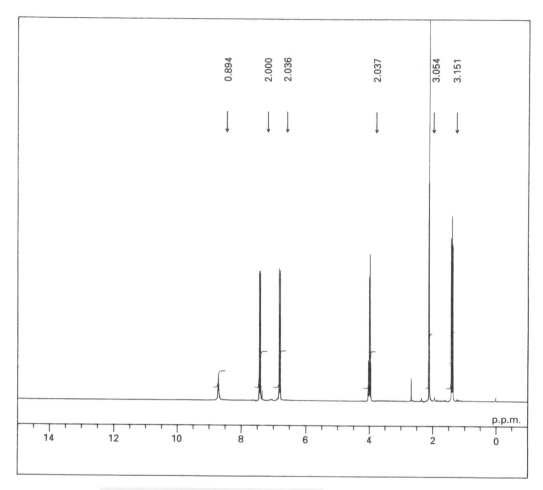

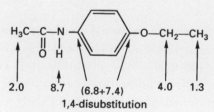

Fig. 10.9. NMR spectrum of phenacetin. The values associated with the downward-pointing arrows, shown slightly to the right of each peak in the upper diagram, indicate the approximate number of protons involved. In the lower diagram the shifts in p.p.m. are shown, indicating which proton is involved. The peak at 1.3 p.p.m. is a triplet because it is next to a -CH_2 group and that at 4.0 is a quadruplet because it is next to a -CH_3 group. The peaks at 6.8 and 7.4 p.p.m. are a pattern characteristic of 1,4 disubstitution in an aromatic ring.

arbitrarily divided into those with relative molecular mass less than 15 000 and those between 15 000 and 30 000. Low resolution NMR has been obtained on the *lac* repressor headpiece and bovine pancreatic trypsin inhibitor (BPTI). High resolution protein structures for antiviral protein BDS-1, the C3a and C5a inflammatory proteins, plastocyanin, thioredoxin, epidermal growth factor and the interleukins are some examples. The application of solid state NMR has been valuable in the study of, for example, Alzheimer's β-amyloid peptide and melanostatin. Much more specialised methods are required to extend the mass range beyond 30 000 but it is now possible and several antibodies have been investigated.

A distinct advantage of NMR is its use in studying molecular behaviour in solution. Any particular state is averaged, of course, but often produces more useful information than the constrained structures available from X-ray crystallographic studies. Results of studies of protein folding are exemplified by ribonuclease A, cytochrome *c*, barnase, α-lactalbumin, lysozyme, ubiquitin and BPTI.

The techniques have been applied to the study of enzyme kinetics both *in vivo* and *in vitro*. Amongst the groups of enzymes studied are: chymotrypsin, trypsin, papain, pepsin, thermolysin; adenylate, creatinine and pyruvate kinases; alkaline phosphatase, ATPase and ribonuclease. Other examples are glycogen phosphorylase, dihydrofolate reductase and triosephosphate isomerase.

Application to the nucleic acids includes not only a variety of structural studies of both DNA and RNA but additionally investigations of interactions between various drugs and DNA and between binding proteins and DNA. Sequence assignments in oligosaccharides have been obtained but work on intact glycoproteins has not been promising, particularly in multidimensional NMR, owing to the difficulty in deconvoluting the data. Interactions between proteins and lipid bilayers in membranes have been observed and the structure of certain membrane proteins has been related to their predicted biological function. Examples of such proteins are gramicidin A, bacteriorhodopsin and rhodopsin, phage coat proteins and alamethicin.

The isotope ^{31}P exhibits nuclear resonance and NMR has been used extensively in studies of phosphate metabolism. The relative and changing concentrations of AMP, ADP and ATP can be measured and hence their metabolism studied in living cells and tissues. Intracellular and extracellular inorganic phosphate concentrations may be measured in living cells and tissues also because the chemical shift of inorganic phosphate varies with pH.

The above list is by no means comprehensive but it is intended to indicate the wide variety of structural, kinetic and molecular dynamics studies that are now available.

Magnetic resonance imaging

The analytical applications described above may be extended into the clinical environment. Physiological material such as urine, blood and cerebrospinal fluid may be studied directly. Appropriate tissue biopsy samples are also amenable to examination. In such cases, biochemical phenomena are being observed. For instance, the measurement of metabolic concentrations at specific sites in tissues

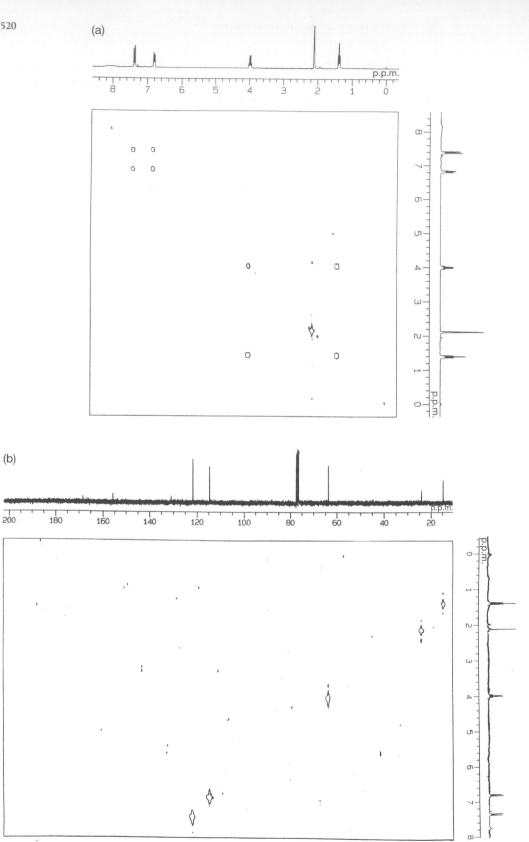

is possible. The extension to small whole animals in pharmacological investigations and the human subject has become possible with the advent of superconducting magnet technology and other improvements. ATP metabolism in healthy and unhealthy individuals and changes during exercise are measurable.

The major direct clinical application, however, is in imaging. Unfortunately, owing to the low energy transitions in the radio frequency region of the electromagnetic spectrum, NMR is a relatively insensitive technique. This imposes limitations and attention is focused almost exclusively on ^{1}H resonance in the development of magnetic resonance imaging (MRI). There are two important reasons for this; first the proton is one of the more sensitive nuclides, and, secondly, it is present in biological systems in considerable abundance. However, not all types of proton in all molecular environments are easily studied. Those protons making a major contribution to the NMR response reside in compounds in rapid physical motion. By far the most important compound in this respect is water, which contains two protons and is a major constituent of biological systems. Lesser contributions from protons in other compounds are measurable in special circumstances.

Fig. 10.10. Two-dimensional NMR spectra may be best imagined as looking down on a forest where all the trees (representing peaks in the spectrum) have been chopped off at the same fixed height. Taller trees would have thicker trunks at a given height. The equivalent is the larger contours observed which derive from larger peaks in the unidimensional spectra.

(a) This figure is the correlated (COSY) NMR spectrum of phenacetin showing the homonuclear ^{1}H–^{1}H interactions. The single spectra along each axis are identical and the contours along the diagonal of the two-dimensional map represent the 'birds-eye view' of the chopped-off peaks. The off-diagonal contours, which are symmetrically distributed as a mirror image about the diagonal, represent new information. As an example of the interpretation, place a rule horizontally at the 1.3 p.p.m. position of the right-hand spectrum (triplet) and another rule vertically at the 4.0 p.p.m. position on the top spectrum (quadruplet). Where these two rules intersect is the location of a contour which represents the interaction between protons located in adjacent -CH$_2$- and -CH$_3$ groups.

(b) This is the heteronuclear ^{13}C – ^{1}H correlation spectrum. The contours in the two-dimensional map here represent interactions between the nuclear magnets of ^{13}C and the associated protons. The ^{1}H spectrum lies vertically along the right-hand axis and the ^{13}C spectrum lies horizontally along the top. The contour positions are located as described in (a) above and the p.p.m. values and interactions are listed below.

p.p.m.			
^{13}C	^{1}H	Interaction	
14	1.3	CH$_3$-	(Ethyl–O)
24	2.1	CH$_3$-	(Acetyl)
63	4.0	CH$_2$-	Ethyl–O
115	6.8	Ring C	(Ethyl–O)
122	7.4	Ring C	(= N–H)
132	—	Ring C	(= N–H)
156	—	Ring C	(Ethyl–O)
167	—	= C = O	
	7.8	= N – H	

A triplet observed at 77 p.p.m. is due to residual chloroform in the solvent.

In NMR, the resonance frequency of the particular nuclide contributing the magnetic spin is proportional to the strength of the applied external magnetic field. If an external magnetic field 'gradient' is applied then a range of resonant frequencies may be observed which reflects the spatial distribution of the spinning nuclei. Three major approaches are in wide use which result in (i) projection reconstruction, (ii) Fourier imaging and (iii) echo-planar imaging. For detailed consideration of these different methods the reader is referred to more specialised texts (see Section 10.6).

A particular advantage of MRI is that there is some flexibility in the choice of physical property that is imaged. The number of spins in a particular, defined spatial region gives rise to the spin density as a measurable parameter. This measure may be combined with measures of the principal relaxation times (T_1 and T_2) to give more meaningful results. The imaging of flux, either as bulk flow or localised diffusion, adds considerably to the options available. In terms of whole-body scanners the 'overall picture' is reconstructed from images generated in contiguous slices and clearly owes much to advances in computing power as well as magnetic resonance technology. Resolution and image contrast are major considerations for the technique and subject to continuing development. Equipment cost and data acquisition time remain other important issues affecting the development of MRI.

Water is distributed differently in different tissues but constitutes, in total, about 55% of body mass in the average human subject. In soft tissues the water distribution varies between 60% and 90% of the total mass. The differences in water content in white and grey matter in the brain and between normal tissue and most tumours generates sufficient contrast to enable high resolution images to be produced. Figure 10.11 reproduces an MRI scan showing a vertical longitudinal section of the human head and brain. In adipose tissue the ^{1}H signal from lipids is measurable and the chemical shift differences for $-CH_2-$ are such that distinction from water may be made. Reproduced in Fig. 10.12 are photographs obtained from MRI scans of fat and thin patients in order that the distribution of adipose tissue may be compared. The thin patient represents the control in the experiment.

It is also possible to distinguish the different relaxation properties. Tissue water behaves quite differently from the pure substance. Transverse relaxation, T_2, does not generally follow a single exponential decay process whereas longitudinal relaxation, T_1, does. T_2 relaxations must be split into at least two exponential decays, having a typical value of 20 to 100 ms. For T_1 decays the range is 100 to 500 ms. These values are significantly less than for pure water and the differences may arise from the presence of hydrophilic macromolecules in the tissue environment. In the case of tumours, however, the T_1 values are elevated compared with normal tissue, adding a further important discriminator, although the elevation is less marked in human tumours compared with laboratory-grown material. Disadvantages with this approach are the overlap of values and also that elevated T_1 decays are not tumour specific but may also be evident in normal rapidly regenerating tissue. Other NMR parameters and observational differential diagnosis of the magnetic resonance image must also be taken into account. The shape, size

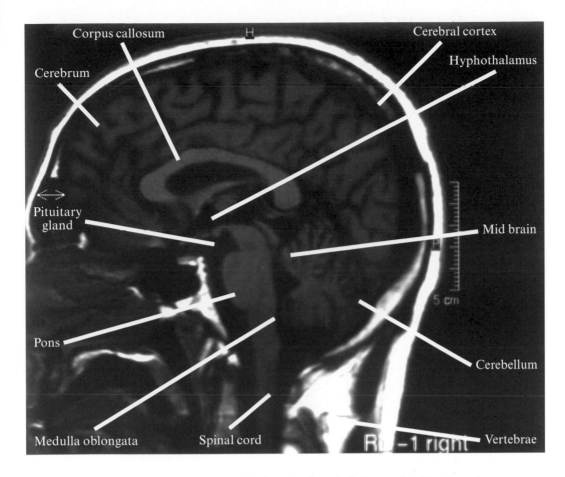

Fig. 10.11. Vertical longitudinal section through the human head by magnetic resonance imaging (MRI). The major features are identified and labelled, although specific items such as the pituitary gland and hypothalamus are barely visible. (This figure is modified from an MRI scan kindly donated by the Radiology Department of the Stepping Hill Hospital, Stockport, Cheshire.)

and location of the abnormal image must be considered by the radiologist when making a diagnosis.

At present there is an almost bewildering array of options available in terms of different pulse sequences, scan protocols, and chemical shift and relaxation time data measurements that can be made. The procedures can be applied to three-dimensional and contiguous slice imaging of whole body or specific organ investigations on head, thorax, abdomen, liver, pancreas, kidney and musculoskeletal regions. Use of contrast agents has enabled 'organ function' such as renal function to be explored, if the agent passes into the urine. If such an agent can be administered intravenously then exploration of blood flow, tissue perfusion, and transport across the blood/brain barrier may be investigated and also defects in vascular anatomy recognised. Contrast agents for use in MRI will generally be

(a)

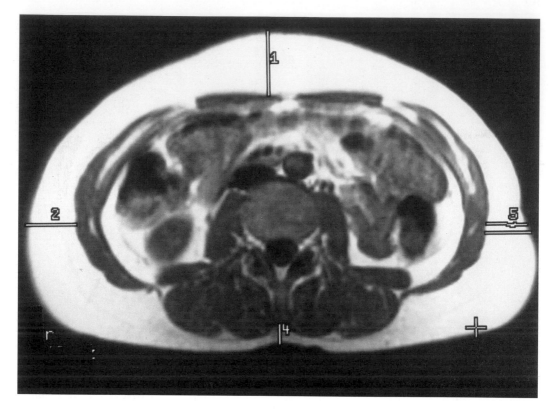

Fig. 10.12. (a) and (b) show MRI scans of transverse sections (contiguous slice) through the abdominal regions of 'fat' and 'obese' subjects. The fatty deposits are indicated by the intense white regions, the resonance arising from the protons of the methylene groups of long-chain fatty acids. (The scans are reproduced by kind permission of the Oxford Lipid Metabolism Group, Nuffield Department of Clinical Medicine, University of Oxford.)

required to show paramagnetic properties. Clearly, as in other invasive methods, they must be non-toxic.

NMR and the associated technique of MRI offer the analytical biochemist and the clinician a phenomenal variety of procedures. Both types of applications continue to challenge almost all alternative approaches. Clearly there are hazards associated with any technique but these magnetic resonance methods appear, on the basis of current knowledge, to be relatively safe, particularly with the absence of ionising radiation.

(b)

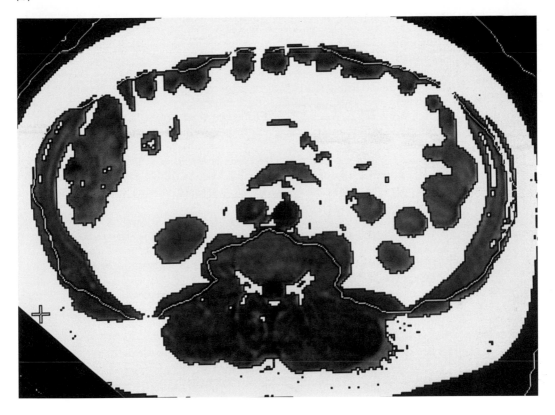

Fig. 10.12. (*cont.*)

10.5 **KEY TERMS**

antiparallel
computer averaging of transients
chemical shift
correlation spectroscopy
dipole moment
distortionless enhancement by
    polarisation transfer
diamagnetism
5,5-dimethylpyrroline-1-oxide
1,1-diphenyl-2′-picrylhydrazyl
electron double resonance
electron nuclear double resonance
electron paramagnetic resonance
electron spin resonance
ferromagnetism
fingerprint
free induction decay
Fourier transform infrared
    spectroscopy

Golay cell
Guoy balance
heteronuclear couplings
heteronuclear chemical shift COSY
homonuclear couplings
imaging
infrared spectrum
interferograph
interferometry
larmor frequency
microwave spectroscopy
multiplicity
NOE difference spectra
nuclear magnetic resonance
nuclear Overhauser effect
nuclear Overhauser effect
    spectroscopy
nuclear paramagnetism
nucleon

Overhauser effect
parallel
paramagnetism
Pauli exclusion principle
proton magnetic resonance
Raman spectroscopy
relaxation
rotating frame ROESY
scan
spectroscopic splitting factor
spin
spin–lattice
spin–spin coupling
spin–spin relaxation
spin–spin splitting
steady-state NOE
2,2,6,6-tetramethylpiperadine-1-oxyl

10.6 SUGGESTIONS FOR FURTHER READING

BREITMEYER, E. (1993). *Structure Elucidation by NMR in Organic Chemistry*. John Wiley and Sons, London. (Contains many worked examples on interpretation of spectra and numerous practice problems. Covers many compounds of biological interest and importance.)

EVANS, J. N. S. (1995). *Biomolecular NMR Spectroscopy*. Oxford University Press, Oxford. (The early chapters cover some deep theoretical concepts but the remainder of the book contains a comprehensive coverage of applications.)

GEORGE, W. O. and MCINTYRE, P. S. (1987). *Infrared Spectroscopy*. ACOL Series. John Wiley and Sons, London. (A valuable learning text for those wishing to pursue the subject in greater depth.)

HARWOOD, L. M. and CLARIDGE, D. W. (1997). *Introduction to Organic Spectroscopy*. Oxford Chemistry Primers **43**, Oxford University Press, Oxford. (Although primarily for students studying chemistry, the text is well suited to biochemists wishing to study the theory in more depth.)

KNOWLES, P. F., MARSH, D. and RATTLE, H. W. E. (1976). *Magnetic Resonance of Biomolecules*. John Wiley and Sons, London. (Contains comprehensive coverage of ESR and NMR.)

MORRIS, P. G. (1986). *Nuclear Magnetic Resonance Imaging in Medicine and Biology*. Oxford University Press, Oxford. (Extensive coverage of the theory and a wide variety of imaging applications.)

WILLIAMS, D. A. R. (1986). *Nuclear Magnetic Resonance Spectroscopy*. ACOL Series. John Wiley and Sons, London. (Offers material for readers wishing to pursue the subject in greater detail.)

WILLIAMS, D. H. and FLEMING, I. (1995). *Spectroscopic Methods in Organic Chemistry*, 5th edn. McGraw-Hill Book Co., New York. (Comments similar to those in previous entry.)

Chapter 11

Mass spectrometric techniques

11.1 INTRODUCTION

In contrast to the spectroscopic techniques described in Chapters 9 and 10, those dealt with here are not dependent on quantum principles. The term mass spectroscopy, though frequently encountered, is in fact incorrect and its use should be discouraged. In spectroscopic techniques it is possible, at least in principle by using quantum mechanical methods, to predict the spectrum. The mass spectrum is essentially dependent upon the thermodynamic stability of the ions produced and collected during a mass spectrometric experiment. Such stability depends essentially on the conditions prevailing during the experiment. In this situation it is difficult to entertain ideas of predicting the mass spectrum, although some attempt has been made to do just this using quasi-equilibrium theory (QET). Usually, to determine the mass spectrum of a compound 'the experiment must be done'.

The variety of mass spectra that may be obtained range from a single peak (generally obtained with so-called soft ionisation methods) to quite complicated patterns of peaks representing various fragments of the original species. Single-peak spectra are of particular value in the determination of very accurate molecular masses. It should be noted at this point that, although 'mass' is a universal property (everything has mass), it is not unique. Isomeric compounds (isomers) are chemical entities that have identical masses but different chemical structures, and hence different properties – they are different things. Examples are shown in Fig. 11.1.

In order to use mass spectrometry to identify the different chemical structures it is necessary to perform the kind of experiment that causes the molecular entity to disintegrate and produce fragment ions, each of which is represented by a peak in the resultant spectrum. It is from these more complicated spectra that skilled interpreters may reconstruct the molecular formulae of the original entity.

11.2 THE MASS SPECTROMETER

11.2.1 Components

All mass spectrometers (Fig. 11.2) are essentially composed of three parts:

(i) an ionisation chamber or source,
(ii) a mass analyser,
(iii) a detector.

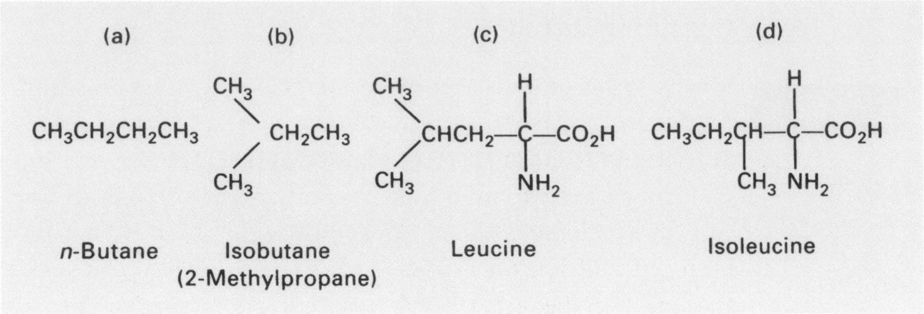

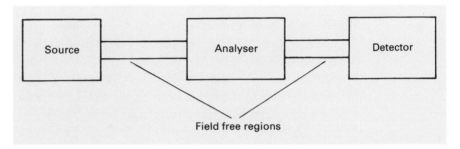

Fig. 11.1. Isomeric pairs: (a) and (b) are isomers, as are (c) and (d). Each has the same mass but different structures and hence are different compounds.

Fig. 11.2. Diagram of a mass spectrometer. The whole system is kept under high vacuum of the order of 10^{-5} torr.

In some cases extra analysers, for example energy analysers, may be included in more sophisticated devices.

In the simplest mass spectrometers, a single mass analyser is used that involves either magnetic or electric fields. The processes involved in separating entities of different masses are different in each of the cases (magnetic or electric fields) and these are explained in detail later (Sections 11.8.1 and 11.8.2). An alternative approach is to measure accurately the times taken for entities of different masses to travel a given distance in space (in a straight line) in the so-called time-of-flight mass spectrometer (Section 11.6.3).

The essential requirements to obtain a mass spectrum are to produce ions in the gas phase, to accelerate them to a specific velocity using electric fields, to project them into a suitable mass analyser, which separates the entities of different masses, and finally to detect each charged entity of a particular mass sequentially in time.

Any material that can be ionised and whose ions can exist in the gas phase (remembering that very low pressures, i.e. high vacua, in the region of 10^{-5} torr are used) can be investigated by mass spectrometry. Almost all compounds of biological interest are 'organic', comprising the elements C, H, N, O and sometimes S and P, although a number of inorganic pollutants are important in environmental studies.

11.2.2 **Ionisation techniques**

Ions may be produced either by removing an electron from the molecule to produce a positively charged cationic species (cation), or conversely by adding an electron to form an anion. Both positive and negative ion mass spectrometry may be carried out, but clearly not at the same time; only one kind of ion may be accelerated out of the source region at any time, despite the fact that both types of ion may have been produced together in the ionisation process. Cations will be accelerated in either an increasing negative gradient field (attracted towards a negative electrode) or a decreasing positive gradient field (repelled from a positive electrode). Exactly the converse is true for anions.

If electrons (Section 11.3.1) are used to effect the ionisation process, however, cations and anions are not produced in equal amounts, because the removal of an electron from a neutral molecule to form a cation is a much more efficient process than electron capture to form an anion (this efficiency depends on the different ionisation energies and electron affinities involved). Many more cations than anions are produced (about 100 to 1) and it is probably for this reason that positive ion electron impact mass spectrometry is more common because there is a natural increase in sensitivity. Nevertheless negative ion spectra may be obtained in appropriate cases and produce important and useful complementary data.

Removal or addition of electrons is not, however, the only means of producing ions. The removal or addition of protons (H atoms) will also produce ions. Whereas the mass of an electron removed from, or added to, a molecular entity may be neglected (insignificant relative to the mass being determined), this is not so in the case of protons. In the latter case the mass of the resultant ion will differ by ± 1 from the mass of the original neutral entity. Furthermore it is possible to produce ions by adduct formation with entities such as NH_4^+ or CH_5^+ in a process known as chemical ionisation (Section 11.4) and here the nominal mass difference from the neutral original is 18 or 17, respectively.

The next sections deal with some of the more common ways of producing ions in a mass spectrometer. The range of ionisation sources is quite large and there are many more ways of producing ions in the gas phase than there are for analysing or detecting them.

Whichever ionisation method is chosen, a successful ionisation process requires the energy is put into the material under investigation. This turns out to be extremely important, because the amount of energy input and the way it is applied dramatically affect the thermodynamic conditions and ultimately the type of mass spectrum produced. It also means that there is no universal ionisation source and the type used is determined by the information required from the experiment.

11.3 **ELECTRON IMPACT IONISATION**

11.3.1 **Source**

Electron impact ionisation (EI) is probably still the most widely used ionisation source in mass spectrometry. In many biological problems involving metabolic studies, drug studies, pollutants, etc. it would probably be the method of choice. It is not appropriate, however, for the study of biological macromolecules, and other sources are described later that are much more important for these types of investigation. EI is a relatively simple source to understand and therefore a description of it serves the useful purpose of elaborating the principles introduced in Section 11.2.

Many metals, when heated to a sufficiently high temperature (approximately 2000 K) lose electrons by diffusion from their surface. This arises from the structural nature of metals; two that are particularly useful are rhenium and tungsten because they can be drawn readily into thin filaments. Tungsten filaments are sometimes coated with thoria (thorium oxide) to increase the ease with which electrons are emitted. If such heated filaments are subjected to an appropriate potential gradient then electrons are removed from the surface more rapidly and gain an energy related directly to the potential applied. Commonly a 70 V potential is applied and the resultant beam contains 70 eV electrons. The electron volt (eV) is a measure of energy. These electrons stream across an evacuated chamber into which molecules of the substance to be analysed are allowed to diffuse. In the electron impact source, the substance to be analysed must be in the vapour state, which obviously limits the applicability to biological materials, although it should be remembered that most substances may have their natural volatility increased by chemical modification.

The stream of 70 eV electrons from the filament interacts with the molecules of the substance to be analysed (which are neutral and in random thermal motion). This interaction results in either loss of an electron from the substance (to produce a cation) or electron capture (to produce an anion). As the positive ionisation potential of most organic molecules is of the order of 20 eV there is ample excess energy in the beam of bombarding electrons. The electron impact source is shown diagrammatically in Fig. 11.3.

The possible events that may occur are shown below. M represents the neutral molecular species:

$$M + e^- \text{ (bombarding electron)} \longrightarrow M^{+\cdot} + 2e^-$$

(one bombarding electron and one removed from M)

or

$$M + e^- \longrightarrow M^{-\cdot}$$

Chemical bonds in organic molecules are formed by the pairing of electrons. Ionisation resulting in a cation requires loss of an electron from one of these bonds (effectively knocked out by the bombarding electrons), but it leaves a bond with a single unpaired electron. This is a radical as well as being a cation and hence the representation as $M^{+\cdot}$, the $(+)$ sign indicating the ionic state and the $(\cdot)$ a radical. Conversely, electron capture results both in an anion but also the addition of an unpaired electron and therefore a negatively charged radical, hence the symbol $M^{-\cdot}$. Such radical ions are termed molecular ions, parent ions or precursor ions and under the conditions of electron bombardment are relatively unstable. The

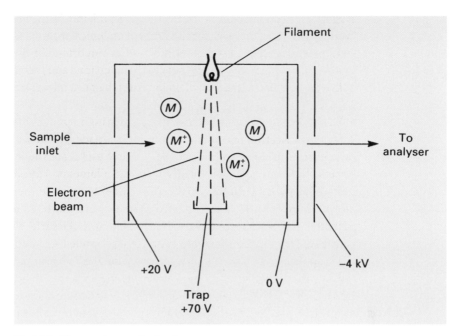

Fig. 11.3. Electron impact ionisation source.

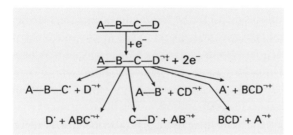

Fig. 11.4. Fragmentation processes in a hypothetical species.

imparted energy in excess of that required for ionisation has to be dissipated and this latter process results in the precursor ion disintegrating into a number of smaller fragments. Also the fragments themselves may be relatively unstable and further fragmentation may occur. This gives rise to a series of daughter ions or product ions, which are eventually recorded as the mass spectrum. The whole process is best shown by a purely hypothetical case shown in Fig. 11.4.

A, B, C, and D represent groups in a molecule linked by electron pair bonds. The example here is for the production of a radical cation. As it is not known where either the positive charge or the unpaired electron actually reside in the molecule, it is usual practice to place the dot signs outside the abbreviated bracket sign '⌐'. This is also true for fragment or product ions and will be used throughout the remainder of this chapter.

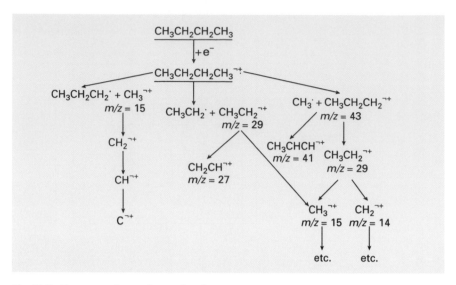

Fig. 11.5. Fragmentation pathways in *n*-butane.

The first thing to note is that, when the precursor ion fragments, one of the possible products carries the charge and the other the unpaired electron, i.e. it splits into a radical and an ion. The product ions are therefore true ions and not radical ions. The radicals produced in the fragmentation process are neutral species and therefore do not take any further part in the mass spectrometry but are pumped away by the vacuum system. Only the charged species may be accelerated out of the source and into the mass analyser. It is also important to recognise that almost all possible bond breakages can occur and any given fragment will arise both as an ion and a radical such as, AB· and AB]+. The distribution of charge and unpaired electron, however, is by no means equal, i.e. it is not usual to get 50% AB· and 50% AB]+. The distribution depends entirely on the thermodynamic stability of the products of fragmentation. Furthermore, any fragment such as AB]+may break down further (until single atoms are obtained) and hence not many ions of a particular type may survive, resulting in a low signal being recorded.

A simple, but non-biological example is given by *n*-butane ($CH_3CH_2CH_2CH_3$) and some of the major fragmentations are shown Fig. 11.5. The resultant EI spectrum that would be obtained is shown in Fig. 11.6. What is actually recorded is the mass to charge ratio spectrum, *m*/*z*, where *m* is the mass and *z* is the number of charges carried by the ion. In ordinary mass spectrometry $z = 1$ and hence in effect a mass spectrum is obtained. It is shown later (Section 11.7.2) that it is possible to produce ions where $z > 1$, enabling much larger species to be analysed

11.3.2 Isotopic composition

In ordinary mass spectrometry satellite peaks are observed at a particular value for *m*/*z* ratio (equation 11.1, below) that arises owing to the isotopic composi-

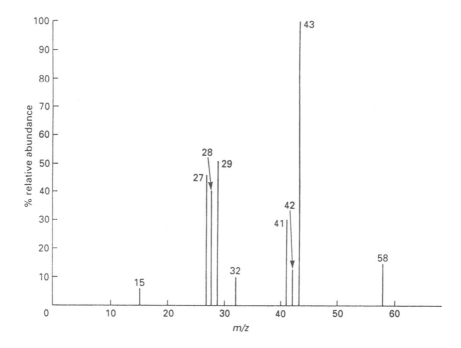

Fig. 11.6. Electron impact ionisation spectrum of *n*-butane. Relative abundance is a scale calibrated from 0 to 100%. The largest peak in the spectrum is set at 100% (base peak) and all the others calculated in proportion as a percentage. Spectra produced in this way are said to be normalised, are machine independent and hence are directly comparable. Conversely, spectra whose ordinates are labelled as intensity are absolute spectra.

tion of the species. For instance, 1.108% of all carbon on the planet is the 13-isotope (designated ^{13}C), the remainder being ^{12}C. Hence if an ion, precursor or product, contained say 12 C atoms, then the approximate percentage probability of at least one of them being the ^{13}C isotope is

$$12 \times 1.108 = 12.96\%$$

At some m/z value (depending on the other atoms present in the ion) there will be a peak in the spectrum corresponding to the ion containing only ^{12}C atoms. The intensity of this peak depends on the thermodynamic stability of the ion. There will also be a satellite isotope peak one atomic mass unit greater owing to the ion containing one ^{13}C atom. The approximate intensity of the satellite peak will be the product of the intensity of the peak representing the ^{12}C only species (I_{12}), the number of carbon atoms in the ion (N) and the natural abundance of the ^{13}C isotope:

$$(I_{12}) \times (N) \times 1.108\%$$

Of course the intensity of this satellite peak may be greater than this if other species contribute to it, but it is possible that any such contributions may be accounted for using high resolution mass spectrometry (Section 11.8.2).

| Table 11.1 | Probability of occurrence of different isotopic compositions |

No of ^{13}C atoms present	% probability of occurrence
0 (all ^{12}C)	95.641
1	4.2863
2	0.0720
3	0.0005
4	0.0000
	99.9998

There have to be four C atoms of one kind or another so that the total percentage adds up to 100.

The probability of more than one ^{13}C atom being present in an ion is finite but of small value, and to obtain this value one has to perform rather more accurate calculations than the approximations carried out above. To do this one has to solve the binomial expansion shown below:

$$(a + b)^m$$

where a is the percentage natural abundance of the light isotope, b is the percentage natural abundance of the heavy isotope, and m is the number of atoms of the element concerned in the molecule.

Consider the earlier simple example of n-butane where $m = 4$. Expansion of $(a + b)^4$ gives

$$a^4 + 4a^3b + 6a^2b^2 + 4ab^3 + b^4$$

(Note that the binomial coefficients may be found from mathematical tables.) Substituting the appropriate values for the relevant isotopic abundances of carbon isotopes gives

$$(98.892)^4 + [4 \times (98.892)^3 \times 1.108] + [6 \times (98.892)^2 \times (1.108)^2)] +$$
$$[4 \times 98.892 \times (1.108)^3] + (1.108)^4 = (9.5641 \times 10^7) + (4.2863 \times 10^6) +$$
$$(7.2036 \times 10^4) + (5.3807 \times 10^2) + 1.5071$$

Dividing throughout by 10^6 (the substituted values are actually percentages so the denominators should be 100^4 or 10^8 and this has to multiplied by 100 to recover a percentage; hence divide by 10^6), the data in Table 11.1 may be constructed. It can be seen that there is now a small but significant probability that natural n-butane will have some molecules containing a ^{13}C atom. The probabilities of there being two, three or four are negligible. However, if the compound contained 100 carbon atoms then there would be a greater chance of any carbon atom being a ^{13}C than a ^{12}C. Biological macromolecules contain several hundred carbon atoms and the isotopic distribution patterns become extremely complicated, the computations unwieldy, and sophisticated computer techniques are necessary to deconvolute the data.

For elements such as chlorine, the isotopic abundances are approximately $3:1$ for $^{35}Cl : ^{37}Cl$. If a compound contains a single chlorine atom and can be ionised to give stable molecular ions, then two such species will be observed, with peak intensities in an approximate ratio of $3:1$. If a compound contained two chlorine atoms, then in order to predict the relative abundances of the three possible peaks that would arise (note that if the number of isotopes of a particular element is n then there are $n+1$ possible peaks predicted by the binomial expansion) is obtained from the expansion of

$$(a+b)^2 = a^2 + 2ab + b^2$$

Substituting $a=3$ and $b=1$ for the isotopic abundances of ^{35}Cl and ^{37}Cl, respectively, we get, for the three possible peaks,

$^{35}Cl^{35}Cl$ 9
$^{35}Cl^{37}Cl$ 6
$^{37}Cl^{37}Cl$ 1

It is left to readers to try as an exercise the calculation of the relative proportions for a compound containing three chlorine atoms. Four peaks are possible with the proportions $27:27:9:1$.

It should be seen that isotope patterns become rather complicated as the possibility of increased numbers of different isotopes being contained within a molecule increases. Nevertheless it is also an aid to interpretation in many cases. Particular interest is being shown by a number of microbiologists in the ability of some microorganisms to metabolise selectively different organohalogen compounds, as these materials are increasingly produced by the heavy-chemical industry. A study of such selective metabolism can be undertaken using even low resolution mass spectrometry, and monitoring the relative consumption of different organohalogen compounds by interpreting the relative isotope abundance patterns obtained.

A rapidly increasing type of mass spectrometry in the biological field is isotope ratio mass spectrometry (IRMS). There is increasing reluctance on the part of clinical research ethical committees to approve metabolic and other studies on human subjects using radioisotopes. The use of the latter in other animals is also diminishing. An alternative approach is to use stable isotopes as labels. Stable isotopes such as ^{13}C, ^{15}N and ^{18}O (for total body water) selectively synthesised into a metabolite may be used as a marker and obviously do not affect the metabolic process in any way that would be different from using the nearest radioisotope. Of course there is no emission of radiation and therefore the concentrations of labelled metabolite cannot be determined by counting methods. Most of the materials used in such investigations, however can be readily combusted in an atmosphere of oxygen to produce gases such as $^{13}CO_2$, $^{15}N_2O$ and $^{15}NO_2$. These compounds can be readily separated by mass spectrometry, and isotope ratios determined from which the metabolic data can be computed.

IRMS involves one of the simplest mass spectrometers available, composed of an EI source (all products are already in the vapour state), a magnetic sector mass

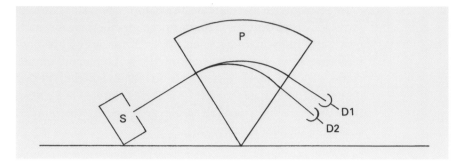

Fig. 11.7. A single-sector mass spectrometer for isotope ratio studies. S, source; P, magnetic pole; D, detectors.

analyser and a Faraday cup detector (Fig. 11.7). The amplified current from the detector is recorded as a peak in the spectrum, whose height is a measure of the particular ion intensity (ion current). The value of the mass to charge ratio is given by

$$m/z = B^2R^2/2V \tag{11.1}$$

where B is the magnetic flux density (of the magnetic analyser), R is the radius of the trajectory (of the ion in the magnetic field), and V is the accelerating voltage (used to accelerate ions out of the source).

Consideration of equation 11.1 should indicate that various values of m/z will be obtained if either B or V is varied (R is a constant for a particular magnetic field). In the IRMS technique a permanent magnet is often used and hence B is also fixed, although modern electromagnets are produced that generate sufficiently stable magnetic fields to be an alternative. By varying V, ions of different masses may be made to traverse the same circular trajectory of radius R slightly separated in time, or for a given appropriate value of V they may be made to traverse two slightly different trajectories of different values for R, i.e. slightly separated in space. In either case, in principle, ions such as $^{13}CO_2$ and $^{15}NO_2$ may be separated.

11.3.3 Applications

IRMS analysis of human breath

Helicobacter pylori (*Campylobacter pylori*) infection is linked with 90% of cases of gastric ulcer. It is also estimated that in the developing world some 80% of children are at risk from life-threatening gastroenteritis arising from *H. pylori* infection. As the bacterium contains urease, a non-invasive test for the presence of the organism may be performed. The patient is required to drink a solution (dose) of 99% ^{13}C labelled urea. The $^{13}CO_2$ produced from the enzyme action is absorbed and eventually exhaled in the patient's breath, which can be collected in a suitable bag. A sample of the breath is then analysed in an IRMS instrument and the amounts of

Table 11.2	Applications of ^{13}C labelling for IRMS measurements
^{13}C compound	Application
Triolein	Fat malabsorption
Bicarbonate	Energy expenditure
Lactose	Lactase deficiency
Glucose	Carbohydrate metabolism
Palmitate	Fatty acid oxidation
Galactose	Liver enzyme function

$^{12}CO_2$ and $^{13}CO_2$ determined. In a typical set of experiments, all *II. pylori*-infected patients showed an increase of $>5\%$ ^{13}C at both 40 and 60 min. Other examples of stable isotope measurements in metabolic studies using ^{13}C labelling are given in Table 11.2. ^{15}N enrichment can also be used to study protein metabolism (turnover) and ^{18}O for total body water and other volume measurements.

11.3.4 Pyrolysis mass spectrometry

The principle is simple in that materials are subjected to a precisely controlled high temperature for a fixed and measured time span. Volatile substances are ejected from the material, under vacuum conditions, and can then be ionised by EI, the mass spectrometric analysis being conducted in any of the usual ways.

The thermal degradation is carried out in a suitable pyrolyser, the most useful of which is the Curie point device in which a specific temperature can be maintained very precisely. This is achieved by taking advantage of the fact that in paramagnetic materials (Section 10.3.1), the magnetic susceptibility is temperature dependent and such materials possess a Curie constant. If the temperature varies then the magnetic susceptibility must vary; conversely, if the susceptibility is maintained by external means, then the temperature is equally maintained. A disadvantage is that only certain temperatures are allowed, depending upon the Curie point properties of the heating material used. A continuum of temperatures is not obtainable, only discrete values.

Inevitably there are mixtures of pyrolysis products, and identification of constituents and relative composition of such mixtures require the use of quite complicated mathematical and statistical procedures such as factor analysis. These methods are readily available on computer programs so should not be a major impediment to the use of such a technique.

A major application is in the identification of microorganisms, which, because such small sample sizes are required, can often be carried out on swab samples. This reduces the need to culture the cells, other than for confirmation by other methods, and eliminates the delays involved. Research into the structures and composition of cell walls can be aided by this technique, particularly in the study of the effects of different growth conditions and in the presence and absence of a variety of antibiotics. However, the most recent developments described later (Section 11.6.4) will probably replace the pyrolysis–MS approach.

Usually the products of pyrolysis are small to medium sized in molecular mass terms. Hence, large mass range spectrometers of the sector type are not necessary and small mass range quadrupoles or ion traps (Section 11.8.3) may be used. This makes the technique portable and it is gaining in importance in field studies. Provided a suitable power supply is available, for example from a generator in a medium-sized off-the-road vehicle, on-site rapid investigations are facilitated. It can be anticipated that the technique will gain increasing applicability in environmental science, ecological studies and more general areas of biological research and monitoring work.

11.4 CHEMICAL IONISATION

Chemical ionisation (CI) is essentially based on the EI source but little fragmentation occurs, giving rise to much cleaner spectra. It is particularly valuable in the determination of molecular masses, as high intensity molecular or pseudomolecular ions are produced.

The construction of the source is essentially the same as described above, but the source is filled, prior to the analytical experiment being carried out, with a suitable reagent gas such as methane (CH_4) or ammonia (NH_3). The normal generation of ions, by EI of these gases, will give rise to species such as $CH_4]^{+\cdot}$ or $NH_3]^{+\cdot}$. However, owing to the relatively high pressure of the reagent gases in the source, the possibility of ion–molecule reactions arises. For example,

$$CH_4]^{+\cdot} + CH_4 \longrightarrow CH_5]^+ + CH_3^{\cdot}, \text{ or,}$$
$$NH_3]^{+\cdot} + NH_3 \longrightarrow NH_4]^+ + NH_2^{\cdot}$$

The species $CH_5]^+$ and $NH_4]^+$ have arisen because the original radical ions have abstracted protons from the corresponding neutral species. These resultant ions are powerful proton donors (Brönsted acids), in the vapour state, and if a material to be analysed is now introduced into the source (the electron beam is switched off) it will be ionised by protonation, giving rise to a thermodynamically relatively stable parent plus one pseudomolecular ion:

$$RCH_2CH_3 + CH_5]^+ (RCH_2CH_3 + H)]^+ + CH_4$$

This type of ionisation is widely used in the study of drugs and secondary metabolites. Negative chemical ionisation is also possible if an appropriate reagent gas is chosen.

However, an increasingly important method for obtaining an anion is by electron capture chemical ionisation. In order to achieve this with increased efficiency the thermodynamics of the process must be changed, or rather the energetics of the process altered. This is done by slowing down the ionising electrons to thermal energies in the presence of a suitable gas, such as methane, hence making the process of electron capture more probable. The temperature of a gas is a measure of the kinetic energy of the motion of its constituent particles and if they can be slowed down there will be a consequent reduction in temperature. The thermal energies referred to above are those associated with approximately room temperature.

11.5 **FIELD IONISATION**

Field ionisation (FI) again requires the sample to be introduced in the vapour state. The molecules are subjected to an intense electric field, or the order of 10^7 to 10^8 V cm^{-1}. Under such conditions the outer bonding electrons are subject to large forces and the energetics are sufficient to overcome the ionisation potential and an electron is removed to generate a molecular radical cation. These ions can then be accelerated out of the source and into the mass analyser in the usual way.

Such a source has several applications, but they tend to be rather specialised. It is probably the case that, for biological applications, other forms of ionisation are more appropriate, either EI or the desorption and evaporation methods discussed below (Sections 11.6 and 11.7).

11.6 **ION DESORPTION METHODS**

It is possible to introduce solid samples into the EI source using various devices, the most common of which is the direct insertion probe (DIP). Of course a required property of the substance under test is that the solid would have to be sufficiently volatile (at the low pressures used) to evaporate, or more strictly volatilise, prior to ionisation in the electron beam. Most biological materials do not possess this property, or, if they do, are fragile or thermally labile. Any decomposition that occurs prior to ionisation means, of course, that what is actually analysed is different from the original.

A number of important desorption methods have been developed that enable solid materials to be introduced into the mass spectrometer, generally with the ionisation process occurring at room temperature or slightly below, hence introducing some degree of protection for thermally labile compounds. In general, the mechanisms of electron removal or capture in desorption methods are a great deal more complicated than for electron impact, field ionisation or the adducts formed in chemical ionisation and will not be considered further here. However, ions are generated abundantly in these methods, hence making available the power of mass spectrometry to the researcher investigating biological materials.

11.6.1 **Field desorption**

The field desorption (FD) source is difficult to prepare, even in expert hands and the source is destroyed each time it is used. The filament of the source has to be prepared in advance. A tungsten wire, 10 μm in diameter, is coated with an appropriate organic material (benzonitrile is commonly used) from which, under suitable conditions, carbon filaments or dendrites may be grown (Fig. 11.8). A solution of the substance to be analysed is then carefully coated onto the dendrites (the

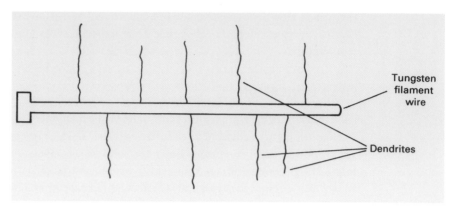

Fig. 11.8. Diagram of field desorption filament.

'filament' is extremely fragile) and allowed to dry. This leaves a solid coat and the filament can be fixed into the source housing, which is then evacuated to the low pressures required. Intense electric fields, again of the order of 10^7 to 10^8 V cm^{-1} can be applied and ions will be desorbed into the evacuated region and accelerated into the mass analyser.

In general, the system is run under such conditions that little fragmentation takes place and hence fairly intense molecular ion peaks may be observed.

11.6.2 Fast atom bombardment ionisation

It is almost certainly true that the advent of the fast atom bombardment (FAB) ionisation method revolutionised mass spectrometry, really opening up the technique to the biologist, and may even have been responsible for the renaissance of the analytical method itself. It certainly has generated a massive interest, stimulated developments in other ionisation sources appropriate for biological materials and, since its invention in 1981, given rise to a whole new field of endeavour that has become known as biological mass spectrometry.

The first important advantage for the investigation of biological materials is that they can be introduced into the ionising beam of neutral atoms, *in solution*. The solution is mixed with a relatively involatile, viscous matrix such as glycerol thioglycerol or *m*-nitrobenzyl alcohol. It is this admixture, placed on a suitable probe, which is then introduced into the source housing, a vacuum applied and the mixture bombarded with atoms travelling at high velocity. One important theory that attempts to describe the ionisation process is that a very short lived transient high temperature spike occurs, too brief to cause thermally induced bond breaking but of sufficient length to allow ionisation to occur. Subsequent fragmentation then allows a mass spectrum to be obtained that contains considerable structural information.

Both positive and negative, complementary, mass spectra may be produced, but pseudomolecular species arise as either protonated or deprotonated entities. For example, if M is the molecular entity then $(M + H)^+$ or $(M - H)^-$ is observed. It is assumed that protonation occurs by abstraction of H^+ from the matrix and deprotonation by donation of H^+ to the matrix. Other charged adducts can also arise (such as $(M + Na)^+$ and $(M + K)^+$), but note that in this ionisation mechanism the radical ion does not occur, indicating that the process is quite different from EI. In addition, cluster ions from the matrix appear, e.g. glycerol clusters, $(C_3H_8O_3)^+$, $(C_3H_8O_3)_2^+$, $(C_3H_8O_3)_3^+ \ldots$ etc. Although the peaks that arise from these appear to complicate the spectrum, they serve as accurate markers because their mass is known. Also, for overall calibration of the analyser, mixtures of alkali metal iodides may be used that produce regular peaks to high mass.

The second important advantage of this method arises from the use of liquid matrices. Most solid surfaces are permanently damaged by a beam of high energy atoms, leading to short-lived samples and spectra, but the mobility of the liquid matrices used allows the surface to be continually replenished. This has distinct advantages for the study of many medium-to-large biological molecules.

Despite the important advantages described above there is one major disadvantage in fast atom bombardment mass spectrometry (FAB–MS) and that is suppression effects. The reader may have guessed from the previous paragraph that the surface is important in this method. In fact there is some evidence to suggest that substances that are surface active in the liquid matrix and reside just in the surface are most readily ionised. Those that reside on the surface seem to be less readily ionised and those that are totally dissolved (i.e. they reside in the bulk of the matrix) seem to be least susceptible of all to ionisation.

The problem arises in analyses such as the so-called peptide mapping technique. Ideally, if a protein, for instance, is subjected to an enzyme digestion and the mixture of peptide products analysed by FAB–MS, it should in principle be possible to detect pseudomolecular ions for each product. However, this possibility is not always achieved because, if the different products possess markedly different surface activities, then one or more of the products may be suppressed by being forced to reside in the bulk matrix. The danger that arises should be obvious because, if the experimenter is dealing with an entirely unknown protein, he or she would have no way of knowing whether or not suppression was occurring. It is possible to relate the hydrophobicity (glycerol has some properties in common with water; Section 6.4.3) of the peptide with surface activity. Hydrophobicity may be expressed in a semiquantitative fashion using, for instance, the Bull and Breeze indices. (Bull and Breeze indices are measures of the water-loving/water-hating (or other solvent) properties of the solute and are expressed as 'hydrophobicities'.) The fundamental measure on which the indices are based is thermodynamic and represents the free energy change when a solute crosses a boundary from an aqueous to a non-aqueous medium.) The problem can sometimes be partially overcome by using different matrices, addition of acid, etc., but this approach is somewhat empirical.

The method described above is known as static FAB. Separating the components of the mixed products prior to FAB–MS largely overcomes the suppression problem. High performance liquid chromatography (HPLC; Section 13.4) and

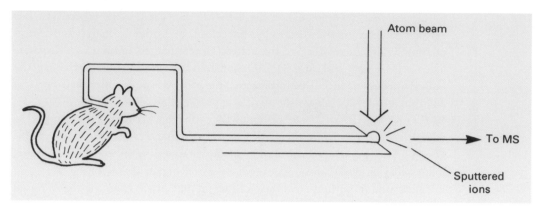

Fig. 11.9. *In vivo* CF–FAB–MS experiment.

electrophoresis (Chapter 12) are powerful methods for achieving such separations. Much greater efficiency can be achieved when these separatory methods are interfaced on-line to the FAB–MS instrument. When this is done the resulting set up is known as a 'hyphenated' technique. Many ingenious ways have been and are being developed for the crucial interface between separatory devices and mass spectrometers. Much of the technology can be transported from the earlier and highly successful hyphenated technique using gas–liquid chromatography (GLC; Section 13.10) and EI–MS, which is represented as GC–EI–MS or GLC–EI–MS.

In the case of FAB, whatever separatory method is used it gives rise to dynamic or continuous flow FAB (CF–FAB). A small quantity of the appropriate matrix is introduced either pre- or postcolumn of the separatory method, depending on the application. The eluent diffuses through a frit or sinter at the end of a flow tube in the FAB source. The aim is to match the flow rate of the eluent to the rate of evaporation in order that a steady-state surface is continually presented to the atom beam. Several of these continuous flow systems are being readily adapted to other ionisation sources described below, particularly the ion evaporation methods.

Perhaps one of the most remarkable recent developments is *in vivo*-CF–FAB–MS. It should be fairly straightforward to recognise the applications to the analysis of body fluids where these have been removed from the animal, perhaps pretreated in some way and then applied to the separatory device coupled on-line to the mass spectrometer. In the *in vivo* approach, the animal is cathetarised, the body fluid sample passed directly into the separatory device and thence to the mass spectrometer (Fig. 11.9). Such small quantities are required for analysis that the animal recovers and suffers no ill effects from the analysis.

During the FAB process, material is said to be sputtered from the surface (Fig. 11.10). The ions of interest are almost certainly solvated with matrix molecules and this helps to stabilise them by dissipating excess energy and limiting fragmentation. This results in reasonable sensitivity for the pseudomolecular ion but still allows sufficient fragmentation to occur as the matrix evaporates.

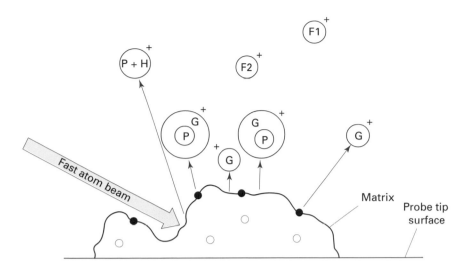

Fig. 11.10. Sputtering phenomenon from liquid matrix during bombardment with fast atoms. G, matrix; P + G$^+$, parent solvated with matrix; P + H$^+$, pseudomolecular ion; F$_1$, F$_2$, fragment ions.

The generation of the atom beam and the angle of impact is fairly critical in FAB. The atoms, usually argon (Ar) or xenon (Xe), are generated in an atom gun. It is not possible to focus neutral atoms in electric or magnetic fields though the beam may be collimated by passing through restriction apertures. The first step is to admit the noble gas into what is essentially an EI-type source that produces cations. No radical ions are produced here as the noble gases are monatomic. These ions are accelerated in the usual way and the ion beam focused into a chamber containing neutral atoms of the same gas. Collisions occur between the fast-moving ions and relatively slow-moving atoms (thermal motion only) and because the same chemical entities are involved, resonant charge exchange takes place. The atoms are knocked out of the collision chamber with virtually the same velocity as the incoming ions, which themselves are slowed down to thermal motion. Just in case any ions manage to get through the chamber without colliding, the emergent atom beam passes between two oppositely charged collector plates. Any positive ions will be deflected from the positively charged plate and attracted to, and collected on, the negatively charged plate. The neutral atoms continue unimpeded to impact with the matrix mixed with sample on the probe (Fig. 11.11). Atom beams are used rather than the original ions in order to eliminate undesirable surface effects that otherwise occur. In fact it is possible to use beams of fast ions such as caesium or gold clusters. In these methods the degree of surface damage is minimised by using a liquid matrix such as glycerol, as in FAB. Some loss of information may be sacrificed because we gain more from using the more massive species, which, owing to their greater mass, have larger kinetic energies. The term liquid secondary ion mass spectrometry (LSIMS) (originally termed fast ion bombardment (FIB) by some groups) has been introduced to distinguish the fast ion tech-

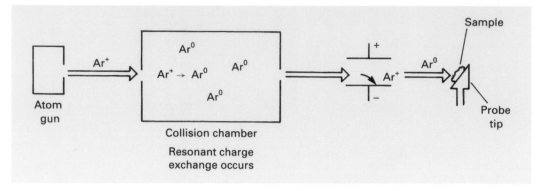

Fig. 11.11. Generation of beams of fast atoms. Ar^0, argon atoms; Ar^+, argon ions.

nique from FAB–MS. FAB/LSIMS–MS have been applied to the structural elucidation of several different kinds of biological macromolecules, including proteins/peptides, nucleic acids, polysaccharides and lipids.

The approach is exemplified by peptide sequencing. It should be recognised that FAB–MS is not meant to be a replacement for conventional Edman-type sequencing methods (Section 6.4.2). There are, however, certain constraints that apply to the Edman method. It does not work at all with peptides containing blocked N-terminal ends, such as pyroglutamic acid. Post-transcriptional and post-translational modifications that remain intact on isolation cannot be determined by Edman-based sequenators, particularly if there are sugar residues present, as the cleavage products are generally too soluble to be extracted and detected. Many of the problems are overcome by using FAB–MS as a complementary technique.

In the case of peptides, although a wide variety of fragmentations may occur, there is a predominance of peptide bond cleavages. This means that the peptide fragments, by losing one amino acid residue at a time, give rise to peaks in the spectrum which differ sequentially by the amino acid residue mass. These sequential mass differences represent exactly the amino acid sequence or primary structure of the peptide. The processes are so reproducible that a set of empirical rules has been devised that enables different series of ions, A, B, C and X, Y, Z, to be recognised, depending upon which mass carries the charge to be recorded in the mass spectrum. Figure 11.12 shows an idealised peptide subjected to FAB. X, Y and Z ions are those that arise by cleavage on the C-terminal side of the peptide bond. For example, the Z_1 ion is the first C-terminal amino acid residue; Y_1 contains the -NH group as well (15 atomic mass units greater) and X_1 includes the carbonyl group. Z_2 is the first two C-terminal amino acid residues, and so on. The A, B, and C ions arise from the N-terminal end, A_1 being the first, A_2 the first two, etc. The superscript double primes represent the number of hydrogen atoms lost or gained by the ion that is collected and recorded. Each series will generally predominate in either positive- or negative-ion FAB so that, in effect, in two experiments the peptide may be sequenced from both ends by obtaining complementary data (Fig. 11.13). Also it

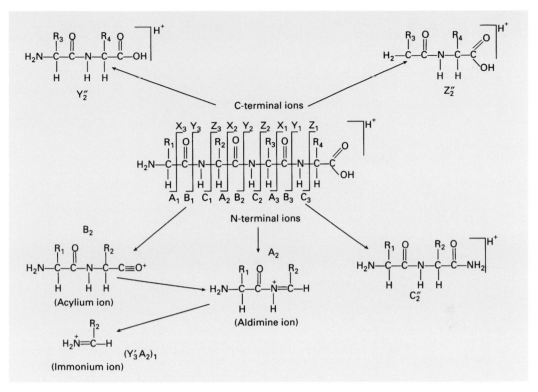

Fig. 11.12. Fragmentation of an idealised peptide (protonated). For explanation, see the text.

is often possible to leave the sample in the source and merely switch operational modes. Furthermore, D- and W-type ions arise, which enable a distinction to be made between isomeric amino acids such as leucine and isoleucine. D-type ions arise from A type and W type from Z type (Fig. 11.14). Substitutions of non-peptidic material may also be detected and identified from the same data but this has been omitted from the description here for clarity.

Figure 11.15a and b shows the FAB mass spectra of the two isomeric tripeptides Gly-Leu-Ala and Ala-Leu-Gly. The mass losses corresponding to the fragments represented by the most prominent peaks are indicated and show how the two sequences can be distinguished.

The power of the FAB method is enormous and many further developments continue to be published. There are, however, limitations to masses that may be transmitted in sector and quadrupole analysers and other sources have been developed to tackle larger species.

11.6.3 Plasma desorption ionisation

Plasma, in this context, is used to describe atomic nuclei stripped of electrons. The source of the plasma is radioactive californium, ^{252}Cf, and two typical emission

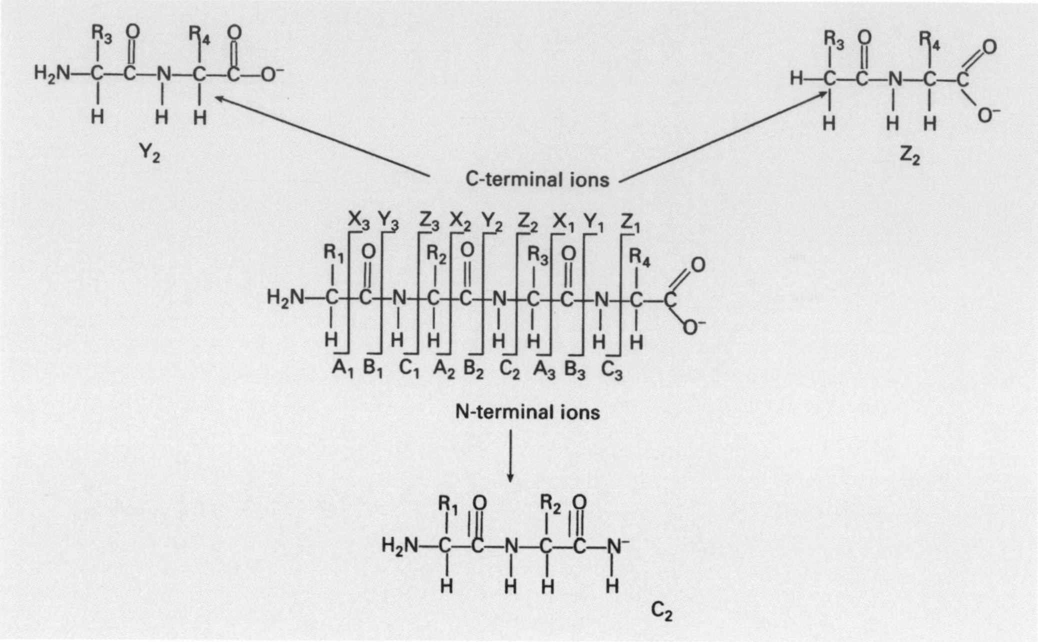

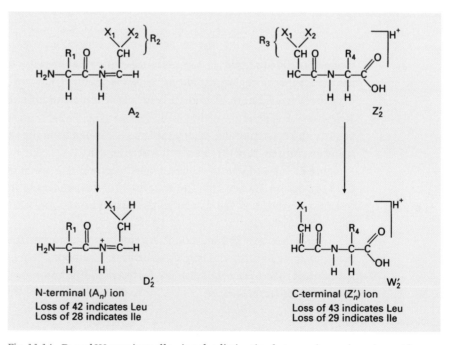

Fig. 11.13. Fragmentation of an idealised peptide (deprotonated). For explanation, see the text.

Fig. 11.14. D- and W-type ions allowing the distinction between isomeric amino acids.

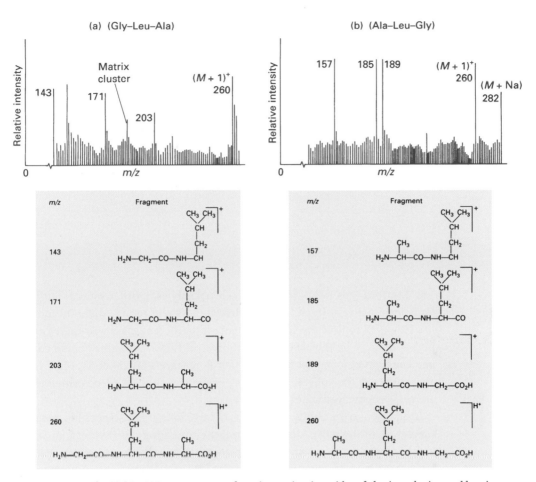

Fig. 11.15. FAB mass spectra of two isomeric tripeptides of alanine, glycine and leucine.

nuclei are the 100 MeV Ba^{20+} and Tc^{18+}, which are ejected in opposite directions, almost colinearly and with equal velocity. This is a pulsed technique, i.e. particles are emitted at discrete time intervals, that requires a different type of mass analysis generally obtained in a time-of-flight (TOF) mass spectrometer.

Samples of large biological molecules, e.g. haemoglobin, can be coated onto a suitable planchette (nickel, mylar or nafion), sometimes in the presence of other additives such as nitrocellulose (which allows the preferential selection of sample against impurities); it is then placed in front of the source. The emitted plasma particle passes through the support foil and imparts sufficient energy to the sample to cause ionisation and project or desorb the sample ion into the gas phase. The ion drifts down the evacuated tube to a suitable collector and is recorded.

In order to be able to measure accurately the time of flight of the ion, the zero point (time from desorption) must be known. It is here that the nature of the disintegration of ^{252}Cf is important because the plasma particle emitted in the opposite direction to that passing through the sample can be used to trigger a time counter.

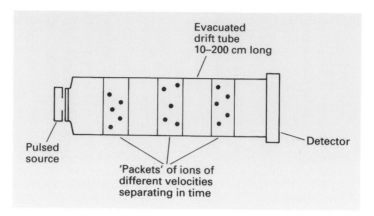

Fig. 11.16. Diagram of the time-of-flight analyser.

The desorbed ions can be accelerated electrically as in other sources but for the same terminal velocity, v, ions of different mass will receive different momenta mv. However, ions of the same momenta but different mass will therefore have higher velocity; i.e. the lower the value of m, the higher the value of v, for constant mv. The lightest (smallest mass) ion therefore travels fastest down the drift tube and arrives at the collector first. Ions of increasing mass (decreasing velocity) arrive successively in time (Fig. 11.16).

In addition to the ability to investigate large ions, it is also possible, because of the nature of the pulsed technique and the time intervals involved, to perform kinetic experiments on the foil or planchette, involving enzymic digestion of large proteins and nucleotides. The parent ions of the digestion products can then be detected. Aberrancies (point substitutions) in haemoglobins have been identified in this way in terms of mass differences (e.g. in sickle-cell anaemia), and if sufficient fragmentation can be induced in the enzyme digestion products the position of substitution may be inferred. To confirm the point of substitution, however, other mass spectrometric analyses should be carried out as fragmentation is limited in PD–MS.

11.6.4 Laser desorption ionisation

Laser beams (being electromagnetic radiation; Section 9.10) can be readily collimated and focused and can be generated with sufficient energy to cause both ionisation and desorption from a sample coated on a suitable probe surface. This gives rise to laser desorption ionisation. Either a continuous stream of ions may be produced but the sample is relatively short lived owing to surface damage by the laser, or the laser may be pulsed and the desorbed ions analysed by TOF–MS.

Matrix-assisted laser desorption ionisation (MALDI), involves a matrix that functions as an energy sink (i.e. a substance absorbing energy at the wavelength of the coherent laser light used then re-emitting appropriate energy levels), resulting in prolonged sample life. The sample is intimately mixed with a solution of the matrix and placed on a suitable metal slide. Cocrystallisation occurs when the mixture is dried in an oven. One of the most recent advances in this method has been the development of surface-enhanced laser desorption ionisation (SELDI) in which the matrix is permanently attached to the surface of a disposable glass-coated metal slide. In the ultraviolet region, substances exhibiting conjugation in their structures make good matrices.

In fact it is possible to choose different matrices that are appropriate for selected wavelengths over the ultraviolet–visible–infrared range of the electromagnetic spectrum. The particular advantage of MALDI is the ability to produce large mass ions, with high sensitivity (which does not appear to diminish with increasing molecular mass), the molecular ions being produced with little fragmentation, hence making it a valuable technique for examining mixtures.

Fragmentation is of course important in the determination of chemical structure. In Section 11.8.2 it is shown how ions arise with different energies and ejection velocities and how an energy analyser is employed in sector machines to overcome this problem. In MALDI and associated methods, the laser pulse generates a plume of material, from the sample, in the form of a jet. Within this plume energy transfers occur between matrix and analyte several tens of micrometres from the probe surface. These ions have to be accelerated or extracted from this region and injected into the analyser. In early systems, ions were continuously extracted by a high electric field. The plume however, occupies a small but finite volume of space and ions arising at different places in this space are subjected to different intensities. An energy spread therefore exists and fragmentation occurring during this initial extraction period usually manifests as 'noise'. If extraction is delayed until all ions have formed, this spread is minimised. The procedure is known as time-lag focusing (TLF) or time-delayed extraction (tDE), where the ions are formed in either a weak or zero-value field during a predetermined time delay, and then extracted by the application of a high voltage pulse. The degree of fragmentation can be controlled, to some extent, by the length of the time delay.

Another problem is post-source decay (PSD), where fragmentation occurs after the precursor ion has been extracted from the source. Many biological macromolecules, particularly peptides, give rise to ions which dissociate over a time span of microseconds and most precursors will have been extracted before this dissociation is complete. The fragments so generated will have the same velocity as the precursor and cause peak broadening and loss of resolution. In a linear TOF analyser (Fig. 11.16), fragment ions arising by PSD, neutral residues and the precursor ions all have the same velocity and reach the detector simultaneously. This prevents a distinction between precursor and PSD fragment being made. The problem is essentially overcome by the use of a reflectron, which is a device in which there exists a gradient electric field. The depth to which ions will penetrate the reflectron field, before reversal of direction of travel, depends upon their energies. Higher energy ions will travel further and lower energy ions a shorter distance. The reflectron is energy dispersive and the flight times become focused. Clearly neutrals are unaffected by the deflection. Figure 11.17 shows a diagrammatic

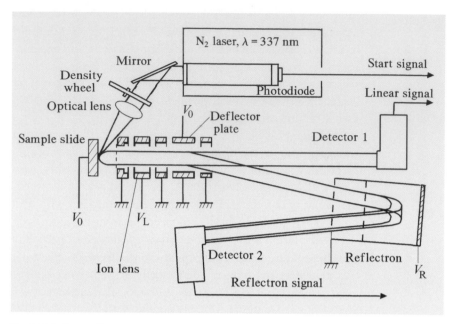

Fig. 11.17. Kratos Kompact MALDI-TOF Instrument. V_o, ground voltage; V_L, lens voltage; V_R, reference voltage; N_2, nitrogen. (Reproduced by permission of Kratos Analytical Ltd, Manchester.)

representation of the Kratos Kompact MALDI III instrument including the facility for both linear and reflectron modes of ion collection.

In Section 11.3.4 (pyrolysis–MS), reference was made to the recent advances in the identification of microorganisms using MALDI–TOF–MS. The use of mass spectrometry in biological science has been mainly in the area of biochemistry. A substantial number of applications in microbiology have also appeared. Until recently the most commonly used approaches that have either involved the use of MS or had the potential for use of MS were as indicated below.

(i) Chemical extraction with suitable solvents, for example fatty acids which may be esterified to their methyl esters (fatty acid methyl ester, FAME) separated by gas chromatography and identified by MS. The method is known as FAME–GC–MS.

(ii) High performance liquid chromatography is appropriate for less volatile or unesterified materials that are still soluble in the extractant. The method has been used in the study of mycolic acids extracted from mycobacteria. Both of the methods in (i) and (ii) suffer from poor resolution of component peaks.

(iii) Suitable extracts may be admitted directly to the mass spectrometer via the electrospray source (Section 11.7.2) or HPLC linked to the MS via this source.

(iv) Pyrolysis–MS, or more usually pyrolysis–GC–MS, has perhaps been the major application of MS in microbiology until very recently. The disadvantage of the pyrolysis approach is that it involves Curie point pyrolytic fragmentation that unfortunately blasts the cell apart, producing very complicated spectra. For extensive interpretation, sophisticated statistical analyses are required.

Provided suitable matrices can be found, producing MALDI–TOF mass spectra directly from a matrix–microorganism admixture has all the advantages of the pyrolysis method, in terms of speed and very small sample loadings, and none of the disadvantages. The spectra produced are very clean and much simpler than those produced by pyrolysis. The microbial cells are held rigidly in the crystal matrix on the surface of the metal carrier and it is presumed that the spectra represent components of the cell wall. The results are highly reproducible and allow classification of organisms at the genus, species and strain levels. It is important to note that this method can be used as a 'fingerprinting' identification – is is not necessary to know the chemical nature of the cell wall constituents giving rise to the spectra. It is sufficient that the patterns are reproducible. Unknown specimens are identified by comparing their spectra with standard patterns obtained from pure culture. Figure 11.18 shows a comparison of spectra obtained from different microorganisms.

11.7 ION EVAPORATION METHODS

These are methods that lend themselves readily to interfacing to other separatory systems to produce 'hyphenated techniques' (cf. CF–FAB).

The essential principle in these methods is that a spray of charged liquid droplets is produced by some form of atomisation or nebulisation. The species to be investigated is solvated by the charged drop. As the solvent evaporates in the high vacuum region, the drop size decreases and the charge eventually resides on the entity under study.

11.7.1 Thermospray ionisation source

As the name thermospray ionisation (TSI) implies, thermal effects are used in this method and may be disadvantageous for thermally labile compounds. In some designs, an electrode and buffers are included to aid the charging of the drop. The mist of drops drifts in an evacuated space where the solvent is removed by evaporation, and the resulting charged species then accelerated into the mass spectrometer (Fig. 11.19).

11.7.2 Electrospray and ion spray ionisation

Electrospray (ESI) and ion spray (IS) ionisation are very similar; the latter uses a gas (usually nitrogen) to cause nebulisation and is sometimes referred to as pneumatically assisted electrospray. Two important features of ESI are:

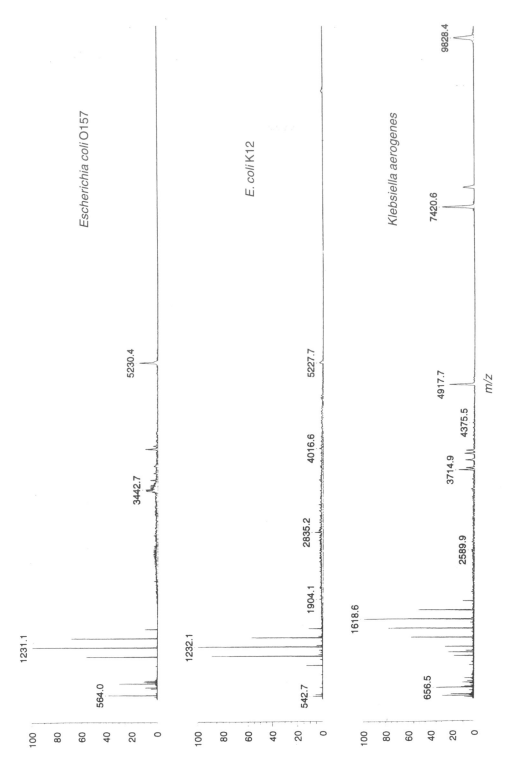

Fig. 11.18. Comparison of MALDI-TOF-mass spectra.

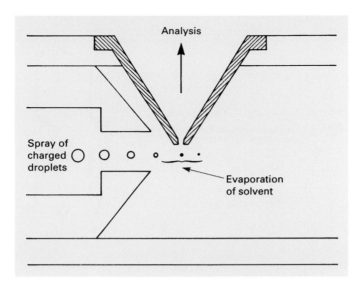

Fig. 11.19. Diagram of the thermospray source. The shading denotes the cross-section through the funnel-shaped orifice.

(i) ionisation can occur at atmospheric pressure (note that this method is also sometimes referred to as atmospheric pressure ionisation (API)),
(ii) the ability to impose multiple charges on the molecular species.

Figure 11.20 shows a diagrammatic representation of the ESI source. In one type, a slowly flowing curtain gas (usually nitrogen) is present to aid the evaporation of the solvent at or below room temperature. This has important advantages for thermally labile materials. The resultant charged species are accelerated through differentially pumped regions where the remaining solvent is removed before entry into the mass spectrometer.

It was noted above (Section 11.3.1) that what is generally referred to as the mass spectrum is strictly an m/z spectrum, where m is the mass of the ion and z the number of charges it carries. When $z = 1$ the spectrum is effectively the mass spectrum. The velocity to which the ions can be accelerated depends only on the total charge and the accelerating force. The momentum of an ion is the product of its mass and this velocity. Hence, as the number of charges are increased for the same accelerating force, the achievable velocity is greater. Furthermore, as z increases, m/z decreases and the effective result of this is that much more massive species can be mass analysed in this situation. All mass analysers have an upper limit (usually termed the mass range) that is dependent on the design characteristics of the instrument. However, if ten charges can be placed on an appropriate species (e.g. for peptides usually the basic amino acids (arginine, lysine, histidine) would be the main carriers of positive charges) then something with a relative mass of 100 000 would behave, in the mass spectrometer, as if it were a 10 000 mass species ($m = 100\,000$, $z = 10$; $m/z = 10\,000$). This brings biological macromolecules into

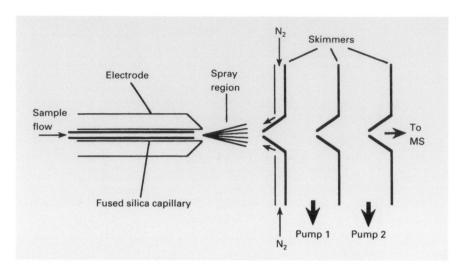

Fig. 11.20. Diagram of the electrospray ionisation source. MS mass spectrometer.

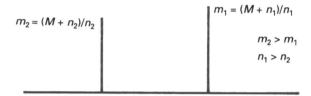

$m_2 = (M + n_2)/n_2$

$m_1 = (M + n_1)/n_1$

$m_2 > m_1$

$n_1 > n_2$

Fig. 11.21. Diagram of two hypothetical multiply charged peaks in an ESI spectrum. It is assumed that the ions are adducts of neutral molecule and protons. If $n_1 = n_2 + 1$; then $n_2 = (m_1 - 1)/(m_2 - m_1)$ and $M = n_2 (m_2 - 1)$, which is equal to the mass of the neutral molecule. m_1 and m_2 are the recorded masses (equivalent to the m/z values). n_1 and n_2 are the number of charges (z values) or protons added, respectively. By taking peaks in pairs, from the recorded masses, n_2 can be calculated and hence M. A range of values may be obtained for M and an average value calculated. (See example associated with Fig. 11.22.)

the range of many existing mass analysers. The main use of ESI at present is to determine very accurate molecular masses (orders of magnitude more accurate than any other method). Little fragmentation occurs but exciting developments are underway that may improve this and produce useful structural information.

The relationship between real relative mass and m/z is shown below. Let m_1, m_2 represent m/z values (peaks in the spectrum) for different ions of the same chemical entity but carrying different multiple charges (Fig. 11.21). The distribution of peaks in the m/z spectrum resulting from multiple charging of the species M forms fingerprint patterns. The data may be deconvoluted using appropriate computer methods to give an average relative molecular mass, M_r, whose accuracy is greater than anything achieved by any other available method. Figures 11.22 and 11.23 show examples of the peak distributions for cytochrome c and insulin B-chain (oxidised). The mass analysers used here are quadrupole devices (Section 11.8.3).

The term relative mass requires some brief explanation. The mass spectrometer does not measure absolute mass. The instrument needs to be calibrated with standard compounds whose M_r values are known accurately. Relative molecular mass, however, relates to the relative scale which is used for calculation and is obviously related to relative atomic mass. Three scales are in current use, the hydrogen, carbon and oxygen scales. In mass spectrometry the carbon scale is used exclusively with $^{12}C = 12.000000$. This level of accuracy is achievable in high resolution double-focusing mass spectrometers (Section 11.8.2). Some confusion may arise, however, on referring to the mass spectrometry literature where M_r is sometimes used to designate relative molar mass instead. Furthermore, molecular weight (which is a force not a mass) is also frequently, and incorrectly used. Also, M_r, because it is a relative measure, has no units. However, M_r is equivalent to M and the latter does have units and, at the very high masses that are encountered in biological macromolecules the familiar dalton may be used as the variations in values between the scales alluded to above is essentially irrelevant. Finally, it is important to note, mass differences that arise from fragmentations may be small and high resolution enables us to distinguish between groups that have the same nominal mass.

It is worth a brief note about the value of carbon as a primary standard. Pure carbon can be obtained easily (as charcoal). It is remarkably stable, is insoluble in water, and cannot be readily reduced or oxidised; in any case the low mass products of oxidation or reduction are gases which may be easily removed.

Another extremely important advantage of this ionisation source is that it lends itself so readily to hyphenation with powerful separatory techniques. The most important of these are capillary electrophoresis, (CE) (Section 12.5) and capillary electrochromatography (CEC) (Section 13.4.9) The second of these two techniques involves packing the capillary with an appropriate stationary phase so that chromatographic separation is achieved as well as electrophoresis. There are two major advantages of these separatory techniques when attempts are made to link them with mass spectrometry. First, the flow rates encountered are highly compatible with the electrospray source. In fact the development of so-called nanospray has eliminated the requirement to dispose of mobile phase (with corresponding loss of sample) before entry into the mass spectrometer. Such fine capillaries are now available that, in certain cases, it proves necessary to add make-up flow before entry into the electrospray source. The second advantage is that the flow is electro-osmotic, driven by the electrical potential across the length of the capillary. This electrodrive gives rise to a flat flow profile, as distinct from the bullet profile shape, characteristic of the Poiseulle flow encountered in mechanically (pump) driven systems (see Fig. 11.24).

11.8 ANALYSERS

Considerable emphasis has been placed on ionisation sources and this is justified because most of the important developments of the last decade that have

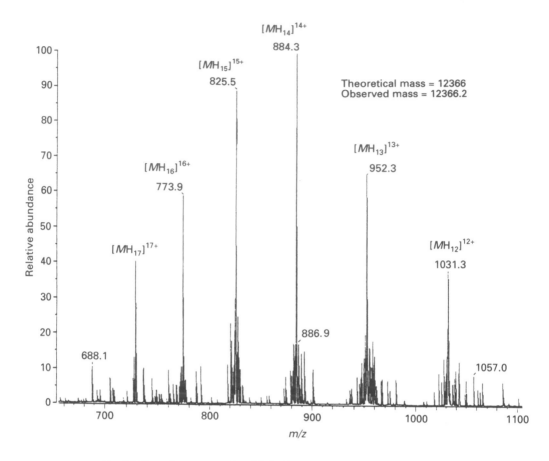

Fig. 11.22. m/z spectrum of multiply charged cytochrome c. Applying the algebra stated in the caption to Fig. 11.21 and remembering that z values must be integers:

$m_1 = 952.3$ and $m_2 = 1031.3$.
Then $n_2 = (m_1 - 1)/m_2 - m_1) = 951.3/(1031.3 - 952.3)$
$= 951.3/79 = 12.04$ or $z = 12$
(12 positive charges associated with relative mass 1031.3).
Consider the two peaks with relative masses:
$m_1 = 884.3$ and $m_2 = 952.3$
then $n_2 = 883.3/(952.3 - 884.3) = 883.3/68$
$= 12.989$ or $z = 13$
(13 positive charges associated with relative mass 952.3).

For practice the reader should calculate the z values for other pairs of peaks, find the series of associated values for M (the mass of the neutral molecule) for each peak (from $M = n_2 (m_2 - 1)$) and find the average value for M. (Reproduced by kind permission of JEOL (UK) Ltd, JEOL House, Welwyn Garden City.)

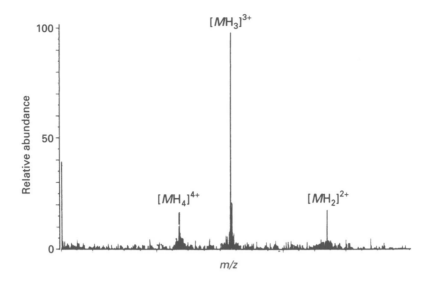

Fig. 11.23. *m/z* spectrum of multiply charged insulin B chain (oxidised). (Reproduced by kind permission of JEOL (UK) Ltd, JEOL House, Welwyn Garden City.)

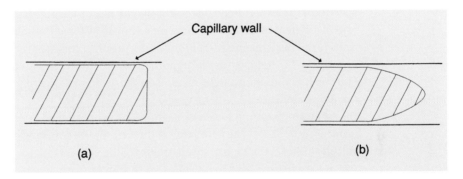

Fig. 11.24. Flow profiles: (a) electroosmotic, flat; (b) Poiseulle, bullet.

influenced the growth of biological mass spectrometry have been in sources. One analyser, the TOF device (Section 11.6.3), is relatively simple in principle. Analysers are of obvious importance and one of the most widely used of these is the magnetic sector.

11.8.1 Magnetic sector analyser

This is shown diagrammatically in Fig. 11.7. Historically the observation of the phenomenon of charged particles following a circular trajectory in a magnetic field dates back to W. Wien (1898), who was the first to demonstrate that a beam of positively charged particles could be deflected using magnetic and electric fields. J. J. Thomson, in 1912, demonstrated the existence of two stable isotopes of neon using a simple magnetic sector device. More elaborate instruments, developed by A. J. Dempster (1918) and F. W. Aston (1919), could be used for isotopic relative abundance measurements.

The term magnetic sector arises because the beam trajectory traverses only a sector of the circular poles of the magnet. The arrangement shown in Fig. 11.7 indicates the sector of only one pole. In a real system, another pole would lie above and parallel to the plane of the diagram. As the whole system must be kept under high vacuum, two possibilities exist. With small permanent magnets it is possible to construct the whole in a sealed box that can be evacuated. As indicated in equation 11.1, for given values of B, V and z, ions of different masses will follow different trajectories (different radii). This is satisfactory in IRMS studies because the actual masses of the ions under investigation are quite close together and R will not differ greatly. In fact they are sufficiently close for separate detectors to be mounted within the system. The situation is quite different with mixtures of ions covering a wide range of masses, as it would prove impractical to have enough separate detectors positioned to accommodate all possible radii. The problem is solved by using the second of the two possibilities, i.e. to make all ions follow the same trajectory of the same radius. There are two ways of achieving this. First, the accelerating voltage V can be varied so as to accelerate ions of different mass to different terminal velocities, v. This type of voltage scanning is used in certain kinds of mass spectrometric experiment. Secondly, by the use of electromagnets (varying B), ions of different mass (but the same velocity) can be forced to follow the particular trajectory. This is magnetic scanning and is the most commonly used form of analysis. Figure 11.25 shows several hypothetical trajectories in a given magnetic field. Only one, R, allows ions to be focused on the detector. If the field is changed, ions travelling along R will be defocused because they do not, in the new field, possess the correct momentum to allow equation 11.1 to be satisfied. A new set of ions will be focused along R at the new value of the field and be collected at the detector. By starting either at the high or low extremes of the magnet range it is possible either to scan down (from high to low mass) or to scan up (from low to high). The whole of this single trajectory resides in a sealed tube, the drift tube, placed between the magnet poles and thus enabling the vacuum to be maintained in this envelope. In this way the mixture of ions, precursor and product, are separated according to m/z and the mass spectrum produced. This design results in low resolution mass spectrometry using single-sector or single focusing.

11.8.2 **Electric sector analyser**

The single-focusing instrument is somewhat limited in application but is still widely used where low resolution is sufficient for the experiment being conducted. In order to understand how the resolution may be improved the simplest approach is to reconsider the EI source. Assuming that the ions have been formed, it is then necessary to accelerate them out of the source. This is achieved by establishing an electric potential across the source, the ions being attracted towards the plate of opposite charge. The ions will emerge through slits or apertures with a

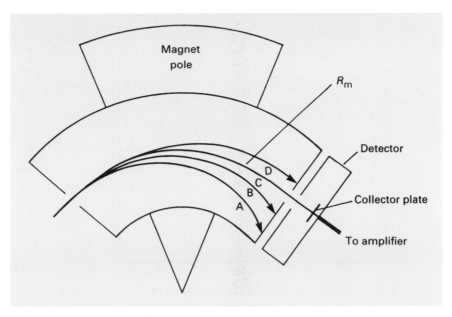

Fig. 11.25. Representative of ion generation between acceleration plates. Only ions following a trajectory of radius R_m will be focused. A, B and D are currently defocused. By altering the field, other ions can be forced to travel along R_m and be focused.

given terminal velocity directly related to the accelerating force applied. However, the terminal velocities differ because not all the ions are subjected to the same force; it depends entirely on where they arise in space (Fig. 11.26).

Ion A arising at the zero plate will experience the full accelerating force; ion B, half way between the plates, will experience only a force related to $-4\,kV$; and ion C, about 10% of the distance from the $-8\,kV$ potential perforated plate, will experience only about 10% of the force. Although this description is considerably oversimplified it should serve to indicate that the ions emerge from the source with varying terminal velocities and hence varying momenta and kinetic energies $(\frac{1}{2}\,mv^2)$. In order to overcome this variation it is necessary to energy analyse the emergent ion beam. This is achieved in the electric sector analyser, which consists of two stainless steel plates bent into segments of concentric circles. The ions follow a circular trajectory, between these plates, whose radius R_e, is given by

$$R_e = 2V/E \qquad\qquad (11.2)$$

where V is the accelerating voltage (in the source), and E is the electrostatic field in the analyser.

The electric sector is usually referred to as the electrostatic analyser (ESA) and packets of ions emerge from this with the whole range of masses but the same velocity. A given packet with the appropriate velocity then enters the magnetic sector analyser to undergo mass analysis. The ESA is solely an energy and not a mass analyser. This type of instrument is the two-sector or double-focusing

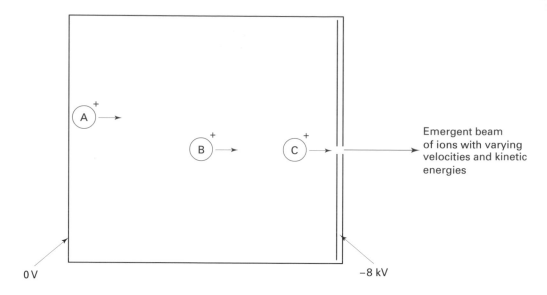

Fig. 11.26. Ions arising at different points in space between the acceleration plates.

device, which enables high resolution mass spectrometry to be performed (Fig. 11.27). The resolving power of these instruments is such that measurements to accuracies of parts per million may be obtained. In Table 11.3 are shown the relative and nominal masses of elements that frequently constitute biological molecules (including drugs, etc., that have biological implications). It can be seen from Table 11.3 that adding up the values for the constituent elements of a compound gives different values, depending on whether nominal or accurate atomic masses are used. This difference increases as the compound increases in size (i.e. contains more atoms). High resolution mass spectrometry can be extremely valuable in distinguishing between compounds that have the same nominal M_r but different accurate M_r.

Another important use of high resolution mass spectrometers is the determination, by accurate mass measurement, of the nature of the chemical group that is

Table 11.3	Relative nominal and accurate masses of some elements	
Element	Nominal mass	Accurate mass
C	12	12.000000
H	1	1.007825
O	16	15.994915
N	14	14.003074
P	31	30.973765
S	32	31.972974
F	19	18.998405

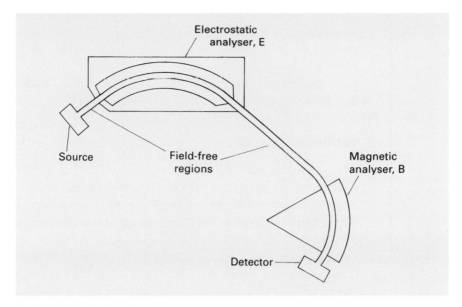

Fig. 11.27. Double focusing mass spectrometer.

Table 11.4 **Nominal and accurate masses of neutral loss groups in fragmentation**

Neutral group lost	Nominal mass	Accurate mass
CO (carbonyl)	28	27.994914
C_2H_4 (double bond fragment)	28	28.031299
N_2 (diazo, in some drugs)	28	28.006158
(CH_2N) (nitrile or isonitrile) (CNH_2) (amino-carbon)	28	28.018732[a]

[a] The last two examples cannot be distinguished by accurate mass measurement.

lost during fragmentation. The reader should recall that much structural information can be gained by considering the mass difference between entities that can show what has to be lost from the greater mass species to give the lesser. Five common groups that may be lost from biological molecules are listed in Table 11.4 together with relative nominal and accurate masses.

Figure 11.27 shows the forward geometry arrangement of what is known as the Nier–Johnson type (after the designers), where the ESA is before the magnetic sector (known as EB; E for electric, B for magnetic). Exactly the same results may be obtained if the reverse geometry (BE) Nier–Johnson type is used. In the latter, the ESA and hence the energy analysis occurs after the mass analysis in the magnetic sector. Different and very sophisticated experiments may be carried out with the different geometries. The regions between the source and analyser, between the analysers and between the last analyser and the collector/detector are the so-called field-free regions. In these regions occur decomposition events; if they can be observed, these give important information regarding structure. Depending on which geometry is employed, certain of the events cannot be observed and there are 'pros' and 'cons' in each case. Also other designs such as the Matteuch–Herzog allow the construction of the mass spectrograph, where the ions all focus in a focal plane (to be recorded by exposure of a photographic plate). Such devices, however, have not found wide application in the biological field.

11.8.3 Quadrupole mass filters

This type of mass analyser is known as a mass filter. It has the advantage of being a smaller and cheaper device than sector systems and is much lighter in weight, hence its widespread use in benchtop-type instruments, particularly many used for 'hyphenated' methods. The disadvantages are the lower mass range and sensitivity.

The theoretical background to these devices is considerably more complicated than that required for sector machines and will not be pursued in any detail here. The underlying idea, however, is simple. The device is generally constructed using four solid cylindrical rods, of circular cross-section, to which are applied both direct current (DC) and radiofrequency (RF) voltages (Fig. 11.28). The only component of motion of ions along the linear z-axis of the filter is that derived from the injection velocity. Both the fixed (DC) and oscillating (RF) fields cause the ions to undergo complicated motion in the x–y plane (cross-section). This, together with the component of motion in the z-direction, results in the ions following complicated trajectories through the quadrupole filter. For a given set of field conditions, only certain trajectories are stable, allowing ions of specific mass to be transmitted through to the collector/detector. Ions whose mass determines that they travel along unstable trajectories are not transmitted, hence the term filter. By careful control of the field conditions, ions of different mass can be successively filtered and transmitted. In an ideal situation, rods with hyperbolic cross-sections would be used. These give pure quadrupole hyperbolic fields. There are, however, cost implications and manufacturing difficulties with symmetry. The circular cross-section rods are a close approximation and satisfactory for most applications.

11.8.4 The ion trap

This is an interesting and versatile device that is rapidly gaining in importance in mass spectrometry. It is a relatively small cylindrical device of some 5 cm diameter and 10 cm length. A longitudinal cross-section is shown in Fig. 11.29, the device being constructed from three separate pieces of metal, two of which (mirror images of each other) form a mathematical figure known as a hyperboloid of two sheets and also form the end cap electrodes. The third, or ring, electrode is a hyperboloid of one sheet and is like a torus or doughnut except that the cross-section of the ring material is hyperbolic, not circular. The end caps (electrically linked) surround the ring electrode (electrically insulated) and together they form the ion trap. Ions are

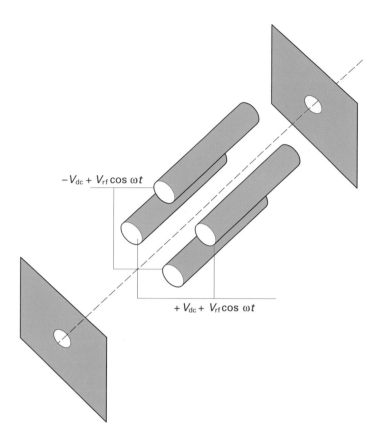

$-V_{\mathrm{dc}} + V_{\mathrm{rf}}\cos \omega t$

$+ V_{\mathrm{dc}} + V_{\mathrm{rf}}\cos \omega t$

Fig. 11.28. Quadrupole mass filter. In the quadrupole mass filter one opposite pair of rods has a negative DC voltage, $-V_{\mathrm{dc}}$, applied and the other pair a positive DC voltage, $+V_{\mathrm{dc}}$. There is also a superimposed radiofrequency (RF) voltage, $V_{\mathrm{rf}}\cos \omega t$, which is 180° out of phase between rod pairs. Mass filtering occurs as these voltages are scanned but the ratio DC to RF is kept constant. In spatial tandem mass spectrometry, Section 11.10.1 and Fig. 11.34, quadrupole collision cells are used which are RF-only devices. No DC voltages are applied and no mass filtering occurs in these cases.

generated, for example by EI, and injected into the trap, where they can be constrained and held in constant motion in the space delineated by the electrodes. The trajectories describe Lissajous' figures, i.e. a two-dimensional display of two frequencies perpendicular to each other and normally with a simple ratio between them. Mass analysis is again performed by careful control of the field conditions, the use of which allows ions of increasing mass to be successively ejected from the trap to an appropriate collector/detector. The ion trap belongs to a group of devices known as *Quadrupole ion storage systems* (QUISTORS). The device is readily adapted as an end detector for GLC instruments and is becoming widely used in toxicological studies and pollution monitoring. Like quadrupole rod systems, they lend themselves to the design of 'portable' instruments, at least in off-the-road vehicles and hence their increasing use in field explorations.

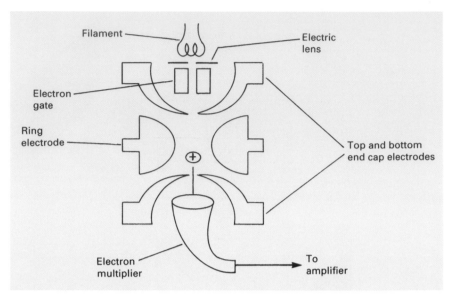

Fig. 11.29. Diagram of the ion trap.

There are several other types of mass spectrometer that have special features: ion cyclotron resonance instruments, in which very high mass range and resolution can be obtained; and Fourier transform devices. Space does not permit any detailed description and, despite their value and importance, their specialised nature is such that they have not gained so widespread a use in the biological field as the designs described above. The ability to obtain mass spectra of compounds with very high M_r (of the order of 10^6), using these types of spectrometer, suggests that they may be of considerable use to the biologist in future. The very high cost of the instrumentation and requirement for highly trained operators has meant that only a few of these devices have been manufactured and are housed in a few specialised research centres.

11.9 DETECTORS

No information could be gained from sources or analysers without a suitable detector being available. Most detectors are of the impact or ion collection type. All types of detector require a surface on which the ions impinge and the charge neutralised, either by collection or donation of electrons. Hence, electron transfer occurs and an electric current flows that may be amplified and ultimately converted into a signal recorded on a chart or processed by a computer. The total ion current (TIC) is the sum of all the currents carried by all the ions.

11.9.1 The Faraday cup

This is probably the simplest device and essentially works as described above and shown in Fig. 11.30. For example, a positive ion striking the surface of the cup

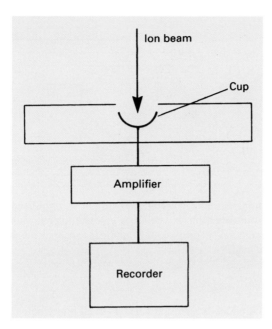

Fig. 11.30. Simplified diagram of the Faraday cup.

abstracts an electron to neutralise its charge and if enough ions strike then a measurable current flows.

11.9.2 **Electron multiplier**

Greater sensitivity can be achieved with this detector and the degree of amplification is large. The original ions cause a shower of new electrons to be produced. These electrons impinge on a second dynode and produce yet more electrons. This process continues until a sufficiently large current for normal amplification is obtained. A diagrammatic representation of the electron multiplier is shown in Fig. 11.31.

Modified photomultipliers may also be used, the advantage being that they are cheaper and more robust than electron multipliers. Here the ions generate a shower of electrons that impinge on a surface that produces photons. The remainder of the device is essentially a photomultiplier.

11.9.3 **Array detectors**

These types of detector are really many detectors arranged in an array or matrix, commonly having 1024 sites for ion collection. Most designs involve the use of microchannel plates (narrow channels along which the ions continually collide with the walls until electrons are produced) as the ion-to-electron converter. Also most array detectors are electrooptical devices in which the electrons strike a suitable surface and produce photons that can be focused and transmitted. Finally, the photons strike a photosensitive plate and an electric current is produced.

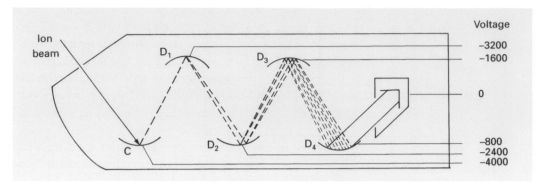

Fig. 11.31. The electron multiplier. The voltages listed on the right-hand side of the diagram are typical. Different manufacturers may produce different values but each dynode has to have a different negative voltage applied to generate the shower of electrons. C, collector; D_1–D_4, dynodes.

Array detectors are ideally suited for use as focal plane detectors and are most easily adapted to the Matteuch–Herzog type of instrument, where all the ions would be collected simultaneously. It is possible, however, to arrange the array in a Nier–Johnson instrument where the focal plane would be if it existed. In Nier–Johnson instruments, however, the ions cannot be collected simultaneously. Portions of the mass range (between 4% and 40%, depending on the design) are collected over, say, 900 of the 1024 sites for a given set of field conditions. For example, for 4% of a mass range of 2000 the field conditions would be such that ions with m/z values between $\pm$ 2% of 2000 ($\pm$ $m/z = 40$) would be detected. The magnetic field then jumps to, say, 1980 and $\pm$ 2% of ions collected at this setting. The process is continued stepwise and it should be noted that an overlap of m/z values is built in at each step. The whole process is under computer control and the data are smoothed so that a continuous spectrum is output and the steps are transparent to the user.

Other specialised variations of detectors are available, but there is nothing like the variety amongst detectors as there is amongst analysers or sources.

11.10 TANDEM MASS SPECTROMETRY

By far the best separatory technique, for charged particles, is the mass spectrometer. However, the observation of a peak in an m/z spectrum does not of itself define the entity it represents in structural terms. Accurate mass measurement may enable us to write down an empirical formula for the species but does not, of itself, confirm any further information. Such difficulties in terms of identifying a peak in a spectrum arise frequently when dealing with mixtures (a situation often encountered with samples from biological sources). In mixed spectra, the facility for identifying the origins of a particular peak are extremely valuable. The experimenter can take several approaches in mass spectrometry, such as linking the scanning modes of the ESA and magnet in sector machines. Referring back to equations 11.1 and 11.2 it can be seen that it is possible to control B, V and E. This enables particular ions to be selected to follow the trajectories through the instrument that allow species to reach the detector. For instance, in a forward geometry instrument, by fixing B, only one species may pass through this analyser and, by linking V and E, only those precursor ions that give rise to this particular product ion can be identified. The converse is also true in that by controlling V and E and allowing a single species through the ESA then the magnet may be scanned for product ions of that single precursor. Additionally it is possible to set up conditions that allow the determination of the mass of the neutral loss fragment. Space does not permit detailed discussion of these topics but the methods can be found in more advanced texts on mass spectrometry.

The ability to select species for transit through the E and B sectors, as described above, allows the technique of tandem mass spectrometry to be used. In these methods a particular peak is selected for further investigation. The ions comprising this peak are made to undergo further fragmentation, usually by a method known as collisionally induced decomposition (CID). As the name implies, the ions are allowed to interact collisionally with atoms or molecules (helium, neon, argon and nitrogen have been used as collision gases). Translational energy (the energy of motion) is transferred between the interacting species, up to 50% in elastic collisions. Energy transferred to the ions under investigation can be distributed in a variety of ways. Some of the transferred energy will remain as translational (involved in direction changes, scattering etc.), whilst some will be distributed into vibrational modes of the chemical bonds of the ion. It is this latter energy that, if sufficient, can cause further degradation, the products of which can be analysed in another mass spectrometric experiment. In principle, the process may be continued and multiple mass spectrometry carried out. It will be seen below that this is only feasible in certain types of instrument but such experiments are performed. In view of this, strictly tandem MS is usually abbreviated to MS^2 and in general the abbreviation would be MS^n.

11.10.1 **MS^2 in space**

This has nothing to do with extraterrestrial exploration (it should be remembered that a mass spectrometer was used on the original Mars probe) but describes the fact that the processes occur sequentially in space. This requires that two mass spectrometers are physically coupled together. Two double-focusing sector machines result in the four-sector device coupled through a collision cell where the CID process occurs. Collision cells are frequently RF-only quadrupoles (no mass filtering occurs here, the RF merely constraining the ions to allow a greater number of collisions to occur), filled with the appropriate collision gas, and such cells are usually designated by the symbol q. All geometries are theoretically possible, although not all are in general use: EBqEB, BEqBE, etc. Figure 11.32 shows what has been described as two-dimensional mass spectrometry, the first axis indicating the m/z spectrum obtained in the first mass spectrometer (MSI) and the

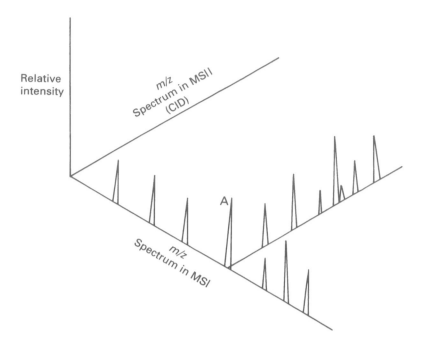

Fig. 11.32. Two-dimensional mass spectrometry spectra obtained in a MSII experiment. The first mass spectrum is generated in mass spectrometer I (MSI) and is shown along the appropriately labelled axis. A particular peak, for example that marked A, is selected and the packet of ions comprising this peak is focused into the collision cell where CID occurs. The m/z spectrum corresponding to these decomposition fragments is analysed in MSII. This CID mass spectrum is shown along the isometric axis parallel to the axis labelled spectrum in MSII.

isometric axis showing the second m/z spectrum obtained in MSII, after CID of the selected peak (packet of ions).

Obviously similar experiments may be performed on other peaks and the amount of information gained is enormous. In Fig. 11.33 is shown the Kratos Concept II H H four-sector instrument. It should be evident to the reader that such instrumentation is extremely expensive and tends to be located only in major research centres.

An alternative approach is to use the triple quadrupole (Q) design (Fig. 11.34), which, although much cheaper, suffers from sensitivity and mass range limitations. The designation here is QqQ or QhQ where, in the latter case, an RF-only hexapole (no mass filtering) is used as the collision cell. The first quadrupole, QI, is used as a mass spectrometer, a selected peak being injected into the collision cell q or h, and the products of decomposition analysed in QII.

Figure 11.35 shows single and multiple mass spectra of phenacetin. The ionisation source was electrospray and the tandem system a triple quadruopole (Micromass UK Ltd, Quattro II) and this combination allows some very sophisticated analyses to be performed. In Fig. 11.35a is shown the single mass spectrum, which indicates only a small degree of fragmentation and is of little help in

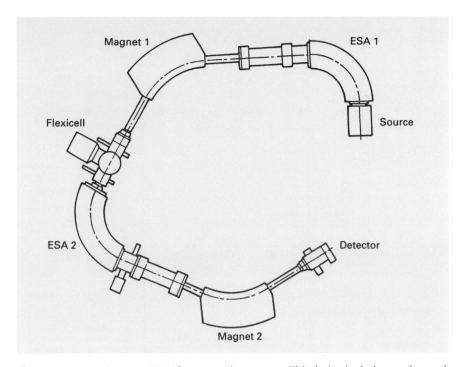

Fig. 11.33. Kratos Concept II H H four-sector instrument. This design includes two forward geometry sector mass spectrometers linked through a collision cell, termed a flexicell by this manufacturer. MSI is represented by ESA 1 and magnet 1 and is where the appropriate first mass spectrum is obtained. Collisionally induced decomposition occurs in the flexicell and the products analysed in MSII, which incorporates ESA 2 and magnet 2. (Reproduced by kind permission of Kratos Analytical, Manchester.)

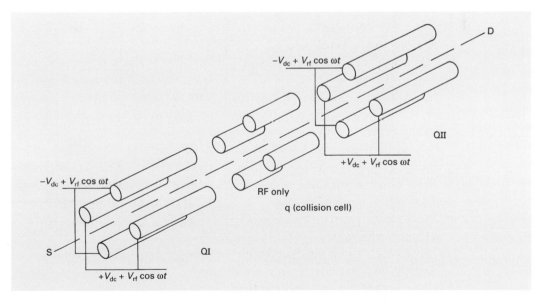

Fig. 11.34. Arrangement in triple quadrupole systems. S, source; D, detector; RF, radiofrequency.

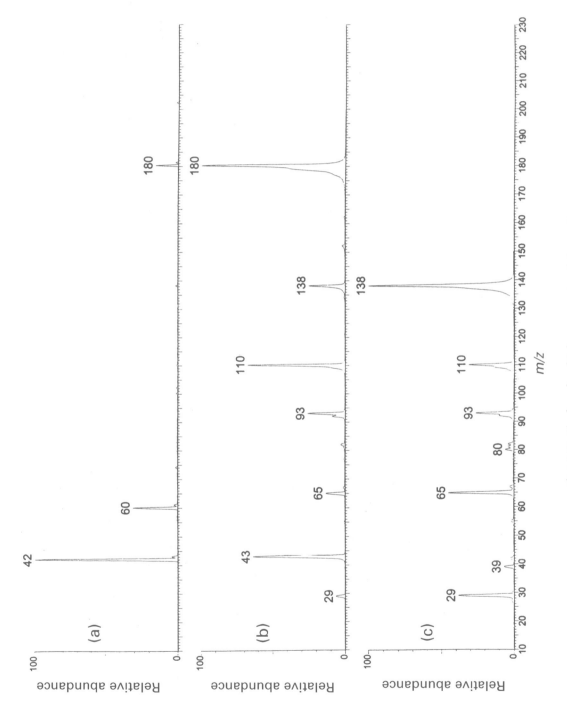

Fig. 11.35. Single and multiple mass spectra of phenacetin.

structural determination. Allowing only the molecular ion to enter the collision chamber, Fig. 11.35b spectrum (MS^2) is obtained after analysis in QII. Considering the mass difference of 42, (180 − 138), this is known to be a classic rearrangement from acetyl moieties that eliminates the stable entity ketene, $CH_2 = C = O$, the methyl hydrogen being transferred to the nitrogen of the ring amino group. This fragmentation, however, results in the elimination of a neutral entity that will not be recorded in the mass spectrum and is probably a most favoured thermodynamic outcome. In spectrum (a), therefore, the large $m/z = 42$ peak is from a different origin, the most likely being protonated solvent acetonitrile $[CH_3CN + H]^+$. The $m/z = 60$ would represent the aquated species $[CH_3CN + H_2O + H]^+$. Spectrum (a) is therefore of little value in determining the structure of phenacetin and it is necessary to resort to multiple mass spectrometry. In electrospray, the fragmentation processes in the collision chamber that give rise to spectrum (b) can be mimicked in the source region by manipulating the cone voltages. Other ions may then be selected to pass QI, enter the collision chamber and undergo CID before analysis in QII. This gives rise to true multiple mass spectrometry. In Fig. 11.35c is shown the result of selecting $m/z = 138$, arising in spectrum (b), subjecting these ions to CID and analysing in QII. The peaks in this spectrum represent decompositions from the ethoxy substituent and ring opening.

Figure 11.36 shows predicted fragmentation pathways for the parent (precursor) species, the protonated drug molecule. These routes are established by considering the mass differences in spectra (b) and (c). Not all routes are equally favoured as indicated by the different peak intensities in the mass spectra.

A useful exercise at this point is to cross refer to the Fourier transformed infrared (Fig. 10.2) and the proton nuclear magnetic resonance (Fig. 10.9) spectra. All of the various spectral absorbances and chemical shift information can be assigned to the appropriate parts of the phenacetin molecule. This information is complemented by the peaks in the mass spectra that were used to construct the fragmentation pathways indicated.

Hybrid instruments exist and are in quite widespread use. In these designs MSI is a two-sector device and MSII (or QII) is a quadrupole. Geometries such as EBqQ and BEqQ are possible. Note that there is still a sensitivity and mass range limitation but as the masses of the products of CID are less than that of the original sample a convenient compromise is achieved. Note also that using Q as MSI would impose severe mass range constraints and is not therefore a feasible option.

CID is not confined to MS^2-type experiments. Collision cells may be placed in any of the field-free regions, leading to a wide variety of experimental methods. Furthermore, in-source CID may be performed in certain situations, for example by using the curtain gas nitrogen in an ESI source.

It will be recognised that a collision cell and a detector cannot occupy the same position in space. In four-sector instruments, for instance, the cell position is critical, hence the detectors are set off-axis at appropriate points. To detect ions after MSI and prior to CID in the cell, the ions must be accelerated round a curved path and into the collector/detector. When the peak has been selected the accelerators are switched off and the ions proceed into the cell to undergo CID.

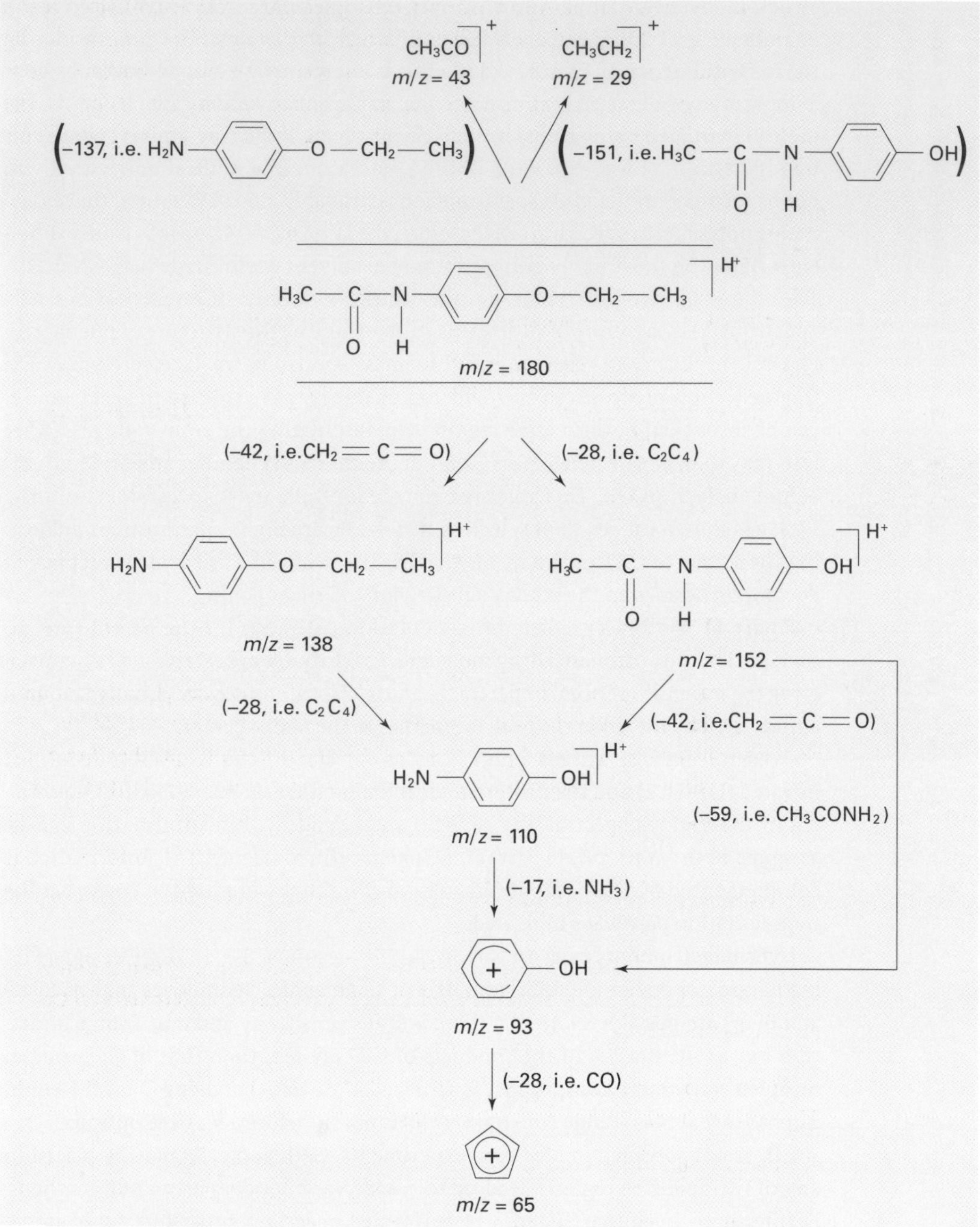

Fig. 11.36. Fragmentation pathways for phenacetin.

11.10.2 MS^n in time

This can be achieved in the ion trap, where all the processes occur in the *same* region of space and the multiple mass spectrometry is distributed in *time*. Owing to the facility of storing ions in the trap, the procedure is to eject all ions except those corresponding to the selected peak. A suitable collision gas is introduced and the CID occurs and MS^2 can be performed. The process can be repeated successively in time, no extra mass spectrometers or collision cells being required. The limitation is sensitivity, as this decreases markedly with each MS experiment, although the claimed world record in an ion trap is currently MS^{14}.

11.11 **KEY TERMS**

atmospheric pressure ionisation	ion spray ionisation	peptide mapping
capillary electrochromatography	isotope ratio mass spectrometry	plasma desorption
capillary electrophoresis	laser desorption ionisation	protonation
chemical ionisation	liquid secondary ion mass	pyrolysis
collisionally induced decomposition	spectrometry	surface-enhanced laser desorption
electron capture	mass spectrum	ionisation
electron impact	mass spectrometry	tandem mass spectrometry
electrospray ionisation	mass-to-charge ratio spectrum	thermospray ionisation
fast atom bombardment	matrix-assisted laser desorption	
field desorption	ionisation	

11.12 **CALCULATIONS**

Question 1
A protein was isolated from human tissue and subjected to a variety of investigations. Relative molecular mass determinations gave values of approximately 12 000 by exclusion chromatography and 13 000 by gel electrophoresis. After purification, a sample was subjected to electrospray ionisation mass spectrometry and the following data obtained.

m/z	773.9	825.5	884.3	952.3	1031.3
Abundance (%)	59	88	100	66	37

Given that $n_2 = (m_1 - 1)/(m_2 - m_1)$ and $M = n_2(m_2 - 1)$ and assuming that the only ions in the mixture arise by protonation, deduce an average molecular mass for the protein by this method.

Answer
M_R by exclusion chromatography = 12 000
M_r by gel electrophoresis   = 13 000

Taking ESI peaks in pairs:

$m_1 - 1$	$m_2 - m_1$	n_2	$m_2 - 1$	M	z
951.3	79.0	12.041	1030.3	12 406.6	12
883.3	68.0	12.989	951.3	12 357.1	13
824.5	58.8	14.022	883.3	12 385.7	14
772.9	51.6	14.978	824.5	12 349.9	15

$\Sigma M = 49\,499.3$
Mean M_r = 12 374.8

Note: Relative abundance values are not required for the determination of the mass.

Question 2

An oligopeptide obtained by tryptic digestion was investigated by ESI–MS and FAB–MS, both in positive mode, and gave the following m/z data:

ESI	178.8	223.2	297.3						
FAB	146	203	260	357	444	591	648	705	802	890

(i) Predict the sequence of the oligopeptide. Use the amino acid residual mass values in the table below.

(ii) Determine the average relative molecular mass.

(iii) Identify the peaks in the ESI spectrum.

Amino acid residual masses

Ala	71	Cys	103	His	137	Met	131	Thr	101
Arg	156	Glu	129	Ile	113	Phe	147	Trp	186
Asn	114	Gln	128	Leu	113	Pro	97	Tyr	163
Asp	115	Gly	57	Lys	128	Ser	87	Val	99

Note: Trypsin cleaves predominantly on the C-terminal side of arginine or lysine.

Answer

(i) The highest mass peak in the FAB spectrum is $m/z = 890$, which represents $(M + H)^+$.

Hence $M = 889$.

m/z	146	203	260	357	444	591	648	705	802	889
Δ		57	57	97	87	147	57	57	97	87
aa		Gly	Gly	Pro	Ser	Phe	Gly	Gly	Pro	Ser

The mass differences (Δ), between sequence ions, represent the amino acid (aa) residual masses. The lowest mass sequence ion, $m/z = 146$ is too low for arginine and must therefore represent Lys + OH. The sequence in conventional order from the N-terminal end would be:

H-Ser-Pro-Gly-Gly-Phe-Ser-Pro-Gly-Gly-Lys-OH

(ii) The summation of the aa residues = 889 daltons, which is a check on the mass spectrometry value for M.

(iii) The m/z values in the ESI spectrum represent multiply charged species and may be identified as follows:

$m/z = 178.8 \equiv (M + 5H)^{5+}$ from $889/178.8 = 4.97$

$m/z = 223.2 \equiv (M + 4H)^{4+}$ from $889/223.2 = 3.98$

$m/z = 297.3 \equiv (M + 3H)^{3+}$ from $889/297.3 = 2.99$

Remember that z must be an integer and hence values need to be rounded to the nearest whole number.

Question 3

Determine the primary structure of the oligopeptide that gave the following, positive mode, FAB–MS data:

....

m/z 149   305   442   529   617

....

Use the amino acid residual mass values in the table in Question 2.

Answer $m/z = 617 \equiv (M + H)^+$

....

m/z	149	305	442	529	616
Δ		156	137	87	87
aa		Arg	His	Ser	Ser

....

Conventional order for the sequence would be:

H-Ser-Ser-His-Arg-?

It is important to note that no assignment has been given for the remaining *m/z* = 149. It may not in fact be a sequence ion and more information would be required, such as an accurate relative molecular mass of the oligopeptide, in order to proceed further. It is, however, possible to speculate as to the nature of this ion. If the *m/z* = 149 ion is the C-terminal amino acid then it would end in -OH and be 17 mass units greater than the corresponding residual mass. The difference between 149 and 17 is 132 which is extremely close to methionine, so this amino acid remains a possibility to end the chain.

Question 4

A peptide metabolite and an enzyme digest of it were analysed by a combination of mass spectrometric techniques giving the data listed below:

(i) The peptide showed two signals at 3841.5 and 1741 in the MALDI spectrum.

(ii) Five signals could be discerned when the peptide was introduced into a mass spectrometer via an electrospray ionisation source:

....

m/z 498.2   581.1   697.1   871.2   1161.2

....

(iii) HPLC-MS of the digest indicated *four* components; the $[M + H]^+$ data for the components being *m/z* = 176, 625, 1229 and 1508. The ions corresponding to the MS of the '625' component appeared at *m/z* = 521, 406, 293, 130, and 113.

(iv) HPLC–MS–MS of the *m/z* = 406 ion of the '625' component identified two ions at *m/z* = 378 and 336 and of the *m/z* = 113 ion gave *m/z* = 85 and 57, in the product ion spectra.

Use the above data to compare and contrast the different ionisation methods, deduce a relative molecular mass for the peptide and determine a sequence for the '625' component.

Use the amino acid residual masses values in the table in Question 2.

Answer | The data in (i) are $m/z = 3481.5$ and $m/z = 1741$. These data could represent either of the following possibilities:

(a) $m/z = 3481.5 \equiv (M + H)^+$
   when $m/z = 1741 \equiv (M + H)^{2+}$, giving $M = 3480.5$
(b) $m/z = 3481.5 \equiv (2M + H)^+$
   when $m/z = 1741 \equiv (M + H)^+$, giving $M = 1740$

Consideration of the data in (ii) allows a choice to be made between these two alternatives. Using $n_2 = (m_1 - 1)/(m_2 - m_1)$ and $M = n_2(m_2 - 1)$.

$m_1 - 1$	$m_2 - m_1$	n_2	$m_2 - 1$	M	z
870.2	290	3.0006	1160.2	3481.2	3
696.1	174.1	3.9982	870.2	3479.3	4
580.1	116	5.0000	696.1	3481.1	5
497.2	82.9	5.9975	580.1	3479.2	6

$\Sigma M = 13920.8$

Mean $M_r = 3480.2$

The mean M_r result confirms set (a) of the conclusions above concerning the data obtained from the MALDI experiments.

The data in (iii) indicate that four products arise from the enzymic digest of the original peptide. As these products arise directly from the original, the sum of these masses will be related to the M_r of the peptide.

Therefore

$176 + 625 + 1229 + 1508 = 3538$

The difference between this mass and the M_r determined above is

$3538 - 3480.2 = 57.8 \approx 58$

The difference of 58 mass units is explained as follows.

Each of the enzyme digest products is protonated (to be 'seen' in the mass spectrometer). Hence this accounts for 4 units. The remaining 54 unit increase arises from the enzymic hydrolysis. From a linear peptide, four products arise from three cleavage points (three cuts in a piece of string give four pieces). Each cleavage point requires the input of one water molecule (hydrolysis, $H_2O = 18$). Three cleavage points require $3 \times 18 = 54$.

The $m/z = 625$, $(M + H)^+$, peak was subjected to further mass spectrometry and sequence ions were observed.

m/z	624	521	406	293	130	113
Δ		103	115	113	163	17
aa		Cys	Asp	Ile/Leu	Tyr	Ile/Leu

The loss of 113 from the $m/z = 406$ ion indicates either Ile or Leu. MS^2 shows consecutive losses of 28 (CO) and 42 ($CH_2 = CH = CH_3$) which is indicative of Leu. The loss of 17 (not a sequence ion) from 130 confirms this as the C-terminal amino acid (OH = 17). The residual mass is again 113 indicating Ile/Leu. MS^2 of this peak shows consecutive losses of 28 (CO) and 28 ($CH_2 = CH_2$) which is indicative of Ile.

The predicted sequence, from the N-terminal end is

H-Cys-Asp-Leu-Tyr-Ile-OH

Question 5 Consider the following mass spectrometric data obtained for a peptide metabolite.

(i) The MALDI spectrum showed three signals at $m/z = 1609, 805$ and 403
(ii) There were two significant signals in the positive ion FAB mass spectrum at $m/z = 805$ and 827; the latter signal being enhanced on addition of sodium chloride.
(iii) Signals at $m/z = 161.8, 202.0, 269.0$ and 403.0 were observed when the sample was introduced into the mass spectrometer via an electrospray ionisation source.

Use these data to give an account of the ionisation methods used. Discuss the significance of the data and deduce a relative molecular mass for the metabolite.
Use the amino acid residual mass values in the table in Question 2.

Answer (i) Signals in the MALDI spectrum were observed at $m/z = 1609, 805$ and 403. These data could represent any of the following possibilities:

(a) $m/z = 1609 \equiv (M + H)^+$
    when $m/z = 805 \equiv (M + 2H)^{2+}$
    and $m/z = 403 \equiv (M + 4H)^{4+}$, giving $M = 1608$
(b) $m/z = 1609 \equiv (2M + H)^+$
    when $m/z = 805 \equiv (M + H)^+$
    and $m/z = 403 \equiv (M + 2H)^{2+}$, giving $M = 804$
(c) $m/z = 1609 \equiv (4M + H)^+$
    when $m/z = 805 \equiv (2M + H)^+$
    and $m/z = 403 \equiv (M + H)^+$, giving $M = 402$

(ii) The distinction between the above options can be made by considering the FAB data. This mode of ionisation gave peaks at $m/z = 805$ and 827, the latter being enhanced on the addition of sodium chloride. This evidence suggests;

$m/z = 805 \equiv (M + H)^+$

$m/z = 827 \equiv (M + Na)^+$

giving $M = 804$ and supports option (b) from the MALDI data.

(iii) The multiply charged ions observed in the electrospray ionisation method allow an average M_r to be calculated. Using the standard formula;

$m_1 - 1$	$m_2 - m_1$	n_2	$m_2 - 1$	M	z
268.0	134	2.0	402.0	804	2
201.0	67	3.0	268.0	804	3
160.8	40.2	4.0	201.0	804	4

The relative molecular mass is clearly 804, confirming the above conclusions.

1 Give an account of the ways in which chromatographs and mass spectrometers have been interfaced, identifying the major problems that had to be overcome and the constraints imposed through the connection of these two methods.

2 An unknown peptide and an enzymic digest of it were analysed by mass spectrometric and chromatographic methods as follows:

   (i) laser desorption mass spectrometry (LDMS) of the peptide gave two signals at $m/z = 3569$ and 1785;

  (ii) LDMS of the hydrolysate showed signals at $m/z = 766, 891, 953$ and 1016;

 (iii) the data obtained from analysis of the peptide using coupled HPLC–MS operating through an electrospray ionisation source were $m/z = 510.7, 595.7, 714.6, 893.0$ and 1190.3;

 (iv) when the hydrolysate was analysed by HPLC, four distinct components could be discerned.

Explain what information is available from these observations and determine a relative molecular mass, using the amino acid residual mass values in the table in Question 2, for the unknown peptide.

Answer

  (i) Signals from LDMS were observed at $m/z = 3569$ and 1785. These data could represent either of the following possibilities:

    (a) $m/z = 3569 \equiv (M + H)^+$
        when $m/z = 1785 \equiv (M + 2H)^{2+}$, giving $M = 3568$

    (b) $m/z = 3569 \equiv (2M + H)^+$,
        when $m/z = 1785 \equiv (M + H)^+$, giving $M = 1784$

  (ii) It is possible to distinguish between these two options by considering the LDMS of the products of hydrolysis. Four m/z values were obtained: 766, 891, 953 and 1016.

      Each is a protonated species and the sum of these masses, 3626, will be of the order of the M_r of the original peptide. The value of this sum supports option (a) in (i) above.

 (iii) Electrospray ionisation data represent multiply charged ions. Using the standard formula the mean M_r may be obtained.

$m_1 - 1$	$m_2 - m_1$	n_2	$m_2 - 1$	M	z
892.0	297.3	3.0003	1189.3	3568.3	3
713.6	178.4	4.0000	892.0	3568.0	4
594.7	118.9	5.0016	713.6	3569.2	5
509.7	85	5.9964	594.7	3566.1	6

      $\Sigma M = 14271.6$
    Mean $M_r = 3567.9$

    This more precise value confirms the conclusions found above. For an explanation of the mass difference between M_r and the sum of the hydrolysate products, refer to the answer to Question 4.

    The data in (iv) are confirmatory chromatographic evidence that only four hydrolysis products were obtained.

11.13 **SUGGESTIONS FOR FURTHER READING**

CHAPMAN, J. R. (1995) *Practical Organic Mass Spectrometry: A Guide for Chemical and Biochemical Analysis*. John Wiley and Sons, London. (Covers theory and applications in depth, with a comprehensive bibliography.)

DAVIES, R. and FREARSON, M. (1988). *Mass Spectrometry*. ACOL Series. John Wiley and Sons, London. (An open learning text for those requiring a deeper understanding of the principles.)

FENSELAU, C. (ed.) (1994). *Mass Spectrometry for the Characterization of Microorganisms*. American Chemical Society Symposium Series **541**. (A collection of published work presented at symposia giving an up-to-date view of research in the subject.)

GASKELL, S. J. (1986). *Mass Spectrometry in Biomedical Research*. John Wiley and Sons, London. (An advanced text on specific methods and applications.)

Many specific applications are published in manufacturers' application notes, which are generally available free on request. Two of particular interest appear in the VG *Monographs in Mass Spectrometry Series*, published by VG Instruments (now Micromass UK Ltd), Tudor Road, Altrincham, WA14 5RZ, UK.

MELLON, F. A. (1991). *Liquid Chromatography/Mass Spectrometry*, vol. 2, no. 1.

ROSE, M. E. (1990). *Modern Practice of Gas Chromatography/Mass Spectrometry*, vol. 1, no. 1.

Chapter 12

Electrophoretic techniques

12.1 GENERAL PRINCIPLES

The term electrophoresis describes the migration of a charged particle under the influence of an electric field. Many important biological molecules, such as amino acids, peptides, proteins, nucleotides and nucleic acids, possess ionisable groups and, therefore, at any given pH, exist in solution as electrically charged species either as cations (+) or anions (−). Under the influence of an electric field these charged particles will migrate either to the cathode or to the anode, depending on the nature of their net charge.

The equipment required for electrophoresis consists basically of two items, a power pack and an electrophoresis unit. Electrophoresis units are available for running either vertical or horizontal gel systems. Vertical slab gel units of the type shown in Fig. 12.1 are commercially available and routinely used to separate proteins in acrylamide gels (Section 12.2). The gel is formed between two glass plates that are clamped together but held apart by plastic spacers. Gel dimensions are typically 12 cm × 14 cm, with a thickness of 0.5 to 1 mm. A plastic comb is placed in the gel solution and is removed after polymerisation to provide loading wells for samples. When the apparatus is assembled, the lower electrophoresis tank buffer surrounds the gel plates and affords some cooling of the gel plates. A typical horizontal gel system is shown in Fig. 12.2. The gel is cast on a glass or plastic sheet and placed on a cooling plate (an insulated surface through which cooling water is passed to conduct away generated heat). Connection between the gel and electrode buffer is made using a thick wad of wetted filter paper (Fig. 12.2: note, however, that agarose gels for DNA electrophoresis are run submerged in the buffer (Section 12.4.1). The power pack supplies a direct current between the electrodes in the electrophoresis unit. All electrophoresis is carried out in an appropriate buffer, which is essential to maintain a constant state of ionisation of the molecules being separated. Any variation in pH would alter the overall charge and hence the mobilities (rate of migration in the applied field) of the molecules being separated.

In order to understand fully how charged species separate it is necessary to look at some simple equations relating to electrophoresis. When a potential difference (voltage) is applied across the electrodes, it generates a potential gradient, E, which is the applied voltage, V, divided by the distance, d, between the

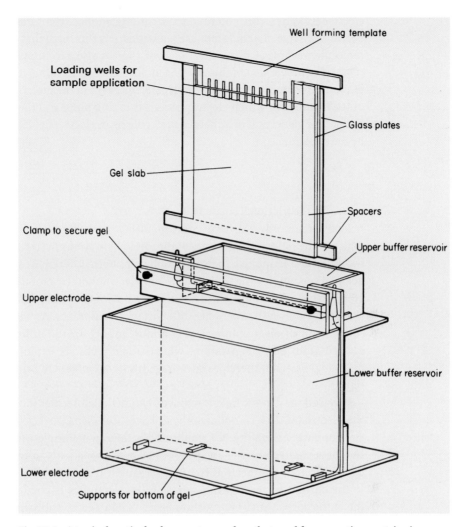

Fig. 12.1. A typical vertical gel apparatus, such as that used for separating proteins in a polyacrylamide gel. Note that, once the gel has set, the lower spacer is removed prior to the gel being run.

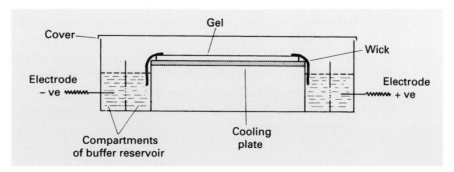

Fig. 12.2. A typical horizontal apparatus, such as that used for immunoelectrophoresis, isoelectric focusing and the electrophoresis of DNA and RNA in agarose gels.

electrodes. When this potential gradient E is applied, the force on a molecule bearing a charge of q coulombs is Eq newtons. It is this force that drives a charged molecule towards an electrode. However, there is also a frictional resistance that retards the movement of this charged molecule. This frictional force is a measure of the hydrodynamic size of the molecule, the shape of the molecule, the pore size of the medium in which electrophoresis is taking place and the viscosity of the buffer. The velocity, v, of a charged molecule in an electric field is therefore given by the equation:

$$v = \frac{Eq}{f} \tag{12.1}$$

where f is the frictional coefficient.

More commonly the term electrophoretic mobility (μ), of an ion is used, which is the ratio of the velocity of the ion to field strength (v/E). When a potential difference is applied, therefore, molecules with different overall charges will begin to separate owing to their different electrophoretic mobilities. Even molecules with similar charges will begin to separate if they have different molecular sizes, since they will experience different frictional forces. As will be seen below, some forms of electrophoresis rely almost totally on the different charges on molecules to effect separation, whilst other methods exploit differences in molecular size and therefore encourage frictional effects to bring about separation.

Provided the electric field is removed before the molecules in the sample reach the electrodes, the components will have been separated according to their electrophoretic mobility. Electrophoresis is thus an incomplete form of electrolysis. The separated samples are then located by staining with an appropriate dye or by autoradiography (Section 14.2.3) if the sample is radiolabelled.

The current in the solution between the electrodes is conducted mainly by the buffer ions, a small proportion being conducted by the sample ions. Ohm's law expresses the relationship between current (I), voltage (V) and resistance (R):

$$\frac{V}{I} = R \tag{12.2}$$

It therefore appears that it is possible to accelerate an electrophoretic separation by increasing the applied voltage, which would result in a corresponding increase in the current flowing. The distance migrated by the ions will be proportional to both current and time. However, this would ignore one of the major problems for most forms of electrophoresis, namely the generation of heat.

During electrophoresis the power (W, watts) generated in the supporting medium is given by

$$W = I^2 R \tag{12.3}$$

Most of this power generated is dissipated as heat. Heating of the electrophoretic medium has the following effects:

(i) An increased rate of diffusion of sample and buffer ions leading to broadening of the separated samples.

(ii) The formation of convection currents, which leads to mixing of separated samples.

(iii) Thermal instability of samples that are rather sensitive to heat. This may include denaturation of proteins or loss of activity of enzymes.

(iv) A decrease of buffer viscosity, and hence a reduction in the resistance of the medium.

If a constant voltage is applied, the current increases during electrophoresis owing to the decrease in resistance (see Ohm's law, equation 12.2) and the rise in current increases the heat output still further. For this reason, workers often use a stabilised power supply, which provides constant power and thus eliminates fluctuations in heating.

Constant heat generation is, however, a problem. The answer might appear to be to run the electrophoresis at very low power (low current) to overcome any heating problem, but this can lead to poor separations as a result of the increased amount of diffusion resulting from long separation times. Compromise conditions, therefore, have to be found with reasonable power settings, to give acceptable separation times, and an appropriate cooling system, to remove liberated heat. While such systems work fairly well, the effects of heating are not always totally eliminated. For example, for electrophoresis carried out in cylindrical tubes or in slab gels, although heat is generated uniformly through the medium, heat is removed only from the edges, resulting in a temperature gradient within the gel, the temperature at the centre of the gel being higher than that at the edges. Since the warmer fluid at the centre is less viscous, electrophoretic mobilities are therefore greater in the central region (electrophoretic mobilities increase by about 2% for each 1 deg.C rise in temperature), and electrophoretic zones develop a bowed shape, with the zone centre migrating faster than the edges.

A final factor that can effect electrophoretic separation is the phenomenon of electroendosmosis (also known as electroosmotic flow), which is due to the presence of charged groups on the surface of the support of the support medium. For example, paper has some carboxyl groups present, agarose (depending on the purity grade) contains sulphate groups and the surface of glass walls used in capillary electrophoresis (Section 12.5) contains silanol (Si-OH) groups. Figure 12.3 demonstrates how electroendosmosis occurs in a capillary tube, although the principle is the same for any support medium that has charged groups on it. In a fused-silica capillary tube, above a pH value of about 3, silanol groups on the silica capillary wall will ionise, generating negatively charged sites. It is these charges that generate electroendosmosis. The ionised silanol groups create an electrical double layer, or region of charge separation, at the capillary wall/electrolyte interface. When a voltage is applied, cations in the electrolyte near the capillary wall migrate towards the cathode, pulling electrolyte solution with them. This creates a net electroosmotic flow towards the cathode.

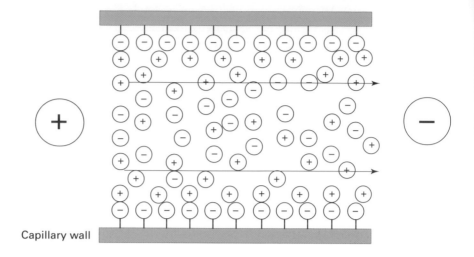

• Acidic silanol groups impart negative charge on wall
• Counter ions migrate toward cathode, dragging solvent along

Fig. 12.3. Electroosmotic flow through a glass capillary. Electrolyte cations are attracted to the capillary walls, forming an electrical double layer. When a voltage is applied, the net movement of electrolyte solution towards the cathode is known as electroendosmotic flow.

12.2 SUPPORT MEDIA

The pioneering work on electrophoresis by A. Tiselius and co-workers was performed in free solution. However, it was soon realised that many of the problems associated with this approach, particularly the adverse effects of diffusion and convection currents, could be minimised by stabilising the medium. This was achieved by carrying out electrophoresis on a porous mechanical support, which was wetted in electrophoresis buffer and in which electrophoresis of buffer ions and samples could occur. The support medium cuts down convection currents and diffusion so that the separated components remain as sharp zones. The earliest supports used were filter paper or cellulose acetate strips, wetted in electrophoresis buffer. Nowadays these media are infrequently used, although cellulose acetate still has its uses (see Section 12.3.6). In particular, for many years small molecules such as amino acids, peptides and carbohydrates were routinely separated and analysed by electrophoresis on supports such as paper or thin-layer plates of cellulose, silica or alumina. Although occasionally still used nowadays, such molecules are now more likely to be analysed by more modern and sensitive techniques such as high performance liquid chromatography (Section 13.4). While paper or thin-layer supports are fine for resolving small molecules, the separation of macromolecules such as proteins and nucleic acids on such supports is poor.

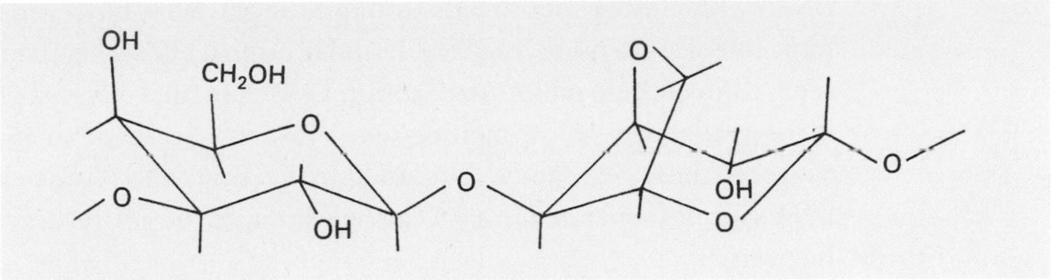

Fig. 12.4. Agarobiose, the repeating unit of agarose.

However, the introduction of the use of gels as a support medium led to a rapid improvement in methods for analysing macromolecules. The earliest gel system to be used was the starch gel and, although this still has some uses, the vast majority of electrophoretic techniques used nowadays involve either agarose gels or polyacrylamide gels.

12.2.1 **Agarose gels**

Agarose is a linear polysaccharide (average relative molecular mass about 12 000) made up of the basic repeat unit agarobiose, which comprises alternating units of galactose and 3,6-anhydrogalactose (Fig. 12.4). Agarose is one of the components of agar that is a mixture of polysaccharides isolated from certain seaweeds. Agarose is usually used at concentrations of between 1% and 3%. Agarose gels are formed by suspending dry agarose in aqueous buffer, then boiling the mixture until a clear solution forms. This is poured and allowed to cool to room temperature to form a rigid gel. The gelling properties are attributed to both inter- and intramolecular hydrogen bonding within and between the long agarose chains. This cross-linked structure gives the gel good anticonvectional properties. The pore size in the gel is controlled by the initial concentration of agarose; large pore sizes are formed from low concentrations and smaller pore sizes are formed from the higher concentrations. Although essentially free from charge, substitution of the alternating sugar residues with carboxyl, methyoxyl, pyruvate and especially sulphate groups occurs to varying degrees. This substitution can result in electro-endosmosis during electrophoresis and ionic interactions between the gel and sample in all uses, both unwanted effects. Agarose is therefore sold in different purity grades, based on the sulphate concentration – the lower the sulphate content, the higher the purity.

Agarose gels are used for the electrophoresis of both proteins and nucleic acids. For proteins, the pore sizes of a 1% agarose gel are large relative to the sizes of proteins. Agarose gels are therefore used in techniques such as immunoelectrophoresis (Section 4.4.1) or flat-bed isoelectric focusing (Section 12.3.4), where the proteins are required to move unhindered in the gel matrix according to their native charge. Such large pore gels are also used to separate much larger molecules such as DNA or RNA, because the pore sizes in the gel are still large enough for

DNA or RNA molecules to pass through the gel. Now, however, the pore size and molecule size are more comparable and frictional effects begin to play a role in the separation of these molecules (Section 12.4). A further advantage of using agarose is the availability of low melting temperature agarose (62 to 65 °C). As the name suggests, these gels can be reliquified by heating to 65 °C and thus, for example, DNA samples separated in a gel can be cut out of the gel, returned to solution and recovered.

Owing to the poor elasticity of agarose gels and the consequent problems of removing them from small tubes, the gel rod system sometimes used for acrylamide gels is not used. Horizontal slab gels are invariably used for isoelectric focusing or immunoelectrophoresis in agarose. Horizontal gels are also used routinely for DNA and RNA gels (Section 12.4), although vertical systems have been used by some workers.

12.2.2 **Polyacrylamide gels**

Electrophoresis in acrylamide gels is frequently referred to as PAGE, being an abbreviation for *poly*acrylamide *g*el *e*lectrophoresis.

Cross-linked polyacrylamide gels are formed from the polymerisation of acrylamide monomer in the presence of smaller amounts of N,N'-methylenebisacrylamide (normally referred to as 'bis'-acrylamide) (Fig. 12.5). Note that bis-acrylamide is essentially two acrylamide molecules linked by a methylene group, and is used as a cross-linking agent. Acrylamide monomer is polymerised in a head-to-tail fashion into long chains and occasionally a bis-acrylamide molecule is built into the growing chain, thus introducing a second site for chain extension. Proceeding in this way a cross-linked matrix of fairly well-defined structure is formed (Fig. 12.5). The polymerisation of acrylamide is an example of free-radical catalysis, and is initiated by the addition of ammonium persulphate and the base N,N,N',N'-tetramethylenediamine (TEMED). TEMED catalyses the decomposition of the persulphate ion to give a free radical (i.e. a molecule with an unpaired electron):

$$S_2O_8^{2-} + e^- \rightarrow SO_4^{2-} + SO_4^{-} \cdot$$

If this free radical is represented as R$^{\cdot}$ (where the dot represents an unpaired electron) and M as an acrylamide monomer molecule, then the polymerisation can be represented as follows:

R$^{\cdot}$ + M → RM$^{\cdot}$

RM$^{\cdot}$ + M → RMM$^{\cdot}$

RMM$^{\cdot}$ + M → RMMM$^{\cdot}$ etc.

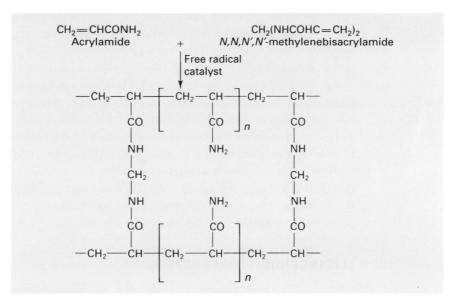

Fig. 12.5. The formation of a polyacrylamide gel from acrylamide and bis-acrylamide

Free radicals are highly reactive species due to the presence of an unpaired electron that needs to be paired with another electron to stabilise the molecule. $R^\bullet$ therefore reacts with M, forming a single bond by sharing its unpaired electron with one from the outer shell of the monomer molecule. This therefore produces a new free radical molecule $R - M^\bullet$, which is equally reactive and will attack a further monomer molecule. In this way long chains of acrylamide are built up, being cross-linked by the introduction of the occasional bis-acrylamide molecule into the growing chain. Oxygen removes free radicals and therefore all gel solutions are normally degassed (the solutions are briefly placed under vacuum to remove loosely dissolved oxygen) prior to use.

Photopolymerisation is an alternative method that can be used to polymerise acrylamide gels. The ammonium persulphate and TEMED are replaced by riboflavin and when the gel is poured it is placed in front of a bright light for 2 to 3 h. Photodecomposition of riboflavin generates a free radical that initiates polymerisation.

Acrylamide gels are defined in terms of the total percentage of acrylamide present, and the pore size in the gel can be varied by changing the concentrations of both the acrylamide and bis-acrylamide. Acrylamide gels can be made with a content of between 3% and 30% acrylamide. Thus low percentage gels (e.g. 4%) have large pore sizes and are used, for example, in the electrophoresis of proteins, where free movement of the proteins by electrophoresis is required without any noticeable frictional effect, for example in flat-bed isoelectric focusing (Section 12.3.4) or the stacking gel system of an SDS-polyacrylamide gel (Section 12.3.1). Low percentage acrylamide gels are also used to separate DNA (Section 12.4). Gels of between 10% and 20% acrylamide are used in techniques such as SDS-gel electrophoresis, where the smaller pore size now introduces a sieving effect that contributes to the separation of proteins according to their size (Section 12.3.1).

Proteins were originally separated on polyacrylamide gels that were polymerised in glass tubes, approximately 7 mm in diameter and about 10 cm in length. The tubes were easy to load and run, with minimum apparatus requirements. However, only one sample could be run per tube and, because conditions of separation could vary from tube to tube, comparison between different samples was not always accurate. The later introduction of vertical gel slabs allowed running of up to 20 samples under identical conditions in a single run. Vertical slabs are now used routinely both for the analysis of proteins (Section 12.3) and for the separation of DNA fragments during DNA sequence analysis (Section 12.4). Note, however, that tube gels are still used for the first dimension of two-dimensional gel electrophoresis (Section 12.3.5).

12.3 ELECTROPHORESIS OF PROTEINS

12.3.1 Sodium dodecyl sulphate-polyacrylamide gel electrophoresis

SDS-polyacrylamide gel electrophoresis (SDS-PAGE) is the most widely used method for analysing protein mixtures qualitatively. It is particularly useful for monitoring protein purification and, because the method is based on the separation of proteins according to size, the method can also be used to determine the relative molecular mass of proteins. SDS (CH_3-$(CH_2)_{10}$-$CH_2OSO_3^-$$Na^+$) is an anionic detergent. Samples to be run on SDS-PAGE are firstly boiled for 5 min in sample buffer containing β-mercaptoethanol and SDS. The mercaptoethanol reduces any disulphide bridges present that are holding together the protein tertiary structure, and the SDS binds strongly to, and denatures, the protein. Each protein in the mixture is therefore fully denatured by this treatment and opens up into a rod-shaped structure with a series of negatively charged SDS molecules along the polypeptide chain. On average, one SDS molecule binds for every two amino acids residues. The original native charge on the molecule is therefore completely swamped by the negatively charged SDS molecules. The rod-like structure remains, as any rotation that tends to fold up the protein chain would result in repulsion between negative charges on different parts of the protein chain, returning the conformation back to the rod shape. The sample buffer also contains an ionisable tracking dye, usually bromophenol blue, that allows the electrophoretic run to be monitored, and sucrose or glycerol, which gives the sample solution density thus allowing the sample to settle easily through the electrophoresis buffer to the bottom when injected into the loading well (see Fig. 12.1). Once the samples are all loaded, a current is passed through the gel. The samples to be separated are not in fact loaded directly into the main separating gel. When the main separating gel (normally about 10 cm long) has been poured between the glass plates and allowed to set, a shorter (approximately 1 cm) stacking gel is poured on top of the separating gel and it is into this gel that the wells are formed and the proteins loaded. The purpose of this stacking gel is to concentrate the protein sample into a sharp band before it enters the main separating gel. This is achieved by utilising differences in ionic strength and pH between the electrophoresis buffer and the stacking gel, and involves a phenomenon known as isotachophoresis. The stacking gel has a very large pore size (4% acrylamide), which allows the proteins to move freely and concentrate, or stack, under the effect of the electric field. The band-sharpening effect relies on the fact that negatively charged glycinate ions (in the electrophoresis buffer) have a lower electrophoretic mobility than do the protein–SDS complexes, which, in turn, have lower mobility than the chloride ions (Cl^-) of the loading buffer and the stacking gel. When the current is switched on, all the ionic species have to migrate at the same speed otherwise there would be a break in the electrical circuit. The glycinate ions can move at the same speed as Cl^- only if they are in a region of higher field strength. Field strength is inversely proportional to conductivity, which is proportional to concentration. The result is that the three species of interest adjust their concentrations so that $[Cl^-] > [\text{protein–SDS}] > [\text{glycinate}]$. There is only a small quantity of protein–SDS complexes, so they concentrate in a very tight band between glycinate and Cl^- boundaries. Once the glycinate reaches the separating gel it becomes more fully ionised in the higher pH environment and its mobility increases. (The pH of the stacking gel is 6.8, that of the separating gel is 8.8). Thus, the interface between glycinate and Cl^- leaves behind the protein–SDS complexes, which are left to electrophorese at their own rates. The negatively charged protein–SDS complexes now continue to move towards the anode, and, because they have the same charge per unit length, they travel into the separating gel under the applied electric field with the same mobility. However, as they pass through the separating gel the proteins separate, owing to the molecular sieving properties of the gel. Quite simply, the smaller the protein the more easily it can pass through the pores of the gel, whereas large proteins are successively retarded by frictional resistance due to the sieving effect of the gels. Being a small molecule, the bromophenol blue dye is totally unretarded and therefore indicates the electrophoresis front. When the dye reaches the bottom of the gel, the current is turned off, and the gel is removed from between the glass plates and shaken in an appropriate stain solution (usually Coomassie Brilliant Blue, see Section 12.3.8) for a few hours and then washed in destain solution overnight. The destain solution removes unbound background dye from the gel leaving stained proteins visible as blue bands on a clear background. A typical gel would take 1 to 1½ h to prepare and set, 3 h to run at 30 mA, and have a staining time of 2 to 3 h with an overnight destain. Vertical slab gels are invariably run, since this allows up to 20 different samples to be loaded onto a single gel. A typical SDS-polyacrylamide gel is shown in Fig. 12.6.

Typically, the separating gel used is a 15% polyacrylamide gel. This gives a gel of a certain pore size in which proteins of relative molecular mass (M_r) 10 000 move through the gel relatively unhindered, whereas proteins of 100 000 can only just enter the pores of this gel. Gels of 15% polyacrylamide are therefore useful for separating proteins in the range 100 000 to 10 000. However, a protein of 150 000, for example, would be unable to enter a 15% gel. In this case a larger-pored gel (e.g. a 10% or even 7.5% gel) would be used so that the protein could now enter the gel

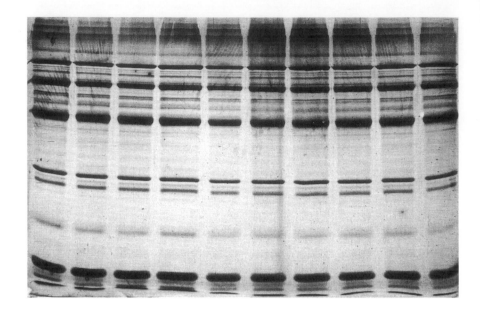

Fig. 12.6. A typical SDS-polyacrylamide gel. All 10 wells in the gel have been loaded with the same complex mixture of proteins. (Courtesy of Bio-Rad Laboratories.)

and be stained and identified. It is obvious, therefore, that the choice of gel to be used depends on the size of the protein being studied.

The M_r of a protein can be determined by comparing its mobility with those of a number of standard proteins of known M_r that are run on the same gel. By plotting a graph of distance moved against log M_r for each of the standard proteins, a calibration curve can be constructed. The distance moved by the protein of unknown M_r is then measured, and then its log M_r and hence M_r can be determined from the calibration curve.

SDS-gel electrophoresis is often used after each step of a purification protocol to assess the purity or otherwise of the sample. A pure protein should give a single band on an SDS-polyacrylamide gel, unless the molecule is made up of two unequal subunits. In the latter case two bands, corresponding to the two subunits, will be seen. Since only submicrogram amounts of protein are needed for the gel, very little material is used in this form of purity assessment and at the same time a value for the relative molecular mass of the protein can be determined on the same gel run (as described above), with no more material being used.

12.3.2 **Native (buffer) gels**

While SDS-PAGE is the most frequently used gel system for studying proteins, the method is of no use if one is aiming to detect a particular protein (often an enzyme) on the basis of its biological activity, because the protein (enzyme) is denatured by the SDS-PAGE procedure. In this case it is necessary to use non-denaturing conditions. In native or buffer gels, polyacrylamide gels are again used (normally a 7.5% gel) but the SDS is absent and the proteins are *not* denatured prior to loading. Since all the proteins in the sample being analysed carry their native charge at the pH of the gel (normally pH 8.7), proteins separate according to their different electrophoretic mobilities *and* the sieving effects of the gel. It is not possible to predict the behaviour of a given protein in a buffer gel but, because of the range of different charges and sizes of proteins in a given protein mixture, good resolution is achieved. The enzyme of interest can be identified by incubating the gel in an appropriate substrate solution such that a coloured product is produced at the site of the enzyme. An alternative method for enzyme detection is to include the substrate in an agarose gel that is poured over the acrylamide gel and allowed to set. Diffusion and interaction of enzyme and substrate between the two gels results in colour formation at the site of the enzyme. Often, duplicate samples will be run on a gel, the gel cut in half and one half stained for activity, the other for total protein. In this way the total protein content of the sample can be analysed and the particular band corresponding to the enzyme identified by reference to the activity stain gel.

12.3.3 Gradient gels

This is again a polyacrylamide gel system, but instead of running a slab gel of uniform pore size throughout (e.g. a 15% gel) a gradient gel is formed, where the acrylamide concentration varies uniformly from, typically, 5% at the top of the gel to 25% acrylamide at the bottom of the gel. The gradient is formed via a gradient mixer (Section 13.3.6) and run down between the glass plates of a slab gel. The higher percentage acrylamide (e.g. 25%) is poured between the glass plates first and a continuous gradient of decreasing acrylamide concentration follows. Therefore at the top of the gel there is a large pore size (5% acrylamide) but as the sample moves down through the gel the acrylamide concentration slowly increases and the pore size correspondingly decreases. Gradient gels are normally run as SDS gels with a stacking gel. There are two advantages to running gradient gels. First, a much greater range of protein M_r values can be separated than on a fixed-percentage gel. In a complex mixture, very low molecular weight proteins travel freely through the gel to begin with, and start to resolve when they reach the smaller pore sizes towards the lower part of the gel. Much larger proteins, on the other hand, can still enter the gel but start to separate immediately due to the sieving effect of the gel. The second advantage of gradient gels is that proteins with very similar M_r values may be resolved, although they cannot otherwise be resolved in fixed percentage gels. As each protein moves through the gel the pore sizes become smaller until the protein reaches its pore size limit. The pore size in the gel is now too small to allow passage of the protein, and the protein sample stacks up at this point as a sharp band. A similar-sized protein, but with slightly lower M_r will be able to travel a little further through the gel before reaching its pore size limit, at which point it will form a sharp band. These two proteins, of slightly different M_r values, therefore separate as two, close, sharp bands.

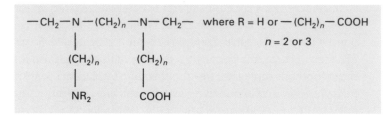

Fig. 12.7. The general formula for ampholytes.

Nowadays the emphasis in protein electrophoresis centres on the speed with which samples can be analysed. For example, the Phast System sold by Pharmacia LKB comes complete with ready-poured native, SDS-added or gradient minigels and the corresponding buffers in agarose strips. The system is programmed to run 0.5 to 1.0 µl samples in about 30 min and to stain the gels with either Coomassie Brilliant Blue or silver stain (Section 12.3.8) in approximately 30 min and 2 h, respectively.

12.3.4 Isoelectric focusing gels

This method is ideal for the separation of amphoteric substances such as proteins because it is based on the separation of molecules according to their different isoelectric points (Section 6.1). The method has high resolution, being able to separate proteins that differ in their isoelectric points by as little as 0.01 of a pH unit. The most widely used system for IEF utilises horizontal gels on glass plates or plastic sheets. Separation is achieved by applying a potential difference across a gel that contains a pH gradient. The pH gradient is formed by the introduction into the gel of compounds known as ampholytes, which are complex mixtures of synthetic polyamino-polycarboxylic acids (Fig. 12.7). Ampholytes can be purchased in different pH ranges covering either a wide band (e.g. pH 3 to 10) or various narrow bands (e.g. pH 7 to 8), and a pH range is chosen such that the samples being separated will have their isoelectric points (pI values) within this range. Commercially available ampholytes include Bio-Lyte and Pharmalyte.

Traditionally 1 to 2 mm thick isoelectric focusing gels have been used by research workers, but the relatively high cost of ampholytes makes this a fairly expensive procedure if a number of gels are to be run. However, the introduction of thin-layer IEF gels, which are only 0.15 mm thick and which are prepared using a layer of electrical insulation tape as the spacer between the gel plates, has considerably reduced the cost of preparing IEF gels, and such gels are now commonly used. Since this method requires the proteins to move freely according to their charge under the electric field, IEF is carried out in low percentage gels to avoid any sieving effect within the gel. Polyacrylamide gels (4%) are commonly used, but agarose is also used, especially for the study of high M_r proteins that may undergo some sieving even in a low percentage acrylamide gel.

To prepare a thin-layer IEF gel, carrier ampholytes, covering a suitable pH range, and riboflavin are mixed with the acrylamide solution, and the mixture is then poured over a glass plate (typically 25 cm × 10 cm), which contains the spacer. The second glass plate is then placed on top of the first to form the gel cassette, and the gel polymerised by photopolymerisation by placing the gel in front of a bright light. The photodecomposition of the riboflavin generates a free radical, which initiates polymerisation (Section 12.2.2). This takes 2 to 3 h. Once the gel has set, the glass plates are prised apart to reveal the gel stuck to one of the glass sheets. Electrode wicks, which are thick (3 mm) strips of wetted filter paper (the anode is phosphoric acid, the cathode sodium hydroxide) are laid along the long length of each side of the gel and a potential difference applied. Under the effect of this potential difference, the ampholytes form a pH gradient between the anode and cathode. The power is then turned off and samples applied by laying on the gel small squares of filter paper soaked in the sample. A voltage is again applied for about 30 min to allow the sample to electrophorese off the paper and into the gel, at which time the paper squares can be removed from the gel. Depending on which point on the pH gradient the sample has been loaded, proteins that are initially at a pH region below their isoelectric point will be positively charged and will initially migrate towards the cathode. As they proceed, however, the surrounding pH will be steadily increasing, and therefore the positive charge on the protein will decrease correspondingly until eventually the protein arrives at a point where the pH is equal to its isoelectric point. The protein will now be in the zwitterion form with no net charge, so further movement will cease. Likewise, substances that are initially at pH regions above their isoelectric points will be negatively charged and will migrate towards the anode until they reach their isoelectric points and become stationary. It can be seen that as the samples will always move towards their isoelectric points it is not critical where on the gel they are applied. To achieve rapid separations (2 to 3 h) relatively high voltages (up to 2500 V) are used. As considerable heat is produced, gels are run on cooling plates (10 °C) and power packs used to stabilise the power output and thus to minimise thermal fluctuations. Following electrophoresis, the gel must be stained to detect the proteins. However, this cannot be done directly, because the ampholytes will stain too, giving a totally blue gel. The gel is therefore first washed with fixing solution (e.g. 10% (v/v) trichloroacetic acid). This precipitates the proteins in the gel and allows the much smaller ampholytes to be washed out. The gel is stained with Coomassie Brilliant Blue and then destained (Section 12.3.8). A typical IEF gel is shown in Fig. 12.8. The technique is strongly similar to the technique of chromatofocusing (Section 13.7.3).

The pI of a particular protein may be determined conveniently by running a mixture of proteins of known isoelectric point on the same gel. A number of mixtures of proteins with differing pI values are commercially available, covering the pH range 3.5 to 10. After staining, the distance of each band from one electrode is measured and a graph of distance for each protein against its pI (effectively the pH at that point) plotted. By means of this calibration line, the pI of an unknown protein can be determined from its position on the gel.

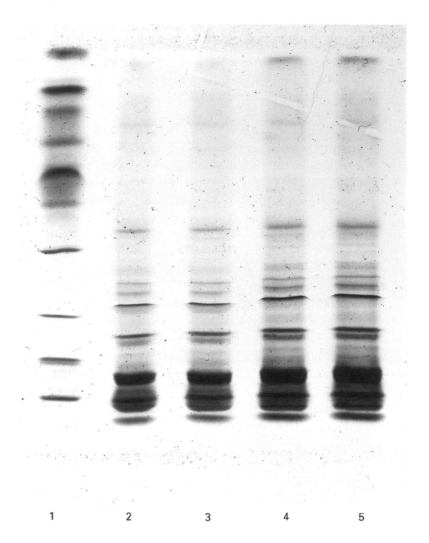

Fig. 12.8. A typical isoelectric focusing gel. Track 1 contains a mixture of standard proteins of known isoelectric points. Tracks 2 to 5 show increasing loadings of venom from the Japanese water moccasin snake. (Courtesy of Bio-Rad Laboratories Ltd.)

IEF is a highly sensitive analytical technique and is particularly useful for studying microheterogeneity in a protein. For example, a protein may show a single band on an SDS-added gel, but may show three bands on an IEF gel. This may occur, for example, when a protein exists in mono-, di- and tri-phosphory-lated forms. The difference of a couple of phosphate groups has no significant effect on the overall relative molecular mass of the protein, hence a single band on SDS-added gels, but the small charge difference introduced on each molecule can be detected by IEF.

The method is particularly useful for separating isoenzymes (Section 6.2), which are different forms of the same enzyme often differing by only one or two amino acid residues. Since the proteins are in their native form, enzymes can be detected in the gel either by washing the unfixed and unstained gel in an appropriate substrate or by overlayering with agarose containing the substrate. The approach has found particular use in forensic science, where traces of blood or other biological fluids can be analysed and compared according to the composition of certain isoenzymes.

Although IEF is used mainly for analytical separations, it can also be used for preparative purposes. In vertical column IEF, a water-cooled vertical glass column is used, filled with a mixture of ampholytes dissolved in a sucrose solution containing a density gradient to prevent diffusion. When the separation is complete, the current is switched off and the sample components run out through a valve in the base of the column. Alternatively, preparative IEF can be carried out in beds of granulated gel, such as Sephadex G-75 (Section 13.8).

12.3.5 **Two-dimensional polyacrylamide gel electrophoresis**

This technique combines the technique of IEF, which separates proteins in a mixture according to charge (pI), with the size separation technique of SDS-PAGE. When combined to give two-dimensional polyacrylamide gel electrophoresis (2-D PAGE), the most sophisticated analytical method for separating proteins available is obtained. The first dimension (isoelectric focusing) is carried out in polyacrylamide gels in narrow tubes (approximately 1 to 2 mm internal diameter) in the presence of ampholytes, 8 M urea and a non-ionic detergent. The denatured proteins therefore separate in this gel according to their isoelectric points. The gel is then extruded from the tube by applying slight pressure to one end, incubated for 15 min in a buffer containing SDS (thus binding SDS to the denatured proteins), then placed along the stacking gel of an SDS-added gel (either linear or gradient), and fixed in place by pouring molten agarose, in electrophoresis buffer, over the gel. Once the agarose has set, electrophoresis is commenced and the SDS-bound proteins run into the gel, stack, and separate according to size, as described in Section 12.3.1. A typical 2-D polyacrylamide gel is shown in Fig. 12.9.

This method is capable of routinely resolving between 1000 and 2000 proteins from a whole cell or tissue extract, and, using large-format (giant) 2-D gels, some workers have been able to resolve between 5000 and 10 000 proteins. Since it is estimated that any given cell type expresses about 10 000 to 20 000 proteins, we are now in a position to be able to 'observe' a significant portion of the total protein component of a given cell using two-dimensional electrophoresis (2-DE). This achievement has led to the introduction of the term proteome, which describes the complete set of proteins expressed by the genome in an organism (the term is of course analogous to 'genome', which describes the full nucleic acid component of a species). However, although the DNA sequence of the genome allows us to deduce which proteins might be made, it cannot tell us what proteins are *actually* expressed in any given tissue, whether they undergo post-translational modifications (e.g. phosphorylation, glycosylation, etc.) or anything about their functions. Analysis of the protein component of a cell or tissue provides this information.

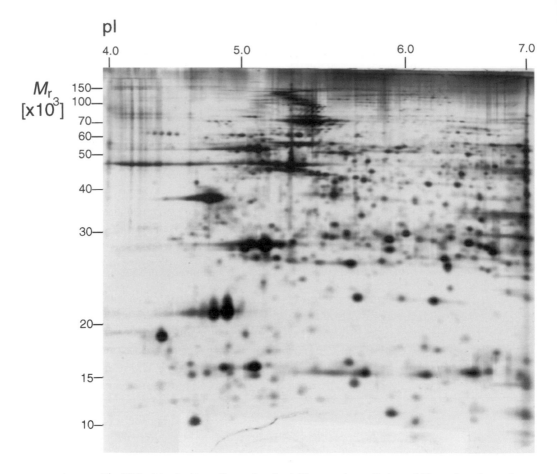

Fig. 12.9. A typical two-dimensional gel. The sample applied was 100 μg of total protein extracted from a normal dog heart ventricle. The first dimension was carried out using a pH 4 to 7 isoelectric-focusing gel. The second dimension was a 12% SDS-PAGE vertical slab gel. The pattern was visualised by silver staining. (Courtesy of Monique Heinke and Dr Mike Dunn, Division of Cardiothoracic Surgery, Imperial College School of Medicine, Heart Science Centre, Harefield, UK.)

As will be seen below, the ability to separate large numbers of proteins by 2-D PAGE, then identify individual proteins by partial sequence analysis, and database searching for this sequence is resulting in a rapid increase in our knowledge of the protein component of cells. Clearly this development goes hand-in-hand with the Human Genome Project, which continues to produce an ever-increasing database of DNA sequences (and hence protein sequences) that can be searched for sequence similarities. The sheer complexity and amount of data available from 2-D gel patterns is daunting, but fortunately there is a range of commercial 2-D gel analysis software, compatible with personal computer workstations, which can provide both qualitative and quantitative information from gel patterns, and can also compare patterns between two different 2-D gels. This has allowed the construction of a range of databases of quantitative protein expression in a range of tissue and cell types. For example, a 2-D protein database of proteins of the cardiovascular system has been constructed by the Heart Sciences Centre, Imperial College School of Medicine at Harefield Hospital, UK, and this can be rapidly accessed via the World Wide Web (WWW). An extensive series of 2-DE databases, known as SWISS-2D PAGE is maintained at Geneva University Hospital and is also accessible via the WWW. This facility therefore allows an individual laboratory to compare their own 2-D protein database with that in another laboratory.

We now have the ability to follow changes in the expression of *all* proteins in a cell or tissue type, rather than just one or two, which has been the situation in the past. The potential applications of proteome analysis are vast. Initially one must produce a 2-D map of the proteins expressed by an organism, tissue or cell under 'normal' conditions. This 2-D reference map and database can then be used to compare similar information from 'abnormal' or treated organisms, tissues or cells. For example, we can compare normal tissue with diseased tissue (e.g. malignant versus non-malignant), analyse the effects of drug treatment, or toxins on cells, observe the changing protein component of the cell at different stages of the cell cycle or during apoptosis, observe the response to extracellular stimuli such as hormones or cytokines, or compare pathogenic and non-pathogenic bacterial strains. As a typical example, a research group studying the toxic effect of drugs on the liver can compare the 2-D gel patterns from their 'damaged' livers with the normal liver 2-D reference map, thus identifying protein changes that occur as a result of drug treatment.

Characterisation of proteins separated by 2-DE

Having compared two 2-DE patterns and identified any protein spot(s) of interest, it is then necessary to identify each specific protein. This is achieved by obtaining partial sequence data and then searching protein sequence databases for sequence identity. Universal databases are available that store information on all types of proteins from all biological species. These databases can be divided into two categories: (a) databases that are a simple repository of sequence data, mostly deduced directly from DNA sequences, for example the Tr EMBL database; and (b) annotated databases where information in addition to the sequence is extracted by the biologist (the annotator) from the literature, review article, etc. for example SWISS-PROT database. At the time of writing, the SWISS-PROT database contains about 65 000 annotated entries from more than 5000 different species (although the majority of entries come from about 30 species that are the focus of most biological studies). The sequence data is obtained in one of two ways:

(i) Direct protein sequencing of the spot using the Edman degradation (Section 6.4.3). In this approach, the proteins in the 2-D gel are electroblotted onto a suitable membrane, for example poly(vinylidine difluoride (PVDF). After staining of the blot, the spot of interest is excised and introduced directly into an automated sequence analyser, thus generating an amino acid sequence from the N-terminus of the protein.

(ii) Peptide mass profiling. This method is based on the observation that the accurate peptide masses obtained by mass spectrometric analysis (see Chapter 11) of a protein digest (e.g. with trypsin) provides a characteristic fingerprint of that protein. The protein spot is therefore either digested *in situ* within the gel matrix or after electroblotting onto a membrane. Following extraction of the peptides produced, these unfractionated peptides can be analysed by MALDI–MS (see Chapter 11) to give accurate relative molecular mass values for the peptides produced. This experimentally derived relative molecular mass data can then be used for comparison with databases of peptide relative molecular masses generated from sequences of known proteins (or predicted sequences deduced from nucleotide sequences).

(iii) Sequence determination by mass spectrometry. Partial sequence data can be determined by mass spectrometry and databases searched for sequence identity. An example of this approach is shown in Fig. 12.10. A lysate of 2×10^6 rat basophil leukaemic (RBL) cells were separated by 2-DE and spot 2 chosen for analysis. This spot was digested *in situ* using trypsin and the resultant peptides extracted. This sample was then analysed by tandem MS using a triple quadrupole instrument (ESI–MS^2). Mass spectrometry of the peptide mixture showed a number of molecular ions relating to peptides. One of these (m/z 890) was selected for further analysis, being further fragmented in a quadrupole mass spectrometer to give fragment ions ranging from m/z 595.8 to 1553.6 (Fig. 12.10). The ions at m/z 1002.0, 1116.8, 1280.0, 1466.2 and 1553.6 are likely to be part of a Y ion series (see Fig. 11.12) as they appear at higher m/z than the precursor at m/z 890. The gap between adjacent Y ions is related directly to an amino acid residue because the two flanking Y ions result from cleavage of two adjacent amide bonds. Therefore, with a knowledge of the relative molecular masses of each of the 20 naturally occurring amino acids, it is possible to determine the presence of a particular residue at any point within the peptide. The position of the assigned amino acid is deduced by virtue of the m/z ratio of the two ions. By reading several amino acids it was possible to assemble a sequence of amino acids, in this case (using the one-letter code) YWS. Database searching was then possible using the peptide M_r 1778, the position of the lower m/z Y ion (1116.8), the proposed amino acid sequence (YWS) and the higher Y ion at m/z 1553. This provides a sequence tag, which is written as (116.8)YWS(1553.6).

A search of the SWISS-PROT database (Fig. 12.11), showed just two 'hits' from 40 000 entries, suggesting the protein is glyceraldehyde-3-phosphate dehydrogenase. The full sequence of this peptide is LISWYDNEYGYSNR and the HS/MS fragmentation data give a perfect match. Other peptides in the sample can also be analysed in the same manner, confirming the identity of the protein.

12.3.6 Cellulose acetate electrophoresis

Although one of the older methods, cellulose acetate electrophoresis still has a number of applications. In particular it has retained a use in the clinical analysis

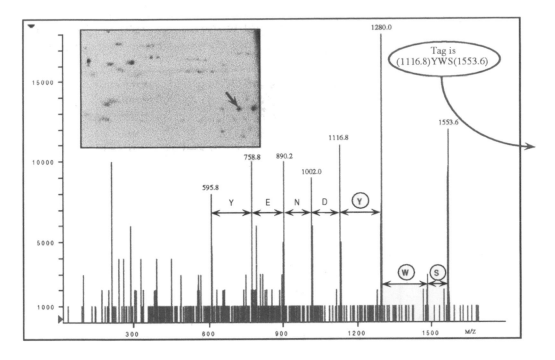

Fig. 12.10. Nano-ESI MS² spectrum of *m/z* 890 from RBL spot 2 showing construction of a sequence tag. The *y*-axis shows relative intensity. (Courtesy of Mr Malcolm Ward, Glaxo Wellcome Research and Development, Stevenage, UK.)

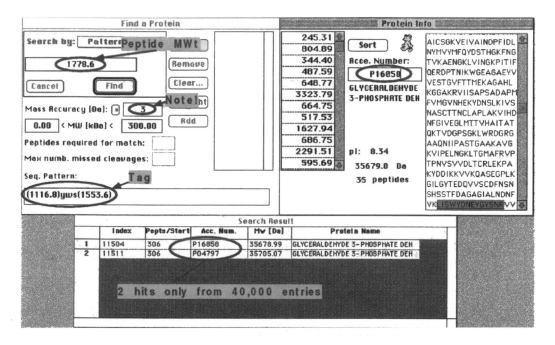

Fig. 12.11. The PeptideSearch™ input form and search result based on data obtained from nano-ESI MS² of *m/z* 890 from RBL spot 2. (Courtesy of Mr Malcolm Ward, Glaxo Wellcome Research and Development, Stevenage, UK.)

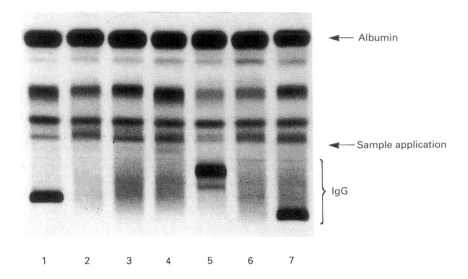

Fig. 12.12. Electrophoresis of human serum samples on an agarose gel. Tracks 2, 3, 4 and 6 show normal serum protein profiles. Tracks 1, 5 and 7 show myeloma patients, who are identified by the excessive production of a particular monoclonal antibody seen in the IgG fraction. (Courtesy of Charles Andrews and Nicholas Cundy, Edgware General Hospital, London.)

of serum samples. Cellulose acetate has the advantage over paper in that it is a much more homogeneous medium, with uniform pore size, and does not adsorb proteins in the way that paper does. There is therefore much less trailing of protein bands and resolution is better, although nothing like as good as that achieved with polyacrylamide gels. The method is, however, far simpler to set up and run. Single samples are normally run on cellulose acetate strips (2.5 cm × 12 cm), although multiple samples are frequently run on wider sheets. The cellulose acetate is first wetted in electrophoresis buffer (pH 8.6 for serum samples) and the sample (1 to 2 μl) loaded as a 1 cm wide strip about one-third of the way along the strip. The ends of the strip make contact with the electrophoresis buffer tanks via a filter paper wick that overlaps the end of the cellulose acetate strip, and electrophoresis conducted at 6 to 8 V cm^{-1} for about 3 h. Following electrophoresis, the strip is stained for protein (see Section 12.3.8), destained, and the bands visualised. A typical serum protein separation shows about six major bands. However, in many disease states, this serum protein profile changes and a clinician can obtain information concerning the disease state of a patient from the altered pattern. Although still frequently used for serum analysis, electrophoresis on cellulose acetate is being replaced by the use of agarose gels, which give similar but somewhat better resolution. A typical example of the analysis of serum on an agarose gel is shown in Fig. 12.12. Similar patterns are obtained when cellulose acetate is used.

Enzymes can easily be detected, in samples electrophoresed on cellulose acetate, by using the zymogram technique. The cellulose strip is laid on a strip of filter paper soaked in buffer and substrate. After an appropriate incubation period, the strips are peeled apart and the paper zymogram treated accordingly to detect enzyme product; hence, it is possible to identify the position of the enzyme activity on the original strip. An alternative approach to detecting and semiquantifying *any* particular protein on a strip is to treat the strip as the equivalent of a protein blot and to probe for the given protein using primary antibody and then enzyme-linked secondary antibody (Section 12.3.9). Substrate colour development indicates the presence of the particular protein and the amount of colour developed in a given time is a semiquantitative measure of the amount of protein. Thus, for example, large numbers of serum samples can be run on a wide sheet, the sheet probed using antibodies, and elevated levels of a particular protein identified in certain samples by increased levels of colour development in these samples.

12.3.7 **Continuous flow electrophoresis**

The continuous flow form of electrophoresis is used for separations in free solution in large-scale productions. Electrophoresis takes place continuously as the

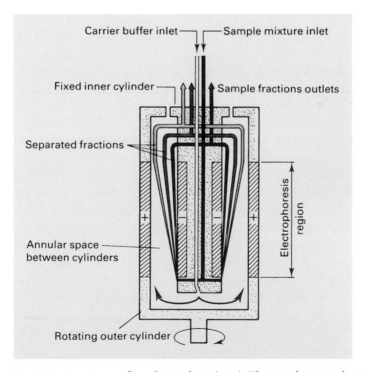

Fig. 12.13. Continuous flow electrophoresis unit. The sample enters the annular space via the sample inlet and is subject to upward movement due to electrophoresis. The result is radial separation into a series of bands (fractions) that may be collected via a series of sample outlets. (Reproduced by permission of AERE Harwell.)

separating material is carried upwards by a flow of carrier buffer through annular space between two vertical concentric cylinders (Fig. 12.13). The outer cylinder is rotated to maintain a stable laminar flow of the buffer solution. An electrical field is applied between the two cylinders, causing the sample material to separate radially as it is carried upwards by the buffer flow. At the top of the inner cylinder a series of radial slits enables the buffer stream to be separated into as many as 30 individual fractions.

Equipment suitable for large-scale separations is now available commercially. However, it would be fair to say that resolution is certainly no better, and often worse, than that which can be achieved just as easily and more cheaply by ion-exchange chromatography, a technique that is also highly amenable to large-scale operation. However, this method does have useful applications in the separation of particles and cells such as human erythrocytes, which otherwise are difficult to separate.

12.3.8 Detection, estimation and recovery of proteins in gels

The most commonly used general protein stain for detecting protein on gels is the sulphated trimethylamine dye Coomassie Brilliant Blue R-250 (CBB). Staining is usually carried out using 0.1% (w/v) CBB in methanol:water:glacial acetic acid (45:45:10, by vol.). This acid–methanol mixture acts as a denaturant to precipitate or fix the protein in the gel, which prevents the protein from being washed out whilst it is being stained. Staining of most gels is accomplished in about 2 h and destaining, usually overnight, is achieved by gentle agitation in the same acid–methanol solution but in the absence of the dye. The Coomassie stain is highly sensitive; a very weakly staining band on a polyacrylamide gel would correspond to about 0.1 μg (100 ng) of protein. The CBB stain is not used for staining cellulose acetate (or indeed protein blots) because it binds quite strongly to the paper. In this case, proteins are first denatured by brief immersion of the strip in 10% (v/v) trichloroacetic acid, and then immersed in a solution of a dye that does not stain the support material, for example Procion blue. Amido black or Procion S.

Although the Coomassie stain is highly sensitive, many workers require greater sensitivity and use a silver stain. Silver stains are based either on techniques developed for histology or on methods based on the photographic process. In either case, silver ions (Ag^+) are reduced to metallic silver on the protein, where the silver is deposited to give a black or brown band. Silver stains can be used immediately after electrophoresis, or, alternatively, after staining with CBB. With the latter approach, the major bands on the gel can be identified with CBB and then minor bands, not detected with CBB, resolved using the silver stain. The silver stain is at least 100 times more sensitive than Coomassie Brilliant Blue, detecting proteins down to 0.1 ng amounts.

Glycoproteins have traditionally been detected on protein gels by use of the periodic acid–Schiff (PAS) stain. This allows components of a mixture of glycoproteins to be distinguished. However, the PAS stain is not very sensitive and often gives very weak, red-pink bands, difficult to observe on a gel. A far more sensitive method used nowadays is to blot the gel (Section 12.3.9) and use lectins to detect the glycoproteins. Lectins are protein molecules that bind carbohydrates, and different lectins have been found that have different specificities for different types of carbohydrate. For example, certain lectins recognise mannose, fucose, or terminal glucosamine of the carbohydrate side-chains of glycoproteins. The sample to be analysed is run on a number of tracks of an SDS-polyacrylamide gel. Coloured bands appear at the point where the lectins bind if each blotted track is incubated with a different lectin, washed, incubated with a horseradish peroxidase-linked antibody to the lectin, and then peroxidase substrate added. In this way, by testing a protein sample against a series of lectins, it is possible to determine not only that a protein is a *glyco*protein, but to obtain information about the type of glycosylation.

Quantitative analysis (i.e. measurements of the relative amounts of different proteins in a sample) can be achieved by scanning densitometry. A number of commercial scanning densitometers are available, and work by passing the stained gel track over a beam of light (laser) and measuring the transmitted light. A graphic presentation of protein zones (peaks of absorbance) against migration distance is produced, and peak areas can be calculated to obtain quantitative data. However, such data must be interpreted with caution because there is only a limited range of protein concentrations over which there is a linear relationship between absorbance and concentration. Also, equal amounts of different proteins do not always stain equally with a given stain, so any data comparing the relative amounts of protein can only be semiquantitative. An alternative and much cheaper way of obtaining such data is to cut out the stained bands of interest, elute the dye by shaking overnight in a known volume of 50% pyridine, and then to measure spectrophotometrically the amount of colour released. More recently gel documentation systems have been developed, which are replacing scanning densitometers. Such benchtop systems comprise a video imaging unit (computer linked) attached to a small 'darkroom' unit that is fitted with a choice of white or ultraviolet light (transilluminator). Gel images can be stored on the computer, enhanced accordingly and printed as required on a thermal printer, thus eliminating the need for wet developing in a purpose built darkroom, as is the case for traditional photography.

Although gel electrophoresis is used generally as an analytical tool, it can be utilised to separate proteins in a gel to achieve protein purification. Protein bands can be cut of protein blots and sequence data obtained by placing the blot in a protein sequencer (see Section 6.4.3). Stained protein bands can be cut out of protein gels and the protein recovered by electrophoresis of the protein out of the gel piece (electroelution). A number of different designs of electroelution cells are commercially available, but perhaps the easiest method is to seal the gel piece in buffer in a dialysis sac and place the sac in buffer between two electrodes. Protein will electrophorese out of the gel piece towards the appropriate electrode but will be retained by the dialysis sac. After electroelution, the current is reversed for a few seconds to drive off any protein that has adsorbed to the wall of the dialysis sac and then the protein solution within the sac is recovered.

12.3.9 **Protein (western) blotting**

Although essentially an analytical technique, PAGE does of course achieve fractionation of a protein mixture during the electrophoresis process. It is possible to
make use of this fractionation to examine further individual separated proteins.
The first step is to transfer or blot the pattern of separated proteins from the gel on
to a sheet of nitrocellulose paper. The method is known as protein blotting, or
western blotting by analogy with Southern blotting (Section 2.10), the equivalent
method used to recover DNA samples from an agarose gel. Transfer of the proteins
from the gel to nitrocellulose can be achieved in one of two ways. In capillary blotting, the gel is placed on a wet pad of buffer-soaked filter paper and a sheet of nitrocellulose placed on the gel. Buffer is then drawn through the gel by placing a pad of
dry absorbent material (usually filter paper) followed by a heavy weight on top of
the nitrocellulose sheet. Passage of buffer by capillary action through the gel
carries the separated proteins on to the nitrocellulose sheet, to which they bind
irreversibly by hydrophobic interaction. The process is carried out overnight, but
because of the small pore size of the acrylamide gel, only a limited amount of
buffer travels through the gel in this time, so that only a fraction (10% to 20%) of
each protein in the gel is transferred in this way. A quicker (a few hours) and more
efficient method of transfer is achieved by electroblotting. In this method a sandwich of gel and nitrocellulose is compressed in a cassette and immersed, in buffer,
between two parallel electrodes (Fig. 12.14). A current is passed at right angles to
the gel, which causes the separated proteins to electrophorese out of the gel and
into the nitrocellulose sheet. The nitrocellulose with its transferred protein is
referred to as a blot. Once transferred on to nitrocellulose, the separated proteins
can be examined further. This involves probing the blot, usually using an antibody to detect a specific protein. The blot is firstly incubated in a protein solution,
for example 10% (w/v) bovine serum albumin, or 5% (w/v) non-fat dried milk (the
so-called blotto technique), which will block all remaining hydrophobic binding
sites on the nitrocellulose sheet. The blot is then incubated in a dilution of an antiserum (primary antibody) directed against the protein of interest. This IgG molecule will bind to the blot if it detects its antigen, thus identifying the protein of
interest. In order to visualise this interaction the blot is incubated further in a
solution of a secondary antibody, which is directed against the IgG of the species
that provided the primary antibody. For example, if the primary antibody was
raised in a rabbit then the secondary antibody would be anti-rabbit IgG. This secondary antibody is appropriately labelled so that the interaction of the secondary
antibody with the primary antibody can be visualised on the blot. Anti-species IgG
molecules are readily available commercially, with a choice of a different labels
attached. One of the most common detection methods is to use an enzyme-linked
secondary antibody (Fig. 12.15). In this case, following treatment with enzyme-
labelled secondary antibody, the blot is incubated in enzyme–substrate solution,
when the enzyme converts the substrate into an insoluble coloured product that is
precipitated onto the nitrocellulose. The presence of a coloured band therefore
indicates the position of the protein of interest. By careful comparisons of the blot

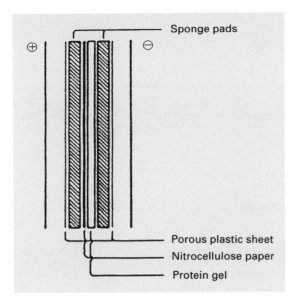

Fig. 12.14. Diagrammatic representation of an electroblotting set-up. The gel to be blotted is placed on top of a sponge pad saturated in buffer. The nitrocellulose sheet is then placed on top of the gel, followed by a second sponge pad. This sandwich is supported between two rigid porous plastic sheets and held together with two elastic bands. The sandwich is then placed between parallel electrodes in a buffer reservoir and an electric current passed. The sandwich must be placed such that the immobilising medium is between the gel and the anode for SDS-polyacrylamide gels, because all the proteins carry a negative charge.

with a stained gel of the same sample, the protein of interest can be identified. The enzyme used in enzyme-linked antibodies is usually either alkaline phosphatase, which converts colourless 5-bromo-4-chloro-indolylphosphate (BCIP) substrate into a blue product, or horseradish peroxidase, which, with H_2O_2 as a substrate, oxidises either 3-amino-9-ethylcarbazole into an insoluble brown product, or 4-chloro-1-naphthol into an insoluble blue product. An alternative approach to the detection of horseradish peroxidase is to use the method of enhanced chemiluminescence (ECL). In the presence of hydrogen peroxide and the chemiluminescent substrate luminol (Fig. 12.16) horseradish peroxidase oxidises the luminol with concomitant production of light, the intensity of which is increased 1000-fold by the presence of a chemical enhancer. The light emission can be detected by exposing the blot to a photographic film. Corresponding ECL substrates are available for use with alkaline-phosphatase-labelled antibodies. The principle behind the use of enzyme-linked antibodies to detect antigens in blots is highly analogous to that used in enzyme-linked immunosorbent assays (Section 4.7).

Although enzymes are commonly used as markers for second antibodies, other markers can also be used. These include:

[125]*I-labelled secondary antibody* Binding to the blot is detected by autoradiography (Section 14.2.3).

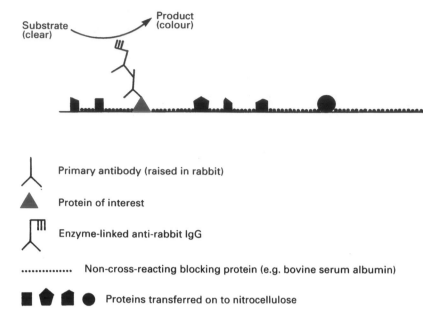

Fig. 12.15. The use of enzyme-linked second antibodies in immunodetection of protein blots. (1) The primary antibody (e.g. raised in a rabbit) detects the protein of interest on the blot. (2) Enzyme-linked anti-rabbit IgG detects the primary antibody. (3) Addition of enzyme substrate results in coloured product deposited at the site of protein of interest on the blot.

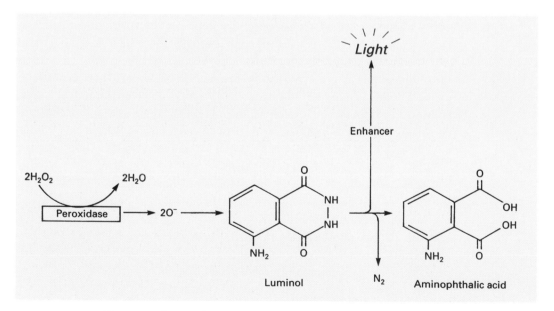

Fig. 12.16. The use of enhanced chemiluminescence to detect horseradish peroxidase.

Fluorescein isothiocyanate-labelled secondary antibody. This fluorescent label is detected by exposing the blot to ultraviolet light.

^{125}I-*labelled protein A.* Protein A is purified from *Staphylococcus aureus* and specifically binds to the Fc region of IgG molecules. ^{125}I-labelled protein A is therefore used instead of a second antibody, and binding to the blot is detected by autoradiography.

Gold-labelled secondary antibodies. Second antibodies (anti-species IgG) coated with minute gold particles are commercially available. These are directly visible as a red colour when they bind to the primary antibody on the blot.

Biotinylated secondary antibodies. Biotin is a small molecular weight vitamin that binds strongly to the egg protein avidin ($K_d = 102^{-5}$ M). The blot is incubated with biotinylated second antibody, then incubated further with enzyme-conjugated avidin. Since multiple biotin molecules can be linked to a single antibody molecule, many enzyme-linked avidin molecules can bind to a single biotinylated antibody molecule, thus providing an enhancement of the signal. The enzyme used is usually alkaline phosphatase or horseradish peroxidase.

In addition to the use of labelled antibodies or proteins, other probes are sometimes used. For example, radioactively labelled DNA can be used to detect DNA-binding proteins on a blot. The blot is first incubated in a solution of radiolabelled DNA, then washed, and an autoradiograph of the blot made. The presence of radioactive bands, detected on the autoradiograph, identifies the positions of the DNA-binding proteins on the blot.

12.4 ELECTROPHORESIS OF NUCLEIC ACIDS

12.4.1 Agarose gel electrophoresis of DNA

For the majority of DNA samples, electrophoretic separation is carried out in agarose gels. This is because most DNA molecules and their fragments that are analysed routinely are considerably larger than proteins and therefore, because most DNA fragments would be unable to enter a polyacrylamide gel, the larger pore size of an agarose gel is required. For example, the commonly used plasmid pBR322 has an M_r of 2.4×10^6. However, rather than use such large numbers it is more convenient to refer to DNA size in terms of the number of base-pairs. Although, originally, DNA size was referred to in terms of base-pairs (bp) or kilo-base-pairs (kbp), it has now become the accepted nomenclature to abbreviate kbp to simply kb when referring to double-stranded DNA. pBR322 is therefore 4.36 kb. Even a small restriction fragment of 1 kb has an M_r of 620 000. When talking about single-stranded DNA it is common to refer to size in terms of nucleotides (nt). Since the charge per unit length (due to the phosphate groups) in any given fragment of DNA is the same, all DNA samples should move towards the anode with the same mobility under an applied electrical field. However, separation in agarose gels is achieved due to resistance to their movement caused by the gel matrix. The largest molecules will have the most difficulty passing through the gel pores (very large molecules may even be blocked completely), whereas the smallest molecules will be relatively unhindered. Consequently the mobility of DNA molecules during gel electrophoresis will depend on size, the smallest molecules moving fastest. This is analogous to the separation of proteins in SDS-polyacrylamide gels (Section 12.3.1), although the analogy is not perfect, as double-stranded DNA molecules form relatively stiff rods and it is not completely understood how they pass through the gel, although it is probable that long DNA molecules pass through the gel pores end-on. While passing through the pores, a DNA molecule will experience drag; so the longer the molecule, the more it will be retarded by each pore. Sideways movement may become more important for very small double-stranded DNA and for the more flexible single-stranded DNA. It will be obvious from the above that gel concentrations must be chosen to suit the size range of the molecules to be separated. Gels containing 0.3% agarose will separate double-stranded DNA molecules of between 5 and 60 kb size, whereas 2% gels are used for samples of between 0.1 and 3 kb. Many laboratories routinely use 0.8% gels, which are suitable for separating DNA molecules in the range 0.5 to 10 kb. Since agarose gels separate DNA according to size, the M_r of a DNA fragment may be determined from its electrophoretic mobility by running a number of standard DNA markers of known M_r on the same gel. This is most conveniently achieved by running a sample of bacteriophage λ DNA (49 kb) that has been cleaved with a restriction enzyme such as *Eco*RI. Since the base sequence of λ DNA is known, and the cleavage sites for *Eco*RI are known, this generates fragments of accurately known size (Fig. 12.17).

DNA gels are invariably run as horizontal, submarine or submerged gels; so named because such a gel is totally immersed in buffer. Agarose, dissolved in gel buffer by boiling, is poured onto a glass or plastic plate, surrounded by a wall of adhesive tape or a plastic frame to provide a gel about 3 mm in depth. Loading wells are formed by placing a plastic well-forming template or comb in the poured gel solution, and removing this comb once the gel has set. The gel is placed in the electrophoresis tank, covered with buffer, and samples loaded by directly injecting the sample into the wells. Samples are prepared by dissolving them in a buffer solution that contains sucrose, glycerol or Ficoll, which makes the solution dense and allows it to sink to the bottom of the well. A dye such as bromophenol blue is also included in the sample solvent; it makes it easier to see the sample that is being loaded and also acts as a marker of the electrophoresis front. No stacking gel (Section 12.3.1) is needed for the electrophoresis of DNA because the mobilities of DNA molecules are much greater in the well than in the gel, and therefore all the molecules in the well pile up against the gel within a few minutes of the current being turned on, forming a tight band at the start of the run. General purpose gels are approximately 25 cm long and 12 cm wide, and are run at a voltage gradient of about 1.5 V cm^{-1} overnight. A higher voltage would cause excessive heating. For rapid analyses that do not need extensive separation of DNA molecules, it is common to use minigels that are less than 10 cm long. In this way information can be obtained in 2 to 3 h.

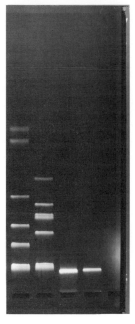

4 3 2 1

Fig. 12.17. Photograph showing four tracks from a 0.8% agarose submarine gel. The gel was run at 40 V in Tris/borate/EDTA buffer for 16 h, stained with ethidium bromide and viewed under ultraviolet light. Sample loadings were about 0.5 μg of DNA per track. Tracks 1 and 2, λ DNA (49 kb). Track 3, λ DNA cleaved with the enzyme EcoRI to generate fragments of the following size (in order from the origin): 21.80 kb, 7.52 kb, 5.93 kb, 5.54 kb, 4.80 kb, 3.41 kb. Track 4, λ DNA cleaved with the enzyme HindIII to generate fragments of the following size (in order from the origin): 23.70 kb, 9.46 kb, 6.75 kb, 4.26 kb, 2.26 kb, 1.98 kb. (Courtesy of Stephen Boffey, University of Hertfordshire.)

Once the system has been run, the DNA in the gel needs to be stained and visualised. The reagent most widely used is the fluorescent dye ethidium bromide. The gel is rinsed gently in a solution of ethidium bromide ($0.5\ \mu g\ cm^{-3}$) and then viewed under ultraviolet light (300 nm wavelength). Ethidium bromide is a cyclic planar molecule that binds between the stacked base-pairs of DNA (i.e. it intercalates) (Section 2.8.3). The ethidium bromide concentration therefore builds up at the site of the DNA bands and under ultraviolet light the DNA bands fluoresce orange-red. As little as 10 ng of DNA can be visualised as a 1 cm wide band. It should be noted that extensive viewing of the DNA with ultraviolet light can result in damage of the DNA by nicking and base-pair dimerisation. This is of no consequence if a gel is only to be viewed, but obviously viewing of the gel should be kept to a minimum if the DNA is to be recovered (see below). It is essential to protect one's eyes by wearing goggles when ultraviolet light is used. If viewing of gels under ultraviolet is carried out for long periods, a plastic mask that covers the whole face should be used to avoid 'sunburn'.

12.4.2 **DNA sequencing gels**

Although agarose gel electrophoresis of DNA is a 'workhorse' technique for the molecular biologist, a different form of electrophoresis has to be used when DNA sequences are to be determined. Whichever DNA sequencing method is used (Section 2.14), the final analysis usually involves separating single-stranded DNA molecules shorter than about 1000 nt and differing in size by only 1 nt. To achieve this it is necessary to have a small-pored gel and so acrylamide gels are used instead of agarose. For example, 3.5% polyacrylamide gels are used to separate DNA in the range 80 to 1000 nt and 12% gels to resolve fragments of between 20 and 100 nt. If a wide range of sizes is being analysed it is often convenient to run a gradient gel, for example from 3.5% to 7.5%. Sequencing gels are run in the presence of denaturing agents, urea and formamide. Since it is necessary to separate DNA molecules that are very similar in size, DNA sequencing gels tend to be very long (100 cm) to maximise the separation achieved. A typical DNA sequencing gel is shown in Fig. 2.37.

As mentioned above, electrophoresis in agarose can be used as preparative method for DNA. The DNA bands of interest can be cut out of the gel and the DNA recovered by: (a) electroelution, (b) macerating the gel piece in buffer, centrifuging and collecting the supernatant; or, (c) if low melting point agarose is used, melting the gel piece and diluting with buffer. In each case, the DNA is finally recovered by precipitation of the supernatant with ethanol.

12.4.3 **Pulsed-field gel electrophoresis**

The agarose gel methods for DNA described above can fractionate DNA of 60 kb or less. The introduction of pulsed-field gel electrophoresis (PFGE) and the further development of variations on the basic technique now means that DNA fragments up to 2×10^3 kb can be separated. This therefore allows the separation of whole chromosomes by electrophoresis. The method basically involves electrophoresis in agarose where two electric fields are applied alternately at different angles for defined time periods (e.g. 60 s). Activation of the first electric field causes the coiled molecules to be stretched in the horizontal plane and start to move through the gel. Interruption of this field and application of the second field force the molecule to move in the new direction. Since there is a length-dependent relaxation behaviour when a long-chain molecule undergoes conformational change in an electric field, the smaller a molecule, the quicker it realigns itself with the new field and is able to continue moving through the gel. Larger molecules take longer to realign. In this way, with continual reversing of the field, smaller molecules draw ahead of larger molecules and separate according to size. Figure 12.18 shows the separation of yeast chromosomes that vary in size from 260 to 850 kb. Needless to say the physics of designing a PFGE system is complex and in recent years a number of different developments on the same basic theme have resulted in a bewildering array of related techniques. Detailed description of these techniques is beyond the scope of this chapter but the names of a few of these techniques

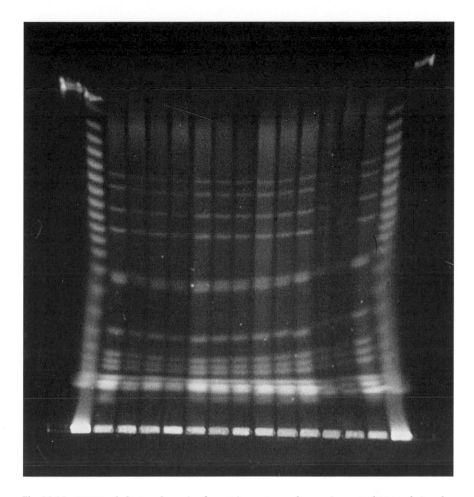

Fig. 12.18. CHEF gel electrophoresis of yeast (repeat samples run in central 13 tracks) and bacteriophage λ multimers (the 'ladders' on the two outside lanes). Every step of the ladder in the two outer lanes is about 43.5 kb and 20 steps are resolved up to 850 kb. The yeast chromosomes are of sizes 260, 290, 370, 460, 580/600, 700, 780, 820 and 850 kb. (Courtesy of Margit Burmeister, University of Michigan.)

indicate the principles involved, for example orthogonal field alternating gel electrophoresis (OFAGE), field inversion gel electrophoresis (FIGE), transverse alternating field gel electrophoresis (TAFE), contour-clamped homogeneous electric field electrophoresis (CHEF), and rotating field electrophoresis (RFE).

12.4.4 Electrophoresis of RNA

Like that of DNA, electrophoresis of RNA is usually carried out in agarose gels, and the principle of the separation, based on size, is the same. Often one requires a rapid method for checking the integrity of RNA immediately following extraction but before deciding whether to process it further. This can be achieved easily by electrophoresis in a 2% agarose gel in about 1 h. Ribosomal RNAs (18 S and 28 S) are clearly resolved and any degradation (seen as a smear) or DNA contamination is seen easily. However, if greater resolution is required, a smaller-pored acrylamide gel is used to enhance resolution, for example to resolve transfer RNAs (4 S) from 5 S ribosomal RNA. This can be achieved on a 2.5% to 5% acrylamide gradient gel with an overnight run. Both these methods involve running native RNA. There will almost certainly be some secondary structure within the RNA molecule owing to intramolecular hydrogen bonding (see e.g. the clover leaf structure of tRNA, Section 2.2). For this reason native RNA run on gels can be stained and visualised with ethidium bromide. However, if the study objective is to determine RNA size by gel electrophoresis, then full denaturation of the RNA is needed to prevent hydrogen bond formation within or even between polynucleotides that will otherwise affect the electrophoretic mobility. There are three denaturing agents (formaldehyde, glyoxal and methylmercuric hydroxide) that are compatible with both RNA and agarose. Either one of these may be incorporated into the agarose gel and electrophoresis buffer, and the sample is heat denatured in the presence of the denaturant prior to electrophoresis. After heat denaturation, each of these agents forms adducts with the amino groups of guanine and uracil, thereby preventing hydrogen bond reformation at room temperature during electrophoresis. It is also necessary to run denaturing gels if the RNA is to be blotted (northern blots, Section 2.10) and probed, to ensure that the base sequence is available to the probe. Denatured RNA stains only very weakly with ethidium bromide, so acridine orange is commonly used to visualise RNA on denaturing gels. However, it should be noted that many workers will be using radiolabelled RNA and will therefore identify bands by autoradiography. An example of the electrophoresis of RNA is shown in Fig. 12.19.

12.5 CAPILLARY ELECTROPHORESIS

The technique has variously been referred to as high performance capillary electrophoresis (HPCE), capillary zone electrophoresis (CZE), free solution capillary electrophoresis (FSCE) and capillary electrophoresis (CE), but the term CE is the one most common nowadays. Capillary electrophoresis can be used to separate a wide spectrum of biological molecules including amino acids, peptides, proteins, DNA fragments (e.g. synthetic oligonucleotides) and nucleic acids, as well as any number of small organic molecules such as drugs or even metal ions (see below). The method has also been applied successfully to the problem of chiral separations (Section 13.6.5).

As the name suggests, capillary electrophoresis involves electrophoresis of samples in very narrow-bore tubes (typically 50 μm internal diameter, 300 μm external diameter). One advantage of using capillaries is that they reduce problems resulting from heating effects. Because of the small diameter of the tubing there is a large surface-to-volume ratio, which gives enhanced heat dissipation. This helps to eliminate both convection currents and zone broadening owing to

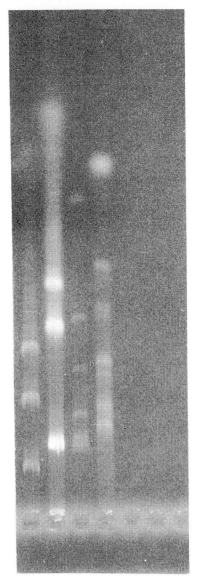

1   2   3   4

Fig. 12.19. Gel electrophoresis of RNA in a 1.4% agarose gel. Track 1 is total RNA from the tobacco plant denatured with glyoxal prior to running. Track 2 is the same sample, *not* denatured. The two faster-running major bands are 18 S and 25 S ribosomal RNA. The slower running major band is nuclear DNA. Tracks 3 and 4 show a mixture of RNA marker fragments, with (track 3) and without (track 4) glyoxal treatment. The sizes of the marker RNA fragments are 0.24, 1.4, 2.4, 4.4, 7.5 and 9.5 kb. Note that, with each sample, denaturation results in lower mobilities for the components of each sample. (Courtesy of Debbie Cook and Robert Slater, Division of Biosciences, University of Hertfordshire.)

increased diffusion caused by heating. It is therefore not necessary to include a stabilising medium in the tube and allows free-flow electrophoresis.

Theoretical considerations of CE generate two important equations:

$$t = \frac{L^2}{\mu V} \qquad (12.4)$$

where t is the migration time for a solute, L is the tube length, μ is the electrophoretic mobility of the solute, and V is the applied voltage.

The separation efficiency, in terms of the total number of theoretical plates, N, is given by

$$N = \frac{\mu V}{2D} \qquad (12.5)$$

where D is the solute's diffusion coefficient.

From these equations it can be seen, first, that the column length plays no role in separation efficiency, but that it has an important influence on migration time and hence analysis time, and, secondly, high separation efficiencies are best achieved through the use of high voltages (μ and D are dictated by the solute and are not easily manipulated).

It therefore appears that the ideal situation is to apply as high a voltage as possible to as short a capillary as possible. However, there are practical limits to this approach. As the capillary length is reduced, the amount of heat that must be dissipated increases owing to the decreasing electrical resistance of the capillary. At the same time the surface area available for heat dissipations is decreasing. Therefore at some point significant thermal effect will occur, placing a practical limit on how short a tube can be used. Also the higher the voltage that is applied, the greater the current, and therefore the heat generated. In practical terms a compromise between voltage used and capillary length is required. Voltages of 10 to 50 kV with capillaries of 50 to 100 cm are commonly used.

The basic apparatus for CE is shown diagrammatically in Fig. 12.20. A small plug of sample solution (typically 5 to 30 μm^3) is introduced into the anode end of a fused silica capillary tube containing an appropriate buffer. Sample application is carried out in one of two ways: by high voltage injection or by pressure injection.

(i) *High voltage injection.* With the high voltage switched off, the buffer reservoir at the positive electrode is replaced by a reservoir containing the sample, and a plug of sample (e.g. 5 to 30 μm^3 of a 1 mg cm^{-3} solution) is introduced into the capillary by briefly applying high voltage. The sample reservoir is then removed, the buffer reservoir replaced, voltage again applied and the separation is then commenced.

(ii) *Pressure injection.* The capillary is removed from the anodic buffer reservoir and inserted through an air-tight seal into the sample solution. A second tube provides pressure to the sample solution, which forces the sample into the capillary. The capillary is then removed, replaced in the anodic buffer and a voltage applied to initiate electrophoresis.

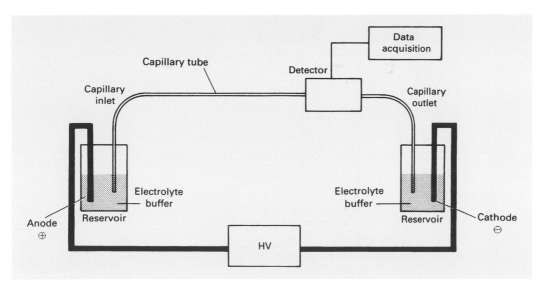

Fig. 12.20. Diagrammatic representation of a typical capillary electrophoresis apparatus.

A high voltage (up to 50 kV) is then put across the capillary tube and component molecules in the injected sample migrate at different rates along the length of the capillary tube. Electrophoretic migration causes the movement of charged molecules in solution towards an electrode of opposite charge. Owing to this electrophoretic migration, positive and negative sample molecules migrate at different rates. However, although analytes are separated by electrophoretic migration, they are all drawn towards the cathode by electroendosmosis (Section 12.1). Since this flow is quite strong, the rate of electroendosmotic flow usually being much greater than the electrophoretic velocity of the analytes, all ions, regardless of charge sign, and neutral species are carried towards the cathode. Positively charged molecules reach the cathode first because the combination of electrophoretic migration and electroosmotic flow cause them to move fastest. As the separated molecules approach the cathode, they pass through a viewing window where they are detected by an ultraviolet monitor that transmits a signal to a recorder, integrator or computer. Typical run times are between 10 and 30 min. A typical capillary electrophoretograph is shown in Fig. 12.21.

This free solution method is the simplest and most widely practised mode of capillary electrophoresis. However, while the generation of ionised groups on the capillary wall is advantageous via the introduction of electroendosmotic flow, it can also sometimes be a disadvantage. For example, protein adsorption to the capillary wall can occur with cationic groups on protein surfaces binding to the ionised silanols. This can lead to smearing of the protein as it passes through the capillary (recognised as peak broadening) or, worse, complete loss of protein due to total adsorption on the walls. Some workers therefore use coated tubes where a neutral coating group has been used to block the silanol groups. This of course

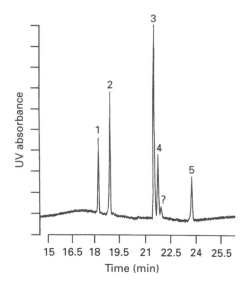

Fig. 12.21. Capillary electrophoresis of five structurally related peptides. Column length was 100 cm and the separation voltage 50 kV. Peptides were detected by their ultraviolet absorbance at 200 nm.

Peptide	
1	Lys-Arg-Pro-Pro-Gly-Phe-Ser-Pro-Phe-Arg
2	Met-Lys-Arg-Pro-Pro-Gly-Phe-Ser-Pro-Phe-Arg
3	Arg-Pro-Pro-Gly-Phe-Ser-Pro-Phe-Arg
4	Ser-Arg-Pro-Pro-Gly-Phe-Ser-Pro--Phe-Arg
5	Ile-Ser-Arg-Pro-Pro-Gly-Phe-Ser-Pro-Phe-Arg

(Courtesy of Patrick Camilleri and George Okafo, SmithKline Beecham Pharmaceuticals Ltd.)

eliminates electroendosmotic flow. Therefore, during electrophoresis in coated capillaries, neutral species are immobile while acid species migrate to the anode and basic species to the cathode. Since detection normally takes place at only one end of the capillary, only one class of species can be detected at a time in an analysis using a coated capillary.

A range of variations on this basic technique also exist. For example, as seen above, in normal CE neutral molecules do not separate but rather travel as a single band. However, separation of neutral molecules can be achieved by including a surfactant such as SDS with the buffer. Above a certain concentration some surfactant molecules agglomerate and form micelles, which, under the influence of an applied electric field, will migrate towards the appropriate electrode. Solutes will interact and partition with the moving micelles. If a solute interacts strongly it will reach the detector later than one which partitions to a lesser degree. This method is known as micellular electrokinetic capillary electrophoresis (MECC). Since ionic solutes will also migrate under the applied field, separation by MECC is due to a combination of both electrophoresis and chromatography.

Original developments in CE concentrated on the separation of peptides and proteins, but in recent years CE has been successfully applied to the separation of a range of other biological molecules. The following provides a few examples.

In the past, peptide analysis has been performed routinely using reversed-phase HPLC, achieving separation based on hydrophobicity differences between peptides. Peptide separation by CE is now also routinely carried out, and is particularly useful, for example as a means of quality (purity) control for peptides and proteins produced by preparative HPLC. Figure 12.21 shows the impressive separation that can be achieved for peptides with very similar structures.

High purity synthetic oligodeoxyribonucleotides are necessary for a range of applications including use as hybridisation probes in diagnostic and gene cloning experiments, use as primers for DNA sequencing and the polymerase chain reaction (PCR), use in site-directed mutagenesis and use as antisense therapeutics. CE can provide a rapid method for analysing the purity of such samples. For example, analysis of an 18-mer antisense oligonucleotide containing contaminant fragments (8-mer to 17-mer) can be achieved in only 5 min.

Point mutations in DNA, such as occur in a range of human diseases, can be identified by CE.

CE can be used to quantify DNA. For example, CE analysis of PCR products from HIV-I allowed the identification of between 200 000 and 500 000 viral particles per cubic centimetre of serum.

Chiral compounds can be resolved using CE. Most work has been carried in free solution using cyclodextrins as chiral selectors.

A range of small molecules, drug and metabolites can be measured in physiological solutions such as urine and serum. These include amino acids (over 50 are found in urine), nucleotides, nucleosides, bases, anions such as chloride and sulphate (NO_2^- and NO_3^- can be separated in human plasma) and cations such as Ca^{2+} and Fe^{3+}.

12.6 KEY TERMS

ampholytes	gradient gel	silver stain
capillary blotting	isoelectric focusing	sodium dodecyl sulphate-
capillary electrophoresis	isotachophoresis	polyacrylamide gel electrophoresis
continuous flow electrophoresis	native gel	stacking gel
electroblotting	photopolymerisation	submarine gel
electroelution	primary antibody	submerged gel
electroendosmosis	protein blotting	two-dimensional polyacrylamide gel
electrophoretic mobility	proteome	electrophoresis
enhanced chemiluminescence	pulsed-field gel electrophoresis	western blotting
flat-bed isoelectric focusing	secondary antibody	zymogram
free-radical catalysis	sequence tag	
gel documentation systems	scanning densitometry	

12.7 CALCULATION

Question 1

The following table shows the distance moved in an SDS-polyacrylamide gel by a series of marker proteins of known relative molecular mass (M_r). A newly purified protein (X) run on the same gel showed a single band that had moved a distance of 45 mm. Construct a calibration graph by plotting log M_r versus distance moved for each of the marker proteins and hence determine the M_r of protein X.

Protein	M_r	Distance moved (mm)
Transferrin	78 000	6.0
Bovine serum albumin	66 000	12.5
Ovalbumin (egg albumin)	45 000	32.0
Glyceraldehyde-3-phosphate dehydrogenase	36 000	38.0
Carbonic anhydrase	29 000	50.0
Trypsinogen	24 000	54.0
Soyabean trypsin inhibitor	20 100	61.0
β-Lactoglobulin	18 400[a]	69.0
Myoglobin	17 800	69.0
Lysozyme	14 300	79.0
Cytochrome c	12 400	86.5

a Note: β-lactoglobulin has a molecular mass of 36 800 but is a dimer of two identical subunits of 18 400 molecular mass. Under the reducing conditions of the sample buffer the disulphide bridges linking the subunits are reduced and thus the monomer chains are seen on the gel.

Answer

From the graph you should determine a relative molecular mass for protein X of approximately 31 000. Note that this method is accurate to $\pm$ 10%, so your answer is 31 000 $\pm$ 3100.

12.8 SUGGESTIONS FOR FURTHER READING

ALTRIA, K. D. (1996). *Capillary Electrophoresis Guide Book*. Humana Press, Totowa, NJ. (Detailed theory and practical procedures for the analysis of proteins, nucleic acids and metabolites.)

ANDREWS, A. T. (1986). *Electrophoresis: Theory, Techniques and Biochemical and Clinical Applications*. Oxford University Press, Oxford. (Very comprehensive text on theory and practical details.)

DUNN, M. J. (1993). *Gel Electrophoresis: Proteins*. Bios Scientific, Oxford. (A good introduction to protein electrophoresis.)

HAWCROFT, D. M. (1996). *Electrophoresis: The Basics*. IRL Press, Oxford. (An excellent book on the theory of electrophoretic techniques.)

WALKER, J. M. (1996). *The Protein Protocols Handbook*. Humana Press, Totowa, NJ. (Detailed theory and laboratory protocols for a range of electrophoretic techniques and blotting procedures.)

Chapter 13

Chromatographic techniques

13.1 INTRODUCTION

13.1.1 Distribution coefficients

The Russian botanist Mikhail Tswett is credited with the original development of a separation technique that we now recognise as a form of chromatography. In 1903 he reported the successful separation of a mixture of plant pigments using a column of calcium carbonate and in the process became the first scientist to recognise that chlorophyll was not a single chemical compound. Modern chromatographic techniques take multiple forms, the majority of which can be automated and adapted to deal with large or very small amounts of substances to be separated and purified.

The basis of all forms of chromatography is the partition or distribution coefficient (K_d), which describes the way in which a compound distributes itself between two immiscible phases. For two such immiscible phases A and B, the value for this coefficient is a constant at a given temperature and is given by the expression:

$$\frac{\text{concentration in phase A}}{\text{concentration in phase B}} = K_d \tag{13.1}$$

The term effective distribution coefficient is defined as the total amount, as distinct from the concentration, of substance present in one phase divided by the total amount present in the other phase. It is in fact the distribution coefficient multiplied by the ratio of the volumes of the two phases present. If the distribution coefficient of a compound between two phases A and B is 1, and if this compound is distributed between 10cm³ of A and 1cm³ of B, the concentration in the two phases will be the same, but the total amount of the compound in phase A will be 10 times the amount in phase B.

Basically, all chromatographic systems consist of the stationary phase, which may be a solid, gel, liquid or a solid/liquid mixture that is immobilised, and the mobile phase, which may be liquid or gaseous and which flows over or through the stationary phase. The choice of stationary and mobile phases is made so that the compounds to be separated have different distribution coefficients. This may be achieved by setting up:

(i) an adsorption equilibrium between a stationary solid phase and a mobile liquid phase (adsorption chromatography; hydrophobic interaction chromatography);

(ii) a partition equilibrium between a stationary liquid phase and a mobile liquid or gas phase (partition chromatography; reversed-phase liquid chromatography; ion-pair chromatography; chiral chromatography; gas–liquid chromatography; countercurrent chromatography);

(iii) an ion-exchange equilibrium between a stationary ion exchanger and mobile electrolyte phase (ion-exchange chromatography; chromatofocusing);

(iv) an equilibrium between a liquid phase trapped inside the pores of a stationary porous structure and a mobile liquid phase (molecular exclusion or permeation chromatography);

(v) an equilibrium between a stationary immobilised ligand and a mobile liquid phase (affinity chromatography; immunoaffinity chromatography; lectin affinity chromatography; metal chelate affinity chromatography; dye–ligand chromatography; covalent chromatography).

In practice it is quite common for two or more of these equilibria to be involved simultaneously in a particular chromatographic separation.

13.1.2 Modes of chromatography

Chromatography separations may be achieved by two basic techniques:

(i) *Column chromatography* in which the stationary phase attached to a suitable matrix (an inert, insoluble support) is packed into a glass or metal column and the mobile phase passed through the column either by gravity feed or by use of a pumping system or applied gas pressure. This is the most commonly used mode of chromatography.

(ii) *Thin-layer or planar chromatography* in which the stationary phase attached to a suitable matrix is coated thinly onto a glass, plastic or metal foil plate. The mobile liquid phase passes across the thin-layer plate, held either horizontally or vertically, by capillary action. This mode of chromatography has the practical advantage over column chromatography that a large number of samples can be studied simultaneously. Planar chromatography includes paper chromatography in which the stationary liquid phase is supported by the cellulose fibres of a paper sheet. As with thin-layer chromatography on a plate, the mobile phase is passed over the immobilised stationary phase by capillary action. This form of chromatography is one of the older forms and has few serious biochemical applications today.

The two chromatographic techniques can be subdivided on the basis of the development mode. This relates to the way the sample and the mobile phase are applied to the stationary phase.

In the zonal or elution development mode, the sample is dissolved in a suitable solvent and applied to the stationary phase as a narrow, discrete band. Mobile phase, commonly referred to as the eluent and normally consisting of an organic solvent or a mixture of solvents possibly incorporating a buffered aqueous system, is then allowed to flow continuously over the stationary phase, resulting in the progressive separation of the sample components (analytes). The analytes with the highest solubility in the mobile phase will move along the stationary phase fastest. To facilitate separation, the composition of the mobile phase may be gradually changed, for example with respect to pH or polarity. Successful zonal separation results in pure samples of all the analytes and is the most common form of chromatography. When a particular analyte has been removed from the column by the mobile phase, it is said to have been eluted.

In displacement or affinity development mode the sample is again applied to the stationary phase as a discrete band but separation of the analytes is achieved not on the basis of the physical characteristics of the mobile phase but rather on the fact that it contains a specific solute that has a higher affinity for the stationary phase than have the analytes. Thus, as the mobile phase is added, this agent displaces the analytes from the stationary phase in a competitive fashion, resulting in their movement along the stationary phase and eventual elution from the column in the order of their affinity for the stationary phase, the one with the lowest affinity moving fastest.

In the frontal development mode the sample is continuously added to the stationary phase thereby forcing the analytes along the stationary phase in the order of their affinity for the stationary phase. The analyte with the lowest affinity accumulates at the front of the moving sample band and, whilst a pure sample of it can be isolated, pure samples of the other analytes cannot. In practice, the technique is effectively restricted to the analysis of a single trace impurity in an otherwise pure sample.

13.1.3 Performance of column chromatography

The principle of a column chromatographic separation may be depicted by considering a column packed with a solid granular stationary phase to a height of 5 cm, surrounded by the mobile liquid phase of which there is 1 cm^3 per cm of column, as shown in Fig. 13.1. If 32 µg of a compound is added to the column in 1 cm^3 of mobile phase, then, as this 1 cm^3 moves on to the column to occupy position A, 1 cm^3 of mobile phase will leave the base of the column. If the compound added has an effective distribution coefficient of 1, it will distribute itself equally between the solid and liquid phases (stage 1). If a further 1 cm^3 of mobile phase is introduced on to the column, the mobile phase in section A will move down to B, taking 16 µg of the compound with it, leaving 16 µg at A (stage 2). At both A and B, a redistribution of the compound will occur so that there is 8 µg in the mobile phase and 8 µg in the solid phase. The addition of a further 1 cm^3 of mobile phase to the column displaces the mobile phase in A to B and that in B to C, giving the distribution of the compound as shown in stage 3. Addition of a further 1 cm^3 of mobile phase leads to the distribution shown at stage 4, and a further 1 cm^3 of mobile phase leads to the distribution shown at stage 5.

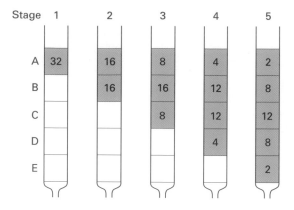

Fig. 13.1. Principle of column chromatographic separation.

It is apparent that after a relatively small number of equilibrations the compound distributes itself symmetrically within a band. It should be equally apparent that if a mixture of two compounds, one having a distribution coefficient of 1 the other a distribution coefficient of 100, was added to the column it would separate rapidly into distinct bands. In a real chromatographic column a very large number of equilibrations occur as the mobile phase passes down the column as a result of more mobile phase being added constantly to the top of the column.

A typical column chromatographic system using a liquid mobile phase consists of the column, a mobile phase reservoir and delivery system, a detector for identifying the separated compounds (analytes) as they emerge in the effluent from the column, a recorder and a fraction collector (Fig. 13.2). The detector and recorder give a continuous record of the presence of the analytes in the effluent, as measured by a physical parameter such as ultraviolet absorption. Each separated analyte is represented by a peak on the chart recorder and the fraction collector allows each individual analyte to be collected separately and studied further if necessary. Liquid column chromatography can be subdivided according to the pressure generated within the column during the separation process. Low pressure liquid chromatography (LPLC) generates pressures of less than 5 bar (1 bar = 14.5 lbf in. $^{-2}$ = 0.1 MPa), since there is little resistance to solvent flow owing to the physical nature of the stationary phase. Medium pressure liquid chromatography (MPLC) generates pressures of between 6 and 50 bar and high pressure liquid chromatography (HPLC) pressures in excess of 50 bar. In practice the distinctions between MPLC and HPLC are often blurred and their equipment and procedures are virtually identical. Both give excellent resolutions and hence the term high performance liquid chromatography is preferred for both of them, since it better describes the chromatography characteristics of the techniques and avoids the misconception that it is the high pressure that is fundamentally responsible for the high performance chromatography.

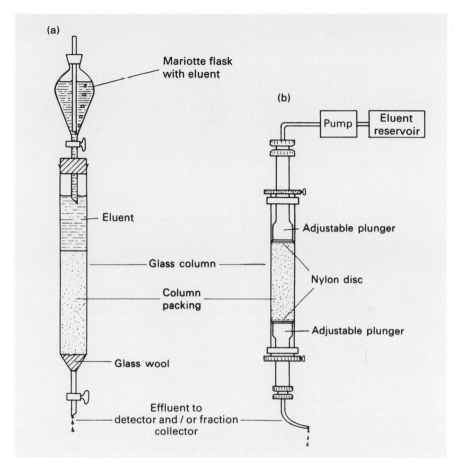

(a)

Mariotte flask
with eluent

(b)

Pump — Eluent reservoir

Eluent

Adjustable plunger

Glass column

Nylon disc

Column packing

Glass wool

Adjustable plunger

Effluent to detector and / or fraction collector

Fig. 13.2. Equipment for column chromatography: (a) simple version; (b) more sophisticated version.

13.2 CHROMATOGRAPHY THEORY AND PRACTICE

13.2.1 Introduction

The successful chromatographic separation of analytes in a mixture depends upon the selection of the most appropriate form of chromatography followed by the optimisation of the experimental conditions associated with the separation. Optimisation requires an understanding of the processes that are occurring during the separation and development and of the calculation of a number of experimental parameters characterising the behaviour of each analyte in the mixture.

In any chromatographic separation two processes occur concurrently to affect the behaviour of each analyte and hence the success of the separation. The first involves the basic mechanisms defining the chromatographic process such as

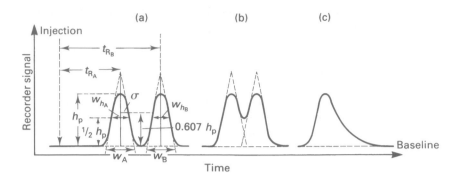

Fig. 13.3. (a) Chromatograph of two compounds showing complete resolution and the calculation of retention times; (b) two compounds giving incomplete resolution and the production of fused peaks; (c) a compound showing excessive tailing.

adsorption, partition, ion-exchange, ion-pairing and molecular exclusion. These mechanisms involve the unique kinetic and thermodynamic processes that characterise the interaction of each analyte with the mobile and stationary phases. The second general process, such as diffusion, tends to oppose the separation and result in non-ideal behaviour of each analyte; such processes are manifest as a broadening or tailing of each analyte band. The challenge is to minimise these secondary processes.

The chromatographic parameters associated with the performance of a given chromatographic system are best illustrated by reference to column chromatography but are equally applicable to planar chromatography.

13.2.2 **The chromatograph: elution time and volume**

A chromatograph is the pictorial record of the detector response as a function of elution time or volume. It consists of a series of peaks, representing the elution of individual analytes, as shown in Fig. 13.3. The retention time t_R for each analyte has two components. The first is the time it takes the analyte molecule to pass through the free spaces between the stationary phase matrix. This space is referred to as the column void volume, V_0, and the time taken to pass through it as the dead time, t_M. The value of t_M will be the same for all analytes and can be measured by using a solute that does not interact with the stationary phase but simply spends all of the elution time in the mobile phase travelling through the void volume. The second component is the time the analyte is retained by the stationary phase, t'_R. This time is characteristic of the analyte. Its value which is referred to as the adjusted retention time, is therefore given by:

$$t'_R = t_R - t_M \tag{13.2}$$

It is common practice to relate the retention time t_R or t'_R for an analyte to a reference internal or external standard (Section 13.2.5). In such cases the relative retention time is often calculated. It is simply the retention time for the analyte divided by that for the standard.

13.2.3 Capacity factor

One of the most important parameters in chromatography is the capacity factor, k'. It is simply the additional time that the analyte takes to elute from the column relative to an unretained or excluded analyte that does not interact with the stationary phase and, by definition, has a k' value of 0. Thus

$$k' = \frac{t_R - t_M}{t_M} = \frac{t'_R}{t_M} \tag{13.3}$$

It is apparent from this equation that if the analyte spends an equal time in the stationary and mobile phases, its t_R would equal $2t_M$ and its k' would be 1, whilst if it spent four times as long in the stationary phases as the mobile phase its k' would equal 4. Note that k' has no units.

If an analyte has a k' of 4 it follows that there will be four times the amount of analyte in the stationary phase than in the mobile phase at any time. It is evident, therefore, that k' is related to the distribution coefficient of the analyte (equation 13.1), which was defined as the relative concentrations of the analyte between the two phases. Since amount and concentration are related by volume, we can write

$$k' = \frac{t'_R}{t_M} = \frac{M_S}{M_M} = k_d \times \frac{V_S}{V_M} \tag{13.4}$$

where M_S is the mass of analyte in the stationary phase, M_M is the mass of analyte in the mobile phase, V_S is the volume of stationary phase, and V_M is the volume of mobile phase.

The ratio V_S/V_M is referred to as the volumetric phase ratio, β. Hence

$$k' = K_d\beta \tag{13.5}$$

Thus the capacity factor for an analyte will increase with both the distribution coefficient between the two phases and the volume of the stationary phase. k' values normally range from 1 to 10. Capacity factors are important because they are independent of the physical dimensions of the column and the rate of flow of mobile phase through it. They can therefore be used to compare the behaviour of an analyte in different chromatographic systems. They are also a reflection of the selectivity of the system which is a measure of its inherent ability to discriminate between two analytes. Such selectivity is expressed by the selectivity or separation factor, α, which can also be viewed as simply the relative retention ratio for the two analytes:

$$\alpha = \frac{k'_A}{k'_B} = \frac{K_{d_A}}{K_{d_B}} = \frac{t'_{R_A}}{t'_{R_B}} \tag{13.6}$$

The selectivity factor is influenced by the chemical nature of the stationary and mobile phases. Some chromatographic mechanisms are inherently highly selective. Good examples are affinity chromatography (Section 13.9) and chiral chromatography (Section 13.6.5).

13.2.4 Column efficiency and resolution

Chromatography columns are considered to consist of a number of adjacent zones in each of which there is sufficient space for an analyte to completely equilibrate between the two phases. Each zone is called a theoretical plate (of which there are N in total in the column) by analogy with distillation columns. The length of column containing one theoretical plate is referred to as the plate height, H, which has units of length normally in micrometres. The numerical value of both N and H for a particular column is expressed by reference to a particular analyte. Plate height is simply related to the width of the analyte peak and the distance it travelled within the column, x, specifically:

$$H = \frac{\sigma^2}{x} \qquad (13.7)$$

where σ is the standard deviation of the Gaussian band (Fig. 13.3). For symmetrical Gaussian peaks, the base width is equal to 4σ and the peak width at the point of inflexion, w_i is equal to 2σ. Hence the value of H can be calculated from the chromatograph by measuring the peak width. The number of theoretical plates in the whole column is therefore given by

$$N = \frac{L}{H} = \frac{Lx}{\sigma^2} \qquad (13.8)$$

where L is the length of the column.

If we consider the position for a peak emerging from the column so that $x = L$ and from knowledge of the fact that the width of the peak at its base, w, obtained from tangents drawn to the two steepest parts of the peak, is equal to 4σ, we can convert equation 13.8 to

$$N = \frac{16L^2}{w^2} \qquad (13.9)$$

If both L and w are measured in units of time rather than length, then equation 13.9 becomes:

$$N = 16\left(\frac{t_R}{w}\right)^2 \qquad (13.10)$$

Equations 13.9 and 13.10 therefore represent alternative ways to calculate the column efficiency in theoretical plates. The value of N, which has no units, can be as high as 50 000 to 100 000 per metre for efficient columns and the corresponding value of H can be as little as a few micrometres. The smaller the plate height (the larger the value of N), the narrower is the analyte peak (Fig. 13.4). However, opposing this narrowing of the analyte peak is the process of diffusion. Fick's law of diffusion (equation 8.10) states that a compound will diffuse from a region of high concentration to one of low concentration at a rate determined by the concentra-

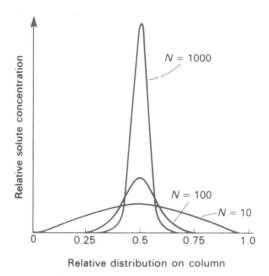

Fig. 13.4. Relationship betweeen the number of theoretical plates (N) and the shape of the analyte peak.

tion gradient and the diffusion coefficient of the analyte. Thus the analyte within a narrow band will tend to diffuse outwards, resulting in band broadening. There are other reasons why bands broaden. First, there is simply the fact that it takes a finite time to apply the analyte mixture to the column, so that the part of the sample applied first will already be moving along the column by the time the final part is applied. The part of the sample applied first will elute at the front of the peak. Secondly, in packed columns there are multiple pathways between the particles for both mobile phase and analytes and these pathways will vary in length and hence elution time. The smaller the particle size the less serious is this problem and in open tubular columns the phenomenon is totally absent, which is one of the reasons why they give shorter elution times and better resolution than packed columns.

In some chromatographic separations, the ideal Gaussian-shaped peaks are not obtained, but rather asymmetrical peaks are produced. In cases where there is a gradual rise and a sharp fall in the peak, a phenomenon known as fronting, the most common cause is overloading the column. Reducing the amount of mixture applied to the column often resolves the problem. In cases where the rise in the peak is normal but the tail is protracted, a phenomenon known as tailing (Fig. 13.3), the probable explanation is the retention of analyte by a few 'active sites' on the stationary phase, commonly on the inert support matrix. Such sites strongly adsorb molecules of the analyte and only slowly release them. The problem can be overcome by chemically removing the sites, most commonly by treating the matrix with a silanising reagent such as hexamethyldisilazine. This process is sometimes referred to as capping.

The success of a chromatographic separation is judged by the ability of the system to resolve one analyte peak from another. Resolution is defined as the ratio of the difference in retention time between the two peaks to the mean of their base widths (w_{av}):

$$R_S = \frac{2(t_{R_A} - t_{R_B})}{w_A + w_B} = \frac{\Delta t_R}{w_{av}} \qquad (13.11)$$

When $R_S = 1.0$, the separation of the two peaks is 97.7% complete (thus the overlap is 2.3%). When $R_S = 1.5$ the overlap is reduced to 0.2%. Unresolved peaks are said to be fused (Fig. 13.3). Provided the overlap is not excessive, the analysis of the individual peaks can be made on the assumption that their characteristics are not affected by the incomplete resolution.

Resolution is influenced by column efficiency, selectivity factor and capacity factors according to the equation:

$$R_S = \frac{\sqrt{N}}{4}\left(\frac{\alpha - 1}{\alpha}\right)\left(\frac{k_2'}{1 + k_{av}'}\right) \qquad (13.12)$$

where k_2' is the capacity factor for the longest retained peak, and k_{av}' is the mean capacity factor for the two analytes.

Equation 13.12 is one of the most important in chromatography as it enables a rationale approach to be taken to the improvement of the resolution between the compounds. For example, it can be seen that resolution increases with $\sqrt{N}$. Since N is linked to the length of the column, doubling the length of the column will increase resolution by $\sqrt{2}$, i.e. by a factor of 1.4. Since both capacity factors and selectivity factors are linked to retention times and retention volumes, altering the nature of the two phases or their relative volumes will impact on resolution. Capacity factors are also dependent upon distribution coefficients, which in turn are temperature dependent, hence altering the column temperature may improve resolution. The capacity of a particular chromatographic separation is a measure of the amount of material that can be resolved into its components without causing peak overlap or fronting. Ion-exchange chromatography (Section 13.7) and chromatofocusing (Section 13.7.3) have a high capacity, which is why they are often used in the earlier stages of a purification process.

13.2.5 Quantification of analytes: internal and external standards

When the column effluent has been monitored to produce a chart recording, then generally the area of each peak can be shown to be proportional to the amount of a given analyte eluting from the column. The area of the peak may be determined by measuring the height of the peak (h_P) and its width at half the height (w_h). The product of these dimensions is taken to be equal to the area of the peak. Alternatively the peak may be cut out of the chart paper and weighed and the assumption made that area and weight are linearly related. These procedures are very time consuming when complex and/or a large number of analyses are involved. The calculations are best performed by dedicated integrators or micro-computers. These can be programmed to compute retention time and peak area and to relate them to those of standards (pure reference compounds), enabling relative retention ratios and relative peak area ratios to be calculated. These may be used to identify a particular analyte and to quantify it using previously obtained and stored calibration data from standards. The data system can also be used to correct problems inherent in the chromatographic system. Such problems can arise either from the characteristics of the detector or from the efficiency of the separation process. Problems that are attributable to the detector are baseline drift, where the detector signal gradually changes with time, and baseline noise, which is a series of rapid minor fluctuations in detector signal, commonly the result of the operator using too high a detector sensitivity or possibly an electronic fault.

When the new peak area has been determined, the amount of the analyte present may be determined by use of a calibration curve obtained by chromatographing, under identical conditions, known amounts of the pure form of the analyte. To aid this assay by attempting to compensate for variations in chromatographic conditions and of any preliminary extraction procedure, use is made of an internal standard. The internal standard is a compound that has physical properties as similar as possible to the test analytes and which chromatographs near to, but distinct from, them. Ideally, it should have the same detector response as those of the analytes. A known amount of the standard is introduced into the test sample as early as possible in the extraction, and is therefore taken through any preliminary procedures with it. Any loss of standard during the analysis will be identical with the loss of the test analytes. The peak area associated with the fixed amount of internal standard is used to calculate the relative peak area ratio for each peak in both the calibration data and the sample under analysis. A calibration curve therefore consists of a plot of relative peak area ratio against the known amount of the analyte, thereby enabling the amount of the analyte in the test sample to be calculated. An alternative procedure is to use an external standard. In this method the standard is added to the test sample immediately before the sample is chromatographed and separate analyte and calibration standard solutions are produced independently. It is therefore not taken through any preliminary extraction procedure and cannot compensate for variations in the efficiency of the extraction procedure. This method is valid only in those cases where the recovery of the analyte from the test sample is virtually quantitative and in those cases where there are no short-term fluctuations in detector response.

13.2.6 Sample preparation

Whilst chromatographic techniques are designed to separate mixtures of compounds this does not mean that no attention has to be paid to the preliminary purification (clean up) of the test sample. On the contrary, it is clear that, for quantitative work using HPLC techniques in particular, such preliminary action is essential particularly if the test compound(s) is in a complex matrix such as plasma, urine, cell homogenate or microbiological culture medium. The extraction and purification of the components from a cell homogenate is often a complex multistage process. The associated principles for protein purification are discussed in Section 6.3. For some forms of analysis, for example the analysis of drugs in biological fluids, sample preparation is relatively much simpler. The simplest and most commonly used clean-up technique is solvent extraction. This is based on the fact that organic compounds can usually be extracted from aqueous mixtures by extraction with a low boiling water-immiscible solvent such as diethylether or dichloromethane. The technique is another example of the application of the principle of partition coefficients. Organic compounds that are weak electrolytes, such as acids and bases, can exist in ionised or unionised forms depending upon their pK_a and the prevailing pH. For extraction into an organic solvent the unionised species is generally required and hence the pH of the test sample must be adjusted to the appropriate value. Organic solvents such as diethylether and dichloromethane also extract significant quantities of water and, in general, this should be removed, for example by the addition of an anhydrous salt such as sodium sulphate or magnesium sulphate, before the extract is evaporated to dryness (often under nitrogen or *in vacuo*), dissolved in an appropriate solvent such as methanol or acetonitrile, and subjected to chromatographic separation. This solvent extraction procedure tends to lack selectivity and is often unsatisfactory for the HPLC analysis of compounds in the $ngcm^{-3}$ or less range. It can sometimes be improved by the technique of ion-pairing (Section 13.6.4).

The alternative to solvent extraction is solid phase extraction. Its advantage over simple solvent extraction is that it exhibits greater selectivity, mainly because it is a form of chromatography. The test solution is passed through a small (few millimetres in length) disposable column (cartridge) packed with relatively large particles of a bonded silica similar to those used for HPLC (Section 13.4.3). These selectively adsorb the analyte under investigation and ideally allow interfering compounds to pass through. Preliminary thought has to be given to the particular bonded silica selected and the test sample should be treated with agents such as trichloroacetic acid, perchloric acid or organic solvents such as acetonitrile to deproteinise it so that the opportunity for protein binding of the analyte is minimised. The pH of the test solution should also be adjusted to maximise the retention of the analyte. Once the test solution has been passed through the column, either by simple gravity feed or by the application of a slight vacuum to the receiver vessel, the column is washed with water and the adsorbed analyte recovered by elution with an organic solvent such as methanol or acetonitrile. The minimum volume of elution solvent is used because the analyte is recovered by evaporating the solution to dryness (under nitrogen or *in vacuo*) and the residue dissolved in the minimum volume of an appropriate solvent prior to chromatographic analysis. Several commercial forms of this solid phase extraction technique are available that facilitate the simultaneous treatment of a large number of test samples.

A more sophisticated procedure for sample preparation, particularly suited to the analysis of analytes in very low concentrations in complex mixtures by HPLC, is the technique of column switching. In this technique, the test solution is applied to a preliminary short column similar to the type used in solid phase extraction. Once the test analyte has been adsorbed and impurities washed through the column, the analyte is eluted with a suitable organic solvent and the column effluent transferred directly to an analytical HPLC column. Technically, this is not easy to achieve and requires several pumps and switching valves and is therefore expensive. One of the main problems with the technique is that unless all interfering compounds are eluted from the preliminary column before the adsorbed analyte is switched to the analytical column they will eventually accumulate in the analytical column and reduce its resolving power. Nevertheless, the technique has achieved many very difficult resolutions.

In recent years, a new approach to sample preparation has been investigated. Termed supercritical fluid extraction (SFE), it exploits the fact that gases such as carbon dioxide exist as a liquid under certain critical conditions. In the case of carbon dioxide, these conditions are 31.1 °C and 7.38 MPa (10.7 ibf in.$^{-2}$) and the resultant liquid carbon dioxide can be used as the extraction solvent, behaving as a low polarity solvent comparable to hexane. By altering the physical conditions of the extract, the carbon dioxide can be made to revert to a gas, thus simplifying the recovery of the extracted analytes.

The technique of analyte pre- or postcolumn derivatisation may facilitate better chromatographic separation and detection. Derivatisation is designed to improve separation and analyte detection using reagents of the type shown in Table 13.1.

13.3 LOW PRESSURE COLUMN CHROMATOGRAPHY

13.3.1 Columns

The glass column used should have a means of supporting the stationary phase as near to the base of the column as possible in order to minimise the dead space below the column support in which postcolumn mixing of separated analytes could occur. Commercial columns possess either a porous glass plate fused onto the base of the column or a suitable device for supporting a replaceable nylon net, which in turn supports the stationary phase. A cheaper alternative to these commercial column supports is to use a small plug of glass wool together with a minimal amount of quartz sand or glass beads. Capillary tubing normally leads the effluent from the column to the detector and/or fraction collection system (Fig. 13.2). For some chromatographic separations, it is necessary for the temperature of the column to be maintained constant during the separation. This is most simply achieved by jacketing the column so that liquid from a thermostatically controlled bath (set at the required working temperature, which may be below room temperature) may be pumped around the outside of the column. More sophisticated methods include placing the column in a heating block or in a thermostatically controlled oven.

13.3.2 Matrix materials

The matrix is the material used to support the stationary phase. The selection of a matrix for a particular stationary phase is vital to the successful chromatographic

| Table 13.1 | Examples of derivatising reagents |

Analyte	Reagent
A. Precolumn	
Ultraviolet detection	
Alcohols, amines, phenols	3,5-Dinitrobenzoyl chloride
Amino acids, peptides	Phenylisothiocyanate, dansyl chloride
Carbohydrates	Benzoyl chloride
Carboxylic acids	1-p-Nitrobenzyl-N,N'-diisopropylisourea
Fatty acids, phospholipids	Phenacyl bromide, naphthacyl bromide
Electrochemical detection	
Aldehydes, ketones	2,4-Dinitrophenylhydrazine
Amines, amino acids	o-Phthalaldehyde, fluorodinitrobenzene
Carboxylic acids	p-Aminophenol
Fluorescent detection	
Amino acids, amines, peptides	Dansyl chloride, dabsyl chloride, fluoroescamine, o-phthalaldehyde
Carboxylic acids	4-Bromomethyl-7-methoxycoumarin
Carbonyl compounds	Dansylhydrazine
B. Postcolumn	
Ultraviolet detection	
Amino acids	Phenylisothiocyanate
Carbohydrates	Orcinol and sulphuric acid
Penicillins	Imidazole and mercuric chloride
Fluorescent detection	
Amino acids	o-Phthalaldehyde, fluorescamine, 6-aminoquinolyl-n-hydroxysuccinimidyl carbamate

use of the phase. Generally speaking, a matrix needs to have: high mechanical stability to encourage good flow rates and to minimise pressure drop along the column; good chemical stability; functional groups to facilitate the attachment of the stationary phase; and high capacity, i.e. density of functional groups to minimise bed volume. It also needs to be available in a range of particle sizes. In addition some forms of chromatography require a matrix with a porous structure, in which case the pores need to be of the correct size and shape. Finally, the surface of a matrix needs to be inert to minimise the non-selective adsorption of analytes.

In practice, the six most commonly used types of matrix are as follows:

Agarose – a polysaccharide made up of D-galactose and 3,6-anhydro-1-galactose units (Fig. 12.4). The unbranched polysaccharide chains are cross-linked with agents such as 2,3-dibromopropanol to give gels that are stable in the pH range 3 to 14. They have good flow properties and high hydrophilicity but should never be allowed to dry out otherwise they undergo irreversible change. Commercial examples include Sepharose and Bio-Gel A.

Cellulose – a polysaccharide of β-1–4-linked glucose units. For matrix use it is cross-linked with epichlorohydrin, the extent of cross-linking dictating the pore size. It is available in bead, microgranular and fibrous forms, has good pH stability and flow properties, and is highly hydrophilic.

Dextran – a polysaccharide consisting of α-1–6-linked glucose units. For matrix use it is cross-linked with epichlorohydrin but is less stable to acid hydrolysis than are cellulose matrices. It is stable up to pH 12 and is hydrophilic. Commercial examples include Sephadex.

Polyacrylamide – a polymer of acrylamide cross-linked with N,N′-methylene-bis-acrylamide (Fig. 12.5). It is stable in the pH range 2 to 11. Commercial examples include Bio-Gel P.

Polystyrene – a polymer of styrene cross-linked with divinylbenzene. Polystyrene matrices have good stability over all pH ranges and are most commonly used for exclusion and ion-exchange chromatography. They have relatively low hydrophilicities.

Silica – a polymeric material produced from orthosilicic acid. The numerous silanol (Si-OH) groups make it hydrophilic. When derivatised, excess silanol groups can be removed by treatment with trichloromethylsilane. The stability of silica matrices is confined to the pH range 3 to 8. Closely related to the silica matrices is controlled pore glass. It is chemically inert but, like the silicas, tends to dissolve above pH 8.

13.3.3 Stationary phases

The chemical nature of the stationary phase depends upon the particular form of chromatography to be carried out. Full details are given in later sections of this chapter. Most stationary phases are available attached to the matrices in a range of sizes and shapes. Both properties are important because they influence the flow rate and resolution characteristics. The larger the particle, the faster the flow rate but, conversely, the smaller the particle the larger the surface area-to-volume ratio and potentially the greater their resolving power. In practice a balance has to be struck. The best packing characteristics are given by spherical particles and most stationary phases now have a spherical or approximately spherical shape. Particle size is commonly expressed by a mesh size, which is a measure of the openings per inch in a sieve; hence the larger the mesh size, the smaller is the particle. A 100 to 120 mesh is most common for routine use, whereas a 200 to 400 mesh is used for higher resolution work.

13.3.4 Column packing

This is one of the most critical factors in achieving a successful separation by any form of column chromatography. Packing a column is normally carried out by gently pouring a slurry of the stationary phase in the mobile phase into a column that has its outlet closed, whilst the upper part of the slurry in the column is stirred and/or the column is gently tapped to ensure that no air bubbles are trapped and that the packing settles evenly. Poor column packing gives rise to uneven flow (channelling) and reduced resolution. The slurry is added until the required height is obtained. Once the required column height has been obtained, the flow of mobile phase through the packed column is started by opening the outlet, and continued until the packing has completely settled. This whole process generally requires considerable practice to achieve reproducible results. To prevent the surface of the packed material from being disturbed either by the addition of mobile phase to the column or during the application of the sample to the column, it is normal to place a suitable protection device, such as filter paper disc or nylon or rayon gauze, on the surface of the column. Some commercial columns possess an adaptor and plunger, which serve the dual purpose of protecting the surface of the column and providing an inlet (often capillary tubing) to carry the mobile phase to the column surface. Once a column has been prepared, it is imperative that no part of it should be allowed to run dry; hence a layer of mobile phase should always be maintained above the column surface.

It is difficult to generalise about the ideal column height-to-diameter ratio and the total bed volume. They both influence the amount of material that can be separated on the column and in practice will need to be determined by systematic trial and error. Experience frequently provides a guide; thus, for example, in exclusion chromatography, a height-to-diameter ratio of 10:1 to 20:1 is normally suitable.

13.3.5 Application of sample

Several methods are available for the application of the sample to the top of the prepared column. A simple way is to remove most of the mobile phase from above the column by suction and *just* to drain the remainder into the column bed. The sample is then carefully applied by pipette and it too is allowed just to run into the column. A small volume of mobile phase is then applied in a similar manner to wash final traces of the sample into the bed. More mobile phase is then carefully added to the column to a height of 2 to 5 cm. The column is then connected to a suitable reservoir that contains more mobile phase so that the height of the phase in the column can be maintained at 2 to 5 cm. An alternative procedure, which avoids the necessity to drain the column to the surface of the bed, is to increase the density of the sample by addition of sucrose to a concentration of about 1%. When this solution is layered onto the liquid above the column bed, it will automatically sink to the surface of the column and hence be quickly passed into the column. This method of sample application is satisfactory, provided that the presence of sucrose in no way interferes with the separation and subsequent analysis of the sample. A third method involves the use of capillary tubing and/or syringe or peristaltic pump to pass the sample directly to the column surface. This latter method is the most satisfactory of the three.

In all cases, care must be taken to avoid overloading the column with sample, otherwise irregular separation will occur. It is also advantageous to apply the sample in as small a volume of mobile phase as possible because this ensures an initial tight band of material when the separation commences.

13.3.6 **Column development and sample elution**

The components of the applied sample are separated by the continuous passage of the mobile phase through the column. This is known as elution development (Section 13.1.2). During the elution process it is essential that the flow of mobile phase is maintained at a stable rate and this is most simply achieved by gravity feed. The flow rate may be regulated by adjusting the operating pressure, which corrresponds to the difference between the level of the liquid in a reservoir situated above the column and the level at the outlet site of the column. An ordinary open reservoir is not satisfactory because the operating pressure will drop in the course of the experiment owing to the drop in level in the reservoir as the mobile phase runs into the column. This can be overcome by the use of a Mariotte flask, which will keep the operating pressure constant (Fig. 13.2). An alternative and more effective method of maintaining stable flow rates is to use a peristaltic pump. The most commonly used pumps are of the roller type (Fig. 13.5). These deliver the mobile liquid phase through silicon, polyvinylchloride or fluororubber tubing by compressing the tubing as the revolving disc is rotated at a rate predetermined according to the flow rate required. Pumps and the tubing of known diameter must be precalibrated to determine the flow rate. Care must be exercised when pumps are used, to ensure that the operating pressure does not compact the column excessively and cause the column structure to change.

Column development using a single liquid as the mobile phase is known as an isocratic elution. However, in many cases in order to increase the resolving power of the mobile phase, it is necessary continuously to change its pH, ionic concentration or polarity. This is known as gradient elution. In order to produce a suitable gradient, two eluents have to be mixed in the correct proportions prior to their entering the column. This may be achieved by use of commercially available gradient mixers or more simply as follows. The two eluents are placed in separate chambers, a recipient chamber linked to the column and a donor chamber, linked to the recipient chamber by a siphon (Fig. 13.6). As eluent enters the column from the recipient chamber, the eluent in the donor chamber replaces it

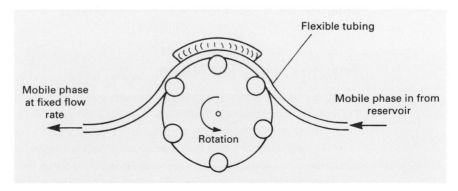

Fig. 13.5. Simple peristaltic pump commonly used in low pressure liquid chromatography.

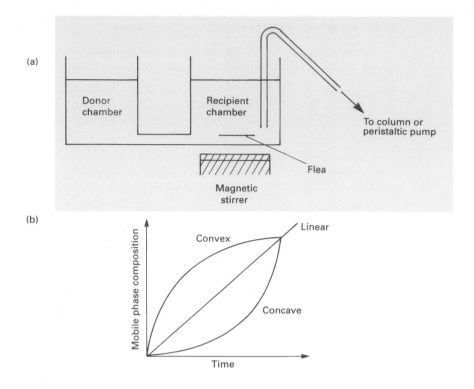

Fig. 13.6. (a) Simple apparatus for producing gradient elution and (b) gradient shapes commonly used.

and is mixed by a stirrer. The relative pH, ionic strength or polarity of the eluent in the donor with respect to that in the recipient chamber will determine the direction in which the gradient will be formed. Moreover, the relative diameters and shapes of the two chambers will determine whether the gradient varies with time in a linear convex, or concave manner (Fig. 13.6b). In more sophisticated systems, two pumps are used to deliver the two eluents at predetermined rates into a mixing area, before application to the column. Convex gradients give better resolution initially, whereas concave gradients give better resolution at the end.

13.3.7 Detectors and fraction collection

As the resolved analytes emerge in the effluent from the column it is necessary to detect their presence. For coloured analytes this can be achieved simply by visual observation but for colourless compounds alternatives are necessary. Detection may be based on ultraviolet absorption, fluorescence spectroscopy, changes in the refractive index of the effluent, the presence of a radioactive emission atom or on the ease of oxidation or reduction of the analytes as measured by an electrochemical detector (Section 15.7).

Ultraviolet detectors are probably the most common form of detector in bio-chemical analysis. The best instruments allow proteins to be detected and quantified at 190 to 220 nm and 260 to 280 nm wavelengths (Section 6.3.2). Fluorescence detectors generally give greater sensitivity if they can be used but tend to be more sensitive to impurities in the mobile phase. All spectrophotomet-ric detectors use continuous flow cells with a small internal volume (typically 8 mm^3) which allow the continuous monitoring of the column effluent (Section 9.4.2).

For studies in which the analyte in the effluent is to be collected and studied further, the effluent has to be divided into fractions. Two approaches are available to achieve this objective: either the effluent can be continuously monitored and the fraction containing a particular analyte collected, or the effluent can be divided into small (1 to 10 cm^3) fractions, which are subsequently analysed and those containing a particular analyte bulked together.

A range of automatic fraction collectors is available commercially. They are designed to collect a certain amount of effluent in each tube before a new tube is placed in position automatically. The amount of effluent in each fraction may be determined in one of several ways. There may be a siphoning or similar system to deliver a predetermined volume into each tube, or there may be an electronic means of allowing a predetermined number of drops of effluent to enter each tube. This latter method has the slight disadvantage that, if the composition of the effluent changes (e.g. during gradient elution), so too may its surface tension and hence droplet size, so that the actual volume collected also changes. A further pos-sibility is that the effluent is allowed to enter each tube for a fixed time interval. In this case, if the flow rate through the column varies, so too will the volume of each fraction, but this is unusual and, in practice, fixed-time collectors are the most common.

13.4 HIGH PERFORMANCE LIQUID CHROMATOGRAPHY

13.4.1 Principle

As can be seen from equations 13.1 to 13.12, the resolving power of a chromato-graphic column increases with column length and the number of theoretical plates per unit length, although there are limits to the length of a column owing to the problem of peak broadening. As the number of theoretical plates is related to the surface area of the stationary phase, it follows that the smaller the particle size of the stationary phase, the better the resolution. Unfortunately, the smaller the particle size, the greater is the resistance to flow of mobile phase. This creates a back-pressure in the column that is sufficient to damage the matrix structure of the stationary phase, thereby actually reducing eluent flow and impairing resolu-tion. In the recent past there has been a dramatic development in column chro-matography technology that has resulted in the availability of new, smaller particle size, stationary phases that can withstand these pressures. This develop-ment, which has occurred in adsorption, partition, ion-exchange, exclusion and

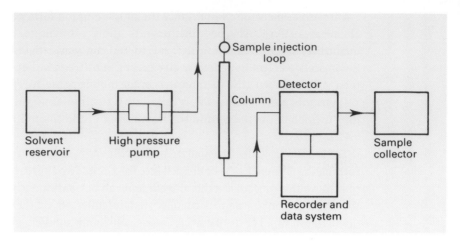

Fig. 13.7. Diagram of the components of an isocratic HPLC system.

affinity chromatography, has resulted in faster and better resolution and explains why HPLC has emerged as the most popular, powerful and versatile form of chromatography. Many commercially available HPLC systems are microprocessor controlled to allow dedicated, continuous chromatographic separations.

13.4.2 Columns

The columns (Fig. 13.7) used for HPLC are generally made of stainless steel and are manufactured so that they can withstand pressures of up to 5.5×10^7Pa (~8000 lbf in.$^{-2}$). Straight columns of 15 to 50 cm length and 1 to 4mm diameter are generally used, although smaller microbore or open tubular columns are available. Microbore columns have an internal diameter of 1 to 2 mm and are generally 25 cm long. They can sustain flow rates of 0.05 to 0.20 cm^3 min^{-1} as opposed to the 2 cm^3 min^{-1} of conventional HPLC columns. Preparative columns are also available commercially, with internal diameters of up to 25 mm; they can sustain flow rates of up to 100 cm^3 min^{-1}. The best columns are precision bored, with an internal mirror finish that allows efficient packing of the column. Porous plugs of stainless steel or Teflon are used in the ends of the columns to retain the packing material. These plugs must be homogeneous to ensure uniform flow of liquid through the column. It is advantageous in some separations involving liquid partition chromatography and ion-exchange chromatography to maintain the column temperature slightly above room temperature (up to 60 °C) during the analysis.

13.4.3 Matrices and stationary phases

Three forms of column packing material are available, based on a rigid solid (as opposed to gel) structure. These are as follows:

Microporous supports in which micropores ramify through the particles which are generally 5 to 10 μm in diameter.

Pellicular (superficially porous) supports in which porous particles are coated onto an inert solid core such as a glass bead of about 40 μm in diameter.

Bonded phases in which the stationary phase is chemically bonded on to an inert support such as silica.

For adsorption chromatography, adsorbents such as silica and alumina are available as microporous or pellicular forms with a range of particle sizes. Pellicular systems generally have a high efficiency but low sample capacity and therefore microporous supports are preferred when available.

In partition chromatographic systems, the stationary phase may be coated onto the inert microporous or pellicular support. One disadvantage of supports coated with liquid phases is that the developing mobile phase may gradually wash off the liquid phase. To overcome this problem, bonded phases have been developed in which the supporting material is silica.

In normal phase liquid chromatography, the stationary phase is a polar compound such as an alkyl nitrile or an alkylamine, and the mobile phase is a non-polar solvent such as hexane. For reversed-phase liquid chromatography, the stationary phase is a non-polar compound such as octasilane (OS) or octadecylsilane (ODS) and the mobile phase is a polar solvent such as water/acetonitrile or water/methanol.

Many different types of ion-exchanger suitable for HPLC are available, of which the cross-linked microporous polystyrene resins are widely used. Pellicular resin forms are also available, as are bonded-phase exchangers covalently bonded to a cross-linked silicone network. These resins are classed as hard gels and readily withstand the pressures generated during analysis.

The stationary phases for exclusion separations are generally porous silica, glass, polystyrene or polyvinylacetate beads and are available in a range of pore sizes. They are generally used where the eluting solvent is an organic system. Semi-rigid gels such as Sephadex or Bio-Gel P, and non-rigid gels such as Sepharose and Bio-Gel A, are of only limited use in HPLC because they can withstand only low pressures. The supports for affinity separations are similar to those for exclusion separations. The spacer arm and ligand are attached to these supports by chemical means similar to those used in conventional low pressure affinity chromatography (Section 13.9). Table 13.2 lists some examples of commonly used HPLC stationary phases.

13.4.4 **Column packing**

HPLC columns may be purchased already packed with specified packing material, structure and dimensions. Many workers, however, prefer to pack their own columns as this is cheaper. Several methods are available for packing columns and the method used will depend on the nature of the packing material and the dimensions of the particles. The major priority in the packing of a column is to obtain a

| Table 13.2 | Some examples of HPLC stationary phases |

Chromatographic separation principle	Commercial name	Nature of stationary phase	Type of support
Adsorption	Partisil C$_8$	Octylsilane	Porous
	Corasil	Silica	Pellicular
	Pellumina	Alumina	Pellicular
	Partisil	Silica	Microporous
	MicroPak A1	Alumina	Microporous
Partition	Bondapak-C$_{18}$/Corasil	Octadecylsilane	Pellicular
	μBondapak-C$_{18}$	Octadecylsilane	Porous
	ULTRApak TSK ODS	Octadecylsilane	Porous
	μBondapak-NH$_2$	Alkylamine	Porous
	ULTRApak TSK NH$_2$	Alkylamine	Porous
Ion-exchange	Partisil-SAX	Strong base	Porous
	MicroPak-NH$_2$	Weak base	Porous
	Partisil-SCX	Strong base	Porous
	AS Pellionex-SAX	Strong base	Pellicular
	Zipak-WAX	Weak base	Pellicular
	Perisorb -KAT	Strong base	Pellicular
Exclusion	Bio-Glas	Glass	Rigid solid
	Styragel	Polystyrene-divinylbenzene	Semi-rigid gel
	Superose	Agarose	Soft gel
	Fractogel TSK	Polyvinylchloride	Semi-rigid gel

uniform bed of material with no cracks or channels. Rigid solids and hard gels should be packed as densely as possible, but without fracturing the particles during the packing process. The most widely used technique for column packing is the high pressure slurrying technique. A suspension of the packing is made in a solvent of density equal to that of the packing material. The slurry is then pumped rapidly at high pressure into a column with a porous plug at its outlet. The resulting bed of packed material within the column can then be prepared for use by running the developing mobile phase through the column. When hard gels are to be used, it is necessary for them to be allowed to swell in the solvent to be used in the chromatographic process before they are packed under pressure. Soft gels cannot be packed under pressure and have to be allowed to pack from a slurry in a way similar to that of the packing of columns for LPLC (Section 13.3.4).

13.4.5 Mobile phases and pumps

The choice of mobile phase to be used in any separation will depend on the type of separation to be achieved. Isocratic separations may be made with a single pump, using a single solvent or two or more solvents premixed in fixed proportions.

Gradient elution (Section 13.3.6) generally uses separate pumps to deliver two solvents in proportions predetermined by a gradient programmer. All solvents for use in HPLC systems must be specially purified because traces of impurities can affect the column and interfere with the detection system. This is particularly the case if the detection system is measuring absorbance below 200 nm. Purified solvents for use in HPLC systems are available commercially, but even with these solvents a 1 to 5 μm microfilter is generally introduced into the system prior to the pump. It is also essential that all solvents are degassed before use otherwise gassing (the presence of air bubbles in the solvent) tends to occur in most pumps. Gassing, which tends to be particularly bad for aqueous methanol and ethanol, can alter column resolution and interfere with the continuous monitoring of the effluent. Degassing may be carried out in several ways; by warming the solvent, by stirring it vigorously with a magnetic stirrer, subjecting it to a vacuum, by ultrasonication, or by bubbling helium gas through the solvent reservoir.

Pumping systems for delivery of the mobile phase are one of the most important features of HPLC systems. The main features of a good pumping system are that it is capable of outputs of at least 5×10^7 Pa ($\sim$7200 lbf in.$^{-2}$) and ideally there must be no pulses (i.e. cyclical variations in pressure) as this may affect the detector response. There must be a flow capability of at least 10 cm^3 min^{-1} and up to 100 cm^3 min^{-1} for preparative separations. Various pumping systems are available that operate on the principle of constant pressure or constant displacement.

Constant displacement pumps maintain a constant flow rate through the column irrespective of changing conditions within the column. One form of constant displacement pump is a motor-driven syringe-type pump that delivers a fixed volume of solvent on to the column by a piston driven by a motor. The constant volume syringe pump contains a screw-jack driven by a stepper motor. On the delivery stroke, the piston is driven at a constant rate, displacing eluent onto the column at the same rate. Two one-way valves control eluent flow in the chamber (Fig. 13.8a). The reciprocating pump is the most commonly used form of constant displacement pump. The piston is moved by a motorised crank, and entry of solvent to the column is regulated by check valves. On the compression stroke solvent is forced from the pump chamber onto the column. During the return stroke the exit check valve closes and solvent is drawn in via the entry valve to the pump chamber ready to be pumped onto the column on the next compression stroke. Such pumps produce small pulses of flow and pulse dampeners are usually incorporated into the system to minimise this pulsing effect. All constant displacement pumps have in-built safety cut-out mechanisms so that if the pressure within the chromatographic systems changes from preset limits the pump is inactivated automatically.

13.4.6 **Application of sample**

The correct application of the sample onto an HPLC column is a particularly important factor in achieving successful separations and one of two methods is generally used. The first method makes use of a microsyringe to inject the sample

(a)

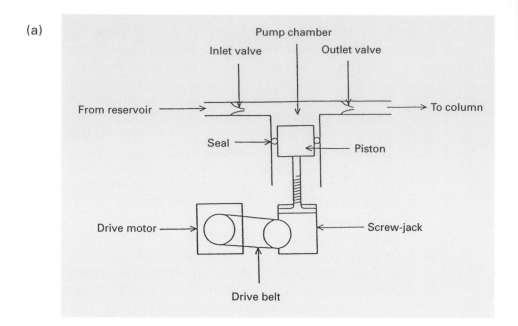

(b)

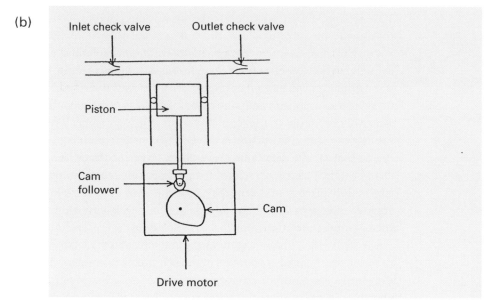

Fig. 13.8. Commonly used constant displacement pumps: (a) constant volume; (b) reciprocating. In both types the down stroke of the piston closes the outlet valve and opens the inlet valve to release eluent into the pump chamber. The upstroke of the piston closes the inlet valve and opens the outlet valve to release the eluent onto the column. (Reproduced by permission of Academic Press Inc. (London) Limited, from R. Newton (1982) in *Food Analysis* edited by R. Macrae.)

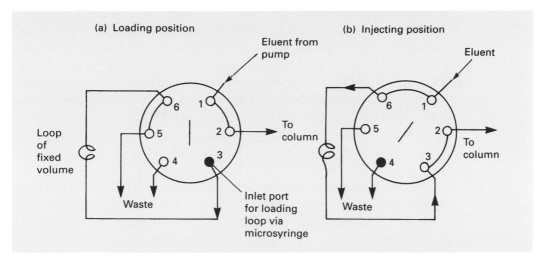

Fig. 13.9. HPLC loop injector: the loop is loaded (a) via port 3 with excess sample going to waste via port 5. In this position the eluent from the pump passes to the column via ports 1 and 2. In the injecting position (b), eluent flow is directed through the loop (ports 1 and 6) and then onto the column.

either directly onto the column packing or onto a small plug of inert material immediately above the column packing. This injection can be done while the system is under pressure or it may require the pump to be turned off and, when the pressure has dropped to near atmospheric, the injection is made and the pump switched on again. This latter approach is termed a stop flow injection. The second method of sample introduction that retains the column pressure is by use of a loop injector (Fig. 13.9). This consists of a metal loop, of fixed small volume, that can be filled with the sample. By means of an appropriate valve switching system, the eluent from the pump is channelled through the loop, the outlet of which leads directly onto the column. The sample is thus flushed onto the column by the eluent without interruption of flow to the column.

Repeated application of highly impure samples such as sera, urine, plasma or whole blood, which have preferably been deproteinated, may eventually cause the column to lose its resolving power. To prevent this occurrence, a guard column is frequently installed between the injector and the analytical column. This guard column is a short (1 to 2 cm) column of the same internal diameter and packed with material similar to that present in the analytical column. The packing in the guard column preferentially retains contaminating material and can be replaced at regular intervals.

13.4.7 Detectors

Since the quantity of material applied to the column is frequently very small, it is imperative that the sensitivity of the detector system is sufficiently high and stable to respond to the low concentrations of each analyte in the effluent. Most commonly the detector is a variable wavelength detector based upon ultraviolet–visible spectrophotometry. This type of detector is capable of measuring absorbances down to 190 nm wavelength and has sensitivities as low as 0.001 absorbance units for full-scale deflection (AUFS). Scanning wavelength detectors have the facility to record the complete absorption spectrum of each analyte, thus aiding identification. Such opportunities are possible either by temporarily stopping the effluent flow or by the use of diode array techniques, which allow the simultaneous measurement of absorbance at many or all wavelengths within 0.01 s (Fig. 13.10).

Fluorescence detectors are extremely valuable for HPLC because of their sensitivity but the technique is limited by the fact that relatively few compounds fluoresce. Electrochemical detectors, which are selective for electroactive species (Section 15.7), are potentially highly sensitive. Two types are available, amperometric and coulometric, the principles of which are similar. A flow cell is fitted with two electrodes – a stable counter electrode (Ag/AgCl or calomel) and a working electrode, which is highly polarisable. A constant potential is applied to the working electrode at such a value that, as an analyte flows through the flow cell, molecules at the electrode surface undergo either an oxidation or a reduction, resulting in a current flow between the two electrodes. The potential applied to the counter electrode is sufficient to ensure that the current detected gives a full-scale deflection on the recorder. Compounds capable of undergoing oxidation include hydrocarbons, amines, amides, phenols, di- and triazines, phenothiazines, catecholamines and quinolines. Compounds capable of undergoing reduction include olefins, esters, ketones, aldehydes, ethers, azo and nitro compounds. The mobile phase should of course be free from compounds capable of responding to the detector. The electrochemical detector has been particularly successful in the assay of catecholamines, vitamins and antioxidants.

Perhaps the greatest advance in detection using HPLC has been made by the coupling of the HPLC to a mass spectrometer. The technical problems associated with the logistics of removing the bulk of the mobile phase before the sample is introduced into the mass spectrometer have been resolved in a number of ways. The direct liquid insertion interface (DLI) consists of a flow of effluent via a capillary into a direct insertion probe in the mass spectrometer. The analyte enters the ionisation source together with an excess of mobile phase molecules and as a consequence the ionisation is weak (soft) and CI (Section 11.3) rather than EI spectra (Section 11.4) predominate. However the $(M + H)^+$ ion of the analyte is clearly visible and this facilitates structure identification. Thermospray ionisation (TSI) (Section 11.7.1) normally requires the use of an aqueous mobile phase commonly containing ammonium acetate. The end of a heated (400 °C) capillary from the effluent flow enters a chamber exposed to electron bombardment and to a vacuum pumping system. The high temperature creates a supersonic expanding jet of droplets that are ionised and gradually reduced in size due to the pumping system. Eventually ions of the analyte are ejected from the droplet into the mass analyser.

(a)

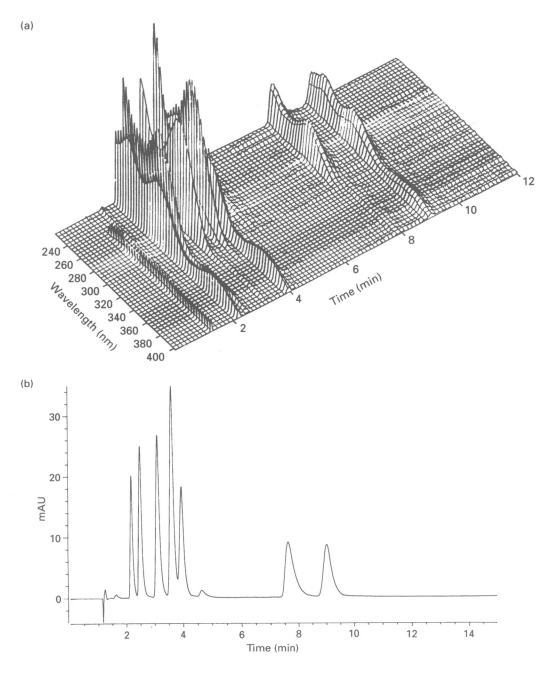

(b)

Fig. 13.10. Separation by HPLC of the dihydropyridine calcium channel blocker lacidipine and its metabolites. Column: ODS Hypersil. Eluent: Methanol/acetonitrile/water (66%, 5%, 29%, by vol.) acidified to pH 3.5 with 1% formic acid. Flow rate: 1 cm^3 min^{-1}. Column temperature: 40 °C. (a) As recorded by diode array detector; (b) as recorded by an ultraviolet detector. (Reproduced by permission of Glaxo Wellcome, Stevenage.)

CI spectra are again recorded as $(M + H)^+$ or $(M + NH_4)^+$ ions. In electrospray ionisation (ESI) (Section 11.7.2) the capillary containing the effluent is held at a high voltage and the effluent mixed with nitrogen gas. The voltage creates a charge on the liquid surface that causes it to disperse into a very fine spray. The solvent in the fine droplets evaporates and is flushed away by the nitrogen gas. The ions of the analyte are swept as a supersonic stream into a vacuum chamber and eventually into the mass analyser. More recently, HPLC has been interfaced with NMR spectroscopy to give structural information about the analytes that is complementary to that obtained via HPLC–MS.

The sensitivity of ultraviolet absorption, fluorescence and electrochemical detectors can often be increased significantly by the process of derivatisation, whereby the analyte is converted pre- or postcolumn to a chemical derivative. Examples are given in Table 13.1.

13.4.8 Applications

The wide applicability, speed and sensitivity of HPLC has resulted in it becoming the most popular form of chromatography and virtually all types of biological molecule have been assayed or purified using the technique. HPLC has had a big impact on the separation of oligopeptides and proteins. Instruments dedicated to the separation of proteins have given rise to the technique of fast protein liquid chromatography (FPLC). There are no unique principles associated with FPLC, it is simply based on reversed-phase, affinity, exclusion, hydrophobic interaction and ion-exchange chromatography and on chromatofocusing. Microbore glass-lined stainless steel columns enable very small amounts of sample to be used, with separation taking as little as 10 min. The technique enables such complex mixtures as tryptic digests of proteins and the culture supernatant of microorganisms to be applied directly to the column, but protein mixtures from cell extracts still need some form of preliminary fractionation (Section 6.3.3) prior to study.

13.4.9 Capillary electrochromatography

This latest development in chromatography is effectively a hybrid of HPLC and capillary electrophoresis (Section 12.5). As its name implies, it is carried out in capillary columns in which the stationary phase is either attached to an inert support and packed, or is coated directly onto the walls of the capillary. As in capillary electrophoresis, a potential is applied across the walls of the capillary, generating solvent flow by electroosmosis (see Section 12.1). This electroosmotic flow (EOF) drives the solvent and the analytes in the applied sample through the capillary column. As the analytes move along the capillary they are subject to the opposing forces of EOF and distribution between the mobile and stationary phases. They will therefore be separated partly on the basis of their differences in distribution coefficients, K_d, between the two phases exactly as in all other forms of chromatography. In addition, however, they will be influenced by differences in their electrophoretic mobility as in capillary electrophoresis. The consequence is that the capacity factor, k', characteristic of chromatography, is not valid in CEC.

To date, CEC has been operated in the reversed-phase mode. The stationary phases used are similar to those of HPLC based on silica matrices. The mobile phase is generally an organic–aqueous system containing an electrolyte. The EOF is generated at the solid/liquid interface. The silica surface is negatively charged owing to deprotonisation of silanol groups and hence the mobile phase molecules carry a net positive charge, thereby forming an electrical double layer. The positively charged molcules near the surface of the silica induce similar changes in the nearby molecules. Under the influence of the applied field, these molecules migrate towards the negative electrode, dragging the bulk of the mobile phase with them. The velocity of the EOF is determined by a number of factors including the applied field and the viscosity and dielectric constant of the mobile phase. It is significantly slower in packed capillary columns than in the open tube variety.

The instrumentation for CEC is similar to that for CE except that both ends of the column are pressurised to ensure no pressure drop. Columns measuring 50 cm × 100 μm are commonly used and, because flow is produced by electroosomosis rather than applied pressure, smaller sized particles (1.5 to 5 μm) can be used than with HPLC, with the result that the column efficiency is much higher in CEC and the resolution time shorter than in HPLC.

CEC is potentially a very attractive form of chromatography because of its miniaturisation and low running cost. It is currently still in the development stage, but within a decade could challenge HPLC as the preferred separation technique.

13.5 ADSORPTION CHROMATOGRAPHY

13.5.1 Principle

This is the classic form of chromatography which is based upon the principle that certain solid materials, collectively known as adsorbents, have the ability to hold molecules at their surface. This adsorption process, which involves weak, non-ionic attractive forces of the van der Waals' and hydrogen-bonding type, occur at specific adsorption sites. These sites have the ability to discriminate between molecules and in the adsorption chromatographic process are occupied by molecules of the eluent or of the analytes present in the mixture in proportions depending upon the relative strengths of their interaction. As eluent is constantly passed down the column, differences in these binding strengths eventually lead to the separation of the analytes. The strength of binding of a particular analyte depends upon the functional groups present in its structure. Hydroxyl groups and aromatic groups tend to increase interaction with the adsorption surface, whereas aliphatic groups of different size usually differ only slightly in their interaction. In general, adsorption chromatography is influenced more by the presence of specific groups than by simple molecular size because only a specific group rather than the whole molecule can interact with the adsorption site.

A typical adsorbent is silica, which has silanol (Si — OH) groups on its surface. These groups, which are slightly acidic, can interact with polar functional groups of the analyte or eluent. The topology (arrangement) of these silanol groups in different commercial preparations of silica explains their different separation properties. Other commonly used adsorbents are alumina and carbon. Materials based on carbon, alumina or silica are available for low pressure chromatography and for HPLC (Table 13.2). Whereas the silicas are acidic and good for the separation of basic materials, the aluminas are more basic and better suited for the resolution of acidic materials.

The selection of the correct eluent (mobile phase) is essential for good resolution because it influences the capacity factor, k', of the analytes (Section 13.2.3). In general, an eluent with a polarity comparable to that of the most polar analyte in the mixture is chosen. Thus, alcohols would be selected if the analytes contained hydroxyl groups, acetone or esters would be selected for analytes containing carbonyl groups, and hydrocarbons such as hexane, heptane and toluene for analytes that are predominantly non-polar. Mixtures of solvents are commonly used in the context of gradient elution (Section 13.3.6). The presence of small amounts of water in the mobile phase is often beneficial when silica is used as the stationary phase, as the water molecules selectively block the more active silanol groups, leaving a more selective population of weaker binding sites.

Adsorption chromatography, which can be carried out in the thin-layer mode as well as the column mode, is most commonly used to separate non-ionic, water-insoluble compounds such as triglycerides, PTH amino acids (Section 6.4.3), vitamins and many drugs.

13.5.2 Hydroxylapatite chromatography

Crystalline hydroxylapatite ($Ca_{10}(PO_4)_6(OH)_2$) is an adsorbent used to separate mixtures of proteins or nucleic acids. The mechanism of adsorption is not fully understood but is thought to involve both the calcium ions and phosphate ions on the surface and to involve dipole–dipole interactions and possibly electrostatic attractions. One of the most important applications of hydroxylapatite chromatography is the separation of single-stranded from double-stranded DNA. Both forms of DNA bind at low phosphate buffer concentrations but as the buffer concentration is increased single-stranded DNA is selectively desorbed. As the buffer concentration is increased further, double-stranded DNA is released. This behaviour is exploited in the technique of Cot analysis (Section 2.3.1). The affinity of hydroxylapatite for double-stranded DNA is so high that the latter can be selectively removed from RNA and proteins in cell extracts by use of this type of chromatography.

Hydroxylapatite is available commercially in a range of forms suitable for LPLC and HPLC. These include crystalline or spheroidal hydroxylapatite and forms bonded to an agarose matrix. The adsorption capacity of all these forms is maximum around neutral pH and the conditions usually include 20 mM phosphate buffer for the adsorption process. Elution is achieved by increasing the phosphate buffer concentration to 500 mM.

13.5.3 **Hydrophobic interaction chromatography**

This type of chromatography was developed to purify proteins by exploiting their surface hydrophobicity, which is related to the presence of non-polar amino acid residues (Section 6.3.4). Groups of hydrophobic residues are scattered over the surface of proteins in a way that gives characteristic properties to each protein. In aqueous solution, these hydrophobic regions on the protein are covered with an ordered film of water molecules that effectively masks the hydrophobic groups. These groups can, however, be exposed by the addition of salt ions, which preferentially take up the ordered water molecules. The exposed hydrophobic regions can then interact with each other and this is the basis of salting-out (Section 6.3.4) using ammonium sulphate. In HIC, rather than facilitating protein–protein interaction by the exposure of the hydrophobic groups, the presence of hydrophobic groups attached to a suitable matrix facilitates protein–matrix interaction. The most commonly used stationary phases are alkyl (hexyl, octyl) or phenyl groups attached to an agarose matrix. Commercial materials include Phenyl Sepharose and Phenyl SPW, both for low pressure HIC, and Bio-Gel TSK Phenyl and Spherogel TSK Phenyl for HPLC.

Since HIC requires the presence of salting-out compounds such as ammonium sulphate to facilitate the exposure of the hydrophobic regions on the protein molecule, it is commonly used immediately after fractionation with ammonium sulphate (Section 6.3.4) as ammonium and sulphate ions are already present in the protein sample. To maximise the process, it is advantageous to adjust the pH of the protein sample to that of its isoelectric point. Once the proteins have been adsorbed to the stationary phase, selective elution can be achieved in a number of ways, including the use of an eluent of gradually decreasing ionic strength or of increasing pH (this increases the hydrophilicity of the protein) or by selective displacement by a displacer that has a stronger affinity for the stationary phase than has the protein. Examples include non-ionic detergents such as Tween 20 and Triton X-100, aliphatic alcohols such as butanol and ethylene glycol, and aliphatic amines such as butylamine. One of the potential problems with HIC is that some of these elution conditions may cause protein denaturation. The other practical problem with the technique is its non-predictability in that it works well for some proteins but not for others and a trial study is invariably necessary. Proteins purified by the technique include aldolase, transferrin, cytochrome c and thyroglobulin.

13.6 **PARTITION CHROMATOGRAPHY**

13.6.1 **Principle**

Like other forms of chromatography separation partition chromatography is based on differences in capacity factors, k', and distribution coefficients, K_d, of the analytes using liquid stationary and mobile phases (Section 13.2.3). It can be subdivided into liquid–liquid chromatography, in which the liquid stationary phase is attached to a supporting matrix by purely physical means, and bonded-phase liquid chromatography, in which the stationary phase is covalently attached to the matrix. An example of liquid–liquid chromatography is one in which a water stationary phase is supported by a cellulose, starch or silica matrix, all of which have the ability to bind physically as much as 50% (w/v) water and remain free-flowing powders. The advantages of this form of chromatography are that it is cheap, has a high capacity and has broad selectivity. Its disadvantage is that the elution process may gradually remove the stationary phase, thereby altering the chromatographic conditions. This problem is overcome by the bonded phases and this explains their more widespread use. Most bonded phases use silica as the matrix, which is derivatised to immobilise the stationary phase by reaction with an organochlorosilane:

$$\equiv Si-OH \;+\; Cl-\underset{\underset{CH_3}{|}}{\overset{\overset{CH_3}{|}}{Si}}-R \longrightarrow Si-O-\underset{\underset{CH_3}{|}}{\overset{\overset{CH_3}{|}}{Si}}-R \;+\; HCl$$

Silica   Organo-
                  chloro-
                  silane

Surplus silanol groups are removed by capping with chlorotrimethylsilane to improve the quality of the chromatography by decreasing tailing (Fig. 13.3c). There are two commonly used modes of partition chromatography that differ in the relative polarities of the stationary and mobile phases and give rise to normal phase liquid chromatography and reversed-phase liquid chromatography.

13.6.2 Normal phase liquid chromatography

In this form of chromatography, the stationary phase is polar and the mobile phase relatively non-polar. The most popular stationary phase is an alkylamine bonded to silica (Table 13.2). The mobile phase is generally an organic solvent such as hexane, heptane, dichloromethane or ethylacetate. The mechanism of separation exploits the ability of the analyte to displace molecules of the mobile phase adsorbed as a monolayer on the surface of the stationary phase, as well as the ability of the analyte to compete with mobile phase molecules in the formation of a bilayer on the stationary phase surface. The order of elution of analytes is such that the *least* polar is eluted *first* and the *most* polar *last*. Indeed, polar analytes generally require gradient elution with a mobile phase of *increasing* polarity, generally achieved by the use of methanol or dioxane. The main advantages of normal phase liquid chromatography are its ability to separate analytes that have low water solubility and those that are not amenable to reversed-phase liquid chromatography.

13.6.3 Reversed-phase liquid chromatography

In this form of liquid chromatography, the stationary phase is non-polar and the mobile phase relatively polar. By far the most commonly used type is the

Table 13.3 Examples of bonded phases for reversed-phase HPLC

Product	Medium	Particle size (μm)	Manufacturer
Sephacil C18	Silica, C18	5	Pharmacia
LiChrsorb PR18	C18	5–10	Merck
Zorbax ODS	C18	6	DuPont
μBonda-Pak	C18	10	Waters
Sephacil C8	C8	5	Pharmacia
Resolve C8	C8	10	Waters
μBonda-Pak Phenyl	Phenyl	10	Waters
μBonda-Pak CN	CN	10	Waters
μBonda-Pak NH$_2$	NH$_2$	10	Waters

bonded-phase form, in which alkylsilane groups are chemically attached to silica. Butyl (C_4), octyl (C_8) and octadecyl (C_{18}) silane groups are invariably used (Table 13.3). The mobile phase is commonly water or aqueous buffers, methanol, acetonitrile, or tetrahydrofuran or mixtures of them. The organic solvent is referred to as an organic modifier. Reversed-phase liquid chromatography differs from most other forms of chromatography in that the stationary phase is essentially inert and only non-polar (hydrophobic) interactions with analytes are possible. Chromatographic separation of analytes is determined principally by the characteristics of the mobile phase and probably involves a combination of adsorption and partition mechanisms. It is believed to have many similarities to hydrophobic interaction chromatography. No simple model has been described to explain reversed-phase chromatography but the solvophobic theory is the one most widely considered. It is based on the consideration of the balance of free energy and entropy changes associated with bonding of the analyte with the stationary phase and with the mobile phase. The attraction of the reversed-phase technique is that small changes in the mobile phase composition such as the addition of salts, change of pH or the amount of organic solvent, profoundly affect the separation characteristics. Moreover, the technique is sensitive to temperature change such that a 10 deg.C increase approximately halves the capacity factor, k' (Section 13.2.3).

In reversed-phase chromatography, *polar* analytes elute *first* and *non-polar* analytes *last*. Non-polar analytes may need gradient elution using increasing proportions of a low polarity solvent such as hexane.

Reversed-phase HPLC is probably the most widely used form of chromatography mainly because of its flexibility and high resolution. It is widely used to analyse drugs and their metabolites, insecticide and pesticide residues, and amino acids. It is also now widely applied to proteins by using FPLC. Octadecylsilane (ODS) phases bind proteins more tightly than do octyl- or methylsilane phases and are therefore more likely to cause protein denaturation because of the more extreme conditions required for the elution of the protein. In non-aqueous form, reversed-phase chromatography can be used to separate lipophilic compounds such as fats.

13.6.4 Ion-pair reversed-phase liquid chromatography

The separation of some highly polar compounds, such as amino acids, peptides, organic acids and the catecholamines, which are difficult to resolve adequately by conventional reversed-phase chromatography, can often be improved by one of two possible approaches. The first is ion suppression in which the ionisation of the compound is suppressed by chromatographing at an appropriately high or low pH. Weak acids, for example, can be chromatographed using an acidified mobile phase. The second is ion-pairing in which a counter ion with charge opposite to that to be separated is added to the mobile phase so that the resulting ion-pair has sufficient lipophilic character to be retained by the non-polar stationary phase of a reversed-phase system. Thus, to aid the separation of acidic compounds, which would be present as their conjugate anions, a quaternary alkylamine ion such as tetrabutylammonium would be used as the counter ion, whereas for the separation of bases, which would be present as cations, an alkyl sulphonate such as sodium heptanesulphonate would be used:

$$RCOO^- \quad + \quad R_4'N^+ \quad \rightleftharpoons \quad [RCOO^-\overset{+}{N}R_4']$$

carboxylic   counter cation   ion-pair
acid anion

$$R\overset{+}{N}H_3 \quad + \quad R'SO_3^- \quad \rightleftharpoons \quad [R\overset{+}{N}H_3{}^-O_3SR']$$

conjugate acid   counter anion   ion-pair
of weak base

The mechanism by which ion-pairing results in better separation is not clear but two theories have been proposed. The first suggests that the ion-pair behaves as a single neutral species, whilst the second suggests that an active ion-exchange surface is produced in which the counter ion, which has considerable lipophilic properties, and the ions to be separated are adsorbed by the hydrophobic, non-polar stationary phase. In practice, the success of the ion-pairing approach is variable and somewhat empirical. The size of the counter ion, its concentration and the pH of the solution are all factors that may profoundly influence the outcome of the separation.

Octyl- and octadecylsilane-bonded phases are used most commonly in conjunction with a water/methanol or water/acetonitrile mobile phase. One of the advantages of ion-pair reversed-phase chromatography is that, if the sample to be resolved contains a mixture of non-ionic and ionic compounds, the two groups of compounds can be separated simultaneously because the ion-pair reagent does not affect the chromatography of the non-ionic species. This is not true of ion-exchange chromatography.

13.6.5 Chiral chromatography

Chiral compounds either contain at least one asymmetric carbon atom or are molecularly asymmetric. They exist in two enantiomorphic forms, related as object and mirror images, have the same physical and chemical properties and differ only in their interaction with plane-polarised light such that one is dextrorotatory ($+$) and the other laevorotatory ($-$). There are a number of conventions for indicating the spatial configuration, as opposed to optical properties, of enantiomers. The classical D and L system for monosaccharides and amino acids cannot be applied easily to other structures and the Cahn–Ingold–Prelog system, which assigns R (*rectus*) or S (*sinister*) configurations to an enantiomer, is of more general use. Until recently it has not been possible to resolve mixtures of enantiomers and this has created problems for the pharmaceutical industry in its development and clinical use of drugs, many of which are chiral, for although enantiomers have identical chemical and physical properties they are distinguishable biologically. Thus they differ in their ability to interact with the receptors involved in a range of physiological responses and they are often metabolised and excreted at different rates.

Chromatographic techniques have now been developed that allow mixtures of enantiomers to be resolved. One of these techniques is based on the fact that diastereoisomers, which are optical isomers that do not have an object–image relationship, do differ in physical properties even though they contain identical functional groups. They can therefore be separated by conventional chromatographic techniques, most commonly reversed-phase chromatography (Section 13.6.3). The diastereoisomer approach requires that the enantiomers contain a function group that can be derivatised by a chemically and optically pure chiral derivatising agent (CDA) to convert them to a mixture of diastereoisomers:

(R + S)	+	R′	→	RR′ + SR′
mixture of enantiomers		chiral derivatising agent		mixture of diastereoisomers

Examples of CDAs include the R or S form of the following:

For amines	*N*-trifluoroacetyl-L-prolylchloride, α-phenylbutyric anhydride
For alcohols	2-Phenylpropionyl chloride, 1-phenylethylisothiocyanate
For ketones	2,2,2-Trifluoro-1-pentylethylhydrazine
For aliphatic and alicyclic acids	1-Menthol, desoxyephedrine

Although this approach to chiral resolution is relatively simple, it is essential that the derivatisation process should be rapid and quantitative. Very often this is not the case and this has restricted its use. An alternative approach to the resolution problem is to use a chiral mobile phase. In this technique a transient diastereomeric complex is formed between the enantiomers and the chiral mobile phase agent. Examples of chiral mobile phase agents include albumin, α_1-acid glycoprotein, α, β- and γ-cyclodextrins, 10-camphorsulphonic acid and *N*-benzoxycarbonylglycyl-L-proline, all of which are used with a reversed-phase chromatographic system.

The most successful approach to chiral chromatography, however, has been the use of a chiral stationary phase. This is based upon the principle that the need for a three-point interaction between the stationary phase (working as a chiral discriminator) and the enantiomer would allow the resolution of racemic mixtures due to the different spatial arrangement of the functional groups at the chiral centre in the enantiomers. One such successful approach uses Pirkle phases, based on dinitrobenzoyl derivatives of amino acids such as phenylglycine that are bonded to silica. These phases are thought to function by allowing transient formation of enantiomer–stationary phase complexes by bonding such as hydrogen bonding and van der Waals' forces. Elution is generally by the reversed-phase technique. Alternative chiral stationary phases include triacetylcellulose and various cyclodextrins bonded to silica. These cyclodextrins are cyclic oligosaccharides that have an open truncated conical structure 6 to 8 Å (0.6 to 0.8 nm) wide at their base. Their inner surface is predominantly hydrophobic, but secondary hydroxyl groups are located around the wide rim of the cone. β-Cyclodextrin has 7 glucopyranose units and contains 35 chiral centres and α-cyclodextrin has 6 glucopryanose units, 30 chiral centres and is smaller than β-cyclodextrin. Collectively they are referred to as chiral cavity phases because they rely on the ability of the enantiomer to enter the three-dimensional cyclodextrin cage while at the same time presenting functional groups and hence the chiral centre for interaction with hydroxyl groups on the cone rim. Enantiomers possessing a five-, six- or seven-membered aromatic ring have been resolved by this approach in conjunction with reversed-phase elution. A more recent innovation has been the use of the macrocyclic antibiotics vancomycin and teicoplanin as chiral stationary phases. Vancomycin has 18 chiral centres and teicoplanin 23. Both have been used successfully in chiral separations using normal and reversed-phase separations.

Since proteins are optically active, they can in principle be used as a chiral stationary phase. Bovine serum albumin and α_1-acid glycoprotein (AGP) have been evaluated and found to be successful for a wide range of separations, but their mechanism of chiral separation is poorly understood. Both albumin and α_1-acid glycoprotein occur in plasma and have long been known to bind drugs (Fig. 13.11). Albumin has at least two distinct binding sites to which acidic and basic drugs may bind. α_1-Acid glycoprotein has a single drug-binding site restricted to the binding of basic drugs such as propranolol. These protein chiral phases are used in conjunction with aqueous buffers and cannot be used at extremes of pH or in the presence of organic solvents.

13.6.6 Countercurrent chromatography

This separation process is based upon the distribution of a compound between two immiscible liquid phases. These phases may be mixtures of organic solvents, buffers, salts and various complexing agents. The technique is atypical of normal partition chromatographic techniques in that neither of the phases is supported by

(a)

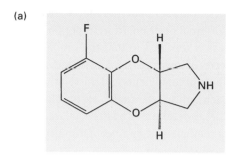

(b)

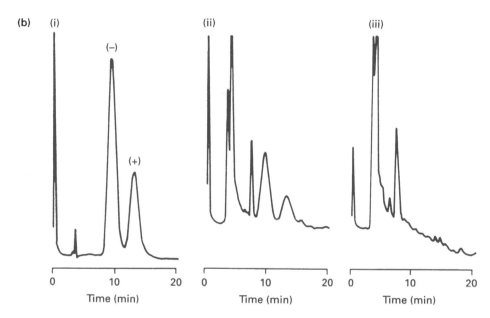

Fig. 13.11. Chiral separation of the enantiomers of GR50360 ((a), M_r 195) in pure solution (b(i)) and in human plasma (b(ii)). (b(iii)) A blank sample of plasma. Resolution was achieved on a bovine serum albumin (Resolvosil 7) column using 0.25 M phosphate buffer, pH 6.2, flow rate 0.8 cm³ min⁻¹ at 35 °C and ultraviolet detection (220 nm wavelength). (Reproduced by permission of Glaxo Wellcome, Stevenage.)

an inert support and the process is not conducted in a simple column. Nevertheless, the separation of compounds is based upon the different distribution coefficients between two immiscible phases and therefore the principle of the separation is the same as that of conventional liquid–liquid partition chromatography.

The apparatus most commonly used is the Craig Countercurrent Distribution apparatus. It consists of between 30 and 1000 interconnected H-shaped vessels (the so-called train), each of which retains a fixed volume of the stationary liquid phase. The solute mixture is introduced to the first vessel in the train and equilibrated with the immiscible and less dense mobile phase by the repeated rocking of the vessel through 90°. After equilibration is complete (1 to 2 min), the mobile phase is transferred to the next vessel as a result of the complete tipping of the first vessel. When this returns to its original position, fresh upper phase is introduced automatically. The whole process is repeated so that the mobile phase is transferred progressively along the series of lower phases. The solutes are transferred at a rate determined by their distribution coefficients and the relative volumes of the two solvents in each vessel. Each solute eventually accumulates in a specific group of vessels, the resolution being determined by the total number of transfers and their differences in partition coefficient. A number of miniaturised versions of the technique are now available commercially.

CCC is one of the few forms of chromatography that have been used successfully for cell organelle fractionation. It has also been used for cell fractionation and membrane receptor isolation.

13.7 ION-EXCHANGE CHROMATOGRAPHY

13.7.1 Principle

This form of chromatography relies on the attraction between oppositely charged particles. Many biological materials, for example amino acids and proteins, have ionisable groups and the fact that they may carry a net positive or negative charge can be utilised in separating mixtures of such compounds. The net charge exhibited by these compounds is dependent on their pK_a and on the pH of the solution in accordance with the Henderson–Hasselbalch equation (Section 1.4.5, equation 1.27).

Ion-exchange separations are carried out mainly in columns packed with an ion-exchanger. There are two types of ion-exchanger, namely cation and anion exchangers. Cation exchangers possess negatively charged groups and these will attract positively charged cations. These exchangers are also called acidic ion-exchange materials because their negative charges result from the ionisation of acidic groups. Anion exchangers have positively charged groups that will attract negatively charged anions. The term basic ion-exchange materials is also used to describe these exchangers, as positive charges generally result from the association of protons with basic groups.

The ion-exchange mechanism is thought to be composed of five distinct steps:

  (i) Diffusion of the ion to the exchanger surface. This occurs very quickly in homogeneous solutions.
 (ii) Diffusion of the ion through the matrix structure of the exchanger to the exchange site. This is dependent upon the degree of cross-linkage of the exchanger and the concentration of the solution. This process is thought to be the feature that controls the rate of the whole ion-exchange process.
(iii) Exchange of ions at the exchange site. This is thought to occur instantaneously and to be an equilibrium process.

Cation exchanger

$$RSO_3^- \quad \ldots Na^+ \; + \; \overset{+}{N}H_3R' \; \rightleftharpoons \; RSO_3^- \ldots \overset{+}{N}H_3R' \; + \; Na^+$$

| exchanger | counter ion | charged molecule to be exchanged | | bound molecular ion | exchanged ion |

Anion exchanger

$$(R)_4\overset{+}{N}\ldots Cl^- \; + \; {}^-OOCR' \; \rightleftharpoons \; (R)_4\overset{+}{N}\ldots{}^-OOCR' + \; Cl^-$$

The more highly charged the ionised molecule to be exchanged, the tighter it binds to the exchanger and the less readily it is displaced by other ions.

(iv) Diffusion of the exchanged ion through the exchanger to the surface.

(v) Selective desorption by the eluent and diffusion of the molecule into the external eluent. The selective desorption of the bound ion is achieved by changes in pH and/or ionic concentration or by affinity elution, in which case an ion that has greater affinity for the exchanger than has the bound ion is introduced into the system.

13.7.2 **Materials and applications**

Low pressure ion-exchange chromatography can be carried out using a variety of matrices and ionic groups. Matrices used include polystyrene, cellulose and agarose. Functional ionic groups include sulphonate ($-SO_3^-$) and quaternary ammonium ($-\overset{+}{N}R_3$), both of which are strong exchangers because they are totally ionised at all normal working pH values, and carboxylate ($-COO^-$) and diethyl-ammonium ($-\overset{+}{H}N(CH_2CH_3)_2$), both of which are termed weak exchangers because they are ionised over only a narrow range of pH values. Examples are given in Table 13.4. Bonded phase ion-exchangers suitable for HPLC, containing a wide range of ionic groups, are now available in pellicular and porous forms. The porous variety, which are based on polystyrene, porous silica or hydrophilic poly-ethers, are particularly valuable for the separation of proteins. They have a particle diameter of 5 to 25 μm. Most HPLC ion-exchangers are stable up to 60 °C and separations are often carried out at this temperature, owing to the fact that the raised temperature decreases the viscosity of the mobile phase and thereby increases the efficiency of the separation.

All exchangers are characterised by a total exchange capacity, which is defined as the number of milliequivalents of exchangeable ions available, either per gram of dried exchanger or per unit volume of hydrated resin. Sometimes available capacity is also used to express the available capacity for an arbitrarily chosen molecule such as haemoglobin. These exchange capacities give an indication of the degree of substitution of the exchanger and are therefore a helpful guide in deciding on the scale of a particular application.

The choice of the ion-exchanger depends upon the stability of the sample components, their relative molecular mass and the specific requirements of the

Table 13.4 Examples of commonly used ion-exchangers

Type	Matrices	Functional groups	Functional group name
Weakly acidic (cation exchanger)	Agarose Cellulose Dextran Polyacrylate	$-COO^-$ $-CH_2COO^-$	Carboxy Carboxymethyl
Strongly acidic (cation exchanger)	Cellulose Dextran Polystyrene	$-SO_3^-$ $-CH_2SO_3^-$ $-CH_2CH_2CH_2SO_3^-$	Sulpho Sulphomethyl Sulphopropyl
Weakly basic (anion exchanger)	Agarose Cellulose Dextran Polystyrene	$-CH_2CH_2\overset{+}{N}H_3$ $-CH_2CH_2\overset{+}{N}H(CH_2CH_3)_2$	Aminoethyl Diethylaminoethyl
Strongly basic (anion exchanger)	Cellulose Dextran Polystyrene	$-CH_2\overset{+}{N}(CH_3)_3$ $-CH_2CH_2\overset{+}{N}(CH_2CH_3)_3$ $-CH_2\overset{+}{N}(CH_3)_2$ $\quad\mid$ $\quad CH_2CH_2OH$ $-CH_2CH_2\overset{+}{N}(CH_2CH_3)_2$ $\quad\quad\mid$ $\quad\quad CH_2CHCH_3$ $\quad\quad\quad\mid$ $\quad\quad\quad OH$	Trimethylaminomethyl Triethylaminoethyl Dimethyl-2-hydroxyethylaminomethyl Diethyl-2-hydroxypropylaminoethyl

separation. Many biological components, especially proteins, are stable within only a fairly narrow pH range so the exchanger selected must operate within this range. Generally, if the sample is most stable below its isoionic points (giving it a net positive charge) a cation exchanger should be used, whereas if it is most stable above its isoionic points (giving it a net negative charge) an anion exchanger should be used. Compounds that are stable over a wide range of pH may be separated by either type of exchanger. The choice between a strong and weak exchanger also depends on sample stability and the effect of pH on sample charge. Weak electrolytes requiring a very low or high pH for ionisation can be separated only on strong exchangers, as only they operate over a wide pH range. In contrast, for strong electrolytes, weak exchangers are advantageous for a number of reasons, including a reduced tendency to cause sample denaturation, their inability to bind weakly charged impurities and their enhanced elution characteristics. Although the degree of cross-linking of an exchanger does not influence the ion-exchange mechanism, it does influence its capacity. The relative molecular mass and hence size of the sample component therefore determines which specific exchanger should be used.

The pH of the buffer used should be at least one pH unit above or below the isoionic point of the compounds being separated. In general, cationic buffers such as Tris, pyridine and alkylamines are used in conjunction with anion exchangers, and anionic buffers such as acetate, barbiturate and phosphate are used with cation exchangers. The precise initial buffer pH and ionic strength should be such as just to allow the binding of the sample components to the exchanger. Equally, a buffer of the lowest ionic strength that effects elution should initially be used for the subsequent elution of the components. This ensures that initially the minimum number of undesired substances bind to the exchanger and that subsequently the maximum number of these impurities remain on the column. The amount of sample that can be applied to a column is dependent upon the size of the column and the capacity of the exchanger. Generally, if the starting buffer is to be used throughout the development of the column (isocratic elution), the sample volume should be 1% to 5% of the bed volume. If, however, gradient elution is to be used, the initial conditions chosen are such that the entire sample is bound by the exchanger at the top of the column. In this case the sample volume is not important and large volumes of dilute solution can be applied, thereby effectively introducing a concentration stage.

Gradient elution is far more common than isocratic elution. Continuous or stepwise pH and ionic strength gradients may be employed but continuous gradients tend to give better resolution with less peak tailing (Section 13.1.3). Generally with an anion exchanger the pH gradient decreases and the ionic strength increases, whereas for cation exchangers both the pH and ionic gradients increase.

The separation of amino acids (e.g. in a protein hydrolysate) can be achieved using a strong acid cation exchanger. The sample is introduced onto the column at a pH of 1 to 2, thus ensuring complete binding of all of the various types of amino acid (Section 6.1). Gradient elution using increasing pH and ionic concentration results in the sequential elution of amino acids. The acidic amino acids, aspartic and glutamic, are eluted first, followed by the neutral amino acids such as glycine and valine. The basic amino acids such as lysine and arginine retain their net positive charge up to pH values of 9 to 11 and are eluted last. These principles are embodied in automatic amino acid analysers. The effluent from the column is mixed with a detection reagent (Section 6.4.2) and nitrogen is also introduced to break the effluent stream into discrete segments and thus avoid axial mixing. The mixture is heated to 105 °C to develop the colour, the intensity of which is then determined by two colorimeters, one set at 570 nm wavelength to monitor the majority of the amino acids and a second set at 440 nm wavelength to monitor specifically the colour produced by proline and hydroxyproline. Alternatively, the amino acids may be detected by conversion to derivatives that undergo fluorescence. Whilst this dispenses with the need for two detectors, the method is more tedious and generally less reproducible than the ninhydrin method. In all cases, the system is calibrated for quantitative work by the use of standards of each amino acid. The separation of amino acids in a protein hydrolysate is increasingly being achieved by reversed-phase chromatography (Section 6.4.2) rather than ion-exchange, because of its greater speed and convenience and also because of the fact that it dispenses with the need for a dedicated amino acid analyser. In contrast, ion-exchange chromatography is commonly chosen for the separation and purification of proteins, peptides, nucleic acids, polynucleotides and other charged molecules, mainly because of its high resolving power and high capacity.

13.7.3 Chromatofocusing

The technique of chromatofocusing, the principle of which is similar to that of isoelectric focusing (Section 12.3.4), is particularly suitable for protein separations. A linear pH gradient is generated in the column by exploiting the high buffer capacity of an ion-exchanger pre-equilibrated to a particular pH. Using an amphoteric buffer that has even buffering capacity over a range of pH, and with a starting pH lower than that at which the ion-exchange column has been pre-equilibrated, the pH gradient, which is 3 to 4 pH units lower at the top of the column than at the bottom, is formed by running the buffer through the column for a predetermined time. When the protein is added to this pH gradient, with a buffer whose pH is similar to that prevailing at the top of the column, it will migrate down the column as a cation, encountering an increasing pH, until it reaches a pH corresponding to its isoelectric point. Just beyond this point it will become an anion and will be able to bind to the positive groups of the exchanger (in this example, an anion exchanger would be in use). As the elution continues with the starting buffer, the prevailing pH will be lowered, causing the binding of the protein to cease. The protein will continue its movement down the column until once again it encounters a pH slightly above its isoelectric point, when again it will bind. This process is repeated continuously until the protein is eluted at a pH slightly above its isolectric point (Fig. 13.12). In a mixture of proteins, each molecule would elute in the order of its isoelectric point. More protein added to the top of the column during this elution process would automatically catch up with the initial protein, thereby producing a focusing effect and enabling large volumes to

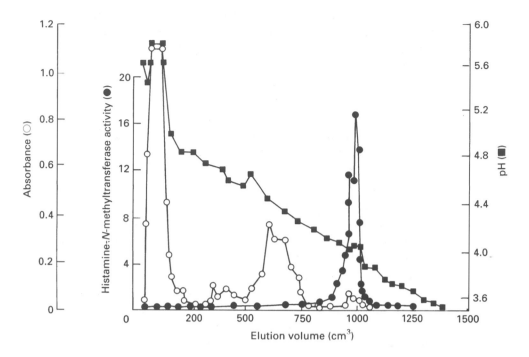

Fig. 13.12. Chromatofocusing elution profile of rat kidney histamine-*N*-methyl transferase. The partially purified sample (approximately 130 mg of protein) was chromatographed on a PBE 94 column (62 cm × 1.6 cm), previously equilibrated with 25 mM piperazine-HCl at pH 5.5. Five cm³ of the eluent Polybuffer™74, pH 3.5, preceded the sample. Elution was carried out at a flow rate of 20 cm³ h⁻¹. The fractions (5.0 cm³) were assayed for pH (■), histamine-*N*-methyl transferase activty (●) expressed as extracted d.p.m. × 10⁻⁴ per 2.5 cm³ chloroform, and absorbance at 600 nm (○) measured after reaction with Coomassie Brilliant Blue. (Reproduced by permission of Glaxo Wellcome, Stevenage.)

be applied to the column, with no deleterious effect. Thus the technique has a high capacity. Chromatofocusing gives a good resolution of quite complex mixtures of proteins, provided that there are discrete differences in their isoelectric point. Proteins possessing very similar isoelectric points tend to be poorly resolved.

13.8 MOLECULAR EXCLUSION (PERMEATION) CHROMATOGRAPHY

13.8.1 Principle

The separation of molecules on the basis of their molecular size and shape utilises the molecular sieve properties of a variety of porous materials. Probably the most commonly used of such materials is a group of polymeric organic compounds that possess a three-dimensional network of pores that confers gel properties upon them. The term gel filtration is used to describe the separation of molecules of varying molecular size utilising these gel materials. Porous glass granules have

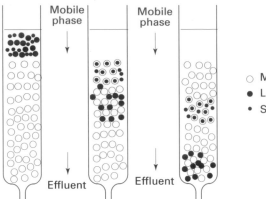

Fig. 13.13.   Separation of different sized molecules by exclusion chromatography. Large (excluded) molecules are eluted first in the void volume.

also been used as molecular sieves and the term controlled-pore glass chromatography introduced to describe this separation technique. The terms exclusion or permeation chromatography describe all molecular separation processes using molecular sieves. This section is devoted mainly to gel filtration, as its principles and applications are best documented, but it must be appreciated that controlled-pore glass chromatography has much in common with gel filtration.

The general principle of exclusion chromatography is quite simple. A column of gel particles or porous glass granules is in equilibrium with a suitable mobile phase for the molecules to be separated. Large molecules that are completely excluded from the pores will pass through the interstitial spaces and will appear in the effluent first. Smaller molecules will be distributed between the mobile phase inside and outside the molecular sieve and will then pass through the column at a slower rate, hence appearing last in the effluent. Three stages in such a column are represented diagrammatically in Fig. 13.13.

The mobile phase absorbed by a gel is available to an analyte to an extent that is dependent upon the porosity of the gel particle and the size of the analyte molecule. Thus, the distribution of an analyte in a column of a gel is determined solely by the total volume of mobile phase, both inside and outside the gel particles, that is available to it. For a given type of gel, the distribution coefficient, K_d, of a particular analyte between the inner and outer mobile phase is a function of its molecular size. If the analyte is large and completely excluded from the mobile phase within the gel, $K_d = 0$, whereas, if the analyte is sufficiently small to gain complete access to the inner mobile phase, $K_d = 1$. Due to variation in pore size between individual gel particles, there is some inner mobile phase that will be available and some that will not be available to analytes of intermediate size; hence K_d values vary between 0 and 1. It is this complete variation of K_d between these two limits that makes possible the separation of analytes within a narrow molecular size range on a given gel.

Table 13.5 Some gels commonly used for low pressure liquid exclusion chromatography

Polymer	Trade name		Fractionation range[a] ($M_R \times 10^{-3}$)
Dextran	Sephadex	G10	< 0.7
		G25	1.0–5
		G50	1.5–30
		G100	4.0–150
		G200	5.0–600
	Sephacryl	S200	5.0–250
		S300	10.0–1500
		S400	20.0–8000
Agarose	Sepharose	6B	10.0–4000
		4B	60.0–20 000
		2B	70.0–40 000
	Bio-Gel	A5m	10.0–5000
		A15m	40.0–15 000
		A50m	100.0–50 000
		A150m	1000.0–150 000
Polyacrylamide	Bio-Gel	P2	0.1–1.8
		P6	1.0–6.0
		P30	2.5–40.0
		P100	5.0–100.0
		P300	60.0–400.0

[a] Determined for globular proteins. The range is approximately the same for single-stranded nucleic acids and smaller for fibrous proteins and double-stranded DNA.

For two substances of different relative molecular mass and K_d values, K'_d and K''_d the difference in their elution volumes, V_S, can be shown to be

$$V_S = (K'_d - K''_d) V_i \qquad (13.13)$$

where V_i is the inner volume within the gel available to a compound whose $K_d = 1$.

In practice, deviations from ideal behaviour, for example owing to poor packing of the column, make it advisable to reduce the sample volume below the value of V_S because the ratio between sample volume and inside gel volume affects both the sharpness of the separation and the degree of dilution of the sample.

13.8.2 Materials

Gels that are commonly used include cross-linked dextrans (e.g. Sephadex), agarose (Sepharose, Bio-Gel A, Sagavac), polyacrylamide (Bio-Gel P), polyacryloyl-morphine (Enzocryl Gel) and polystyrene (Bio-Beads S). Examples of materials for LPLC are shown in Table 13.5 and examples of materials suitable for HPLC are shown in Table 13.2. The latter type are semi-rigid cross-linked polymers or rigid controlled-pore glasses or silicas.

Exclusion chromatography requires a single mobile phase and isocratic elution. It is most commonly used with ultraviolet absorption spectrophotometric detectors. Exclusion chromatography columns tend to be longer than those for other forms of chromatography in order to increase the amount of stationary phase and hence pore volume.

13.8.3 Applications

Purification.   The main application of exclusion chromatography is in the purification of biological macromolecules by facilitating their separation from larger and smaller molecules. Viruses, enzymes, hormones, antibodies, nucleic acids and polysaccharides have all been separated and purified by use of appropriate gels or glass granules.

Relative molecular mass determination.   The elution volumes of globular proteins are determined largely by their relative molecular mass (M_r). It has been shown that, over a considerable range of relative molecular masses, the elution volume or K_d is an approximately linear function of the logarithm of M_r. Hence the construction of a calibration curve, with proteins of a similar shape and known M_r, enables the M_r values of other proteins, even in crude preparations, to be estimated (See section 6.4.1).

Solution concentration.   Solutions of high M_r substances can be concentrated by the addition of dry Sephadex G-25 (coarse). Water and low M_r substances are absorbed by the swelling gel, whereas the high M_r substances remain in solution. After 10 min the gel is removed by centrifugation, leaving the high M_r material in a solution whose concentration has increased but whose pH and ionic strength are unaltered.

Desalting.   By use of a column of Sephadex G-25, solutions of high M_r compounds may be desalted. The high M_r substances move with the void volume, whereas the low M_r components are distributed between the mobile and stationary phases and hence move slowly. This method of desalting is faster and more efficient than dialysis. Applications include removal of phenol from nucleic acid preparations, ammonium sulphate from protein preparations and salt from samples eluted from ion-exchange chromatography columns.

Protein-binding studies.   Exclusion chromatography is one of a number of methods commonly used to study the reversible binding of a ligand to a macromolecule such as a protein, including receptor proteins (Section 8.2.3). A sample of the protein/ligand mixture is applied to a column of a suitable gel that has previously been equilibrated with a solution of the ligand of the same concentration as that in the mixture. The sample is eluted with buffer in the standard way and the concentration of ligand and protein in the effluent determined. The early fractions will contain unbound ligand, but the subsequent appearance of the protein will result in an increase in the total amount of ligand (bound plus unbound). If the experiment is repeated at a series of ligand concentrations, the appropriate binding constants can be calculated (Section 8.2.2).

13.9 **AFFINITY CHROMATOGRAPHY**

13.9.1 **Principle**

Purification by affinity chromatography is unlike most other forms of chromatography and such techniques as electrophoresis and centrifugation in that it does not rely on differences in the physical properties of the molecules to be separated. Instead, it exploits the unique property of extremely specific biological interactions to achieve separation and purification. As a consequence, affinity chromatography is theoretically capable of giving absolute purification, even from complex mixtures, in a single process. The technique was originally developed for the purification of enzymes, but it has since been extended to nucleotides, nucleic acids, immunoglobulins, membrane receptors and even to whole cells and cell fragments.

The technique requires that the material to be isolated is capable of binding reversibly to a specific ligand that is attached to an insoluble matrix:

$$
\begin{array}{ccccc}
\text{M} & + & \text{L} & \overset{k_{+1}}{\underset{k_{-1}}{\rightleftharpoons}} & \text{ML} \\
\text{macromolecule} & & \text{ligand} & & \text{complex} \\
& & \text{(attached} & & \\
& & \text{to matrix)} & &
\end{array}
$$

Under the correct experimental conditions, when a complex mixture containing the specific compound to be purified is added to the immobilised ligand, generally contained in a conventional chromatography column, only that compound will bind to the ligand. All other compounds can therefore be washed away and the compound subsequently recovered by displacement from the ligand (Fig. 13.14).

The method requires a detailed preliminary knowledge of the structure and biological specificity of the compound to be purified so that the separation conditions that are most likely to be successful may be carefully planned. In the case of an enzyme, the ligand may be the substrate, a reversible inhibitor or an allosteric activator. The conditions chosen would normally be those that are optimal for enzyme–ligand binding. Since the success of the method relies on the reversible formation of the complex and on the numerical values of the first-order rate constants k_{+1} and k_{-1}, as the enzyme is added progressively to the insolubilised ligand in a column, the enzyme molecules will be stimulated to bind and a dynamic situation develops in which the concentration of the complex and the strength of the binding increase. It is because of this progressive increase in effectiveness during the addition of the sample to the column that column procedures are invariably more successful than batch-type methods. Nevertheless, alternative forms have been developed and are particularly suitable for large-scale work. They include:

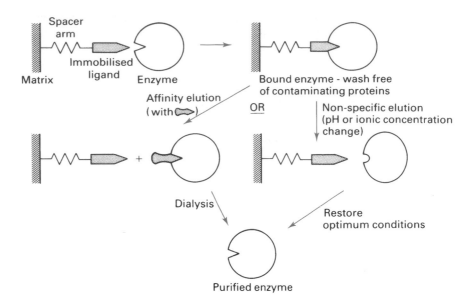

Fig. 13.14. Diagram of purification of an enzyme by affinity chromatography.

(a) affinity precipitation, in which the ligand is attached to a soluble carrier that can be subsequently precipitated by, for example, a pH change; and (b) affinity partitioning in which the ligand is attached to a water-soluble polymer such as polyethylene glycol and which, with the ligand bound, preferentially partitions into an aqueous polymer phase that is in equilibrium with a pure aqueous phase. In all cases, for effective chromatography, the association constant, K_a, for the complex should be in the region 10^4 to 10^8 M^{-1}.

13.9.2 Materials

Matrix

An ideal matrix for affinity chromatography must possess the following characteristics:

(i) It must contain suitable and sufficient chemical groups to which the ligand may be covalently coupled and it must be stable under the conditions of the attachment.
(ii) It must be stable during binding of the macromolecule and its subsequent elution.
(iii) It must at the most interact only weakly with other macromolecules to minimise non-specific adsorption.
(iv) It should exhibit good flow properties.

In practice, particles that are uniform, spherical and rigid are used. The most common ones are the cross-linked dextrans (Sephacryl S), agarose (Sepharose,

BioGel A), polyacrylamide gels (Bio-Gel P), polystyrene (Bio-Beads S), cellulose and porous glass and silica.

Selection and attachment of ligand

The chemical nature of a ligand is determined by the prior knowledge of the biological specificity of the compound to be purified. In practice it is frequently possible to select a ligand that displays absolute specificity in that it will bind exclusively to one particular compound. Alternatively, it is possible to select a ligand that displays group selectivity in that it will bind to a closely related group of compounds that possess a similar in-built chemical specificity. An example of the latter type of ligand is 5′-AMP, which can bind reversibly to many NAD^+-dependent dehydrogenases because it is structurally similar to part of the NAD^+ molecule. It is essential that the ligand possesses a suitable chemical group that will not be involved in the reversible binding of the ligand to the macromolecule, but which can be used to attach the ligand to the matrix. The most common of such groups are $-NH_2$, $-COOH$, $-SH$ and $-OH$ (phenolic and alcoholic). To prevent the attachment of the ligand to the matrix interfering with its ability to bind the macromolecule, it is generally advantageous to interpose a spacer arm between the ligand and the matrix. The optimum length of this spacer arm is six to ten carbon atoms or their equivalent. In some cases, the chemical nature of this spacer is critical to the success of separation. Some spacers are purely hydrophobic, most commonly consisting of methylene groups, others are hydrophilic, possessing carbonyl or imido groups. Spacers are most important for small immobilised ligands but generally are not necessary for macromolecular ligands (e.g. in immunoaffinity chromatography, Section 13.9.5) as their binding site for the mobile macromolecule is well displaced from the matrix.

The most common method of attachment of the ligand to the matrix involves the preliminary treatment of the matrix with cyanogen bromide (CNBr) (Fig. 13.15). The reaction conditions and the relative proportion of the reagents will determine the number of ligand molecules that can be attached to each matrix particle. Alternative coupling procedures involve the use of bis-epoxides, *N,N′*-disubstituted carbodiimides, sulphonyl chloride, sodium periodate, *N*-hydroxysuccinide esters and dichlorotriazines. Many preactivated matrices, prepared using these coupling reagents, are available commercially.

A number of different spacer arms are used. Examples include 1,6-diaminohexane, 6-aminohexanoic acid and 1,4-bis-(2,3-epoxypropoxy)butane. They must possess a second functional group to which the ligand may be attached by conventional organosynthetic procedures, which frequently involve the use of succinic anhydride and a water-soluble carbodiimide. A number of supports of the agarose, dextran and polyacrylamide type are commercially available, with a variety of spacer arms and ligands preattached ready for immediate use. Examples of ligands are given in Table 13.6.

Practical procedure

The procedure for affinity chromatography is similar to that used in other forms of liquid chromatography. The ligand-treated matrix is packed into a column in the

Table 13.6 Examples of group-specific ligands commonly used in affinity chromatography

Ligand	Affinity
Nucleotides	
5′-AMP	NAD$^+$-dependent dehydrogenases, some kinases
2′5′-ADP	NADP$^+$-dependent dehydrogenases
Calmodulin	Calmodulin-binding enzymes
Avidin	Biotin-containing enzymes
Fatty acids	Fatty-acid-binding proteins
Heparin	Lipoproteins, lipases, coagulation factors, DNA polymerases, steroid receptor proteins, growth factors, serine protease inhibitors
Proteins A and G	Immunoglobulins
Concanavalin A	Glycoproteins containing α-D-mannopyranosyl and α–D-glucopyranosyl residues
Soybean lectin	Glycoproteins containing N-acetyl-α-(or β)-D-galactopyranosyl residues
Phenylboronate	Glycoproteins
Poly(A)	RNA containing poly(U) sequences, some RNA-specific proteins
Lysine	rRNA
Cibacron Blue F3G-A	Nucleotide-requiring enzymes, coagulation factors

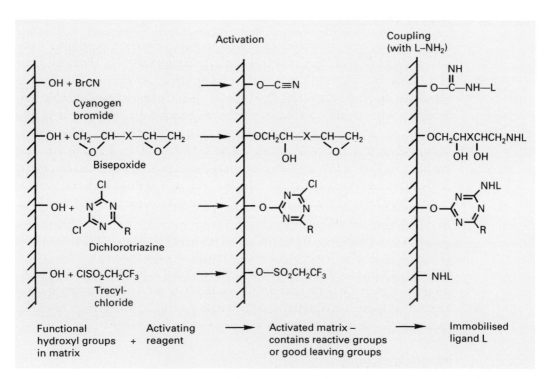

Fig. 13.15. Examples of coupling reactions used to immobilise ligands (L) for affinity chromatography. If a spacer arm is to be introduced between the immobilised ligand and the matrix, the coupling chemistry is similar.

normal way for the particular type of support. The buffer used must contain any cofactors, such as metal ions, necessary for ligand–macromolecule interaction. Once the sampe has been applied and the macromolecule bound, the column is eluted with more buffer to remove non-specifically bound contaminants.

The purified compound is recovered from the ligand by either specific or non-specific elution. Non-specific elution may be achieved by a change in either pH or ionic strength. pH shift elution using dilute acetic acid or ammonium hydroxide results from a change in the state of ionisation of groups, in the ligand and/or the macromolecule, that are critical to ligand–macromolecule binding. A change in ionic strength, not necessarily with a concomitant change in pH, also causes elution due to a disruption of the ligand–macromolecule interaction; 1 M NaCl is frequently used for this purpose. If elution is achieved by a pH change, the pH of the collected fractions must be readjusted to the optimum value to minimise the opportunity for protein denaturation. Affinity elution involves the addition of a high concentration of substrate, or reversible inhibitor of the macromolecule if it is an enzyme, or the addition of ligands for which the macromolecule has a higher affinity than it has for the immobilised ligand. The purified material is eventually recovered in a buffered solution that may be contaminated with specific eluting agents or high concentrations of salt and these must be removed by techniques such as exclusion chromatography before the isolation is complete.

13.9.3 Applications

A wide range of enzymes and other proteins, including receptor proteins and immunoglobulins, has been purified by affinity chromatography. The application of the technique is limited only by the availability of immobilised ligands. The principles have been extended to nucleic acids and have made a considerable contribution to developments in molecular biology. Messenger RNA, for example, is routinely isolated by selective hybridisation on poly(U)-Sepharose 4B by exploiting its poly(A) tail. Immobilised single-stranded DNA can be used to isolate complementary RNA and DNA. Whilst this separation can be achieved on columns, it is usually performed using single-stranded DNA immobilised on nitrocellulose filters. Immobilised nucleotides are useful for the isolation of proteins involved in nucleic acid metabolism.

A valuable development of affinity chromatography is its use for the separation of a mixture of cells into homogeneous populations. The technique relies on the antigenic properties of the cell surface or the chemical nature of exposed carbohydrate residues on the cell surface or on a specific membrane receptor–ligand interaction. The immobilised ligands used include protein A, which binds to the Fc region of IgG, a lectin or the specific ligand for a membrane receptor.

13.9.4 Lectin affinity chromatography

The lectins are a group of proteins produced by animals, plants and slime moulds that have the ability to bind carbohydrate and hence glycoproteins. They have a polymeric structure, most being tetrameric. Their subunits may be either identical, in which case they recognise a single specific saccharide, or of two types in which case they recognise two different saccharides. They all have an Mr in the range 40 000 to 400 000. Their ability to recognise and bind specific saccharides has made them highly valuable in the purification of glycoproteins, particularly membrane receptor proteins.

The most widely used lectins for lectin chromatography are those from leguminous plants (pea, castor bean, soybean) due to their abundance. They can be immobilised to agarose matrices by conventional techniques and many are now available commercially. If the nature of the saccharide component of a glycoprotein is not known, the lectin of choice is selected by a simple screening procedure. Once the glycoproteins have been bound to the immobilised lectin, elution can be achieved in a number of ways: for example, affinity elution using the simple monosaccharide for which the lectin has an affinity; use of a borate buffer, which forms a complex with glycoprotein; by the careful change of pH (not below pH 3 or above pH 10) or by the addition of a reagent such as ethylene glycol to reduce ligand hydrophobic interaction. One of the attractions of lectin affinity chromatography is that it can be carried out in the presence of relatively high salt concentrations because it does not rely on ionic interactions. In principle, therefore, it can be applied directly after salt fractionation. It has also been used to separate mixtures of cells by taking advantage of the saccharide components of their outer membranes. Most lectin affinity chromatography has been carried out using conventional LPLC.

13.9.5 Immunoaffinity chromatography

The use of antibodies as the immobilised ligand has been exploited in the isolation and purification of a range of proteins including membrane proteins of viral origin. Monoclonal antibodies may be linked to agarose matrices by the cyanogen bromide technique. Protein binding to the immobilised antibody is achieved in neutral buffer solution containing moderate salt concentrations. Elution of the bound protein quite often requires forceful conditions because of the very tight binding with the antibody ($K_d = 10^{-8}$ to 10^{-12} M) and this may lead to protein denaturation. Examples of elution procedures include the use of high salt concentrations with or without the use of detergent and the use of urea, sodium dodecyl sulphate or guanidine hydrochloride, all of which cause denaturation. The use of chaotropic agents such as thiocyanate, perchlorate and trifluoracetate or lowering the pH to about 3 may avoid denaturation.

13.9.6 Metal chelate chromatography (immobilised metal affinity chromatography)

This is a special form of affinity chromatography in which an immobilised metal ion such as Cu^{2+}, Zn^{2+}, Hg^{2+} or Cd^{2+} or a transition metal ion such as Co^{2+}, Ni^{2+}, or Mn^{2+} is used to bind proteins selectively by reaction with imidazole groups of histidine residues, thiol groups in cysteine residues and indole groups in tryptophan residues. The immobilisation of the protein involves the formation of a coordinate bond that must be sufficiently stable to allow protein attachment and retention during the elution of non-binding contaminating material. The subsequent release of the protein can be achieved either by simply lowering the pH, therefore destabilising the protein–metal complex, or by the use of complexing agents such as EDTA. Most commonly the metal atom is immobilised by attachment to an iminodiacetate- or tris(carboxymethyl)ethylenediamine-substituted agarose. Proteins purified by this technique include fibrinogen, superoxide dismutase and the non-histone nuclear proteins.

13.9.7 Dye–ligand chromatography

A number of triazine dyes that contain both conjugated rings and ionic groups, fortuitously have the ability to bind to some proteins. The term pseudo-ligands has therefore been used to describe the dyes. It is not possible to predict whether a particular protein will bind to a given dye as the interaction is not specific but is thought to involve interaction with ligand-binding domains via both ionic and hydrophobic forces. Dye binding to proteins enhances their binding to materials such as Sepharose 4B and this is exploited in the purification process. The attraction of the technique is that the dyes are cheap, readily couple to conventional matrices and are very stable. The most widely used dye is Cibacron Blue F3G-A. Dye selection for a particular protein purification is empirical and is made on a trial-and-error basis. Attachment of the protein to the immobilised dye is generally achieved at pH 7 to 8.5. Elution is most commonly brought about either by a salt gradient or by affinity (displacement) elution.

13.9.8 Covalent chromatography

This form of chromatography has been developed specifically to separate thiol (-SH) containing proteins by exploiting their interaction with an immobilised ligand containing a disulphide group. The principle is illustrated in Fig. 13.16. The most commonly used ligand is a disulphide 2′-pyridyl group attached to an agarose matrix such as Sepharose 4B. On reaction with the thiol-containing protein, pyridine-2-thione is released. This process can be monitored spectrophotometrically at 343 nm wavelength, thereby allowing the adsorption of the protein to be followed. Once the protein has been attached covalently to the matrix, non-thiol containing contaminants are eluted and unreacted thiopyridyl groups removed by use of 4 mM dithiothreitol or mercaptoethanol. The protein is then released by displacement with a thiol-containing compound such as 20 to 50 mM dithiothreitol, reduced glutathione or cysteine. The matrix is finally regenerated by reaction with 2,2′-dipyridyldisulphide. The method has been used successfully for many proteins but its use is limited by its cost and the rather difficult regeneration stage. It can, however, be applied to very impure protein preparations.

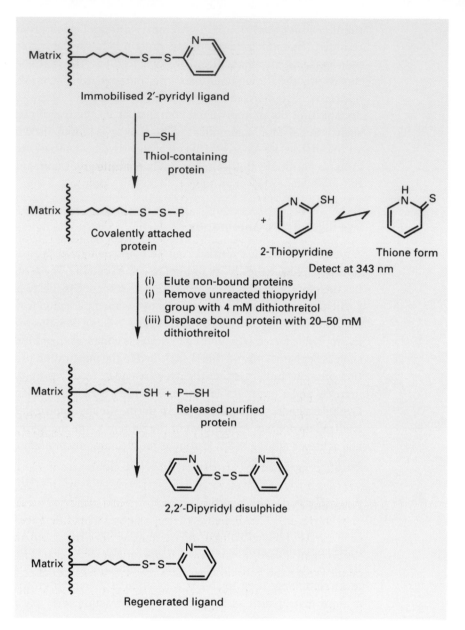

Fig. 13.16. Principles of covalent chromatography.

13.10 GAS–LIQUID CHROMATOGRAPHY

13.10.1 Apparatus and materials

This technique, which is based upon the partitioning of compounds between a liquid and a gas phase, is a widely used method for the qualitative and quantitative analysis of a large number of compounds because it has high sensitivity,

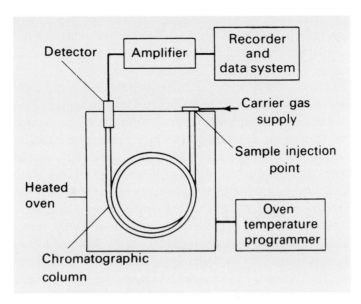

Fig. 13.17. Diagram of a GLC system.

reproducibility and speed of resolution. It has proved to be most valuable for the separation of compounds of relatively low polarity. A stationary phase of a high boiling point liquid material such as silicone grease is supported on an inert granular solid. This material is packed into a narrow coiled glass or steel column 1 to 3 m long and 2 to 4 mm internal diameter, through which an inert carrier gas (the mobile phase) such as nitrogen, helium or argon is passed. The column is maintained in an oven at an elevated temperature, which ensures that the compounds to be separated are kept in the vapour state and that analysis times are reasonable (Section 13.10.3). The basis for the separation is the difference in the partition coefficients of the volatilised compounds between the liquid and gas phases as the compounds are carried through the column by the carrier gas. As the compounds leave the column they pass through a detector that is linked via an amplifier to a chart recorder, which, in turn, records a peak as each analyte passes through the detector (Fig. 13.17).

Gas–liquid chromatography (GLC) may also be performed using capillary columns, which are made of glass or metal with diameters of between 0.03 and 1.0 mm and which may be up to 100 m in length. There are two types of capillary column system known as wall-coated open tubular (WCOT) columns and support-coated open tubular (SCOT), also known as porous layer open tubular (PLOT) columns, for adsorption work. In WCOT columns the stationary phase is coated directly onto the walls of the capillary tubing. As there is only a small amount of stationary phase present, only very small amounts of sample may be chromatographed. Consequently a splitter system has to be used at the sample injection port so that only a small fraction of the injected sample reaches the column. The remainder of the sample is vented to waste. The design of the splitter is critical in quantitative analyses in order to ensure that the ratio of sample chromatographed to sample vented is always the same. Some instruments are equipped with on-column injectors that require considerable skill in their operation.

In SCOT columns a support material is bonded to the walls of the capillary column, and the stationary phase is coated onto the support. The capacity of SCOT columns is considerably higher than that of WCOT columns and consequently small samples can be injected directly onto such columns without the need for a splitter system. SCOT systems are therefore considerably simpler to use for quantitative analyses than are WCOT systems. Their efficiency is less than that of WCOT systems but considerably better than that of conventional GLC columns. Generally speaking, PLOT columns have little biochemical use.

The efficiency of a GLC column is determined by the principles outlined in Section 13.2. There is an optimum carrier gas flow rate for maximum column efficiency (minimum H). For capillary columns, the maximum number of theoretical plates that can be obtained is independent of the carrier gas used. In these cases, a decrease in column diameter should give a proportional increase in the number of plates per unit length, i.e. H. As the length of these columns is very much greater than that of conventional columns, very high efficiencies are obtained (equations 13.8 to 13.12) and these systems are very useful for the analysis of complex mixtures.

Matrix

Since this is used to provide a supporting surface on which is coated the film of stationary phase, it is important that the support should be inert to the sample. This is generally no problem when the support is holding a high percentage coating of stationary phase, but when the percentage coating is low, exposure of the support to the sample often hinders separation. The most commonly used support is Celite (diatomaceous silica), which because of the problem of support–sample interaction is often treated so that the hydroxyl groups that occur in the Celite are modified. This is normally achieved by silanisation of the support with such compounds as hexamethyldisilazane. In addition to the support, the glass column, the glass wool plug located at the base of the column and any other surface that may come into contact with the sample are also silanised. The support particles have an even size, which, for the majority of practical applications, is 60 to 80, 80 to 100, or 100 to 120 mesh (Section 13.3.3).

Stationary phase

The requirements for any GLC stationary phase are that it must be involatile and thermally stable at the temperature used for analysis. Often the phases used are high boiling point organic compounds, and these are coated onto the support to give from 1% to 25% loading, depending upon the analysis. Such phases are of two types, either selective, where separation occurs by utilisation of different chemical characteristics of components, or non-selective, where separation is achieved on the basis of differences in boiling points of the sample components. The operating temperature for the analysis must be compatible with the phase chosen for use. Too high a temperature results in excessive column bleed owing to the phase being volatilised off, contaminating the detector and giving an unstable recorder baseline. The choice of phase for analysis depends on the compound under investigation and is best chosen after reference to the literature. Commonly used stationary phases include the polyethylene glycols, methylphenyl- and methylvinylsilicone gums (so-called OV phases), Apiezon L and esters of adipic, succinic and phthalic acids. β-Cyclodextrin-based phases are available for chiral separations (Section 13.6.5).

The columns are dry-packed under a slight positive gaseous pressure and after packing must be conditioned for 24 to 48 h by heating to near the upper working temperature limit, whilst the carrier gas at normal flow rates is passed through the column. During this conditioning, the column should not be connected to the detector, to prevent contamination. With good-quality liquid phases, column conditioning can be simplified to flushing with carrier gas at 100 °C.

13.10.2 Preparation and application of sample

The majority of non- and low-polar compounds are directly amenable to GLC, but other compounds possessing such polar groups as -OH, $-NH_2$, -COOH are generally retained on the column for excessive periods of time if they are applied directly. This excessive retention is inevitably accompanied by poor resolution and peak tailing (Section 13.2.4). This problem can be overcome by derivatisation of the polar groups. This increases the volatility and effective distribution coefficients of the compounds. Methylation, silanisation and perfluoracylation are common derivatisation methods for fatty acids, carbohydrates and amino acids.

The sample for chromatography is dissolved in a suitable solvent such as acetone, heptane or methanol. Chlorinated organic solvents are generally avoided as they contaminate the detector. The sample is injected onto the column using a microsyringe through a septum in the injection port that is attached to the top of the column. Normally 0.1 to 10 mm^3 of solution is injected. It is common practice to maintain the injection region of the column at a slightly higher temperature than the column itself as this helps to ensure rapid and complete volatilisation of the sample. Sample injection is automated in many commercial instruments.

13.10.3 Separation conditions

Nitrogen, helium and argon are the three most commonly used carrier gases. They are passed through the column at a flow rate of 40 to 80 cm^3 min^{-1}. The column temperature must be within the working range of the particular stationary phase and is chosen to give a balance between peak retention time and resolution. In GLC, partition coefficients are particularly sensitive to temperature so that analysis times may be regulated by adjustment of the column oven, which can be operated in either of two modes. In isothermal analysis a constant temperature is employed. In the separation of compounds of widely differing polarity or M_r it may be advantageous to increase the temperature gradually. This is referred to as temperature programming. This, however, often results in excessive bleed of the stationary phase as the temperature is raised, giving rise to baseline variation. Consequently some instruments have two identical columns and detectors, one set of which is used as a reference. The currents from the two detectors are opposed; hence, assuming equal bleed from both columns, the resulting current gives a steady baseline as the column temperature is raised.

13.10.4 Detectors

By far the most widely used detector is the flame ionisation detector (FID). It responds to almost all organic compounds, can detect as little as 1 ng and has a wide linear response range (10^6). A mixture of hydrogen and air is introduced into the detector to give a flame, the jet of which forms one electrode, whilst the other electrode is brass or platinum wire mounted near the tip of the flame (Fig. 13.18). When the sample components emerge from the column they are ionised in the flame, resulting in an increased signal being passed to the recorder:

$$\text{Organic compound} + H_2 + O_2 \rightarrow \text{combustion products} + H_2O + \text{ions} + \text{radicals} + \text{electrons}$$

$$\Sigma(\text{ions})^- + \Sigma(\text{electrons})^- \rightarrow \text{current}$$

The carrier gas passing through the column and the detector gives a small background signal, that can be offset electronically to give a baseline. An FID has a minimum detection quantity of the order of $5 \times 10^{-12}\,\text{g s}^{-1}$ and an upper temperature limit of $400\,^\circ\text{C}$.

The nitrogen-phosphorus detector (NPD), which is also called a thermionic detector, is similar in design to an FID but has a crystal of a sodium salt fused onto the electrode system, or a burner tip embedded in a ceramic tube containing a

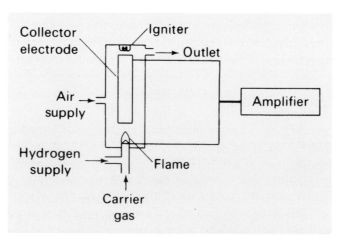

Fig. 13.18. Diagram of a flame ionisation detector.

sodium salt, or a rubidium chloride tip. The NPD has excellent selectivity towards nitrogen- and phosphorus-containing compounds and shows a poor response to compounds possessing neither of these two elements. Its linearity (10^4), upper temperature limit (300 °C) and detection limits (10^{-11} g s^{-1}) are not quite as good as an FID. It is widely used in organophosphorus pesticide residue analysis.

The electron capture detector (ECD) responds only to substances that capture electrons, particularly halogen-containing compounds. This detector is widely used in the analysis of polychlorinated compounds, such as the pesticides DDT, dieldrin and aldrin. It has very high sensitivity (10^{-11} g s^{-1}) and an upper temperature limit of 300 °C but its linear range (10^2 to 10^4) is much lower than that of the FID. The detector works by means of a radioactive source (^{63}Ni) ionising the column gas (e.g. $N_2 \rightarrow \overset{+}{N_2} + e^-$), the electrons so produced giving a current across the electrodes to which a suitable voltage is applied. When an electron-capturing compound (generally one containing a halogen atom) emerges from the column, the ionised electrons are captured, the current drops and this change in current is recorded. The carrier gas most commonly used in conjunction with an ECD is nitrogen or an argon +5% methane mixture.

The volatile solvent used to introduce the test sample gives rise to a solvent peak at the beginning of the chromatograph. The three main forms of detector respond to this solvent with varying sensitivity, thereby affecting the detection and resolution of rapidly eluting analytes. In cases where authentic samples of the test compounds are not available for calibration purposes or in cases where the identity of the analytes is not known, the detector may be replaced by a mass spectrometer. Special separators are available for removing the bulk of the carrier gas from the sample emerging from the column and prior to its introduction in the mass spectrometer (Section 11.7). More recently, GLC has been linked to other types of detector, including an infrared spectrophotometer, a nuclear magnetic resonance spectrometer and an atomic emission spectrometer, the resulting spectra aiding in the identification of unknown compounds.

13.10.5 **Applications**

Until the development of HPLC, GLC was probably the most commonly used form of chromatography. Its use nowadays is confined to volatile, non-polar compounds that do not need derivatisation. Analytes are characterised by their retention time or preferably by their retention time relative to a standard reference compound. In the analysis of compounds that form a homologous series, for example the methyl esters of the saturated fatty acids, there is a linear relationship between the logarithm of the retention time and the number of carbon atoms. There are similar but parallel lines for mono- and di-unsaturated fatty acids. This can be exploited, for example, to identify an unknown fatty acid ester in a fat hydrolysate. A widely used system for quantitative analysis is the retention index (RI), which is based on the retention of a compound relative to n-alkanes. The compound is chromatographed with a number of n-alkanes and a semilogarithmic plot constructed of retention time against number of carbon atoms. Each n-alkane is assigned an RI of 100 times the number of carbon atoms it contains (pentane therefore has an RI of 500), allowing the RI for the compound to be calculated. Many commercially available GLC systems with data-processing facilities have the capacity to calculate RI values automatically.

13.11 THIN-LAYER (PLANAR) CHROMATOGRAPHY

13.11.1 Principle

A thin layer of the stationary phase is formed on a suitable flat surface. Since the layer is so thin, the movement of the mobile phase across the layer, generally by simple capillary action, is rapid, there being little resistance to flow. As the mobile phase moves across the layer from one edge to the opposite, it transfers any analytes placed on the layer at a rate determined by their distribution coefficients, K_d, between the stationary and mobile phases. In practice, the principle of the distribution process may be based on that of adsorption, partition, chiral, ion-exchange or molecular exclusion chromatography. Analyte movement ceases either when the mobile phase (solvent front) reaches the end of the layer and capillary action flow ceases or when the plate is removed from the mobile phase reservoir.

The movement of the analyte is expressed by it retardation factor, R_F such that

$$R_F = \frac{\text{distance moved by analyte from origin}}{\text{distance moved by solvent front from origin}} \qquad (13.14)$$

The efficiency of a thin-layer plate is expressed by its number of theoretical plates, N, and plate height, H, (Section 13.2.4) with the appropriate form of equations 13.8 and 13.9:

$$N = 16 \left(\frac{d_A}{w} \right)^2 \qquad (13.15)$$

where d_A is the distance moved by the analyte from the origin and w is the width of the spot (Fig. 13.19), and

$$H = \frac{d_A}{N} \qquad (13.16)$$

The capacity factor, k' (Section 13.2.3), for the analyte, is given by

$$k' = \frac{1 - R_F}{R_F} = \frac{d_F}{d_A} - 1 \qquad (13.17)$$

where d_F is the distance moved by the solvent front from the origin.

13.11.2 Thin-layer preparation

A slurry of the stationary phase, generally in water, is applied to a glass, plastic or foil plate, generally 20 cm square, as a uniform thin layer by means of a plate spreader starting at one end of the plate and moving progressively to the other. The thickness of the slurry layer used is dictated by the nature of the desired chromatographic separation. For analytical separations the layer is of the order of 0.25 mm thick and for preparative separations it may be up to 2 mm. Where the stationary phase is to be used for adsorption chromatography, a binding agent such as calcium sulphate is incorporated into the slurry in order to facilitate the adhesion of the adsorbent to the plate. With the exception of thin-layer exclusion chromatography (Section 13.8.1), once the slurry layer has been prepared, the plates are dried to leave the coating of stationary phase. In the case of adsorbents, drying is carried out in an oven at 100 to 120 °C. This also serves to activate the adsorbent. A range of preprepared plates is available commercially. So-called polyamide layer sheets, which consist of poly-ε-caprolactam coated onto *both* sides of a solvent-resistant polyester sheet, are unusual in that they are semitransparent, allowing unknowns and standards run on opposite sides of the plate to be compared. They can also be reused if cleaned immediately with ammonia–acetone, and are widely used in protein sequencing studies by the dansyl-Edman method (Section 6.4.3).

13.11.3 **Sample application**

The sample is applied to the plate 2.0 to 2.5 cm from the edge by means of a micropipette or microsyringe. Transparent templates to facilitate the correct location of the samples are available commercially and it is possible for the application process to be automated. The solvent may be removed from the spot by gentle heating or by use of an air blower, care being taken in the case of volatile or thermolabile compounds. It is then possible to apply more sample to the spot if necessary. In the case of adsorption chromatography, diffusion of the sample from the applied spot may be minimised by using a solvent in which components have a low R_F value. For preparative thin-layer chromatography, the sample is applied as a band across the plate rather than as a single spot.

13.11.4 **Plate development**

Separation most commonly takes places in a glass tank that contains the developing solvent (mobile phase) to a depth of about 1.5 cm. This is allowed to stand for at least 1 h with a lid over the top of the tank to ensure that the atmosphere within the tank becomes saturated with solvent vapour (equilibration). Unless this is done, irregular running of the solvent will occur as it ascends the plate by capillary action, resulting in poor separations being achieved. After equilibration, the lid is removed, and the thin-layer plate is then placed vertically in the tank so that it stands in the solvent. The lid is replaced and separation of the compounds then occurs as the solvent travels up the plate. It is also possible to develop the plate in a horizontal plane by connecting the sample end of it to a reservoir of mobile phase by means of a suitable wick. It is preferable to keep the system at a constant temperature whilst the development is occurring, to avoid anomalous solvent-running effects. One of the biggest advantages of TLC is the speed at which separation is achieved. This is commonly about 30 min and is hardly ever greater than 90 min.

In order to improve the resolution of partition and adsorption separations, the technique of two-dimensional chromatography may be used. The material to be chromatographed is placed towards one corner of the plate as a single spot and the plate developed in one direction and then removed from the tank and allowed to dry. It is then developed by another solvent system, in which the compounds to be separated have different K_d values, in a direction at right angles to the first development.

13.11.5 **Analyte detection**

Several detection methods are available. Examination of the plate under ultraviolet light will show the position of ultraviolet-absorbing or fluorescent compounds. Many commercially available thin-layer adsorbents contain a fluorescent dye so that, when the plate is examined under ultraviolet light, the separated compounds show up as blue, green or black areas against a fluorescent background. Subjecting the plate to iodine vapour is useful if unsaturated compounds are being investigated. Spraying of plates with specific colour reagents will stain certain compounds, for example ninhydrin will locate amino acids and peptides. If the compounds are radiolabelled, the plates may be subjected to autoradiography (Section 14.2.3), which will detect the spots as dark areas on X-ray film, or the plate may be scanned by a radiochromatograph scanner (Section 14.2.3). A general, non-specific technique is to spray the plate with 50% (v/v) sulphuric acid or 25% (v/v) sulphuric acid in ethanol and heating at 110 °C, which will result in most compounds becoming charred and showing up as brown spots. Great care has to be taken when this latter method is performed.

Although the movement of compounds on TLC may be characterised by specific R_F values, these measurements are not always reproducible. Component identification is therefore most commonly made on the basis of a comparison of the movement of the components with those of reference compounds chromatographed alongside the sample on the TLC plate.

The amount of compound present in a given spot may be determined in a number of ways. On-plate quantification may be achieved by use of radiochromatograph scanning in the case of radiolabelled compounds or more generally by means of densitometry (Fig. 13.19). Precision densitometers are commercially available that measure the ultraviolet or visible absorption of the compound as well as simultaneously giving a complete absorption spectrum of the compound for identification purposes. Off-plate quantification may be carried out by scraping off the spot and the immediate surrounding stationary phase from the plate and eluting the compound with a suitable solvent. The amount of compound in solution can then be determined by standard methods, most commonly colorimetry or fluorimetry.

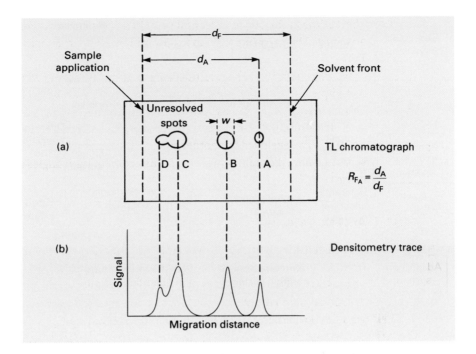

Fig. 13.19. TLC chromatograph of a mixture of compounds A to D (a) and the corresponding densitometer trace (b) from which quantitative data can be calculated.

13.12 SELECTION OF A CHROMATOGRAPHIC SYSTEM

It is possible to rationalise to some extent the type of system most likely to be applicable to the separation of compounds for which the physical characteristics are known (Fig. 13.20).

The majority of chromatographic procedures exploit differences in physical properties of compounds, the exception being affinity chromatography, which is based upon the specific ligand-binding properties of biological macromolecules. If this form of chromatography can be applied, it is the most likely to be successful. Volatile compounds are best separated by GLC, whereas non-volatile compounds that are soluble in organic solvents are generally best separated either by adsorption or normal phase liquid chromatography. If the compounds have different functional groups, adsorption chromatography on silica with non-polar solvent is probably the better method. To separate low polarity compounds in a homologous series, normal phase liquid systems are preferred. If water soluble compounds are non-ionic or weakly ionic, reversed-phase liquid chromatography is preferable where a non-polar stationary phase such as a hydrocarbon is used together with a polar mobile phase such as water/acetonitrile or water/methanol mixtures. Water-soluble compounds that are strongly ionic are best chromatographed by an ion-exchange system, using either an anionic or cationic resin, together with a suitable buffer system for elution. Ionic compounds can, however, be chromatographed by

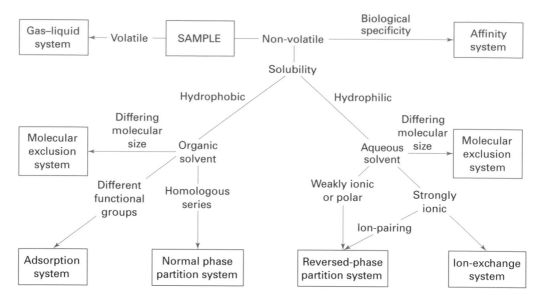

Fig. 13.20. Rationale for the choice of a chromatographic system.

reversed-phase partition systems by the technique of ion-pairing. Compounds differing in molecular size are best separated by molecular exclusion chromatography.

Whatever form of liquid chromatography is chosen for a particular biochemical study, the decision to use LPLC or HPLC depends on many factors including the availability of apparatus, cost, the scale of the separation, and whether the separation is to be qualitative or quantitative. The modern trend is to select HPLC, which is certainly capable of giving fast, accurate and precise data. Reversed-phase HPLC, in particular, is proving to be an extremely versatile technique. The application of HPLC techniques to protein separations, via FPLC, is also proving to be a quick, robust technique, particularly in cases where protein denaturation is not a problem. The simplicity of TLC, especially for qualitative work, with its facility for concurrent investigation of many samples including standards, remains a considerable attraction. Equally, the recent developments in capillary gas chromatography make it a fast and sensitive system for volatile compounds. Capillary electrochromatography is another important recent development but its potential remains to be fully evaluated.

13.13 KEY TERMS

absolute specificity	affinity development	analytes
acidic ion-exchange material	affinity elution	anion exchanger
adjusted retention time	affinity partitioning	available capacity
adsorption chromatography	affinity precipitation	band
affinity chromatography	amino acid analysers	basic ion-exchange material

13.14 **CALCULATIONS**

Question 1 Calculate the capacity factor for an analyte in a column in which the volume of the stationary phase is one-fifth of that of the mobile phase if:

(i) $K_d = 1$; (ii) $K_d = 50$.

Answer $k' = K_d \dfrac{V_S}{V_M}$

(i) $k' = 1 \times \dfrac{1}{5}$, therefore $k' = 0.2$

(ii) $k' = 50 \times \dfrac{1}{5}$, therefore $k' = 10$

Question 2

An analyte eluted from a chromatographic column as a Gaussian peak with a retention time of 7 min 45 s and a base peak width of 30 s.

Calculate:

(i) the number of theoretical plates in the column;
(ii) the plate height if the column was 7.5 cm long.

Answer $N = 16 \left(\dfrac{t_R}{w} \right)^2$

(i) $N = 16 \left(\dfrac{465}{30} \right)^2$, therefore $N = 3844$

(ii) $H = \dfrac{L}{N} = \dfrac{7.5 \times 10^4}{3844}$, therefore $H = 19.5 \ \mu m$

Question 3

Two compounds (1 and 2) with distribution coefficients of 10 and 12 are to be separated on a column in which the volume of the stationary phase is one-fifth that of the mobile phase. Calculate the number of theoretical plates required to give a resolution of 1.5.

Answer $k' = K_d \dfrac{V_S}{V_M}$

$k'_1 = 10 \times \dfrac{1}{5}$, therefore $k'_1 = 2$

$k'_2 = 12 \times \dfrac{1}{5}$, therefore $k'_2 = 2.4$

$\alpha = \dfrac{k'_2}{k'} = \dfrac{2.4}{2} = 1.2$

$R_S = \left(\dfrac{\sqrt{N}}{4} \right) \left(\dfrac{\alpha - 1}{\alpha} \right) \left(\dfrac{k'_2}{1 + k'_{av}} \right)$

$1.5 = \left(\dfrac{\sqrt{N}}{4} \right) \left(\dfrac{0.2}{1.2} \right) \left(\dfrac{2.4}{1 + 2.2} \right)$

Therefore $N = 2304$

Question 4

Two compounds A and B were separated on a 25 cm long column. The observed retention times were 7 min 20 s and 8 min 20 s, respectively. The base peak width for analyte B was 10 s. When a reference compound, which was completely excluded from the stationary phase under the same elution conditions, was studied, its retention time was 1 min 20 s.

Calculate:

(i)   the adusted retention time for A and B;
(ii) the capacity factor for A and B;
(iii) the selectivity factor for the two compounds;

(iv) the number of theoretical plates in the column;

(v) the resolution of the two compounds;

(vi) the required column length to double the resolution.

Answer   (i) $t_R' = t_R - t_M$

(A) $t_R' = 440 - 80 = 360\,\text{s}$

(B) $t_R' = 500 - 80 = 420\,\text{s}$

(ii) $k' = \dfrac{t_R}{t_M}$

(A) $k_A' = \dfrac{360}{80} = 4.5$

(B) $k_B' = \dfrac{420}{80} = 5.25$

(iii) $\alpha = \dfrac{k_B'}{k_A'} = \dfrac{5.25}{4.5} = 1.167$

$$N = \left(\dfrac{t_R}{w}\right)^2$$

(iv) For B $N = \left(\dfrac{420}{10}\right)^2 = 1764$

(v) $R_S = \left(\dfrac{\sqrt{N}}{4}\right)\left(\dfrac{\alpha - 1}{\alpha}\right)\left(\dfrac{k_B}{1 + k_{\text{av}}}\right)$

$= \left(\dfrac{\sqrt{1764}}{4}\right)\left(\dfrac{0.167}{1.167}\right)\left(\dfrac{5.25}{1 + 4.875}\right)$

$= 1.34$

(vi) $H = \dfrac{L}{N} = \dfrac{250}{1764} = 0.14\,\text{mm}$

For $R_S = 2.68$, $N = 7025$

$0.14 = \dfrac{L}{7025}$, therefore $L = 983.5\,\text{mm}$ or $98.35\,\text{cm}$

Question 5   The relative molecular mass (M_r) of a protein was investigated by exclusion chromatography using a Sephacryl S300 column and using aldolase, catalase, ferritin, thyroglobulin and Blue Dextran as standard. The following elution data were obtained.

	M_r	Retention volume $V_r\,(\text{cm}^3)$
Aldolase	158 000	22.5
Catalase	210 000	21.4
Ferritin	444 000	18.2
Thyroglobulin	669 000	16.4
Blue Dextran	2 000 000	13.6
Unknown		19.5

Calculate M_r of the protein.

Answer | A plot of the logarithm of the relative molecular mass of individual proteins versus their retention volume has a linear section from which it can be deduced that the unknown protein with a retention volume of 19.5 cm^3 must have a relative molecular mass of 330 000.

13.15 SUGGESTIONS FOR FURTHER READING

GROB, R. L. (ed.) (1995). *Modern Practice of Gas Chromatography*, 3rd edn. Wiley Interscience, New York. (An excellent, comprehensive coverage of this chromatographic technique.)

JINNO, K. (ed.) (1996). *Chromatographic Separations Based on Molecular Recognition.* Wiley VCH, New York. (Particularly good on the application to protein purification.)

LOUGH, W. J. (1990). *Chiral Liquid Chromatography.* Blackie, New York. (An excellent review of this specialist area of chromatography.)

ROBARDS, K., HADDAD, P. R. and JACKSON, P. E. (1994). *Principles and Practice of Modern Chromatographic Methods.* Academic Press, London. (A recommended general textbook with a good chapter on supercritical fluid chromatography.)

SYNDER, L. R., KIRKLAND, J. J. and GLAJCH, J. L. (1997). *Practical HPLC Method Development*, 2nd edn. Wiley Interscience, New York. (A good practical guide to the applications of HPLC.)

Chapter 14

Radioisotope techniques

14.1 THE NATURE OF RADIOACTIVITY

14.1.1 Atomic structure

An atom is composed of a positively charged nucleus that is surrounded by a cloud of negatively charged electrons. The mass of an atom is concentrated in the nucleus, even though it accounts for only a small fraction of the total size of the atom. Atomic nuclei are composed of two major particles, protons and neutrons. Protons are positively charged particles with a mass approximately 1850 times greater than that of an orbital electron. The number of orbital electrons in an atom must be equal to the number of protons present in the nucleus, since the atom as a whole is electrically neutral. This number is known as the atomic number (Z). Neutrons are uncharged particles with a mass approximately equal to that of a proton. The sum of protons and neutrons in a given nucleus is the mass number (A). Thus

$$A = Z + N$$

where N is the number of neutrons present.

Since the number of neutrons in a nucleus is not related to the atomic number, it does not affect the chemical properties of the atom. Atoms of a given element may not necessarily contain the same number of neutrons. Atoms of a given element with different mass numbers (i.e. different numbers of neutrons) are called isotopes. Symbolically, a specific nuclear species is represented by a subscript number for the atomic number, and a superscript number for the mass number, followed by the symbol of the element. For example:

$$^{12}_{6}C \quad ^{14}_{6}C \quad ^{16}_{8}O \quad ^{18}_{8}O$$

However, in practice it is more conventional just to cite the mass number (e.g. ^{14}C). The number of isotopes of a given element varies: there are 3 isotopes of hydrogen, ^{1}H, ^{2}H and ^{3}H, 7 of carbon ^{10}C to ^{16}C inclusive, and 20 or more of some of the elements of high atomic number.

14.1.2 Atomic stability and radiation

In general, the ratio of neutrons to protons in the nucleus will determine whether an isotope of a given element is stable enough to exist in nature. Stable isotopes for elements with low atomic numbers tend to have an equal number of neutrons and protons, whereas stability for elements of higher atomic numbers is associated with a neutron:proton ratio in excess of 1. Unstable isotopes, or radioisotopes as they are more commonly known, are often produced artificially, but many occur in nature. Radioisotopes emit particles and/or electromagnetic radiation as a result of changes in the composition of the atomic nucleus. These processes, which are known as radioactive decay, arise, either directly or as a result of a decay series, in the production of a stable isotope.

14.1.3 Types of radioactive decay

There are several types of radioactive decay; only those most relevant to biochemists are considered below.

Decay by negatron emission

In this case a neutron is converted to a proton by the ejection of a negatively charged beta (β) particle called a negatron (β^-):

neutron $\rightarrow$ proton + negatron

To all intents and purposes a negatron is an electron, but the term negatron is preferred, although not always used, since it serves to emphasise the nuclear origin of the particle. As a result of negatron emission, the nucleus loses a neutron but gains a proton. The N/Z ratio therefore decreases while Z increases by 1 and A remains constant. An isotope frequently used in biological work that decays by negatron emission is ^{14}C.

$$^{14}_{6}C \rightarrow {}^{14}_{7}N + \beta^-$$

Negatron emission is very important to biochemists because many of the commonly used radionuclides decay by this mechanism. Examples are: ^{3}H and ^{14}C, which can be used to label any organic compound; ^{35}S used to label methionine, for example to study protein synthesis; and ^{32}P, a powerful tool in molecular biology when used as a nucleic acid label.

Decay by positron emission

Some isotopes decay by emitting positively charged β-particles referred to as positrons (β^+). This occurs when a proton is converted to a neutron:

proton $\rightarrow$ neutron + positron

Positrons are extremely unstable and have only a transient existence. Once they have dissipated their energy they interact with electrons and are annihilated. The mass and energy of the two particles are converted to two γ-rays emitted at 180° to each other. This phenomenon is frequently described as back-to-back emission.

As a result of positron emission the nucleus loses a proton and gains a neutron, the N/Z ratio increases, Z decreases by 1 and A remains constant. An example of an isotope decaying by positron emission is ^{22}Na:

$$^{22}_{11}Na \rightarrow {}^{22}_{10}Ne + \beta^+$$

Positron emitters are detected by the same instruments used to detect γ-radiation. They are used in biological sciences to spectacular effect in brain scanning with the technique positron emission tomography (PET scanning) used to identify active and inactive areas of the brain.

Decay by alpha particle emission

Isotopes of elements with high atomic numbers frequently decay by emitting alpha (α) particles. An α-particle is a helium nucleus; it consists of two protons and two neutrons ($^4\text{He}^{2+}$). Emission of α-particles results in a considerable lightening of the nucleus, a decrease in atomic number of 2 and a decrease in the mass number of 4. Isotopes that decay by α-emission are not frequently encountered in biological work. Radium-226 (^{226}Ra) decays by α-emission to radon-222 (^{222}Rn), which is itself radioactive. Thus begins a complex decay series, which culminates in the formation of ^{206}Pb:

$$^{226}_{88}\text{Ra} \rightarrow {}^{4}_{2}\text{He}^{2+} + {}^{222}_{86}\text{Rn} \rightarrow \rightarrow \rightarrow {}^{206}_{82}\text{Pb}$$

Alpha emitters are extremely toxic if ingested, due to the large mass and the ionising power of the atomic particle.

Electron capture

In this form of decay a proton captures an electron orbiting in the innermost K shell:

proton + electron → neutron + X-ray

The proton becomes a neutron and electromagnetic radiation (X-rays) is given out. Example:

$$^{125}_{53}\text{I} \rightarrow {}^{125}_{52}\text{Te} + \text{X-ray}$$

Decay by emission of γ-rays

In contrast to emission of α- and β-particles, γ-emission involves electromagnetic radiation similar to, but with a shorter wavelength than, X-rays. These γ-rays result from a transformation in the nucleus of an atom (in contrast to X-rays, which are emitted as a consequence of excitation involving the orbital electrons of an atom) and frequently accompany α- and β-particle emission. Emission of γ-radiation in itself leads to no change in atomic number or mass.

γ-Radiation has low ionising power but high penetration. For example, the γ-radiation from ^{60}Co will penetrate 15 cm of steel. The toxicity of γ-radiation is similar to that of X-rays.
Example:

$$^{131}_{53}\text{I} \rightarrow {}^{131}_{54}\text{Xe} + \beta^- + \gamma$$

14.1.4 Radioactive decay energy

The usual unit used in expressing energy levels associated with radioactive decay is the electron volt. (One electron volt (eV) is the energy acquired by one electron in accelerating through a potential difference of 1 V and is equivalent to 1.6×10^{-19} J.) For the majority of isotopes, the term million or mega electron volts (MeV) is more applicable. Isotopes emitting α-particles are normally the most energetic, falling in the range 4.0 to 8.0 MeV, whereas β- and γ-emitters generally have decay energies of less than 3.0 MeV.

14.1.5 Rate of radioactive decay

Radioactive decay is a spontaneous process and it occurs at a definite rate characteristic of the source. This rate always follows an exponential law. Thus the number of atoms disintegrating at any time is proportional to the number of atoms of the isotope (N) present at that time (t). Expressed mathematically, the exponential curve (Fig. 14.1) gives the equation.

$$\frac{-\,\mathrm{d}N}{\mathrm{d}t} \propto N$$

$$\text{or} \frac{-\,\mathrm{d}N}{\mathrm{d}t} = \lambda N \tag{14.1}$$

where λ is the decay constant, a characteristic of a given isotope defined as the fraction of an isotope decaying in unit time (t^{-1}). By integrating equation 14.1 it can be converted to a logarithmic form:

$$\ln \frac{N_t}{N_o} = -\lambda t \tag{14.2}$$

where N_t is the number of radioactive atoms present at time t, and N_o is the number of radioactive atoms orginally present. In practice it is more convenient

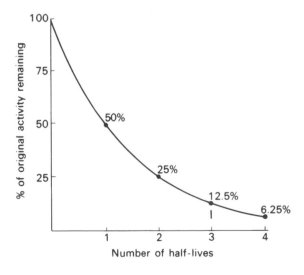

Fig. 14.1. Demonstration of the exponential nature of radioactive decay.

Table 14.1	Half-lives of some isotopes used in biological studies

Isotope	Half-title
^{3}H	12.26 years
^{14}C	5760 years
^{22}Na	2.58 years
^{32}P	14.20 days
^{35}S	87.20 days
^{42}K	12.40 h
^{45}Ca	165 days
^{59}Fe	45 days
^{125}I	60 days
^{131}I	8.05 days
^{135}I	9.7 h

to express the decay constant in terms of half-life $\left(t_{\frac{1}{2}}\right)$. This is defined as the time taken for the activity to fall from any value to half that value (Fig. 14.1). If N_t in equation 14.2 is equal to one-half of N_o then t will equal the half-life of the isotope. Thus

$$\ln\frac{1}{2} = -\lambda t_{\frac{1}{2}} \tag{14.3}$$

$$\text{or } 2.303 \log(1/2) = -\lambda t_{\frac{1}{2}} \tag{14.4}$$

$$\text{or } t_{\frac{1}{2}} = 0.693/\lambda \tag{14.5}$$

The values of $t_{\frac{1}{2}}$ vary widely from over 10^{19} years for lead-204 (^{204}Pb) to 3×10^{-7} s for polonium-212 (^{212}Po). The half-lives of some isotopes frequently used in biological work are given in Table 14.1. Note that two important elements, oxygen and nitrogen, are missing from the table. This is because the half-lives of radioactive isotopes of these elements are too short for most biological studies (^{15}O has a $t_{\frac{1}{2}}$ of 2.03 min, whereas ^{13}N has a $t_{\frac{1}{2}}$ of 10.00 min).

14.1.6 Units of radioactivity

The Système International d'Unités (SI system) uses the becquerel (Bq) as the unit of radioactivity. This is defined as one disintegration per second (1 d.p.s.). However, this unit has still not been widely adopted and a commonly used unit is still the curie (Ci). This is defined as the quantity of radioactive material in which the number of nuclear disintegrations per second is the same as that in 1 g of radium, namely 3.7×10^{10} (or 37 GBq, see Table 14.7). For biological purposes this unit is too large and the microcurie (μCi) and millicurie (mCi) are used. It is important to realise that the curie refers to the number of disintegrations actually occurring in a sample (i.e. d.p.s.) not to the disintegrations detected by the radiation counter, which will generally be only a proportion of the disintegrations occurring and are referred to as counts (i.e. c.p.s.).

Normally, in experiments with radioisotopes, a carrier of the stable isotope of the element is added. It therefore becomes necessary to express the amount of radioisotope present per unit mass. This is the specific activity. It may be expressed in a number of ways including disintegration rate (d.p.s. or d.p.m.), count rate (c.p.s. or c.p.m.) or curies (mCi or μCi) per unit of mass of mixture (units of mass are normally either moles or grams). An alternative method of expressing specific activity, which is not very frequently used, is atom percentage excess. This is defined as the number of radioactive atoms per total of 100 atoms of the compound. For quick reference, a list of units and definitions frequently used in radiobiology is provided in Table 14.7, p. 725.

14.1.7 Interaction of radioactivity with matter

α-Particles

These particles have a very considerable energy (3 to 8 MeV) and all the particles from a given isotope have the same amount of energy. They react with matter in two ways. Firstly, they may cause excitation. In this process energy is transferred from the α-particle to orbital electrons of neighbouring atoms, these electrons being elevated to higher orbitals. The α-particle continues on its path with its energy reduced by a little more than the amount transferred to the orbital electron. The excited electron eventually falls back to its original orbital, emitting energy as photons of light in the visible or near visible range. Secondly, α-particles may cause ionisation of atoms in their path. When this occurs the target orbital electron is removed completely. Thus, the atom becomes ionised and forms an ion-pair, consisting of a positively charged ion and an electron. Because of their size, slow movement and double positive charge, α-particles frequently collide with atoms in their path. Therefore they cause intense ionisation and excitation and their energy is rapidly dissipated. Thus, despite their inital high energy, α-particles are not very penetrating.

Negatrons

Compared with α-particles, negatrons are very small and rapidly moving particles that carry a single negative charge. They interact with matter to cause ionisation and excitation exactly as with α-particles. However, due to their speed and size, they are less likely than α-particles to interact with matter and therefore are less ionising and more penetrating than α-radiation. Another difference between α-particles and negatrons is that, whereas for a given α-emitter all the particles have the same energy, negatrons are emitted over a range of energy, i.e. negatron emitters have a characteristic energy spectrum (Fig. 14.5). The maximum energy level (E_{max}) varies from one isotope to another, ranging from 0.018 MeV for ^{3}H to 4.81 MeV for ^{38}Cl. The difference in E_{max} affects the penetration of the radiation: β-particles from ^{3}H can travel only a few millimetres in air, whereas those from ^{32}P can penetrate over 1 m of air. The reason for negatrons of a given isotope being emitted within an energy range was explained by W. Pauli in 1931, when he postulated that each radioactive event occurs with an energy equivalent to E_{max} but that the energy is shared between a negatron and a neutrino. The proportion of total energy taken by the negatron and the neutrino varies for each disintegration. Neutrinos have no charge and negligible mass and do not interact with matter.

γ-Rays

The γ-rays (and X-rays) are electromagnetic and therefore have no charge or mass. They rarely collide with neighbouring atoms and travel great distances before dissipating all their energy (i.e. they are highly penetrating). They interact with matter in many ways. The three most important ways lead to the production of secondary electrons, which in turn cause excitation and ionisation. In photoelectric absorption, low energy γ-rays interact with orbital electrons, transferring all their energy to the electron, which is then ejected as a photoelectron. The photoelectron subsequently behaves as a negatron. In contrast, Compton scattering, which is caused by medium energy γ-rays, results in only part of the energy being transferred to the target electron, which is ejected. The γ-ray is deflected and moves on with reduced energy. Again the ejected electron behaves as a negatron. Pair production results when very high energy γ-rays react with the nucleus of an atom and all the energy of the γ-ray is converted to a positron and a negatron.

14.2 DETECTION AND MEASUREMENT OF RADIOACTIVITY

There are three commonly used methods of detecting and quantifying radioactivity. These are based on the ionisation of gases, on the excitation of solids or solutions, and the ability of radioactivity to expose photographic emulsions, i.e. autoradiography.

14.2.1 Methods based upon gas ionisation

The effect of voltage upon ionisation

As a charged particle passes through a gas, its electrostatic field dislodges orbital electrons from atoms sufficiently close to its path and causes ionisation (Fig. 14.2). The ability to induce ionisation decreases in the order

$$\alpha > \beta > \gamma \qquad (10\,000{:}100{:}1)$$

Accordingly, α- and β-particles may be detected by gas ionisation methods, but these methods are poor for detecting γ-radiation. If ionisation occurs between a pair of electrodes enclosed in a suitable chamber, a pulse (current) flows, the magnitude of which is related to the applied potential and the number of radiation particles entering the chamber (Fig. 14.3). The various 'regions' shown in Fig. 14.3 will now be considered.

In the ionisation chamber region of the curve, each radioactive particle produces only one ion-pair per collision. Hence the currents are low, and very sensitive measuring devices are necessary. This method is little used in quantitative work, but various types of electroscopes, which operate on this principle, are useful in demonstrating the properties of radioactivity. At a higher voltage level

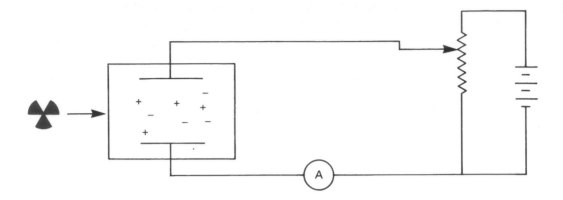

Fig. 14.2. Detection based on ionisation.

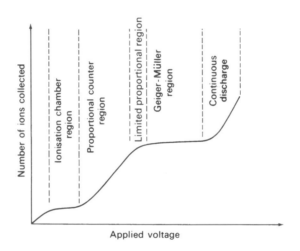

Fig. 14.3. Effect of voltage on pulse flow.

than that of the simple ionisation chambers, electrons resulting from ionisation move towards the anode much more rapidly; consequently they cause secondary ionisation of gas in the chamber, resulting in the production of secondary ionisation electrons, which cause further ionisation and so on. Hence from the original event a whole torrent of electrons reach the anode. This is the principle of gas amplification and is known as the Townsend avalanche effect, after its discoverer. As a consequence of this gas amplification, current flow is much greater. As can be seen in Fig. 14.3, in the proportional counter region the number of ion-pairs collected is directly proportional to the applied voltage until a certain voltage is reached, when a plateau occurs. Before the plateau is reached there is a region known as the limited proportional region, which is not often used in detection and quantification of radioactivity and hence will not be discussed.

The main drawback of counters that are manufactured to operate in the proportional region is that they require a very stable voltage supply because small fluctuations in voltage result in significant changes in amplification. Proportional counters are particularly useful for detection and quantification of α-emitting isotopes, but it should be noted that relatively few such isotopes are used in biological work.

In the Geiger–Müller region all radiation particles, including weak β-particles, induce complete ionisation of the gas in the chamber. Thus the size of the current is no longer dependent on the number of primary ions produced. Since maximal gas amplification is realised in this region, the size of the output pulse from the detector will remain the same over a considerable voltage range (the so-called Geiger–Müller plateau). The number of times this pulse is produced is measured rather than its size. Therefore it is not possible to discriminate between different isotopes using this type of counter.

Since it takes a finite time for the ion-pairs to travel to their respective electrodes, other ionising particles entering the tube during this time fail to produce ionisation and hence are not detected, thereby reducing the counting efficiency. This is referred to as the dead time of the tube and is normally 100 to 200 μs. When the ions reach the electrode they are neutralised. Inevitably some escape and produce their own ionisation avalanche. Thus, if unchecked, a Geiger–Müller tube would tend to give a continuous discharge. To overcome this, the tube is quenched by the addition of a suitable gas, which reduces the energy of the ions. Common quenching agents are ethanol, ethyl formate and the halogens.

Instrumentation

Counters based on gas ionisation used to be the main method employed in the quantification of radioisotopes in biological samples. Currently, scintillation counting (Section 14.2.2) has virtually taken over. However, all laboratories use small hand-held radioactivity monitors based on gas ionisation; the end-window design being the most popular type (Fig. 14.4). These counters have a thin end window made from aluminium and can detect β-radiation from high energy (^{32}P) and weak emitters (^{14}C), but are incapable of detecting ^{3}H because the radiation cannot penetrate the end-window. For the same reason they are not very efficient detectors of α-radiation.

End-window ionisation counters are used for routine monitoring of the radioactive laboratory to check for contamination. They are also useful in experimental situations where the presence or absence of radioactivity needs to be known rather than the absolute quantity, for example quick screening of radioactive gels prior to autoradiography or checking of chromatographic fractions for labelled components.

The inability of end-window counters to detect weak β-emitters presents a problem in biosciences because ^{3}H is a very commonly used radioisotope. The problem can be overcome by using a so-called windowless counter where a gas flow is used. These instruments are rather cumbersome and need to be carried

(a)

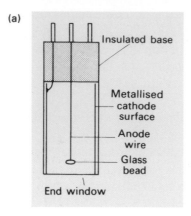

Insulated base

Metallised cathode surface

Anode wire

Glass bead

End window

(b)

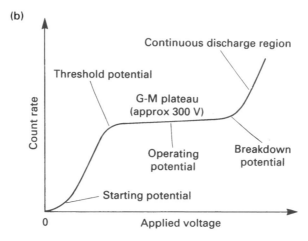

Fig. 14.4. (a) The Geiger–Müller (G–M) tube and (b) the effect of applied voltage on count rate.

around on an object that resembles a golf trolley. They are useful for mass screening of premises for ^{3}H contamination but are rarely used as routine. Most laboratories monitor for ^{3}H by doing a wipe test regularly, i.e. using wet tissues or cotton wool to take swabs for scintillation counting.

14.2.2 Methods based upon excitation

As outlined in Section 14.1.7, radioactive isotopes interact with matter in two ways, causing ionisation, which forms the basis of Geiger–Müller counting, and excitation. The latter effect leads the excited compound (known as the fluor) to emit photons of light. This fluorescence can be detected and quantified. The process is known as scintillation and when the light is detected by a photomultiplier, forms the basis of scintillation counting. The electric pulse that results from the conversion of light energy to electrical energy in the photomultiplier is directly proportional to the energy of the original radioactive event. This is a

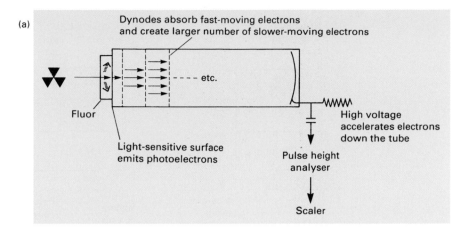

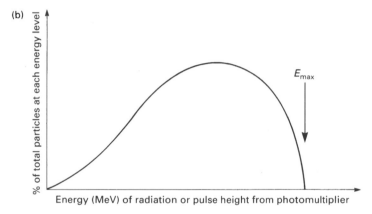

Fig. 14.5. (a) The mode of action of a photomultiplier and (b) the energy spectrum of a typical β-emitter.

considerable asset of scintillation counting, since it means that two, or even more, isotopes can be separately detected and measured in the same sample, provided they have sufficiently different emission energy spectra (see below). The mode of action of a photomultiplier is shown in Fig. 14.5.

In summary, scintillation counting provides information of two kinds:

(i) *Quantitative*, the number of scintillations is proportional to the rate of decay of the sample, i.e. the amount of radioactivity;
(ii) *Qualitative*, the intensity of light given out and therefore signal from the photomultiplier is proportional to the energy of radiation.

Types of scintillation counting

There are two types of scintillation counting, which are illustrated diagrammatically in Fig. 14.6. In solid scintillation counting the sample is placed adjacent to a crystal of fluorescent material. The crystal that is normally used for γ-isotopes is

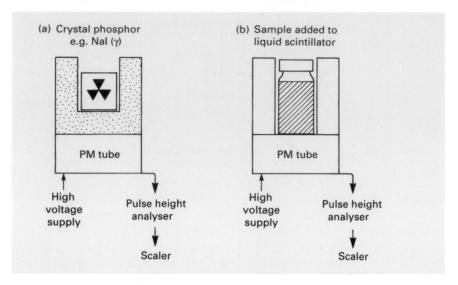

Fig. 14.6. Diagrammatic illustration of solid (a) and liquid (b) scintillation counting methods.

sodium iodide, whereas for α-emitters zinc sulphide crystals are preferred and for β-emitters organic scintillators such as anthracene are used. The crystals themselves are placed near to a photomultiplier, which in turn is connected to a high voltage supply and a scaler (Fig. 14.6a). Solid scintillation counting is particularly useful for γ-emitting isotopes. This is because, as explained in Section 14.1.7, these rays are electromagnetic radiation and collide only rarely with neighbouring atoms to cause ionisation or excitation. Clearly, in a crystal the atoms are densely packed, making collisions more likely. Conversely, solid scintillation counting is generally unsuitable for weak β-emitting isotopes such as ^{3}H and ^{14}C, because even the highest energy negatrons emitted by these isotopes would have hardly sufficient energy to penetrate the walls of the counting vials in which the samples are placed for counting. As many of the isotopes used in radioimmunoassay (Section 4.7) are γ-emitting isotopes, solid scintillation counting is frequently used in biological work.

In liquid scintillation counting (Fig. 14.6b), the sample is mixed with a scintillation cocktail containing a solvent and one or more fluors. This method is particularly useful in quantifying weak β-emitters such as ^{3}H, ^{14}C and ^{35}S, which are frequently used in biological work. For these isotopes, liquid scintillation counting is the usual counting method. Thus the remainder of this section will place particular emphasis on this technique, though it should be pointed out that most of what follows applies equally to solid scintillation counting used in the quantification of γ-emitters.

Energy transfer in liquid scintillation counting

A small number of organic solvents fluoresce when bombarded with radioactivity. The light emitted is of very short wavelength (Fig. 14.7) and is not efficiently

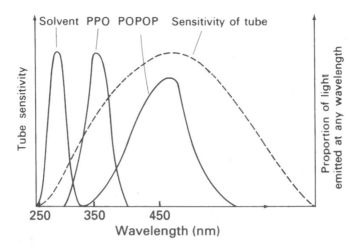

Fig. 14.7. Emission spectra of various fluors in relation to sensitivity of phototubes.

detected by most photomultipliers. However, if a compound is dissolved that can accept the energy from the solvent and itself fluoresce at a longer wavelength, then the light can be more efficiently detected. Such a compound is known as a primary fluor and the most frequently used example is 2,5-diphenyloxazole (PPO). Unfortunately the light emitted by PPO is not always detected with very high efficiency (depending on the photomultiplier detector) but this can be overcome by including a secondary fluor or wavelength shifter such as 1,4-bis(5-phenyloxazol-2-yl) benzene (POPOP). Thus, the energy transfer process becomes

$$\text{Radiation} \longrightarrow \begin{pmatrix} \text{Solvent} \\ \text{Excited} \end{pmatrix} \begin{pmatrix} \text{Excited} \\ \text{Primary} \\ \text{fluor} \end{pmatrix} \begin{pmatrix} \text{Secondary} \\ \text{fluor} \\ \text{Excited} \end{pmatrix} \longrightarrow \textit{Light}$$

The question obviously arises as to why a primary fluor *and* a secondary fluor are necessary when it is the latter that emits light at the best wavelength for detection. The answer is simply that the solvent cannot transfer its energy directly to the secondary fluor.

PPO and POPOP were among the original fluors used in liquid scintillation counting and remain a favourite choice. However compounds such as 2-(4'-*t*-butylphhenyl)-5-(4"-biphenylyl)-1,3,4-oxadiazole (BUTYL-PBD) is a better primary fluor but is quite expensive and is affected by extremes of pH.

Most laboratories now buy their scintillation cocktails already prepared and there are many different makes and recipes on the market. Competition and an increasing awareness of health and safety mean that scintillation cocktails are gradually becoming less toxic and have a lower fire hazard. A final point: some cocktails are designed for aqueous samples and others for organic samples; it is important that the appropriate formulation is used.

Advantages of scintillation counting

The very fact that scintillation counting is widely used in biological work indicates that it has several advantages over gas ionisation counting. These advantages are listed below.

(i) The rapidity of fluorescence decay (10^{-9} s), which, when compared to dead time in a Geiger–Müller tube (10^{-4} s), means much higher count rates are possible.

(ii) Much higher counting efficiencies particularly for low energy β-emitters; over 50% efficiency is routine in scintillation counting and efficiency can rise to over 90% for high energy emitters. This is partly due to the fact that the negatrons do not have to travel through air or pass through an end-window of a Geiger–Müller tube (thereby dissipating much of the energy before causing ionisation) but interact directly with the fluor; energy loss before the event that is counted is therefore minimal.

(iii) The ability to accommodate samples of any type, including liquids, solids, suspensions and gels.

(iv) The general ease of sample preparation (see below).

(v) The ability to count separately different isotopes in the same sample, which means dual labelling experiments can be carried out (see below).

(vi) Scintillation counters are highly automated, hundreds of samples can be counted automatically and built-in computer facilities carry out many forms of data analysis, such as efficiency correction, graph plotting, radioimmunoassay calculations, etc.

Disadvantages of scintillation counting

It would not be reasonable, having outlined some of the advantages of scintillation counting, to disregard the disadvantages of the method. Fortunately, however, most of the inherent disadvantages have been overcome by improvement in instrument design. These disadvantages include the following.

(i) The cost per sample of scintillation counting is not insignificant; however, other factors including versatility, sensitivity, ease and accuracy outweigh this factor for most applications.

(ii) At the high voltages applied to the photomultiplier, electronic events occur in the system that are independent of radioactivity but contribute to a high background count. This is referred to as photomultiplier noise and can be partially reduced by cooling the photomultipliers. Since temperature affects counting efficiency, cooling also presents a controlled temperature for counting, which may be useful. Low noise photomultipliers, however, have been designed to provide greater temperature stability in ambient temperature systems. Also the use of a pulse height analyser can be set so as to reject, electronically, most of the noise pulses that are of low energy (the threshold or gate setting). The disadvantage here is that this also rejects the low energy pulses resulting from low energy radioactivity (e.g. ^3H). Another method of reducing noise, which is incorporated into most scintillation counters, is to use coincidence counting. In this system two photomultipliers are used. These as set in coincidence such that only when a pulse is generated in both tubes at the same time is it allowed to pass to the scaler. The chances of this happening for a pulse generated by a radioactive event is very high compared to the chances of a noise event occurring in both photomultipliers during the so-called resolution time of the system, which is commonly of the order of 20 ns. In general, this system reduces photomultiplier noise to a very low level.

(iii) The greatest disadvantage of scintillation counting is quenching. This occurs when the energy transfer process described earlier suffers interference. Correcting for this quenching contributes significantly to the cost of scintillation counting. Quenching can be any one of three kinds.

(a) *Optical quenching* occurs if inappropriate or dirty scintillation vials are used. These will absorb some of the light being emitted, before it reaches the photomultiplier.

(b) *Colour quenching* occurs if the sample is coloured and results in light emitted being absorbed within the scintillation cocktail before it leaves the sample vial. When colour quenching is known to be a major problem, it can be reduced, as outlined later.

(c) *Chemical quenching*, which occurs when anything in the sample interferes with the transfer of energy from the solvent to the primary fluor or from the primary fluor to the secondary fluor, is the most difficult form of quenching to accommodate. In a series of homogeneous samples (e.g. $^{14}CO_2$ released during metabolism of [^{14}C]glucose and trapped in alkali, which is then added to the scintillation cocktail for counting), chemical quenching may not vary greatly from sample to sample. In these cases relative counting using sample counts per minute can be compared directly. However, in the majority of biological experiments using radioisotopes, such homogeneity of samples is unlikely and it is not sufficiently accurate to use relative counting (i.e. counts per minute). Instead, an appropriate method of standardisation must be used. This requires the determination of the counting efficiency of each sample and the conversion of counts per minute to absolute counts (i.e. disintegrations per minute), as described later. It should be noted that quenching is not such a great problem in solid (external) scintillation counting.

(iv) Chemiluminescence can also cause problems during liquid scintillation counting. It results from chemical reactions between components of the samples to be counted and the scintillation cocktail, and produces light emission unrelated to excitation of the solvent and fluor system by radioactivity. These light emissions are generally low energy events and are rejected by the threshold setting of the photomultiplier in the same way as photomultiplier noise. Chemiluminescence, when it is a problem, can usually be overcome by storing samples for some time before counting, to permit the chemiluminescence to decay. Many contemporaneous instruments are able to detect chemiluminescence and substract it or flag it on the printout.

(v) Phospholuminescence results from components of the sample, including the vial itself, absorbing light and re-emitting it. Unlike chemiluminescence, which is a once-only effect, phospholuminescence will occur on each exposure of a sample to light. Samples that are pigmented are most likely to phosphoresce. If this is a problem, samples should be adapted to dark prior to counting and the sample holder should be kept closed throughout the counting process.

Despite all the complications described above, scintillations counters are universal in biosciences departments. This is because the instruments have automated systems for calculating counting efficiency; in other words the instruments do all the hard work!

Using scintillation counting for dual-labelled samples

A feature of the scintillation process is that the size of electric pulse produced by the conversion of light energy in the photomultiplier is related directly to the energy of the original radioactive event. Because different β-emitting isotopes have different energy spectra, it is possible to quantify two isotopes separately in a single sample, provided their energy spectra are sufficiently different. Examples of pairs of isotopes that have sufficiently different energy spectra are ^3H and ^{14}C, ^3H and ^{35}S, ^3H and ^{32}P, ^{14}C and ^{32}P, ^{35}S and ^{32}P. The principle of the method is illustrated in Fig. 14.8, where it can be seen that the spectra of two isotopes (S and T) overlap only slightly. By setting a pulse height analyser to reject all pulses of an energy below X (threshold X) and to reject all pulses of an energy above Y (window Y) and also to reject below a threshold of A and a window of B, it is possible to separate the two isotopes completely. A pulse height analyser set with a threshold and window for a particular isotope is known as a channel (e.g. a ^3H channel).

Most modern counters operate with a so-called multichannel analyser. These are based on an analogue-to-digital converter; electronic signals from the photomultiplier are converted to digital signals stored in a computer. Thus the entire energy spectrum is analysed simultaneously. This greatly facilitates multi-isotope counting and in particular allows the effect of quenching on dual-label counting to be assessed adequately.

Dual-label counting has proved to be useful in many aspects of molecular biology (e.g. nucleic acid hybridisation and transcription), metabolism (e.g. steroid synthesis) and drug development.

Determination of counting efficiency

As outlined above, a major problem encountered in scintillation counting is that of quenching, which makes it necessary to determine the counting efficiency of

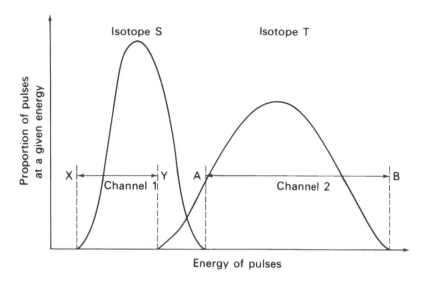

Fig. 14.8. Diagram to illustrate the principle of counting dual-labelled samples.

some, if not all, of the samples in a particular experiment. This can be done by one of several methods of standardisation, all of which apply to both solid and liquid scintillation counting, though again in this section emphasis is placed on the latter method.

Internal standardisation. The sample is counted (and gives a reading of say A c.p.m.), removed from the counter and a small amount of standard material of known disintegrations per minute (B d.p.m.) is added. The sample is then recounted (C c.p.m.) and the counting efficiency of the sample calculated:

counting efficiency $= [100\,(C - A)/B]\,\%$

It is obviously necessary in this method to use an internal standard (the spike) that contains the same isotope as the one being counted and also to ensure that the standard itself does not act as a quenching agent. Suitable ^{14}C-labelled standards include [^{14}C]toluene, [^{14}C]hexadecane, [^{3}H]benzoic acid and ^{3}H$_2$O (benzoic acid and water are themselves quenching agents and must be used in only very small amounts). Internal standardisation is simple and reliable and corrects adequately for all types of quenching. Carefully carried out, it is the most accurate way of correcting for quenching. On the other hand it demands very accurate pipetting when the standard is added, and it is time consuming because each sample must be counted twice. It also means that the sample cannot be recounted in the event of error because it will be contaminated with the standard. Moreover, time elapses between the first and second count and changes in sample quenching characteristics can also occur, which can lead to considerable inaccuracies. However, it is the means by which the following two methods are calibrated.

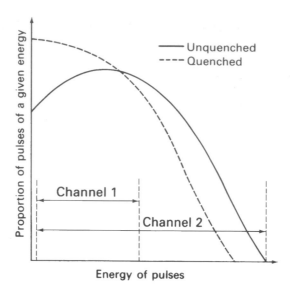

Fig. 14.9. The effect of quenching of a β-energy spectrum.

Channels ratio.   When a sample in a scintillation counter is quenched, the scintillation process is less efficient: less light is produced for a given quantum energy of radiation. Thus the energy spectrum for a quenched sample appears to be lower than for an unquenched sample (Fig. 14.9). The higher the degree of quenching, the more pronounced is the resulting decrease in the spectrum. This fact is made use of in the channels ratio method for determining counter efficiency. This method involves the preparation of a calibration curve based on counting in two channels that cover different, but overlapping, parts of the spectrum. As a sample is quenched, and the spectrum shifts to gradually lower apparent energies, the ratio of counts in each channel will vary. To prepare the standard curve, a set of quenched standards is counted: the absolute amount of radioactivity is known and therefore the efficiency of counting in each channel can easily be determined.

The efficiency is then plotted against channels ratio to form the standard curve (Fig. 14.10). Typical data for a set of ^{14}C quenched standards are given in Table 14.2. It is important to realise that a standard curve applies to only one set of circumstances – one radioisotope, counter and scintillation fluid.

Once the standard curve has been prepared, the efficiency of counting experimental samples can be determined. Samples are counted in the same two channels, the ratio is calculated, put into the graph and the efficiency read. In practice all the data can be stored in the counter's computer and corrected values printed automatically.

Multichannel scintillation counters operate on the same principle but the whole shape and position of the spectrum is analysed. This is given a digital parameter that relates to counting efficiency. Manufacturers have developed their own titles for such parameters, for example LKB Instruments' Spectral Quench

Table 14.2 **Radioactivity recorded with gradually increasing quench in two channels of a scintillation counter**

Sample	c.p.m.		Ratio	Counting efficiency in channel 2 (%)
	Channel 1	Channel 2	Ch1: Ch2	
^{14}C standard (203 600 d.p.m.) unquenched	171 930	184 250	0.93	90.5
^{14}C standard (203 600 d.p.m.) with increasing quench	146 610	168 840	0.87	82.9
	94 240	135 090	0.70	66.3
	52 260	102 030	0.51	50.1
	16 030	58 320	0.27	28.6
	5920	34 740	0.17	17.1
	2060	20 270	0.10	9.9
	1130	13 260	0.08	6.5

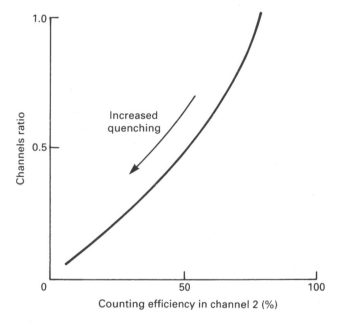

Fig. 14.10. Channels ratio quench correction curve.

Parameter of Isotope (or SQP(I)) or Packard's Spectral Index Sample. These systems have greater precision than the two-channel approach, as the whole of the spectrum is used for analysis. The channels ratio method is suitable for all types and even high degrees of quenching. Furthermore, counting in more than one channel is simultaneous and this method is, therefore, less time consuming than either internal or external standardisation. It is also, in practice, an acceptably accurate method for determining counting efficiency, provided care is taken in the preparation of the calibration curve. However, it is notoriously inaccurate at low count

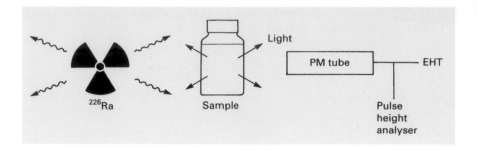

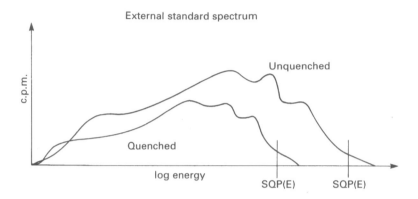

Fig. 14.11. The external standard for estimating counting efficiency. The external source irradiates the sample. The counter analyses the spectrum, which shifts to lower energies if the sample is quenched. The SQP(E), i.e. standard quench parameter (external), expressed without units, is derived from the energy axis and relates to the extent of quench. The greater the quench in the sample, the lower the SQP(E) and the lower the counting efficiency (see Table 14.3).

rates, because the error on the counts per minute is high and there will be a larger error on the channels ratio because it is calculated from two values of the counts per minute. It is also inaccurate for very highly quenched samples. For these reasons the method that follows is most frequently the procedure of choice.

External standardisation. Instruments have a γ-emitting external standard built into the counter. Under the control of the counter each sample to be counted is exposed to this external source, which is automatically shifted from a lead shield to the counting chamber. The γ-radiation penetrates the vial and excites the scintillation fluid. The resulting spectrum is unique to the source and is significantly different from that produced by the sample in the vial. The γ-source used (e.g. ^{137}Cs, ^{133}Ba or ^{226}Ra) varies according to the make of instrument. The spectrum obtained by ^{226}Ra is shown in Fig. 14.11.

Quenching agents present in the scintillation fluid will significantly affect the spectrum obtained. The instrument analyses this spectrum and assigns a quench parameter to it. The precise method used depends on the make of counter; LKB

Table 14.3 **Recorded radioactivity from a ^{14}C standard sample with increasing quench detected by an external standard**

Sample	c.p.m.	External quench parameter[a]	Counting efficiency (%)
^{14}C standard (203 600 d.p.m.) unquenched	194 930	810	95.7
^{14}C standard (203 600 d.p.m.) with increasing quench	146 141	422	93.5
	181 171	207	89.0
	167 731	126	82.4
	145 879	76	71.6
	126 913	55	62.3
	108 641	42	53.3
	96 103	37	47.2

[a] e.g. SQP(E), see Fig. 14.11.

Instruments refer to a standard quench parameter based on a point on the energy axis (Fig. 14.11). Other manufacturers use slightly different approaches but the principle is the same: the spectrum for the external standard varies according to the degree of quench in the vial and, therefore, the efficiency of counting of the internal experimental sample.

As for the channels ratio method, a standard curve is required, i.e. a range of quenched standards is counted and the external standard spectrum analysed in each case. The resulting data (Table 14.3) are used to prepare a standard curve that is held in the instrument's computer. Unknown samples are then counted in the same way, the efficiency read from the standard curve and the sample counts corrected.

The external standard approach is now routine in most laboratories, the main advantage over the channels ratio method being that it is suited to samples with low count rates. However, it is not without disadvantages: a standard curve is required for each set of circumstances (as with the channels ratio) and the user can be lulled into a false sense of security. The system is so highly automated that it is easy to lose sight of the basic principles and the method is not always appropriate. A case in point is the counting of ^3H precipitated onto filters counted in scintillation fluid. The external standard method will calculate the degree of quench in the fluid (which will probably be very low) but will not take into account the poor penetration of ^3H β-particles from the filter into the scintillation fluid: artificially high efficiencies will be recorded.

In all cases where an automated procedure for calculating counting efficiencies is employed it is prudent to count a few prepared samples in which the true amount of radioactivity is known.

Sample preparation

It is impossible here to give details of all aspects of sample preparation for scintillation counting. However, major considerations are outlined below and the reader is referred to books cited in Section 14.9 for further details.

Sample vials.   In solid scintillation counting, sample preparation is easy and only involves transferring the sample to a glass or plastic vial (or tube) compatible with the counter. In liquid scintillation counting, sample preparation is more complex and starts with a decision on the type of sample vial to be used. These may be glass, low potassium glass (with low levels of ^{40}K that reduce background count) or polyethylene. The last of these types are cheaper but are not suitable for cleaning and reuse, whereas glass vials can be reused many times provided they are thoroughly cleaned. Polyethylene vials give better light transfer and result in slightly higher counting efficiencies, but are inclined to exhibit more phosphorescence than do glass vials. The recent trend is towards mini-vials, which use far smaller volumes of expensive scintillation cocktails. Modern counters are able to accept many types of vial; the smallest vial possible should be used (within the obvious constraints of sample volume) to save costs and in consideration of environmental issues, as scintillation fluids are toxic. Some counters are designed to accept very small samples in special polythene bags split into an array of many compartments; these are particularly useful to, for example, the pharmaceutical industry where there are laboratories that do large numbers of receptor binding assays.

Scintillation cocktails.   Toluene-based cocktails are the most efficient, but will not accept aqueous samples, because toluene and water are immiscible and massive quenching results. Cocktails based on 1,4-dioxane and naphthalene that can accommodate up to 20% (v/v) water can be used, but they have largely been phased out due to toxicity. Emulsifier-based cocktails are the most frequently used for counting aqueous samples. They contain an emulsifier such as Triton X-100 and can accept up to 50% water (v/v); however, phase transitions occur from single phase to two phase or gel, as the water content increases. Accurate counting cannot be done if the samples are in the two-phase state. Many ready-made cocktails are on the market and are sold with precise instructions regarding sample condition.

Volume of cocktail.   It should be noted that the efficiency of scintillation counting varies with sample volume, though this is less of a problem in modern counters. Nevertheless, care should be taken that sample vials in a given series of counts contain the same volume of sample and that all instrument calibration is done using the same volume as for experimental samples.

Overcoming major colour quenching.   If colour quenching is a problem it is possible to bleach samples before counting. Care should be taken, however, since bleaching agents such as hydrogen peroxide can give rise to chemiluminescence in some scintillation cocktails.

Tissue solubilisers.   Solid samples, such as plant and animal tissues, may be best counted after solubilisation by quaternary amines such as NCS solubiliser or Soluene. Not surprisingly these solutions are highly toxic and great care is required. The sample is added to the counting vial containing a small amount of

Table 14.4   Some isotopes suitable for Čerenkov counting

Radioisotope	E_{max} (MeV)	% of spectrum above 0.5 MeV	Counting efficiency (%)
^{22}Na	1.39	60	30
^{32}P	1.71	80	40
^{36}Cl	0.71	30	10
^{42}K	3.5	90	80

solubiliser and digestion is allowed to proceed. When digestion is complete, scintillation cocktail is added and the sample counted. Again, chemiluminescence can be a problem with tissue solubilisers.

Combustion methods.   A suitable alternative to bleaching of coloured samples or digestion of tissues is the use of combustion techniques. Here samples are combusted in an atmosphere of oxygen, usually in a commercially available combustion apparatus. Thus, samples containing ^{14}C would be combusted to ^{14}CO$_2$, which is collected in a trapping agent such as sodium hydroxide and then counted; ^{3}H-containing samples are converted to ^{3}H$_2$O for counting.

As indicated earlier, only important considerations in sample preparation are discussed above and details are not given. However, it is worthy of comment that almost any type of radioactive sample containing β-emitting istopes can be prepared for counting in a liquid scintillation counter by one method or another, including cuttings from paper chromatographs or membrane filters, again illustrating the versatility and importance of this technique for quantifying radioactivity.

Čerenkov counting

The Čerenkov effect occurs when a particle passes through a substance with a speed higher than that of light passing through the same substance. If a β-emitter has a decay energy in excess of 0.5 MeV, then this causes water to emit a bluish white light usually referred to as Čerenkov light. It is possible to detect this light using a typical liquid scintillation counter.

Since there is no requirement for organic solvents and fluors, this technique is relatively cheap, sample preparation is very easy, and there is no problem of chemical quenching. Table 14.4 lists some isotopes that are suitable for this detection method. Most work has been done on ^{32}P, which has 80% of its energy spectrum above the Čerenkov threshold and which can be detected at around 40% efficiency. It may be noted from Table 14.4 that, as the proportion of the energy spectrum above 0.5 MeV increases, so too does the detection efficiency.

14.2.3 **Methods based upon exposure of photographic emulsions**

Ionising radiation acts upon a photographic emulsion to produce a latent image much as does visible light. For a photograph, a radiation source, an object to be

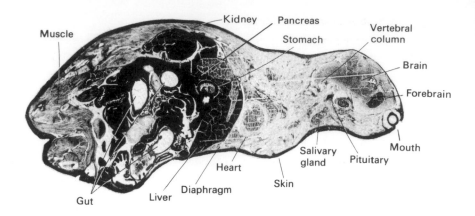

Fig. 14.12. Whole-body autoradiograph of a mouse treated with [L-^{14}C]dopa. The dark areas indicate the presence of radioactive isotope and show high concentrations in the liver, pancreas, kidney, skin and forebrain.

imaged and photographic emulsion are required. For an autoradiograph, a radiation source (i.e. radioactivity) emanating from within the material to be imaged (the object) is required, along with a sensitive emulsion. The emulsion consists of a large number of silver halide crystals embedded in a solid phase such as gelatin. As energy from the radioactive material is dissipated in the emulsion, the silver halide becomes negatively charged and is reduced to metallic silver, thus forming a particulate latent image. Photographic developers are designed to show these silver grains as a blackening of the film, and fixers to remove any remaining silver halide. Thus, a permanent image of the location of the original radioactive event remains.

This process, which is known as autoradiography, is very sensitive and has been used in a wide variety of biological experiments. These unusally involve a requirement to locate the distribution of radioactivity in biological specimens of different types. For instance, the sites of localisation of a radiolabelled drug throughout the body of an experimental animal can be determined by placing whole-body sections of the animal in close contact with a sensitive emulsion such as an X-ray plate. After a period of exposure, the plate, upon development, will show an image of the section in tissues and organs in which radioactivity was present (Fig. 14.12). Similarly, radioactive metabolites isolated and separated by chromatographic or electrophoretic techniques during metabolic studies can be located on the chromatograph or electrophoretograph and the radioactive spots can subsequently be recovered for counting and identification (counting may be carried out on the original chromatograph by using a chromatograph scanner, the design of which is generally based on Geiger–Müller tubes, or by elution from the paper, plate or gel for counting by liquid scintillation counting).

The techniques of autoradiography have become more important with recent developments in molecular biology (Chapters 2 and 3). Consequently more detail is given below on some important aspects of the technique.

Suitable isotopes

In general, weak β-emitting isotopes (e.g. ^{3}H and ^{14}C and ^{35}S) are most suitable for autoradiography, particularly for cell and tissue localisation experiments. This is because, as a result of the low energy of the negatrons, the ionising track of the isotope will be short and a discrete image will result. This is particularly important when radioactivity associated with subcellular organelles is being located. For this, ^{3}H is the best radioisotope, since its energy will all be quickly dissipated within the emulsion. Electron microscopy can then be used to locate the image in the developed film. For location within whole organisms or tissues, either ^{14}C or ^{3}H is suitable; more energetic isotopes (e.g. ^{32}P) are less suitable because their higher energy negatrons produce much longer track lengths and result in less discrete images that are not sufficiently discriminatory for microscopic location. Conversely, for location of, for example, DNA bands in an electrophoretic gel, ^{32}P is useful. In this case low energy ^{3}H negatrons would largely dissipate their energy within the gel (and in the wrapping around the gel, which is usually necessary to prevent the gel sticking to the emulsion), thereby reducing sensitivity to a low level. However, the more energetic ^{32}P negatrons will leave the gel and produce a strong image. If very thin gels are prepared, then ^{35}S or ^{14}C can be detected with high resolution, for example in DNA sequencing gels where ^{35}S is used as the label.

Choice of emulsion and film

A variety of emulsions is available with different packing densities of the silver halide crystals. Care must be taken to choose an emulsion suitable for the purposes of the experiment, since the sensitivity of the emulsion will affect the resolution obtained. Manufacturers' literature should be consulted and their advice sought if one is in any doubt. X-ray film is generally suitable for macroscopic samples such as whole-body sections of small mammals, chromatographs or electrophoretographs. When light or electron microscopic detection of the location of the image in the emulsion is required (cellular and subcellular localisation of radioactivity), very sensitive films are necessary, as is a very close apposition of sample and film. In these cases a stripping film technique can be used in which the film is supplied attached to a support. It is stripped from this and applied directly to the sample. Alternatively, liquid emulsions are prepared by melting strips of emulsion by heating them to around 60 °C. Then either the emulsion is poured onto the sample or the sample attached to a support is dipped into the emulsion. The emulsion is then allowed to set before being dried. Such a method is often referred to as a dipping-film method and is preferred when very thin films are required.

Background

Accidental exposure to light, chemicals in the sample, natural background radioactivity (particularly ^{40}K in glass) and even pressure applied during handling and storage of film will cause a background fog (i.e. latent image) on the developed film. This can be problematic, particularly in high resolution work (e.g. involving microscopy) and care must be taken at all times to minimise its effect. Background will always increase during exposure time, which should therefore always be kept to a minimum.

Time of exposure and film processing

The time of exposure depends upon the isotope, sample type, level of activity, film type and purpose of the experiment. The same applies to the processing of the film in order to display the image. Generally the process must be adapted to a given purpose, and a great deal of trial and error is often involved in arriving at the most suitable procedures.

Direct autoradiography

In direct autoradiography, the X-ray film or emulsion is placed as close as possible to the sample and exposed at any convenient temperature. Quantitative images are produced until saturation is reached. The approach provides high resolution but limited sensitivity: isotopes of energy equal to, or higher than, ^{14}C ($E_{max} = 0.156$ MeV) are required.

Fluorography

Many of the currently popular methods in molecular biology involve separation of macromolecules or fractions of macromolecules by gel electrophoresis (Sections 12.3 and 12.4). The separated macromolecules or fractions form bands in the electrophoretograph that must be located. This is often achieved by radio-labelling the macromolecules with ^3H or ^{14}C and subjecting the gel to autoradiography. Because these are weak β-emitters, much of their energy is lost in the gel and long exposure times are necessary even when very high specific activity sources are used. However, if a fluor (e.g. PPO or sodium silicate) is infiltrated into the gel, and the gel dried and then placed in contact with a pre-flashed film (see below), sensitivity can be increased by several orders of magnitude. This is because the negatrons emitted from the isotope will cause the fluor to become excited and emit light, which will react with the film. Thus, use is made of *both* the ionising and the exciting effects of radioactivity in fluorography.

Intensifying screens

When ^{32}P-labelled or γ-isotope-labelled samples (e.g. [^{32}P]DNA or ^{125}I-labelled protein fractions in gels) are to be located, the opposite problem to that presented by low energy isotopes prevails. These much more penetrating particles and rays cause little reaction with the film as they penetrate right through it, producing a poor image. The image can be greatly improved by placing, on the other side of the film from the sample, a thick intensifying screen consisting of a solid phosphor. Negatrons penetrating the film cause the phosphor to fluoresce and emit light, which superimposes its image on the film. There is, therefore, an increase in sensitivity but a parallel reduction in resolution due to the spread of light emanating from the screen.

Low temperature exposure

If the energy of ionising radiation is converted to light (i.e. with fluorography or intensifying screens) the kinetics of the film's response are affected. The light is of low intensity and a back reaction occurs that cancels the forming latent image.

Exposure at low temperature ($-70°$C) slows this back reaction and will therefore provide higher sensitivity. There is no point in doing direct autoradiography at low temperature as the kinetics of the film response are different. There is nothing to be gained by exposing preflashed film (see below) at low temperature.

Preflashing

As described above, the response of a photographic emulsion to radiation is not linear and usually involves a slow initial phase (lag) followed by a linear phase. Sensitivity of films may be increased by preflashing. This involves a millisecond light flash prior to the sample being brought into juxtaposition with the film and is often used where high sensitivity is required or if results are to be quantified.

Quantification

As indicated earlier, autoradiography is usually used to locate rather than to quantify radioactivity. However, it is possible to obtain quantitative data directly from autoradiographs by using a densitometer, which records the intensity of the image. This in turn is related to the amount of radioactivity in the original sample. There are many varieties of densitometers available and the choice made will depend on the purpose of the experiment. Quantification is not reliable at low or high levels of exposure because of the lag phase (i.e. the back reaction, as described above) or saturation, respectively; however, preflashing combined with fluorography or intensifying screens obviates the problem for small amounts of radioactivity. In this case all photons contribute equally to the image of the pre-exposed film.

14.3 OTHER PRACTICAL ASPECTS OF COUNTING RADIOACTIVITY AND ANALYSIS OF DATA

14.3.1 Counter characteristics

Background count

Radiation counters of all types always register a count, even in the absence of radioactive material in the apparatus. This may be due to such sources as cosmic radiation, natural radioactivity in the vicinity, nearby X-ray generators, and/or circuit noises. By means of the various methods already outlined and the use of lead shielding, this background radiation may be considerably reduced, but its value must always be recorded and accounted for in all experiments. Some commercial instruments have automatic background subtraction facilities.

Dead time

At very high count rates in Geiger–Müller counting, counts are lost due to the dead time of the Geiger–Müller tube. Correction tables are available and these should be used when necessary to correct for lost counts. Dead time is not a problem in scintillation counting.

Geometry

When samples with an end-window ionisation counter, such as a Geiger–Müller tube, are compared, it is important to standardise the position of the sample in relation to the tube, otherwise the fraction of the emitted radiation entering the tube may vary and hence so will the observed count.

14.3.2 Sample and isotope characteristics

Self-absorption

Self-absorption is primarily a problem with low energy β-emitters: radiation is absorbed by the sample itself. Self-absorption can be a serious problem in the counting of low energy radioactivity by scintillation counting if the sample is particulate or is, for instance, stuck to a membrane filter. Care should be taken to ensure comparability of samples because the methods of standardisation outlined earlier will not correct for self-absorption effects. Where homogeneity is not possible, particulate samples should be digested or otherwise solubilised prior to counting. Self-absorption is a major problem with Geiger–Müller counting and significantly reduces sensitivity and reliability. It is very difficult to count low energy emitters reliably with these counters and this was a major factor in the switch to scintillation counting.

Half-life

The half-life of an isotope (Section 14.1.5) may be short and, if so, this must be allowed for in the analysis of data.

Statistics

The emission of radioactivity is a random process. This can be demonstrated readily by making repeated measurements of the activity of a long-lived isotope, each for an identical period of time. The resulting counts will not be the same but will vary over a range of values, with clustering near the centre of the range. If a sufficiently large number of such measurements is made and the data are plotted, a normal distribution curve will be obtained. For a single count, therefore, we cannot obtain a true count. Instead, we take the mean of a large number of counts as being very close to the true count. However, the accuracy of this mean will depend on the spread or standard deviation (σ) for the data. Statistical theory states that, for a normal distribution such as that shown in Fig. 14.13, 68% of values obtained lie $\pm 1\ \sigma$, and 95% lie $\pm 2\ \sigma$ from the mean ($\bar{x}$).

Clearly, if we wish to compare samples, and in particular to state that two samples contain different amounts of radioactivity, then we need to take account of the counting statistics. Fortunately Poisson mathematics makes the task relatively easy as

$$\sigma = \sqrt{\text{total counts taken}}$$

$$\text{or } \sigma = \sqrt{\left(\frac{\text{count rate}}{\text{time}} \right)}$$

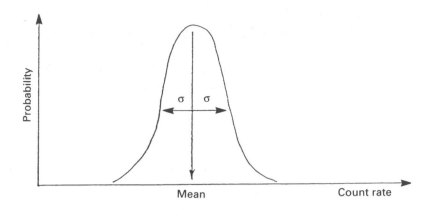

Fig. 14.13. The distribution of count rates around a mean, showing the standard deviation, σ.

Therefore to quote a figure with 95% certainty, state

total counts $\pm 2\sqrt{\text{total counts}}$

For example, if 1600 counts are recorded this can be expressed as 1600 ± 80. There is, therefore, a 95% chance that the true figure lies between 1520 and 1680.

When data are expressed as d.p.m. or c.p.m., again using 95% certainty, then

$$\text{error on count rate} = 2\sqrt{\left(\frac{\text{count rate}}{\text{time}}\right)}$$

Using the same example, if the 1600 counts were obtained in 1 min

$$\text{error on count rate} = 2\sqrt{\left(\frac{1600}{1}\right)} = 80$$

and therefore 1600 c.p.m. $\pm$ 80 c.p.m.

If the 1600 counts were obtained in 10 min:

$$\text{error on count rate} = 2\sqrt{\left(\frac{160}{10}\right)} = 8$$

and therefore 160 c.p.m. $\pm$ 8 c.p.m. Note that the error is the same. This is because effectively the same number of measurements, i.e. counts, has been taken in each case.

If we had recorded 160 counts in only 1 min, then

$$\text{error on count rate} = 2\sqrt{\left(\frac{160}{1}\right)} = 25$$

and therefore 160 c.p.m. $\pm$ 25 c.p.m.

Consider these other simple examples for a series of 1 min counts:

counts = 100 $\sigma = \sqrt{100}$,   therefore $\pm 10\%$ error at 68% certainty
counts = 1000 $\sigma = \sqrt{1000}$,   therefore $\pm 3\%$ error at 68% certainty
counts = 10 000 $\sigma = \sqrt{10\,000}$,   therefore $\pm 1\%$ error at 68% certainty

In summary, the counts per minute data become more accurate for *higher count rates* and/or *longer counting times*. It is common practice to count to 10 000 counts or for 10 min, whichever is the quicker, although for very low count rates longer counting times are required.

14.3.3 **Supply, storage and purity of radiolabelled compounds**

There are several suppliers of radiolabelled compounds, the main ones being Amersham Pharmacie Biotech, Du Pont, NEN and ICN. The suppliers usually include details of the best storage conditions and quality control data with their products. This is because several types of decomposition can occur; for example internal decomposition resulting from radioactive decay such as $^{14}C \rightarrow {}^{14}N$, and external decomposition where emitted radiation is absorbed by other radioactive molecules, causing impurities. The extent to which decomposition occurs is dependent on many factors such as temperature, energy of radiation, concentration and the formulation of the compound. It is, therefore, imperative to store radioisotopes by the method recommended by the supplier and to maintain sterility of the stock. If necessary, chromatographic procedures will be required to check on the purity of the labelled compounds.

14.3.4 **Specific activity**

The specific activity of a radioisotope defines its radioactivity related to the amount of material (e.g. Bq mol^{-1}, Ci mmol^{-1} or d.p.m. μmol^{-1}). Suppliers offer a range of specific activities for their compound, the highest often being the most expensive. The advantages of using a very high specific activity are as follows:

> Products of a reaction using the labelled precursor can be produced at high specific activity (e.g. for DNA probes, see Section 2.11).
> Small quantities of radiolabelled compound can be added such that the equilibrium of metabolic concentrations is not unduly perturbed.
> Calculating the amount of substance required to make up radioactive solutions of known specific activity is simplified, as the contribution to concentration made by the stock radiolabelled solution is often negligible (see below).

Sometimes, however, it is not necessary to purchase the highest specific activity available. For example, enzyme assays *in vitro* often require a relatively high substrate concentration and so specific activity may need to be lowered. Consider the example below (for definitions of units see Table 14.7):

[^{3}H]Leucine is purchased with a specific activity of 5.55 TBq mmol^{-1} (150 Ci mmol^{-1}) and a concentration of 9.25 MBq 250 mm^{-3} (250 μCi 250 mm^{-3}). A 10 cm^3 solution of 250 mmol dm^{-3} and 3.7 kBq cm^{-3} (0.1 μCi cm^{-3}) is required. It is made up as follows:

> 10 cm³ at 3.7 kBq cm⁻³ is 37 kBq (1 μCi), therefore pipette 1 mm³ of stock
> radioisotope into a vessel (or, to be more accurate, pipette 100 mm³ of a ×100
> dilution of stock in water).
>
> Add 2.5 cm³ of a 1 mol dm⁻³ stock solution of cold leucine, and make up to 10
> cm³ with distilled water.

There is no need to take into account the amount of unlabelled leucine in the
[³H]leucine preparation; it is a negligible quantity due to the high specific activity.
If necessary (e.g. to manipulate solutions of relatively low specific activity),
however, the following formula can be applied:

$$W = Ma[(1/A') - (1/A)]$$

where W is the mass of cold carrier required (mg), M is the amount of radioactivity
present (MBq), a is the molecular weight of the compound, A is the original specific
activity (MBq mmol⁻¹), and A' is the required specific activity (MBq mmol⁻¹).

14.3.5 The choice of radionuclide

This is a complex question depending on the precise requirements of the experiment. A summary of some of the key features of radioisotopes commonly used in
biological work is shown in Table 14.5.

14.4 INHERENT ADVANTAGES AND RESTRICTIONS OF RADIOTRACER EXPERIMENTS

Perhaps the greatest advantage of radiotracer methods over most other chemical
and physical methods is their sensitivity. For example, a dilution factor of 10^{12} can
be tolerated without the detection of ³H-labelled compounds being jeopardised. It
is thus possible to detect the occurrence of metabolic substances that are normally
present in tissues at such low concentrations as to defy the most sensitive chemical methods of identification. A second major advantage of using radiotracers is
that they enable studies *in vivo* to be carried out to a far greater degree than can any
other technique.

In spite of these significant advantages, certain restrictions have to be appreciated. First, although they undergo the same reactions, different isotopes may do so
at different rates. This effect is known as the isotope effect. The different rates are
approximately proportional to the differences in mass between the isotopes. The
extreme case is the isotopes ¹H and ³H, the effect being small for ¹²C and ¹⁴C and
almost insignificant for ³¹P and ³²P. Secondly, the amount of activity employed
must be kept to the minimum necessary to permit reasonable counting rates in
the samples to be analysed, otherwise the radiation from the tracer may elicit a
response from the experimental organism and hence distort the results. A third
consideration is that, in order to administer the tracer, the normal chemical level
of the compound in the organism is automatically exceeded. The results are therefore always open to question.

Table 14.5 The relative merits of commonly used β-emitters

Isotope	Advantages	Disadvantages
^{3}H	Safety High specific activity possible Wide choice of positions in organic compounds Very high resolution in autoradiography	Low efficiency of detection Isotope exchange with environment Isotope effect
^{14}C	Safety Wide choice of labelling position in organic compounds Good resolution in autoradiography	Low specific activity
^{35}S	High specific activity Good resolution in autoradiography	Short half-life Relatively long biological half-life
^{32}P	Ease of detection High specific activity Short half-life simplifies disposal Čerenkov counting	Short half-life affects costs and experimental design External radiation hazard Poor resolution in autoradiography

Taken from *Radioisotopes in Biology, A Practical Approach*, ed. R. J. Slater, Oxford University Press, with permission.

14.5 SAFETY ASPECTS

The greatest practical disadvantages of using radioisotopes is their toxicity: they produce ionising radiations. When absorbed, radiation causes ionisation and free radicals form that interact with the cell's macromolecules, causing mutation of DNA and hydrolysis of proteins. The toxicity of radiation is dependent not simply on the amount present but on the amount absorbed by the body, the energy of the absorbed radiation and its biological effect. There are, therefore, a series of additional units used to describe these parameters. Originally, radiation hazard was measured in terms of exposure, i.e. a quantity expressing the amount of ionisation in air. The unit of exposure is the roentgen (R), which is the amount of radiation that produces 1.61×10^{15} ion-pairs (kg air)$^{-1}$ (or 2.58×10^{-4} coulombs (kg air)$^{-1}$).

The amount of energy required to produce an ion-pair in air is 5.4×10^{-18} joules (J) and so the amount of energy absorbed by air with an exposure of 1 R is:

$$1.61 \times 10^{15} \times 5.4 \times 10^{-18} = 0.00869 \, \text{J (kg air)}^{-1}$$

Although the roentgen has been used as a unit of radiation hazard, it is now considered inadequate for two reasons: first, it is defined with reference to X-rays (or γ-rays) only; and, secondly, the amount of ionisation or energy absorption in different types of material, including living tissue, is likely to be different from that in air.

The concept of radiation absorbed dose (rad) was introduced to overcome these restrictions. The rad is defined as the dose of radiation that gives an energy absorption of 0.01 J (kg absorber)$^{-1}$; this has now been changed to the gray, an SI unit, representing absorption of 1 J kg^{-1} (i.e. 100 rads).

The gray (Gy) is a useful unit, but it still does not adequately describe the hazard to living organisms. This is because different types of radiation are associated with differing degrees of biological hazard. It is, therefore, necessary to introduce a correction factor, known as the weighting factor (W), which is calculated by comparing the biological effects of any type of radiation with that of X-rays. The unit of absorbed dose, which takes into account the weighting factor is the sievert (Sv) and is known as the equivalent dose. Thus:

equivalent dose (Sv) = Gy × W

The majority of isotopes used in biological research emit β-radiation. This is considered to have a biological effect that is very similar to X-rays and has a weighting factor of 1. Therefore, for β-radiation, Gy = Sv. Alpha particles, with their stronger ionising power, are much more toxic and have a weighting factor of 20. Therefore, for α-radiation, 1 Gy = 20 Sv. It is likely that, as our knowledge of the biological effectiveness of different forms of radiation progresses, so the quality factor for different types of radiation may change in the future. Absorbed dose from known sources can be calculated from knowledge of the rate of decay of the source, the energy of radiation, the penetrating power of the radiation and the distance between the source and the laboratory worker. As the radiation is emitted from a source in all directions, the level of irradiation is related to the area of a sphere, $4\pi r^2$. Thus the absorbed dose is inversely related to the square of the distance from the source (r); or, put another way, if the distance is doubled the dose is quartered. A useful formula is

$$\text{dose}_1 \times \text{distance}_1^2 = \text{dose}_2 \times \text{distance}_2^2$$

The relationship between radioactive source and absorbed dose is illustrated in Fig. 14.14.

The rate at which dose is delivered is referred to as the dose rate, expressed in Sv h^{-1}. It can be used to calculate your total dose. For example, a source may be delivering 10 μSv h^{-1}. If you worked with the source for 6 h, your total dose would be 60 μSv.

Currently, the dose limit for workers exposed to radiation is 50 mSv in a year to the whole body and, importantly, this exposure cannot be permitted to occur several years running. Limits are set for individual organs. The most important of these to know are for hands (500 mSv year^{-1}) and for lens of the eye (150 mSv year^{-1}). Dose limits are constantly under review and although dose limits are set,

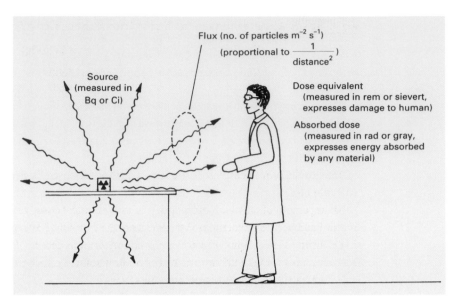

Fig. 14.14. The relationship between radioactivity of source and absorbed dose.

it is against internationally agreed guidelines to work to such a limit, i.e. to assume that all is satisfactory if the limit is not exceeded. Instead, the ALARA principle is applied, to work always to a dose limit that is as low as reasonably achievable. Work that may cause a worker to exceed three-tenths or one-tenth of the dose limit must be carried out in a controlled area or a supervised area, respectively. In practice, work in the biosciences rarely involves a worker receiving a measurable dose. Supervised areas are common but not always required (e.g. for ^{3}H or ^{14}C experiment). Controlled areas are required in only certain circumstances, for example for isotope stores or radioiodination work. A major problem, however, in biosciences is the internal radiation hazard. This is caused by radiation entering the body, for example by inhalation, ingestion, absorption or puncture. This is a likely source of hazard where work involves open sources, i.e. liquids and gases; most work in biology involves manipulations of radioactive liquids. Control of contamination is assisted by:

(i)   complying with local rules, written by an employer,
(ii) conscientious personal conduct in the laboratory,
(iii) regular monitoring,
(iv) carrying out work in some kind of containment.

Calculating the dose received following the ingestion of a radioisotope is complex. Detailed information is published by the International Commission on Radiological Protection and assessments, for example for experiments on human volunteers, can be obtained from the National Radiological Protection Board. However, one relatively simple concept is the annual limit on intake (ALI). The ingestion of one ALI results in a person receiving a dose of either

Table 14.6	Annual limits in intake (ALI) for some commonly used isotopes
Nuclide	ALI (MBq)
^{3}H	3000
^{14}C	90
^{32}P	10
^{125}I	1

50 mSv to the whole body or 500 mSv to a particular organ. Some ALIs are shown in Table 14.6.

Management of radiation protection is similar in most countries. In the UK there is the Radioactive Substances Act 1960 and the Ionising Radiations Regulations 1985. Every institution requires certification, monitored by the Environment Agency and employs a Radiation Protection Advisor in compliance with the Act.

When handling radioisotopes the rule is to:

maximise the distance between yourself and the source,
minimise the time of exposure and
maintain shielding at all times.

14.6 APPLICATIONS OF RADIOISOTOPES IN THE BIOLOGICAL SCIENCES

14.6.1 Investigating aspects of metabolism

Metabolic pathways

Radioisotopes are frequently used for tracing metabolic pathways (see Section 1.3.3). This usually involves adding a radioactive substrate, taking samples of the experimental material at various times, extracting and chromatographically, or otherwise, separating the products. Radioactivity detectors can be attached to gas–liquid chromatography or high performance liquid chromatography columns to monitor radioactivity coming off the column during separation. Alternatively, radioactivity can be located on paper or thin-layer chromatography with either a Geiger–Müller chromatograph scanner or with autoradiography. If it is suspected that a particular compound is metabolised by a particular pathway, then radioisotopes can also be used to confirm this. For instance, it is possible to predict the fate of individual carbon atoms of [^{14}C]acetate through the tricarboxylic acid, or Krebs, cycle. Methods have been developed whereby intermediates of the cycle can be isolated and the distribution of carbon within each intermediate can be ascertained. This is the so-called specific labelling pattern. Should the actual pattern coincide with the theoretical pattern, then this is very good evidence for the mode of operation of the Krebs cycle.

Another example of the use of radioisotopes to confirm the mode of operation, or otherwise, of a metabolic pathway is in studies carried out on glucose catabolism. There are numerous ways whereby glucose can be oxidised, the two most important ones in aerobic organisms being glycolysis followed by the Krebs cycle together with the pentose phosphate pathway. Frequently, organisms or tissues possess the necessary enzymes for both pathways to occur and it is of interest to establish the relative contribution of each to glucose oxidation. Both pathways involve the complete oxidation of glucose to carbon dioxide, but the origin of the carbon dioxide in terms of the six carbon atoms of glucose is different (at least in the initial stages of respiration of exogenously added substrate). Thus, it is possible to trap the carbon dioxide evolved during the respiration of specifically labelled glucose (e.g. [6-^{14}C]glucose or [1-^{14}C]glucose in which only the stated atom is radioactive) and obtain an evaluation of the contribution of each pathway to glucose oxidation.

The use of radioisotopes in studying the operation of the Krebs cycle or in evaluating the pathway of glucose catabolism are just two examples of how such isotopes can be used to confirm metabolic pathways. Further details of these and other examples, including use of dual-labelling methods, can be found in the various texts recommended in Section 14.9.

Metabolic turnover times

Radioisotopes provide a convenient method of ascertaining turnover times for particular compounds. As an example, the turnover of proteins in rats will be considered. A group of rats is injected with a radioactive amino acid and left for 24 h, during which time most of the amino acid is assimilated into proteins. The rats are then killed at suitable time intervals and radioactivity in organs or tissues of interest is determined. In this way it is possible to ascertain the rate of metabolic turnover of protein. Using this sort of method, it has been shown that liver protein is turned over in 7 to 14 days, while skin and muscle protein is turned over every 8 to 12 weeks, and collagen is turned over at a rate of less than 10% per annum.

Studies of absorption, accumulation and translocation

Radioisotopes have been very widely used in the study of the mechanisms and rates of absorption, accumulation and translocation of inorganic and organic compounds by both plants and animals. Such experiments are generally simple to perform and can also yield evidence on the route of translocation and sites of accumulation of molecules of biological interest.

Pharmacological studies

Another field where radioisotopes are widely used is in the development of new drugs. This is a particularly complicated process, because, besides showing whether a drug has a desirable effect, much more must be ascertained before it can be used in the treatment of clinical conditions. For instance, the site of drug accumulation, the rate of accumulation, the rate of metabolism and the metabolic products must all be determined. In each of these areas of study, radiotracers are extremely useful, if not indispensable. For instance, autoradiography on whole sections of experimental animals (Section 14.2.3 and Fig. 14.12) yields information on the site and rate of accumulation, while typical techniques used in metabolic studies can be used to follow the rate and products of metabolism.

14.6.2 **Analytical applications**

Enzyme and ligand binding studies

Virtually any enzyme reaction can be assayed using radiotracer methods, as outlined in Section 7.4.3, provided that a radioactive form of the substrate is available. Radiotracer-based enzyme assays are more expensive than other methods, but frequently have the advantage of a higher degree of sensitivity. Radioisotopes have also been used in the study of the mechanism of enzyme action and in ligand binding studies (Section 8.2.3).

Isotope dilution analysis

There are many compounds present in living organisms that cannot be accurately assayed by conventional means because they are present in such low amounts and in mixtures of similar compounds. Isotope dilution analysis offers a convenient and accurate way of overcoming this problem and avoids the necessity of quantitative isolation. For instance, if the amount of iron in a protein preparation is to be determined, this may be difficult using normal methods, but it can be done if a source of ^{59}Fe is available. This is mixed with the protein and a sample of iron is subsequently isolated, assayed for total iron and the radioactivity determined.

If the original specific activity was 10 000 d.p.m. (10 mg)$^{-1}$ and the specific activity of the isolated iron was 9000 d.p.m. (10 mg)$^{-1}$ then the difference is due to the iron in the protein (x), i.e.

$$\frac{9000}{10} = \frac{10\,000}{10 + x}$$

therefore $x = 1.1$ mg

This technique is widely used in, for instance, studies on trace elements.

Radioimmunoassay

One of the most significant advances in biochemical techniques in recent years has been the development of radioimmunoassay. This technique is discussed in Section 4.7 and is not elaborated upon here.

Radiodating

A quite different analytical use for radioisotopes is in the dating (i.e. determining the age) of rocks, fossil and sediments. In this technique it is assumed that the proportion of an element that is naturally radioactive has been the same throughout time. From the time of fossilisation or deposition the radioactive isotope will decay. By determining the amount of radioisotope remaining (or by examining the amount of a decay product) and from a knowledge of the half-life, it is possible to date the sample. For instance, if the radioisotope normally composes 1% of the element and it is found that the sample actually contains 0.25% then two half-lives can be assumed to have elapsed since deposition. If the half-life is one million years then the sample can be dated as being two million years old.

For long-term dating, isotopes with long half-lives are necessary, such as ^{235}U, ^{238}U and ^{40}K, whereas for shorter-term dating ^{14}C is widely used. It cannot be overemphasised that the assumptions made in radiodating are sweeping and hence palaeontologists and anthropologists who use this technique can give only approximate dates to their samples.

14.6.3 Other applications

Molecular biology techniques

Recent advances in molecular biology that have led to advances in genetic manipulation have depended heavily upon use of radioisotopes in DNA and RNA sequencing, DNA replication, transcription, synthesis of complementary DNA, recombinant DNA technology and many similar studies. Many of these techniques are more fully discussed in Chapters 2 and 3.

Clinical diagnosis

Radioisotopes are very widely used in medicine, in particular for diagnostic tests. Lung function tests routinely made using xenon-133 (^{133}Xe) are particularly useful in diagnosis of malfunctions of lung ventilation. Kidney function tests using [^{133}I]iodohippuric acid are used in diagnoses of kidney infections, kidney blockages or imbalance of function between the two kidneys. Thyroid function tests using ^{131}I are employed in the diagnosis of hypo- and hyperthyroidism.

Various aspects of haematology are also studied by using radioisotopes. These include such aspects as blood cell lifetimes, blood volumes and blood circulation times, all of which may vary in particular clinical conditions.

Ecological studies

The bulk of radiotracer work is carried out in biochemical, clinical or pharmacological laboratories, nevertheless, radiotracers are also of use to ecologists. In particular, migratory patterns and behaviour patterns of many animals can be monitored using radiotracers. Another ecological application is in the examination of food chains where the primary producers can be made radioactive and the path of radioactivity followed throughout the resulting food chain.

Sterilisation of food and equipment

Very strong γ-emitters are now widely used in the food industry for sterilisation of prepacked foods such as milk and meats. Normally either ^{60}C or ^{137}Ce is used, but care has to be taken in some cases to ensure that the food product itself is not affected in any way. Thus doses often have to be reduced to an extent where sterilisation is not complete but nevertheless food spoilage can be greatly reduced. ^{60}Co and ^{137}Ce are also used in sterilisation of plastic disposable equipment such as Petri dishes and syringes, and in sterilisation of drugs that are administered by injection.

Mutagens

Radioisotopes may cause mutations, particularly in microorganisms (Section 3.8.5). In various microbiological studies mutants are desirable, especially in industrial microbiology. For instance, development of new strains of a microorganism that produce higher yields of a desired microbial product frequently involve mutagenesis by radioisotopes.

Table 14.7 **Units commonly used to describe radioactivity**

Unit	Abbreviation	Definition
Counts per minute per second	c.p.m. c.p.s.	The *recorded* rate of decay
Disintegrations per minute or second	d.p.m. d.p.s.	The *actual* rate of decay
Curie	Ci	The number of d.p.s. equivalent to 1 g of radium (3.7×10^{10} d.p.s.)
Millicurie	mCi	$Ci \times 10^{-3}$ or 2.22×10^9 d.p.m.
Microcurie	μCi	$Ci \times 10^{-6}$ or 2.22×10^6 d.p.m.
Becquerel (SI unit)	Bq	1 d.p.s.
Terabecquerel (SI unit)	TBq	10^{12} Bq or 27.027 Ci
Gigabecquerel (SI unit)	GBq	10^9 Bq or 27.027 mCi
Megabecquerel (SI unit)	MBq	10^6 Bq or 27.027 μCi
Electron volt	eV	The energy attained by an electron accelerated through a potential difference of 1 volt. Equivalent to 1.6×10^{-19} J
Roentgen	R	The amount of radiation that produces 1.61×10^{15} ion-pairs kg^{-1}
Rad	rad	The dose that gives an energy absorption of 0.01 J k^{-1}
Gray	Gy	The dose that gives an energy absorption of 1 J k^{-1}. Thus 1 Gy = 100 rad
Rem	rem	The amount of radiation that gives a dose in humans equivalent to 1 rad of X rays
Sievert	Sv	The amount of radiation that gives a dose in humans equivalent to 1 Gy of X-rays. Thus 1 Sv = 100 rem

14.7 **KEY TERMS**

α-particles
ALARA
annual limit on intake
atomic number
atom percentage excess
autoradiography
back-to-back emission
background radiation
becquerel
β-particles
Čerenkov counting
Čerenkov light
channel
chemical quenching
chemiluminescence
coincidence counting
colour quenching
Compton scattering
controlled area
counts
curie
dating
dead time
decay series
dipping-film method
dose rate
dual-labelling experiments
electron volt
energy spectrum
equivalent dose

excitation
exposure
external standard
fluor
fluorography
γ-emission
γ-rays
gate setting
Geiger–Müller plateau
Geiger–Müller region
half-life
intensifying screen
internal radiation hazard
internal standard
ionisation chamber
isotope effect
isotopes
limited proportional region
liquid scintillation counting
mass number
negatron
neutrons
open sources
optical quenching
pair production
phospholuminescence
photoelectron
photons
positron
positron emission tomography

primary fluor
proportional counter
protons
pulse height analyser
quenching
radiation absorbed dose
radioactive decay
radioisotopes
resolution time
roentgen
scintillation cocktail
scintillation counting
secondary fluor
sievert
solid scintillation counting
specific activity
specific labelling pattern
spike
stable isotopes
standardisation
stripping film technique
supervised area
threshold
total dose
Townsend avalanche effect
weighting factor
wipe test
X-rays

14.8 **CALCULATIONS**

Question 1

An experimental sample of ^{3}H on a filter paper in scintillation fluid gave a count rate of 1450 c.p.m. in a liquid scintillation counter. The filter was removed and 5064 d.p.m. added to it. On recounting, the filter gave a reading of 2878 c.p.m. What was the d.p.m. of the experimental sample?

Answer

The efficiency can be calculated as
$[2878 - 1450 / 5064] \times 100\%$
This can be used to correct the figure of 1450 c.p.m. to give 5142 d.p.m.

Question 2

Given $\ln(N_t/N_o) = -\lambda t$ and that the half-life of ^{32}P is 14.2 days, how long would it take a solution containing 42 000 d.p.m. of ^{32}P to decay to 500 d.p.m.?

Answer

Use equation 14.4 to obtain λ. Then, using the equation given in question 2, substitute 42 000 for N_o and 500 for N_t. This gives an answer of 90.6 days.

Question 3

A 1 litre of [^{3}H]uridine with a concentration of 100 μmol cm^{-3} and 50 000 c.p.m. cm^{-3} is required. If all measurements are made on a scintillation counter with an efficiency of 40%, how would you make up this solution if the purchased supply of [^{3}H]uridine has a specific activity of 20/Ci mol^{-1}?

[NB: M_r uridine = 244; 1 Ci = 22.2 × 10^{11} d.p.m.]

Repeat the calculation in becquerels.

Answer See the example on p. 716. Correcting for efficiency: 50 000 c.p.m. is 125 000 d.p.m. Multiplying this by 10^3 for a litre gives a d.p.m. equivalent of 56.3 µCi (125 × 10^6/22.2 × 10^5 = 56.3 µCi). Given 20 Ci mol^{-1}, work out how many moles there are in 56.3 µCi (56.3/20 × 10^6 = 2.815 µmoles). 100 000 µmoles of uridine are required in a litre; from the molecular mass this is 24.4 g. The 2.815 µmoles from the radioactive input is only 0.685 mg and so can effectively be ignored. The answer is, therefore, 56.3 µCi (2.08 MBq) of [^{3}H]uridine plus 24.4 g of uridine.

Question 4 The efficiency of counting 100 000 d.p.m. of a [^{14}C]leucine solution was estimated in a scintillation counter using two channels, A and B, in scintillation fluid containing increasing amounts of chloroform. The following data were obtained:

Chloroform (cm^3)	c.p.m. A	c.p.m. B
0	48 100	54 050
1	31 612	42 150
2	17 608	28 400
3	7400	15 000

An unknown sample of [^{14}C]leucine gave the following data:

Channel A   1890 c.p.m.
Channel B   2700 c.p.m.

How much radioactivity is present in the unknown sample?

Answer Plot efficiency in channel A or B (e.g. 48 000 × 100/100 000 or 54 050 × 100/100 000, then 31 612 × 100/100 000 or 42 150 × 100/100 000 etc.) against c.p.m. A/c.p.m. B (e.g. 48 000/54 050, then 31 612/42 150 etc.). Calculate c.p.m. A/c.p.m. B for the experimental sample (1890/2700), put this into your graph and read off the efficiency. Correct the c.p.m. in channel A or B (depending on which one you chose to calculate efficiencies) for the efficiency (e.g. 1890 × 100/26.5 if you used channel A or 2700 × 100/37.8 if you used channel B).

Try plotting two graphs (efficiency in A or B versus c.p.m. A/c.p.m. B) and work out the answer using both in turn; you should get the same answer of 7130 d.p.m. each time.

Question 5 The efficiency of detecting ^{14}C in a scintillation counter was determined by counting a standard sample containing 105 071 d.p.m. at different degrees of quench analysed by the external standard approach:

c.p.m.	SQP
87 451	0.90
62 361	0.64
45 220	0.46
21 014	0.21

SQP, standard quench parameter

An experimental sample gave 2026 c.p.m. at an SQP of 0.52. What is the true count rate?

Answer Plot the efficiency (e.g. (87 451 × 100/105 071)%) versus SQP. Obtain the efficiency for the experimental sample and correct 2026 to give an answer of 4221 d.p.m.

Question 6 A sample recording 564 c.p.m. was counted over 10 min. What is the accuracy of the measurement for 95% confidence?

Answer 564 ± 15 ($\pm 2\sigma = \pm\sqrt{(564/10)}$). The square root of 564/10 is the standard deviation (σ). $2 \times \sigma$ gives the range in which 95% of the readings are expected to fall.

Question 7 To determine the nutritional quality of protein in a foodstuff the content of lysine was determined by isotope dilution analysis. To an acid hydrolysate of the protein (1 mg), 0.5 μmole of [^{3}H]lysine (1 Ci mol^{-1}) was added. A sample of lysine was purified from the hydrolysate by chromatography and the specific activity determined by scintillation counting at 25% efficiency. The value obtained was 2071 c.p.m. μg^{-1}. What is the % (w/w) lysine content of soybean protein? 1 Ci = 22.2 × 10^{11} d.p.m.; M_r lysine = 148.

Answer 0.5 μmole = 74 μg; 0.5 μCi = 1.11 × 10^6 d.p.m. If x = unknown lysine then:

$$\frac{2071 \times 4}{1} = \frac{1.11 \times 10^6}{74 + x}$$

$x = 60$ μg; 6% of 1 mg.

14.9 SUGGESTIONS FOR FURTHER READING

BILLINGTON, D., JAYSON, G. G. and MALTBY, P. J. (1992). *Radioisotopes*. Bios Scientific, Oxford. (A description of principles and applications in the biosciences, for undergraduates and research workers.)

CHAPMAN, J. M. and AVERY, G. (1981). *The Use of Radioisotopes in the Life Sciences*. George Unwin, London. (A good undergraduate text on the use and detection of radioactivity.)

CONNOR, K. J. and MCLINTOCK, I. S. (1994). *Radiation Protection Handbook for Laboratory Workers*. HHSC, Leeds. (A safety manual for laboratory work.)

SLATER, R. J. (2000). *Radioisotopes in Biology – A Practical Approach*, 2nd edn. IRL Press, Oxford. (A more detailed account of the handling and use of radioactivity in biological research.)

SLATER, R. J. (1995). *Radioisotopes in molecular biology*. In *Molecular Biology and Biotechnology, A Comprehensive Desk Reference*, ed. R. A. Myers, pp. 209–20. VCH, New York. (A summary of the application of radioisotopes to molecular biology.)

Chapter 15

Electrochemical techniques

15.1 INTRODUCTION

15.1.1 Biological interest in electrochemistry

Frequently biologists are interested in the electrical properties and behaviour of biological substances or with the transformation of chemical energy into electrical energy (and vice versa), i.e. the electrochemistry of living systems (Section 15.1.2). In addition, biologists may often utilise electrochemical techniques to measure the concentrations of a great number and diversity of biologically important substances such as oxygen, catecholamines and glucose, and to determine important parameters of biological environments such as pH (Section 15.1.3).

Electrochemistry is, in fact, one of the oldest specialities of classical physical chemistry, tracing its origins to the mid-nineteenth century. However, electrochemical techniques have developed over the years through advances in a number of scientific disciplines, including chemistry, physics, electronics and most recently biology (in the development of biosensors). Consequently the terminology surrounding the subject may, at times, be confusing, or clearly inconsistent. In addition, the sheer number of techniques can be bewildering, and whereas fundamental differences might exist between some groups of techniques (which need to be appreciated before such techniques can be sensibly applied to biological situations) numerous techniques may differ from others only in minor detail. The names of the techniques themselves have been applied historically with little or no semblance of a systematic approach, and only recently has there been any effort to bring some sort of coherence to the nomenclature. This has been done, not by renaming techniques, but by grouping them together in logical sets. This approach has been used in Section 15.2.3. However, this may still leave the student of the subject at a loss to understand why, for example, the Clark oxygen electrode (Section 15.6) may be called an amperometric device by some authors, a voltammetric device by others and a polarographic device by yet others (including Clark himself).

15.1.2 Electrochemistry and energy transduction

The energy contained in many molecules can be released by living organisms through oxidation to produce free energy (i.e. that available to do work). The rates of

729

such oxidation reactions are controlled by enzymes in order to supply the energetic demands of the organism (see Section 1.2.4). The relationship between the oxidised and reduced forms of a molecule may be expressed by the general equation:

reduced form $\rightleftharpoons$ oxidised form $+\ ne^-$

Oxidation in this sense thus means the loss of electrons from a substance, and this loss can occur in three main ways:

(i) *Direct loss.* Electrons may be lost directly and passed on to a second electron acceptor molecule, e.g.

cytochrome(Fe^{2+}) $\rightarrow$ cytochrome(Fe^{3+}) $+\ e^-$ (to acceptor)

This may make up part of an electron transport chain, where the electrons are shuttled down the chain, passing from one carrier to the next. Alternatively single reactions of this type may occur, catalysed by oxidases, where oxygen is not incorporated into the molecule but is used as the electron acceptor to form hydrogen peroxide or occasionally water.

(ii) *Removal of hydrogen.* Electrons are lost during dehydrogenation. Most biological oxidations occur in this fashion rather than by the addition of oxygen. In nearly all cases two electrons plus two protons ($2e^- + 2H^+$) are removed, e.g.

$$[CH_3CH_2OH + NAD^+ \xrightarrow{\text{alcohol dehydrogenase}} CH_3CHO + NADH + H^+$$

ethanol   acetaldehyde

though occasionally loss may occur as a hydride ion and a proton ($H^- + H^+$). Dehydrogenases have a coenzyme requirement (e.g. NAD^+ or $NADP^+$) or have a flavoprotein (FAD or FMN) prosthetic group to serve as the electron and hydrogen acceptor.

(iii) *Addition of oxygen.* In terms of movement of electrons, it is more difficult to understand why addition of oxygen is in fact an oxidation. Closer inspection of the mechanism of such reactions reveals that the first stage of such reactions involves the loss of electrons to molecular oxygen, though this subsequently shares its electrons with the donor molecule when the covalent bond forms. Alternatively, it may be argued that the addition of a highly electronegative oxygen atom to a molecule results in electrons being pulled away from the rest of the atoms in the molecule, i.e. in a partial form of oxidation. Oxidations of this type are catalysed by oxygenases. Dioxygenases catalyse the incorporation of both atoms of molecular oxygen into a structure, whereas monooxygenases (often called hydroxylases) introduce only one atom. The oxidation of natural compounds by oxygenases is rather uncommon.

Within living cells, oxidation reactions in the glycolytic pathway and in the Krebs cycle are catalysed by dehydrogenases. Such reactions yield NADH and $FADH_2$, which then pass their electrons on to the respiratory electron transport

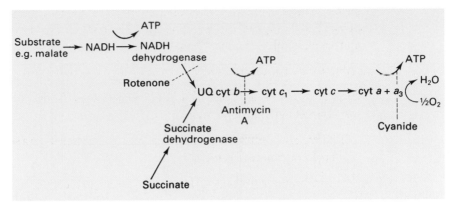

Fig. 15.1. The mitochondrial respiratory chain, showing the site of action of inhibitors, and sites of ATP production by oxidative phosphorylation. UQ, ubiquinone; cyt, cytochrome.

chain found on the inner membrane of the mitochondria. This chain is represented in Fig. 15.1. Electron transport from NADH to oxygen results in the phosphorylation of three molecules of ADP to ATP per atom of oxygen consumed, whereas electron transport from $FADH_2$ bypasses the first phosphorylation site and thus produces only two molecules of ATP per atom of oxygen. The number of molecules of ATP produced from a particular substrate can be found by comparing the rate of phosphorylation with the rate of electron transport, i.e. with the rate of oxygen uptake. Phosphorylation can be measured by the disappearance of either ADP or inorganic phosphorus, whilst oxygen consumption can be measured using a Clark oxygen electrode (Section 15.6) and this can be used to calculate the phosphorylation : oxidation (P : O) ratio (Section 15.6.3).

An explanation for the mechanism of oxidative phosphorylation was proposed by Peter Mitchell in 1961, and is now accepted. Mitchell's chemiosmotic theory proposes that an electrochemical gradient is set up across the inner mitochondrial membrane during the electron transport process. The FMN and ubiquinone function as hydrogen carriers, able to carry both H^+ and e^-, whereas the Fe-sulphur proteins and the cytochromes are able to carry only electrons. These carriers are arranged such that hydrogen and electron carriers alternate. A third hydrogen carrier, X, was also included to account for the third H^+ translocation site (Fig. 15.2). However, in 1975 Mitchell refined his theory and accepted that X really did not exist, but suggested that its function was actually carried out by a complex cyclic series of exchanges involving ubiquinone and cytochrome b, now commonly known as the Q-cycle.

The functioning of the electron transport chain thus ensures that, as electrons pass down the electron transport chain, protons are translocated from the inner matrix of the mitochondrion into the intermembrane space between the inner and outer mitochondrial membranes. A proton gradient is thus set up across the inner membrane and, as protons flow back across the inner membrane through a membrane-bound ATPase, ADP is phosphorylated to ATP.

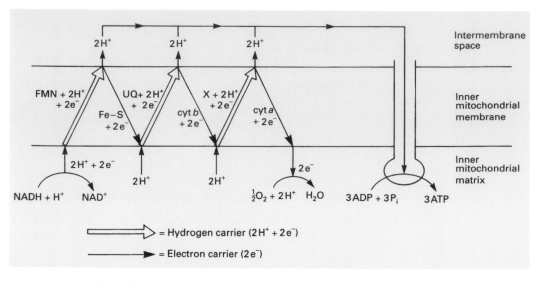

Fig. 15.2. Arrangement of electron transport chain.

Most mitochondria in tissues and carefully prepared samples of isolated mitochondria show respiratory control, in that in the absence of ADP the rate of electron transport slows down so NADH is not wasted. If ADP is added, then ATP synthesis can occur and the rate of electron transport increases (Section 15.6.3, Fig. 15.9) Such mitochondria would be said to be tightly coupled. In uncoupled mitochondria, electrons pass down the electron transport chain whether or not there is ADP to phosphorylate. Naturally uncoupled mitochondria are found in brown adipose tissue where they serve an important function of generating heat. Coupled mitochondria can be deliberately uncoupled by adding uncoupling agents such as 2,4-dinitrophenol. This renders the membrane permeable, such that the proton gradient is abolished, leaving no available power source to drive the ATPase. These phenomena can be demonstrated using a Clark oxygen electrode (Section 15.6).

A second electron transport chain is found within the chloroplasts of higher plants. This photosynthetic electron transport chain (Fig. 15.3) is responsible for the trapping of energy from sunlight to form NADPH, which is then used in the Calvin cycle for the fixation of atmospheric CO_2 to form carbohydrate. Within the photosynthetic electron transport chain, light energy is absorbed at two distinct sites such that an electron is passed from one carrier to another with a more negative redox potential (see Section 15.3 for a description of this term). This is an endergonic process requiring the expenditure of energy. Electrons travel from water to $NADP^+$ via photosystem II and photosystem I, producing oxygen and NADPH; this is known as non-cyclic electron transport and produces ATP by non-cyclic photophosphorylation. Electrons can also undergo cyclic electron transport around photosystem I, releasing no oxygen from water and producing no NADPH, but producing ATP by cyclic photophosphorylation.

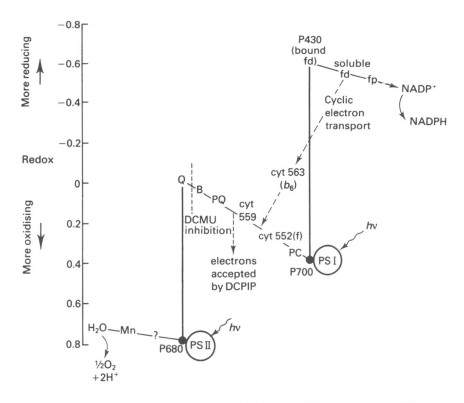

Fig. 15.3. Photosynthetic electron transport in chloroplasts. PSI, photosystem I; PSII, photosystem II; PQ, plastoquinone; cyt, cytochrome; Q, B, postulated intermediates; P680, P700, reaction centre chlorophylls; fd, ferredoxin; fp, flavoprotein (fd NADP oxidoreductase); ?, unknown component.

Many aspects of photosynthetic electron transport and photophosphorylation are similar to mitochondrial electron transport and oxidative phosphorylation. As in mitochondria, when electrons or hydrogen atoms travel along the series of carriers a proton gradient becomes established. However, protons move inwards in response to photosynthetic electron transport, not outwards as in mitochondrial electron transport. Thus the interior of the chloroplast is considerably more acidic than the outside. The chloroplast ATPase is structurally very similar in its general shape and subunit structure to that found in the mitochondria, but is orientated differently because of the reversal of the direction of the proton gradient, such that the ATPase is on the outer rather than the inner face of the membrane. Photosynthetic uncouplers such as NH_4^+ are known to have effects similar to those of respiratory uncouplers. They speed up the rate of photosynthetic electron flow but abolish phosphorylation because they carry protons across the membrane. Inhibitors of photophosphorylation are also known that, like inhibitors of oxidative phosphorylation, combine with the ATPase at a specific site; one example is the antibiotic Dio-9.

15.1.3 **The range of electrochemical techniques**

Whereas at one time the only piece of electrochemical apparatus a biology or bio-chemistry undergraduate might ever actually use would be the pH electrode (Section 15.4), nowadays this is certainly not the case. Various ions other than H⁺ may be measured using special electrodes termed ion-selective electrodes (Section 15.5). Most undergraduate students will also probably come into contact with the Clark oxygen electrode (Section 15.6), which has numerous biological applications, particularly in the study of chloroplast and mitochondrial activity. Biosensors (Section 15.8) are also becoming more common in clinical, industrial and environmental applications. Electrochemical detection of the effluent from HPLC columns (Section 13.4.7 and 15.7) is now a real alternative to the more classical ultraviolet detection techniques, and is the method of choice for the analysis of some important drugs (e.g. morphine) and biomolecules (e.g. neurotransmitters, such as adrenaline and noradrenaline).

Thus, since there is now such a great number of electroanalytical techniques available to the biologist, an understanding of their basic principles, and of the similarities and differences between various groups, is of paramount importance.

15.2 **PRINCIPLES OF ELECTROCHEMICAL TECHNIQUES**

15.2.1 **Electrochemical cells and reactions**

An electrochemical cell consists of two electrode–electrolyte systems termed half-cells, joined internally either by means of a common electrolyte or by means of a relatively concentrated solution of indifferent ions (often saturated or 4 M KCl or KNO_3) called a salt bridge.

It is convenient to consider electrochemical cells by the reactions that take place at only one of the two electrode surfaces (i.e. within one half-cell). Consider, for example, a copper wire dipping into a solution of $CuSO_4$. Within this system the metal electrode may throw off its ions into solution, leaving the electrons behind on the metal:

$$Cu_{solid} \rightarrow + Cu^{2+}_{(aqueous)} + 2e^-$$

The metal thus loses electrons – i.e. it is oxidised. This leaves the metal electrode negatively charged with respect to the surrounding solution. Alternatively, the metal ions in solution may combine with electrons at the metal surface (i.e. be reduced) to deposit metal atoms:

$$Cu^{2+}_{(aqueous)} + 2e^- \rightarrow Cu_{solid}$$

This leads to a deficit of electrons in the metal electrode leaving it positively charged with respect to the surrounding solution. Thus, a potential difference called the electrode potential is established across the electrode/electrolyte interface.

Many electrode reactions are of this type. There is, however, another type of

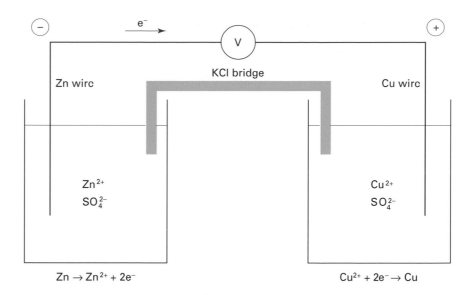

Fig. 15.4. Diagram of a Daniell cell.

half-cell in which both the oxidised and reduced forms of the substance exist in solution. For example, if a platinum wire is immersed in a solution of ferrous and ferric ions the equilibrium would be:

$$Fe^{3+} + e^- \rightleftharpoons Fe^{2+}$$

Although there is no fundamental difference between this half-cell and the $Cu/CuSO_4$ half-cell described above, an electrode in which the oxidised and reduced forms both exist in solution is called a redox electrode and its potential is known as a redox potential. Further consideration of such reactions is included in Section 15.3.

15.2.2 Schematic representation of electrochemical cells

To simplify the description of electrochemical cells, a standardised shorthand has evolved. Consider a simple electrochemical cell as shown in Fig. 15.4. This cell (the Daniell cell) consists of a strip of zinc and a strip of copper immersed in solutions of $ZnSO_4$ and $CuSO_4$ respectively. If the Zn^{2+} and Cu^{2+} concentrations are approximately equal, then reactions will result in the oxidation of the zinc metal in one half-cell and the reduction of the copper ions in the other half-cell. If the two strips are then connected by a wire the solution in the first half-cell will show an increase in zinc ion concentration, whilst the solution in the second half-cell will show a depletion in cupric ion concentration. A salt bridge between the two compartments allows migration of ions between the two compartments but prevents gross mixing of the two solutions. Electrons will thus flow from the zinc anode to the copper cathode. Such an electrochemical cell can be described as follows:

$$- Zn \,|\, Zn^{2+} \,\|\, Cu^{2+} \,|\, Cu +$$

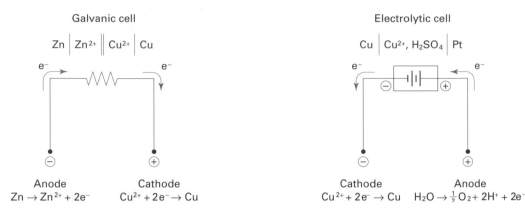

Fig. 15.5. Galvanic and electolytic cells.

where the single vertical bars represents a phase boundary (electrode/electrolyte interface) and the double bars represent the KCl bridge. Such shorthand notation is in common usage.

15.2.3 A classification of electrochemical techniques

An electrochemical cell can be either a galvanic cell or an electrolytic cell (Fig. 15.5). A galvanic cell is one in which reactions occur spontaneously at the electrodes when they are connected externally by a conductor (such as the Daniell cell described in Section 15.2.2). Well-known examples of such cells include both non-rechargeable (e.g. Zn-MnO_2 cell) and rechargeable batteries. In contrast, an electrolytic cell is one in which reactions are effected by the imposition of an external voltage greater than the spontaneous potential of the cell. Well-known applications of electrolytic cells include the electrolytic synthesis of chlorine and aluminium, electrorefining of copper, and electroplating of silver and gold. (In addition, a rechargeable battery when it is being recharged is an electrolytic cell.)

It is unfortunately rather confusing that the anode in a galvanic cell is negatively charged, whereas that in the electrolytic cell is positively charged (Fig. 15.5). However, the reactions at the electrode surfaces are the same in both cases. In both types of cell, oxidation events occur at the anode and reduction events occur at the cathode.

Electoanalytical techniques can be subdivided into two main groups, according to whether the electrochemical cell is galvanic or electrolytic:

(i) *Potentiometry* involves the use of galvanic cells, with the measurement of the potential of an electrode without current flow.
(ii) *Voltammetry* involves the use of electrolytic cells, with the measurement of the current passing through an electrode at constant potential, or as the potential varies under potentiostatic control.

Potentiometry is discussed in Section 15.2.4. The commonest application of potentiometry is the pH electrode (Section 15.4), and in ion-selective and gas-sensing electrodes (Section 15.5). Electrolytic cells are discussed in Section 15.2.5. These are involved in all other forms of measurement (amperometric, polarographic and voltammetric). The commonest of these instruments likely to be encountered by biologists is the amperometric oxygen electrode (Section 15.6), though polarographic and voltammetric applications such as those discussed in Section 15.2.5 are becoming more popular for the measurement of low concentrations of molecules, particularly in environmental and medical situations. One very useful application of voltammetry is in the field of HPLC (Section 13.4), where electrochemical detectors frequently offer better precision and higher selectivity than the more conventional spectrophotometric detectors (Section 15.7).

15.2.4 Introduction to potentiometry

Reference electrodes

Potentiometric measurements that involve an electrode that responds to a particular experimental situation by giving a spontaneous potential require a second so-called reference electrode of constant potential to be present so that the difference between the two can be measured. A reference electrode is necessary when pH electrodes, ion-selective electrodes and redox electrodes are used. Historically, one of the most important reference electrodes has been the standard hydrogen electrode (SHE), which contains an inert metal electrode (e.g. platinum coated with platinum black) in a solution of a fixed concentration of hydrochloric acid (which supplies that H^+). Hydrogen gas at 10^5Pa (1450 lbf in. ^{2}) pressure is bubbled over the electrode, enabling the following equilibrium to be established:

$$\tfrac{1}{2}H_2 \rightleftharpoons H^+ + e^-$$

However, this electrode is highly inconvenient to use because the hydrogen has to be supplied at a constant pressure and must be oxygen free, and the platinum black is also readily contaminated. In practice, therefore, although oxidation reduction potentials (Section 15.3) are expressed relative to the SHE, other reference electrodes are used. Calomel electrodes (Fig. 15.6a) are commonly used as a reference. They consist of a solution of potassium chloride in contact with solid mercurous chloride (calomel) and mercury. This part of the circuit may be written as:

$$Hg\,|\,Hg_2Cl_2\,|\,KCl\,\|\,\text{test solution}$$

The double lines indicating the presence of a salt bridge.

An alternative to the calomel electrode is the silver/silver chloride electrode. A deposit of silver chloride is present on metallic silver in a chloride solution such as KCl.

$$Ag\,|\,AgCl\,|\,KCl\,\|\,\text{test solution}$$

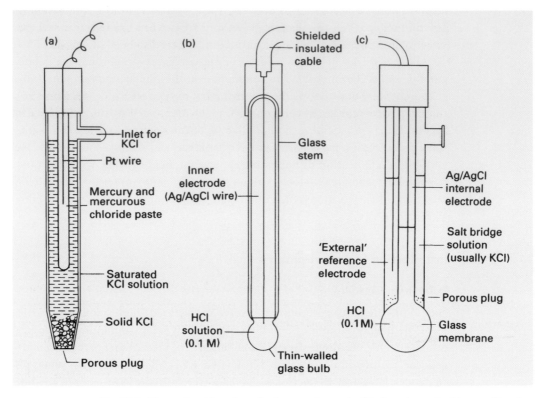

Fig. 15.6. Electrodes: (a) a calomel reference electrode; (b) glass electrode; (c) a combination electrode.

Any reference electrode must be in contact with the test solution via a liquid junction. These generally involve potassium chloride that slowly diffuses out of the electrode, giving electrical continuity. Unfortunately the liquid junction is likely to give an unknown junction potential, which cannot be eliminated completely. In using liquid junctions, care must be taken to ensure that it is the potassium chloride solution that diffuses out slowly, and not the test solution that diffuses in. Although outward diffusion does involve some contamination of the sample, this is not normally important, but, if either potassium or chloride is being measured, then a specially designed reference electrode called a double junction reference electrode must be used to prevent contamination.

There are several types of junction through which KCl diffuses: ceramic or fritted material, fibrous junctions and sleeve junctions. Fritted material is a collection of small particles pressed closely together, allowing some of the filling solution to leak through the gaps between the particles. Fibrous junctions can consist of woven fibres or of straight fibres, the latter giving an increased flow. The sleeve-type reference electrode has a narrow ring-shaped junction formed by the gap between an outer sleeve and the inner body of the electrode. The space between the sleeve and the electrode widens above the tip and forms a reservoir for the fluid. Flow occurs in some areas of the narrow ring junction but not in others. A sleeve junction is easier to clean than the other types (because the sleeve can be removed); it is also faster flowing, which means it is less likely to get clogged.

The Nernst equation

This equation is relevant to equipment that produces a potential, e.g. pH glass electrodes and ion-selective electrodes. Sections 1.2.4, 15.3 and 15.4 discuss the Nernst equation more fully; however, essentially it describes electrode behaviour and can be expressed in the simplified form

$$E = E_{constant} + 2.303 \frac{RT}{nF} \log A \tag{15.1}$$

or even better as

$$E = E_{constant} + \frac{S}{n} \log C \tag{15.2}$$

where E is the total potential (V) developed between the sensing and reference electrodes, $E_{constant}$ is a constant potential that depends mainly on the reference electrode, $2.303 RT/F (= S)$ is the Nernst factor or slope (R being the molar gas constant and T the absolute temperature), n is the number of charges on the ion, A is the activity of the ion, and C is the concentration of the ion.

Activity is an important physicochemical concept. It is the true measure of the ion's ability to affect chemical equilibria and reaction rates, and is its effective concentration in solution. In most biological situations the concentrations of ions are rather low and consequently the activity and concentration are equal. At higher concentrations, however, the activity becomes less than the concentration.

The Nernst equation shows clearly that the electrode response depends on both temperature and the number of charges on the ion. At 25 °C the Nernst factor $2.303 RT/F$ becomes 0.059, thus equation 15.2 becomes:

$$E = E_{constant} + \frac{0.059}{n} \log C \tag{15.3}$$

There is thus a 59 mV change in potential for a 10-fold change in the activity of a monovalent ion, and a 29.5 mV change if the ion is divalent. An electrode is said to have Nernstian characteristics if it obeys Nernst's law. If the changes in potential relative to activity (slopes) are less than the theoretical values (in the operating range) this indicates either interference from other ions or an electrode malfunction.

15.2.5 Introduction to voltammetry

Voltammetric techniques involve reactions effected by an imposed external voltage greater than the spontaneous potential of the cell. The reactions occurring within such an electrolytic half-cell can be considered as reactions occurring at the surface of an electrode in which the electrode supplies electrons (reduction) or

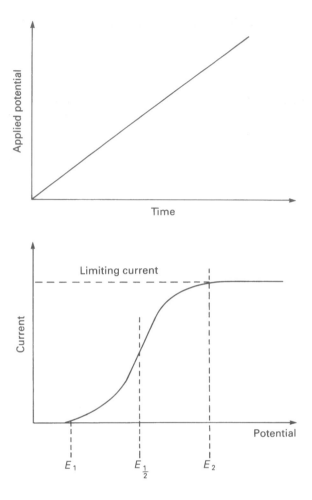

Fig. 15.7. Resultant polarographic wave as applied potential is increased linearly with time.

removes electrons (oxidation) in the same way as a chemical reagent may do so. Many biological substances are thus electroactive in that they can be relatively easily oxidised or reduced by applying a suitable potential to generate the necessary energy to drive the electrochemical reaction. Take, for example, a half-cell containing a solution of an electroreducible species; then, as the potential of the electrode is made progressively more negative, a point will be reached when reduction of the species will begin at the electrode and a small current will flow (E_1 in Fig. 15.7). As the potential is made even more negative, the current will increase dramatically as more reduction of the species occurs, until a potential is reached where the species is reduced at the electrode surface as quickly as it is able to reach the electrode surface by diffusion. At this point the maximum or limiting current is achieved, and further increases in potential will not affect the current (E_2 in Fig. 15.7).

The resulting plot (Fig. 15.7) of current against voltage (I versus E) known as the polarographic wave has two important properties:

(i) The midpoint of the wave (called the half-wave potential, $E_{\frac{1}{2}}$) is characteristic for each species being reduced.
(ii) Since the magnitude of the limiting current is controlled by the rate of diffusion of the reducible species, it will be directly proportional to the concentration of this species.

These features enable voltammetric techniques to be used both to identify and to quantify electroactive materials in solution. Unfortunately, voltammetric terminology remains rather confusing, and, although some authors do not use the term amperometry at all, a fairly standard classification includes:

(i) amperometry – measurement of the current passing through an electrode at constant potential;
(ii) voltammetry/polarography – measurement of the current while the potential varies under potentiostatic control.

Amperometry involves the reduction or oxidation of electroactive species, usually at the limiting current, such that the current is proportional to the concentration of the species of interest. The commonest application of amperometry is the Clark oxygen electrode (Section 15.6), where the reduction of oxygen at a platinum cathode gives rise to a current that is proportional to the oxygen tension in the solution, provided that an applied voltage maintains the platinum cathode at $-0.6\,\text{V}$ versus a silver anode. Amperometry may also be encountered by biologists using electrochemical detectors for the detection of solutes in the effluent from chromatography columns, especially HPLC (Section 15.7).

Polarography and voltammetry are used almost synonymously by some authors. Most modern texts, however, restrict the use of the term polarography to those techniques which use mercury, in the form of the dropping mercury electrode (DME), as the working electrode. This electrode consists of small droplets of mercury generated at the lower end of a glass capillary tube. The lifetime of each drop of mercury is usually arranged to be 0.5 to 5 s, the mass of each drop being around 5 mg. The DME is thus being continuously and reproducibly renewed; its past history is unimportant, giving rise to very reproducible responses. Polarography is used almost exclusively for the analysis of reducible species, usually metallic cations.

In contrast to polarography, voltammetric measurements involve no renewal of the working electrode surface. Instead a stationary hanging mercury drop electrode (HMDE) or a solid electrode made of platinum, gold, silver or carbon is employed. The advantage of this type of electrode over the DME is that a preconcentration step may be included in the measurement. The analyte is then usually stripped from the electrode surface during the potential scan; therefore the technique is often referred to as stripping voltammetry. Using these voltammetric techniques, oxidation reactions may be studied as readily as reduction reactions. Anodic stripping voltammetry involves a negative or oxidation current, whereas cathodic stripping voltammetry involves a positive or reduction current passing through the circuitry. These techniques are greatly superior to polarography in terms of sensitivity; however, the solid electrodes are generally more prone to contamination than is the mercury of the DME and, because they are not renewed, demonstrate poorer surface reproducibility.

Rather than apply a continuously increasing voltage, as in DC voltammetry, pulse voltammetry, differential pulse voltammetry, and AC voltammetry all produce more complex voltage changes, generally resulting in increased sensitivity over DC polarographic techniques. However, these are essentially advanced analytical techniques.

15.3 REDOX REACTIONS

15.3.1 Principles

Compounds capable of existing in an oxidised and a reduced form can be represented by the general equation:

$$\text{oxidised form} + ne^- \rightleftharpoons \text{reduced form}$$

A mixture of the reduced and oxidised form of a substance (e.g. Fe^{2+}/Fe^{3+} or $NADH/NAD^+$) is known as a redox couple. If an inert electrode (such as platinum) is put into a solution of a redox couple, the metal will become charged, and the potential difference set up between the metal and the solution can be compared with the steady potential produced by a reference electrode.

The scale of oxidation–reduction (redox) potentials is based on values obtained with the standard hydrogen electrode used as the reference electrode, and compared with the standard potential (E_0), which is produced by a platinum electrode dipping into 1 M concentrations of both the oxidised and reduced forms of a substance at 25 °C. Redox couples have positive or negative redox potentials according to whether they are more oxidising (positive) or reducing (negative) than the standard hydrogen electrode. The experimental potential measured (E) depends on the ratio of oxidised to reduced forms (i.e. their *relative* concentrations) and frequently on pH, but does not depend to a great extent on the actual concentrations involved. The measured redox potential E is related to the standard potential E_0 by the Nernst equation:

$$E = E_0 + 2.303\,\frac{RT}{nF}\log\left(\frac{[\text{oxid}]}{[\text{red}]}\right)$$

where E is the measured redox potential of a couple of known composition (e.g. a mixture of 0.03 M oxidised form and 0.1 M reduced form), E_0 is the standard redox potential with components of 1 M concentration at 25 °C and pH 0, [oxid] is the concentration of the oxidised form (oxidant = electron acceptor), [red] is the concentration of the reduced form (reductant = electron donor).

Additionally, if H^+ are involved in the reaction (i.e. the couple generates a pH change), then the equation must take this into account to become

Table 15.1 Standard redox potentials of interest to biologists (E_0' determined at pH 7 and 25 °C)

	Reaction	
E_0' (V)	Oxidant + ne^-	$\rightarrow$ Reductant
-0.42	$2H^+ + 2e^-$	$\rightarrow$ H_2
-0.32	$NAD^+ + H^+ + 2e^-$	$\rightarrow$ NADH
-0.22	$FAD + 2H^+ + 2e^-$	$\rightarrow$ $FADH_2$
-0.19	Pyruvate + $2H^+ + 2e^-$	$\rightarrow$ Lactate
-0.17	Oxaloacetate + $2H^+ + 2e^-$	$\rightarrow$ Malate
-0.03	Fumarate + $2H^+ + 2e^-$	$\rightarrow$ Succinate
$+0.05$	Ubiquinone + $2H^+ + 2e^-$	$\rightarrow$ Ubiquinol
$+0.08$	Cytochrome b (Fe^{3+}) + e^-	$\rightarrow$ Cytochrome b (Fe^{2+})
$+0.25$	Cytochrome c (Fe^{3+}) + e^-	$\rightarrow$ Cytochrome c (Fe^{2+})
$+0.29$	Cytochrome a (Fe^{3+}) + e^-	$\rightarrow$ Cytochrome a (Fe^{2+})
$+0.30$	$\frac{1}{2}O_2 + H_2O + 2e^-$	$\rightarrow$ H_2O_2
$+0.82$	$\frac{1}{2}O_2 + 2H^+ + 2e^-$	$\rightarrow$ H_2O

$$E = E_o + 2.303\frac{RT}{nF}\log\left(\frac{[\text{oxid}]}{[\text{red}]}\right) + 2.303\frac{RT}{nF}\log[H^+]^a$$

where a is the number of protons involved in the reaction.

In practice, the standard redox potential (E_o) used by chemists is little used by biologists because it involves pH 0 as one of the standard conditions. Instead biologists adopt pH 7 as a standard condition, and consequently this standard redox potential is given the symbol E_0' to discriminate it from the E_o determined at pH 0. These two commonly used standard redox potentials can cause great confusion unless the pH is clearly stated and uniformity is maintained in comparisons of the potentials of different systems.

Table 15.1 includes some of the E_0' values of interest in biology. Note, for example, that the hydrogen ion E_0' is -0.42 V, whereas the standard value used by chemists (determined at pH 0) is by definition 0.00 V. Thus a redox couple can theoretically be oxidised by (lose electrons to) a couple with a more positive E_0', and in turn will oxidise a couple with a more negative E_0'.

The free energy change in a coupled oxidation–reduction reaction is related to the redox potential of the couple and the number of electrons involved:

$$\Delta G^{0\prime} = -nF\Delta E_0'$$

where $\Delta G^{0\prime}$ is the standard free energy change, and $-nF\Delta E_0'$ is the potential difference between the two participating redox systems, provided n is the same for each system (see also Section 1.2.4).

If $\Delta E_0'$ is positive, then $\Delta G^{0\prime}$ will be negative and the coupled reaction will be exergonic, i.e. free energy will be released and the coupled reaction is thermodynamically favoured (this is often called a spontaneous reaction). If $\Delta E_0'$ is negative, $\Delta G^{0\prime}$ will be positive and the reaction will be termed endergonic; it will thus require an input of free energy to proceed in the direction stated (though the reverse reaction will be spontaneous).

It is difficult to predict the outcome of an interaction in a living cell of two redox couples whose E_0' values are very similar, since this may depend on the conditions within the cell. Factors that may influence the interaction include pH, the relative concentrations of the two molecules or ions, and the presence of chelating agents.

15.3.2 Applications of redox couples

Redox couples have numerous biological applications. Many are useful for investigating electron transport in that the reduced form of the redox couple can donate electrons to the electron transport chain and thus bypass the site of action of inhibitors such as rotenone and antimycin A, or can restart electron transport when an essential component has been removed. The precise site of action of inhibitor or the component can then be accurately pinpointed. Ascorbate is often used as an artificial electron donor, but is usually used in conjunction with another compound. With chloroplasts it has been found that ascorbate alone, or ascorbate with phenylenediamine, can replace water as electron donor to photosystem II, whereas ascorbate with 2,6-dichlorophenolindophenol donates an electron just before photosystem I, i.e. at a totally different site. With mitochondria, ascorbate is often used with cytochrome c or with N,N,N',N'-tetramethyl-p-phenylenediamine (TMPD); in both cases electrons are donated at cytochrome c.

Some redox couples are particularly useful in biochemical investigations because they change colour upon oxidation or reduction. Most of these oxidation–reduction indicators (redox dyes) are brightly coloured when oxidised and colourless when reduced, exceptions being the tetrazoliums and viologens. Examples are shown in Table 15.2. The rate of reduction of a redox dye as measured in a spectrophotometer can be used as the basis of an enzyme assay (Section 7.4.2); for example, the activity of succinate dehydrogenase isolated from mitochondria can be linked to methylene blue as follows:

succinate + methylene blue $\rightarrow$ fumarate + methylene blue
$\qquad$ (oxidised = blue) $\qquad\qquad\qquad$ (reduced = colourless)

Table 15.2 Standard redox potentials of useful artificial redox couples (E_0' determined at pH 7 and 25 °C)

E_0' (V)	Redox dye
− 0.45	Methyl viologen
− 0.36	Benzyl viologen
− 0.08	TTC (2,3,5-triphenyltetrazolium chloride)
− 0.01	Methylene blue
− 0.08	PMS (phenazine methosulphate)
− 0.22	DCPIP (2,6-dichlorophenol indophenol)
− 0.36	Potassium ferricyanide

The rate of decolorisation of methylene blue, i.e. the rate of reaction, can thus be followed spectrophotometrically. However, oxygen must be excluded from the system or else the methylene blue will be reoxidised. The electron transport processes in chloroplasts, mitochondria and bacteria can also be studied using indicator dyes. Provided they have an appropriate oxidation–reduction potential, the electrons are accepted by the indicators instead of being passed on to the next electron carrier in the chain. Unfortunately the vast majority of indicator dyes are not very specific and may receive electrons from several points in the electron transport chain. Care must be taken to interpret correctly the results of experiments using redox dyes because the dyes have been known to influence the nature of the reactions taking place and can inhibit enzymes or act as poisons for microorganisms. pH changes can also cause a change in colour, or in the ease of reduction. There is also the problem that the dye may not be readily able to cross membranes and may, therefore, not be able to reach the appropriate subcellular site. However, in the case of organelles or artificial vesicles, the fact that many dyes cannot penetrate the membrane can be exploited. Thus the extent of interaction of an electron transport component within the membrane and the external solution containing redox dyes indicates on which surface of the membrane the component is situated. The experiment can then be repeated with inverted vesicles, so that the other face of the membrane is then exposed to the dye. The subcellular localisation of enzymes can be ascertained by using carefully prepared tissue slices and staining them with dyes (a histochemical technique). Tetrazolium chloride is frequently used for this purpose because it gives an insoluble precipitate that does not readily diffuse from the site of formation.

15.4 **THE pH ELECTRODE**

15.4.1 **Principles**

Perhaps the most convenient and accurate way of determining pH is by using a glass electrode. Developed in 1919, this device did not become popular until the 1930s, when reliable amplifiers became available. Nowadays, however, the pH electrode/pH meter is one of the most basic items of equipment found in biology laboratories.

The pH electrode depends on ion exchange in the hydrated layers formed on the glass electrode surface. Glass consists of a silicate network amongst which are metal ions coordinated to oxygen atoms, and it is the metal ions that exchange with H^+. The glass electrode acts like a battery whose voltage depends on the H^+ activity of the solution in which it is immersed. The size of the potential (E) due to H^+ is given by the equation:

$$E = 2.303 \frac{RT}{F} \log\left(\frac{[H^+]_i}{[H^+]_o}\right)$$ (15.4)

where $[H^+]_i$ and $[H^+]_o$ are the molar concentrations of H^+ inside and outside the glass electrode (see also Section 1.2.5).

In practice $[H^+]_i$ is fixed and is generally 10^{-1} because the electrode contains 0.1 M HCl. Since $pH = -\log[H^+]$, it follows that the developed potential is directly proportional to the pH of the solution outside the electrode. Glass electrodes are particularly useful because of the lack of interference from the components of the solution. On the whole these electrodes are not readily contaminated by molecules in solution, and if other ions are present they do not cause significant interference. However, at high pH they do respond to sodium. Inaccuracies also occur under very acid conditions.

A glass electrode (Fig. 15.6b) consists of a thin, soft glass membrane that is situated at the end of a hard glass tube, or sometimes an epoxy body. Also present in the glass electrode is an internal reference electrode of the silver/silver chloride (Ag/AgCl) type described in Section 15.2.4 surrounded by an electrolyte of 0.1 M HCl. This internal reference electrode gives rise to a steady potential. Thus, the varying potential of the glass electrode can be compared with a steady potential produced by an external reference electrode such as the standard calomel electrode by joining the internal and external reference electrodes to give

Glass electrode			Test solution	Reference electrode
Refence electrode (internal)	H⁺ (internal) i:e. 0.1 M HCl	Glass membrane	H⁺ (external) i.e. analyte	Refence electrode (external)

The external reference electrode can either be a separate probe (Fig. 15.6a) or built around the glass electrode giving a combination electrode (Fig. 15.6c). If a combination electrode is used, the level of the test solution must be high enough to cover the porous plug (liquid junction) but not so high as the level of the salt bridge solution (KCl) in the external electrode because it is essential for KCl to diffuse out slowly into the test solution.

Whatever reference electrode is used, the measured voltage is the result of the difference between that of the reference and the glass electrode. In practice, however, there are other potentials present in the system. These include the so-called asymmetry potential, which is poorly understood but which is present across the glass membrane even when the H^+ concentration is the same on both sides. Also included are the potentials due to the Ag/AgCl and to the liquid junction to the reference electrode, which gives a potential because the K^+ and Cl^- do not diffuse at exactly the same rate and therefore generate a small potential at the boundary between the sample and the KCl in the reference electrode.

The measured potential of a glass electrode is thus based on equation 15.4 but includes constants to account for the additional potentials within the device:

$$E = E^* + 2.303\frac{RT}{F}\log\left(\frac{[H^+]_i}{[H^+]_o}\right) \tag{15.5}$$

where E^* includes the standard electrode potential of the glass electrode, and the constant junction potentials present in the system.

At 25 °C this becomes

$$E = E^* + 0.059 \, \text{pH} \tag{15.6}$$

where E^* now also includes a term to account for the internal H^+ concentration. As described in Section 15.2.4, at 25 °C, there is a 59 mV change for a 10-fold change in the activity of a monovalent ion; this means that a change of one pH unit produces a 59 mV change.

A pH electrode is used in conjunction with a pH meter. This records the potential due to the H^+ concentration but is designed to take little current from the circuit. A large current flow would cause changes in the ion concentration and hence pH changes; this is prevented by having a high resistance present. The pH meter, glass electrode and reference calomel electrode are designed so that pH 7 gives a zero potential.

15.4.2 Operation of the pH electrode/meter

pH electrodes are available in a variety of shapes and sizes suitable for many different applications. These include electrodes for the measurement of the pH of blood, the mouth, flat moist surfaces such as isoelectric focusing gels, and equipment for field work. Intracellular pH can also be measured using miniature probes (microelectrodes). However, all of these devices rely on the same principle of measurement, and the vast majority will be operated in the same way.

It is important that the outer layer of glass on the glass electrode remains hydrated, and so it is normally immersed in solution. The thin glass membrane is fragile and care must be taken not to break or scratch it, or to cause a build-up of static electric charge by rubbing it. Many modern pH electrodes have a plastic casing surrounding the glass electrode to protect it from damage. Gelatinous and protein-containing solutions should not be allowed to dry out on the glass surface as they would inhibit response.

As can be seen from equation 15.5, the potential produced is dependent on the temperature (each pH unit change represents 54.2 mV at 0 °C and 61.5 mV at 37 °C). This effect is entirely predictable and can be compensated for. The further away from the pH 7 (the isopotential point, where temperature has no effect on potential) the more important it is that the temperature compensation is applied accurately because of the accumulation of errors. The pH meter will thus have a temperature compensation dial that must be correctly set before the meter is calibrated.

Calibration will necessitate the use of two solutions of widely differing pH. Usually calibration is first carried out with a pH 7 buffer, followed by a pH 4 buffer (if the sample is expected to be acidic) or a pH 9 buffer (if the sample is expected to be basic). Once the pH electrode is calibrated it can simply be immersed in the solution to be measured and a rapid and accurate estimate of pH can be made.

15.4.3 The pH-stat

The pH-stat is a form of of automatic titrator that can be used to maintain a constant pH during a reaction that involves either the production or removal of H^+

from solution. The rate of reaction can thus be determined because a recorder draws a curve representing the volume of reagent added by the titrator, against time. A glass pH electrode, pH meter, recorder, controller, burette and magnetic stirrer are necessary; the burette can be an ordinary burette with a magnetic valve or, better still, a motor-driven burette syringe. A controller is necessary to break the current to the burette motor when the end-point is reached. The best sorts of titrator are arranged so that less and less reagent is added as the end-point is approached. This avoids the danger of overshoot. The kind of pH glass electrode used needs to be very accurate and stable for kinetic work.

The pH-stat has some limitations in that, for example, the solution in the reaction vessel has to be stirred constantly, and this may cause denaturation of proteins and introduce atmospheric components that may affect either the pH or the reaction proceeding in the vessel. Other problems are the existence of an unknown junction potential and the tendency of the liquid from the burette tip (under the surface of the solution in the reaction vessel) to leak. The latter effect can be counteracted in part by making the density of the burette liquid lower than that of the reaction mixture.

15.5 ION-SELECTIVE AND GAS-SENSING ELECTRODES

15.5.1 Principles

The glass pH electrode is really a kind of ion-selective electrode (ISE) that is sensitive to H^+. Similar potentiometric electrodes have been developed which are responsive to other ions, for example Na^+, NH_4^+, Cl^-, and NO_3^-. The active material within these devices may be glass, an insoluble organic salt or an ion-exchange material. Glass is the active material within the pH electrode, but modified aluminosilicate glasses can also be used to produce a variety of monovalent cation-responsive electrodes (e.g. Na^+, Li^+ and NH_4^+). Insoluble inorganic salts such as silver sulphide may be used to produce electrodes responsive to Cu^{2+}, Pb^{2+}, and Cd^{2+}, whereas lanthanum fluoride may be used to produce electrodes responsive to F^-. Ion-exchange materials may be dissolved in a water-immiscible solvent, then absorbed on to a Millipore filter to produce a liquid membrane or may be incorporated into PVC to give a solid membrane. The most frequently used electrodes of this type are those responsive to Ca^{2+}, K^+ and NO_3^-.

Ion-selective electrodes respond to the activity of a particular ion. However, if the instrument is calibrated with a standard of known concentration then, provided the ionic strengths of the solutions are similar, the concentration of the test solution will be recorded. To ensure that the ionic strengths are similar an ionic strength adjustor may be added. Ionic strength adjustors contain a high concentration of ions and sometimes pH adjustors and decomplexing agents or agents to remove species that interfere with the measurement. If, however, some of the ion is not free, but exists in a complex or an insoluble precipitate, then ion-selective electrodes will give a much lower reading than will a method that detects all of the ions present. Thus, atomic absorption spectrophotometry (Section 9.12) measures concentration and, for an ion such as calcium that readily forms calcium phosphate, it will give a significantly higher reading than that which would be obtained with an ISE. The ISE results, however, are significant because it is often the free ions that are responsible for clinical/biological effects.

An electrode may be ion selective, but not necessarily ion specific. Manufacturers' instructions will give information about this and will also mention chemicals that can poison the electrode. As with pH glass electrodes, ion-selective electrodes can be fouled by protein forming a surface film.

Many ions can be measured directly by the use of ISEs, or indirectly by titration. One form of indirect measurement is the use of the electrode as the end-point indicator of a titration. The electrode can be sensitive either to the species being determined or to the titrant ion. Titrations are ten times more accurate than direct measurement because the procedure requires accurate measurement of a *change* in potential rather than the absolute *value* of the potential. This is an important point because ISEs are not intrinsically very accurate. For example, the determination of the concentration of calcium ions is best carried out by titrating the solution with EDTA, which is a strong complexing agent for calcium, using a calcium ISE. Since the electrode responds to the logarithm of the concentration of calcium ions in solution, as the EDTA is added a sharp end-point is observed, giving a precision of 0.1% or better.

The response of ion-selective electrodes is (similar to the pH electrode) logarithmic, with 10-fold changes in ion activity giving equal increments on the meter scale. As with pH electrodes, the actual potential produced from an ISE is temperature dependent (Section 15.2.4), except at the isopotential point, which varies depending on the type of electrode. It is therefore important that temperature compensation is used. A reference electrode is also needed so that the varying potential of the ISE can be compared with the steady potential produced by a reference electrode (Section 15.2.4). If either K^+ or Cl^- are being measured, then a double junction reference electrode is needed to prevent contamination of the sample by the internal solution of the reference electrode.

Gas-sensing electrodes usually estimate the concentration of a gas by its interaction in a thin layer surrounding an ion-selective electrode, commonly a pH electrode. Carbon dioxide, ammonia, sulphur dioxide and nitrogen oxide can all be measured by their dissolution in a thin layer surrounding a pH electrode, and measuring the resultant pH of the layer.

The miniaturisation of ion-selective electrodes has been achieved by the modification of field effect transistors to respond to specific ions. Such ion-selective field effect transistors (ISFETs) are likely to have great clinical value. Multifunction ISFETs able to measure pH, Na^+, K^+, and Ca^{2+} are already available, and it is likely that such devices will become commonplace for the analysis of blood parameters either during surgery or in aftercare. ISFETs also make a suitable miniature transducer for incorporation into biosensors (Section 15.8).

15.5.2 **Applications**

ISEs are easy to use, economical, easily transportable, capable of continuous monitoring without hazard, and require little power. Because of these advantages, they

Table 15.3   Application of ion-selective and gas-sensing electrodes

Ions or gas detected	Application
Na^+	Analysis of sea water, serum, soil, skin
K^+	Analysis of serum (often combined with Na^+ electrode)
Ca^{2+}	Analysis of serum, beer
Cl^-	Quick test for cystic fibrosis; food analysis
NO_3^-	Analysis of drinking water, fertilisers, microbial growth
NH_3	Analysis of solutions produced by Kjeldahl digestion of proteins (Section 6.3.2)
CO_2	Analysis of blood
Nitrogen oxides	Air pollution monitoring

are widely used, as shown in Table 15.3. Miniaturised electrodes called spearhead microelectrodes have been manufactured and are used to determine the ion contents of single cells, muscle and nerves.

Unlike measurements by atomic absorption spectrophotometry, ISEs respond over a wide range of concentrations, do not destroy the test sample, and are rapid in use. However, for clinical use where high precision is required, and where the normal range of blood cations is so small. ISEs are less commonly used than is atomic absorption or emission spectrophotometry.

15.6 THE CLARK OXYGEN ELECTRODE

15.6.1 Principles

In 1956 L. C. Clark Jr described a compact oxygen probe that has been found to be suitable in a great variety of biological applications. The electrode consists of a platinum cathode and a silver anode, both immersed in the same solution of saturated potassium chloride, and separated from the test solution by an oxygen-permeable membrane. When a potential difference of -0.6 V is applied across the electrodes such that the platinum cathode is made negative with respect to the silver anode, electrons are generated at the anode and are then used to reduce oxygen at the cathode. The oxygen tension at the cathode then drops and this acts as a sink so that more oxygen diffuses towards it to make up the deficit. Since the rate of diffusion of oxygen through the membrane is the limiting step in the reduction process, the current produced by the electrode is proportional to the oxygen tension in the sample. These electrode reactions may be summarised as:

at silver anode $4Ag + 4Cl^- \rightarrow 4AgCl + 4e^-$
at platinum cathode $O_2 + 4H^+ + 4e^- \rightarrow 2H_2O$

There are many variants of the Clark electrode, the Rank electrode (produced by Rank Bros Ltd, Bottisham, Cambridge, England) being perhaps the most commonly used (Section 15.6.2). Probe-type Clark oxygen electrodes are also available

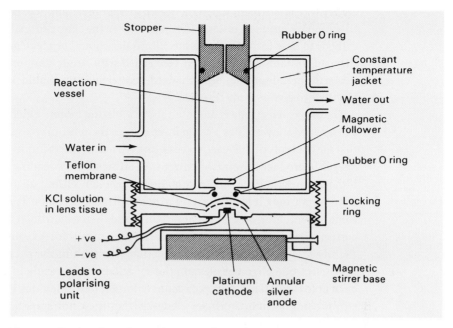

Fig. 15.8. Section through a Rank oxygen electrode.

and are of particular value in fermentation (so called pO_2 probes) and in environmental monitoring (Section 15.6.4). These probes generally need to be physically robust and in the case of fermenter probes need to be capable of withstanding the high temperatures necessary to sterilise the fermenter. Additionally, leaf disc electrodes capable of measuring gaseous oxygen concentrations have important biological applications (Section 15.6.5).

15.6.2 Operation of the Rank oxygen electrode (Clark electrode)

The Rank electrode (Fig. 15.8) allows a sample (usually about 3 cm³) to be placed in an upper reaction vessel, which is separated from the electrode chamber by an oxygen-permeable, ion-impermeable, membrane. Teflon (12 μm thick) is the usual choice of membrane, though Cellophane, polythene, silicone rubber and Cling Film have been used with varying degrees of success. Care must be taken to ensure that the membrane does not become contaminated, for example it should not be touched by hand; creasing and twisting can also cause problems. Thinner membranes give a quicker response but are more fragile. The membrane covers the electrodes and allows oxygen to diffuse towards them whilst preventing other reaction ingredients reaching the electrodes and poisoning them. The electrodes are maintained in electrical continuity with each other via the potassium chloride solution. A square piece of microscope lens tissue is immersed in the potassium chloride to keep the solution in place, to provide some physical support for the thin membrane above it, and to make it easier to exclude air bubbles from the electrode compartment when the Teflon membrane is applied. However, the lens tissue square needs a 1 to 2 mm diameter hole in the centre to enable the platinum cathode to pass through the tissue. Electrodes should be clean and bright, and if they are contaminated they can be cleaned with dilute ammonium hydroxide. When the membrane has been changed, several minutes should be allowed for the electrode to give a steady response.

The oxygen electrode is mounted above a stirring motor, which is able to rotate a magnetic follower ('flea') when inserted into the reaction vessel. It is important that the contents of the reaction vessel are stirred as the platinum cathode reduces oxygen to produce the electric current. An artificially low reading will be obtained if the magnetic stirrer should stop. However, when setting up an electrode (and after calibration), it is often useful to demonstrate the responsiveness of the electrode by switching off the magnetic stirrer and then restarting it after 10 to 15 s. A correctly set up electrode will show a reduction in current (oxygen tension) when the stirrer is switched off due to depletion of oxygen in the potassium chloride-filled electrode chamber. Resumption of stirring will result in a return of the current (oxygen tension in potassium chloride) to its previous level prior to the stirrer being switched off. An electrode that does not respond in this way is unlikely to be of any value – the electrode should be disassembled and a fresh membrane applied. Since both the solubility and the rate of diffusion of oxygen are affected by temperature, then some form of temperature control is necessary for best results. Water from a thermocirculator may therefore be pumped through the water jacket surrounding the reaction vessel. During experimentation care should be taken to ensure that all reagents reach the required temperature before experimentation commences; if ice-cold reagents are pipetted into the reaction vessel and insufficient time is allowed for the reagents to reach the required temperature, incorrect results will be obtained. Calibration should also be carried out at the same temperature as that of the experiment.

The Rank oxygen electrode has a polarising module that enables the correct polarising voltage between the electrodes to be set, and also allows adjustment of the current for the 0% and 100% oxygen values so that output can be made directly to a chart recorder. One hundred per cent oxygen can be set with a gain (sensitivity) control using distilled water or appropriate reaction buffer that has stood in air at the temperature of the reaction vessel for several hours. The concentration of dissolved oxygen at that temperature and pressure can be found from various scientific tables. Some useful values are presented in Table 15.4. However, a more accurate calibration of the instrument can be obtained by using mitochondrial fragments to oxidise a known amount of NADH, the amount of this having been accurately determined by spectrophotometric means (Section 7.4.2). Zero per cent oxygen can be achieved by adding a few crystals of sodium dithionite, which removes oxygen from solution, by using yeast respiring sugars, or by bubbling nitrogen gas through the solution in the reaction vessel. At 0% oxygen, there should be no current flowing, but small faults in insulation of the platinum electrode may mean that a small leakage current is present.

The calibration solutions are removed from the reaction vessel (usually by a

Table 15.4	Oxygen content of air-saturated water	
Temp. (°C)	Oxygen (μmol l^{-1})	Oxygen (p.p.m.)
15	305	9.8
20	276	8.8
25	253	8.1
30	230	7.5
35	219	7.0

suction pump or Pasteur pipette) and the experimental samples pipetted in. The stopper is then put in position, so that oxygen from the air cannot enter. Air bubbles should be excluded from the reaction vessel whilst experimentation is in progress. Addition of small amounts of solutions such as inhibitors is best achieved using a Hamilton syringe to inject the addition through the small hole in the stopper. Many chemicals are adsorbed onto the surface of the membrane and reaction vessel; hence, it is important that the apparatus is thoroughly cleaned after each experiment. In addition, care must be taken when organic solvents are present in the reaction vessel because they may give an incorrect response. If the electrode is going to be reused without the membrane being changed, then it is essential that water is left in the reaction vessel to prevent the membrane from drying.

15.6.3 Applications of the Rank oxygen electrode

Due to their ability to give a continuous trace, oxygen electrodes have largely replaced manometric techniques in the study of reactions involving oxygen uptake and evolution.

Mitochondrial studies

The study of respiratory control and the effects of inhibitors on mitochondrial respiration and the measurement of phosphorylation : oxidation (P : O) ratios are best done by means of the oxygen electrode (Section 15.1.2). As shown in Fig. 15.9, a slow rate of respiration occurs with a mitochondrial suspension until ADP is added, whereupon ATP production starts and an enhanced rate of electron transport occurs. This produces an increased rate of loss of oxygen (the terminal electron acceptor in the mitochondrial electron transport chain) from solution as it is reduced to water (Fig. 15.1); the slope of the oxygen electrode trace thus increases (rate X in Fig. 15.9). Once the mitochondria have used up all of the available ADP (i.e. they have phosphorylated it to ATP) they can no longer phosphorylate and this causes a reduction in electron transport and in the rate of oxygen reduction; the slope of the oxygen electrode trace thus decreases (rate Y in Fig. 15.9). The respiratory control ratio (shown as the ratio of rates X : Y in Fig. 15.9) is a measure of the extent of coupling of respiration and phosphorylation. The P : O ratio, the

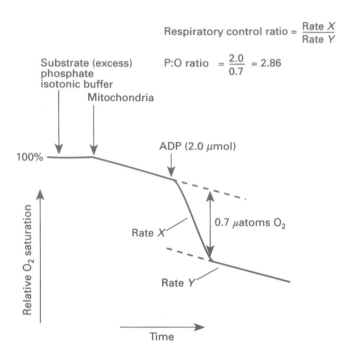

Fig. 15.9. A typical experimental trace of oxygen consumption for intact mitochondria obtained using an oxygen electrode.

number of molecules of ATP formed (P) per atom of oxygen consumed (O), can be calculated from the trace if the amount of ADP added and the amount of oxygen reduced (Fig. 15.9) are known. If an uncoupler such as 2,4-dinitrophenol (DNP) is added, the respiratory rate (electron transport rate) is not regulated by ADP.

The sites of action of electron transport inhibitors can also be determined using an oxygen electrode. A typical result is shown in Fig. 15.10. Inhibition of respiration by rotenone can be overcome by use of succinate as an electron donor (it donates electrons below the site of action of rotenone on the electron transport chain). Antimycin A can still, however, inhibit respiration, which can be restarted by tetramethylphenylenediamine (TMPD) and ascorbate. However, even this rate can be inhibited by cyanide. These results enable the sites of action of the inhibitors to be placed as in Fig. 15.1.

Microorganism and chloroplast studies

Microorganisms that use oxygen as the terminal electron acceptor of respiratory electron transport can be studied using an oxygen electrode, and the effects of electron transport inhibitors determined. Respiration of yeast and other microorganisms can be studied using different sugars. The most readily used sugars speed up the rate of respiration in starved yeast, which gives a steep slope on the oxygen electrode trace. The results also show that the sugar can enter the organism through the cell membrane. Oxygen evolution from cyanobacteria, algae, chloroplasts and

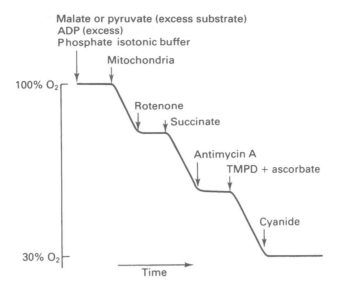

Fig. 15.10. Oxygen electrode trace showing the effect of inhibitors of electron transport and electron donors on mitochondrial respiration.

chloroplast fractions enriched in photosystem II can be studied utilising a suitably illuminated Clark oxygen electrode. The oxygen content of the suspension medium must normally be reduced below 100% by bubbling nitrogen through the system. This ensures that the oxygen produced stays in solution and is recorded.

Enzyme assays

Enzymes are readily studied using a Clark oxygen electrode, provided oxygen is involved in the reaction (Section 7.4.5). Glucose oxidase, D-amino acid oxidase and catalase are examples of enzymes whose properties can be studied in this way.

15.6.4 **Probe-type Clark electrodes**

Probe-type Clark oxygen electrodes have a variety of uses. These devices rely on the same principle of operation as the Rank electrodes; however, the cathode and retaining membrane are arranged at the end of a probe to enable insertion into a liquid phase. With such a configuration, however, problems may arise because of lack of stirring in the device.

Measurement of oxygen in bulk liquids

Oxygen concentrations are routinely monitored in fermentation processes, sewage and industrial waste treatment, and in inland, coastal and oceanic waters. This may involve a variant of the Clark electrode called flush top sensor, which has a large cathode that gives a high current (but a negligible current at zero oxygen concentration). The equipment is rugged and easily manufactured, but to eliminate stirring effects the fluid must flow over the electrode. Oxygen solubility is different in fresh and salt water; hence such instruments have an adjustment for the degree of salinity of the sample. With respect to fermentation, dissolved oxygen probes (usually called pO_2 probes) need to be physically robust and capable of withstanding the high temperatures necessary to sterilise the fermenter. A popular electrode of this type is the Ingold pO_2 electrode, which may be autoclaved *in situ* within the dermenter and may operate maintenance-free for five to ten sterilisation/fermentation cycles or, in terms of time, for six to eight weeks. After this time, the internal electrolyte needs to be replaced before further use of the probe.

Clinical uses

An early clinical use of oxygen electrodes was in monitoring heart–lung machines during open-heart surgery. Because of their speed of response and ease of operation, oxygen electrodes have been used for testing patients who are being treated with oxygen. Some oxygen electrodes have been specially modified to be small enough to be inserted into a blood vessel, but frequently this is avoided because of the danger of infection or of blood clot formation. Often it is considered preferable to remove small samples of blood from a warmed earlobe or a finger-tip and measure the oxygen content of the blood in a small Clark-type pO_2 electrode.

15.6.5 The leaf disc electrode

Whilst the Rank oxygen electrode is ideally suited to many applications requiring a measurement of oxygen in aqueous samples, a leaf disc electrode such as the Hansatech LD2 is of more use if gaseous oxygen measurements are required. Since the measurement of oxygen evolution is one of the easiest ways of following photosynthetic processes in leaves, this instrument has found many biological applications.

This device measures oxygen amperometrically using the same principle as the Rank electrode. However, instead of being a liquid-filled reaction vessel, the reaction chamber is designed to allow a leaf to be held in place and provided with saturating carbon dioxide (or bicarbonate as a source of carbon dioxide). Illumination is usually provided by an array of light-emitting diodes (which produce little heat), and the oxygen emitted by the leaf during photosynthesis can be measured.

Calibration is slightly more complex than with the Rank electrode. A zero oxygen signal can be produced by passing nitrogen through the reaction chamber of the electrode. Once this is stopped, and air is passed into the chamber, the signal corresponding to 21% oxygen (i.e. the oxygen content of air) can be determined. However, in the closed chamber the amount of oxygen is related both to the oxygen concentration and the chamber volume. Thus, if the chamber volume is only $1\,cm^3$ then it will contain $210\,mm^3$ oxygen. In practice, because the leaf disc itself may reduce the effective volume of the chamber (i.e. that available to the oxygen), calibration involves injecting known volumes of air into the chamber and measuring the voltage response to obtain the effective volume of the chamber and thence a precise calibration of the electrode.

The leaf disc electrode has been used extensively for the study of the relationship between photosynthetic oxygen evolution under saturating carbon dioxide and the intensity of illumination, enabling calculation of quantum yield. The inclusion of probes to measure emitted fluorescence from the leaf disc at the same time as measurements of oxygen evolution are being made has resulted in a device that provides a variety of information useful to the plant physiologist or biochemist. Applications of those devices are diverse, ranging from studies of micropropagated plants to those of plants suffering from atmospheric pollution.

Although the leaf disc electrode was clearly designed for whole-leaf studies, photosynthetic rates of microalgae have also been studied in such electrodes. However, this demands that the algal suspension is first filtered, and the filter paper (with a covering of algal cells) used in the same way as a leaf in the electrode.

15.7 ELECTROCHEMICAL DETECTORS FOR HPLC

15.7.1 Principles

Electrochemical detectors (ECDs) can be used in the same way as other detectors to detect and quantify analytes in the effluent from HPLC columns (Section 13.4.7). A variety of ECDs are commercially available, most working on the same principle of amperometric detection. Normally, when an ECD is used the potential is chosen so that it is sufficiently high to cause the reaction to occur. This information can be obtained from the polarographic wave of the compound determined, as described in Section 15.2.5. The selected potential is then maintained at that level and a trace of current against time is recorded. As the effluent containing the analyte comes off the end of the HPLC column it flows through the detector and a peak is obtained, which may look very similar to those produced by ultraviolet or fluorescence detectors.

Not all compounds in the liquid give rise to a current at a particular chosen potential. This means that if two analytes have not been separated by chromatographic means, and one alone gives a current at the selected potential, then the ECD will give only one peak and it will be easy to make quantitative measurements despite the presence of the second analyte. In order to make use of this feature, it is important to know the reaction potentials of the various analytes in the mixture being injected onto the column. Such information can be found in the literature or, with modern detectors, by examining the compound under the same analytical conditions but at varying electrode potentials.

ECDs require an electrolyte to be present in the mobile phase so that a current may flow. This means that reversed-phase and ion-exchange chromatography (Sections 13.6.3 and 13.7), which both use aqueous solvents, can be coupled to ECDs if sufficient electrolytes are present. When the mobile phase is an organic solvent or a mixed organic/aqueous solvent, it is usual to add some inert salt such as potassium nitrate, ammonium thiocyanate or tetrabutylammonium perchlorate

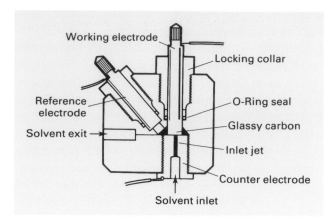

Fig. 15.11. A wall jet electrochemical detector.

(which dissolves in pure organic solvents) to act as the electrolyte. ECDs are very sensitive to flow changes; hence they can be used only with pulse-free pumps (Section 13.4.5).

Whilst there are a great many configurations of ECD, they all comprise the same essential elements. One of the commonest detector types is the wall jet electrochemical detector (Fig. 15.11), in which the electrodes are mounted in a fluorocarbon block. The liquid flows under pressure up to the electrodes and through a jet to impinge on the surface of the working electrode. A high current efficiency ensues and the working electrode stays clean as the products of the electrochemical reaction are washed off in the flow. As well as the glassy carbon working electrode, there are two other electrodes present. One is the counter or auxiliary electrode, which is stainless steel and forms part of the inlet. Any deviation from the preset voltage of the working electrode can be corrected by the auxiliary electrode. The Ag/AgCl reference electrode gives a steady potential, and is in contact with the liquid as it leaves the wall jet flow cell.

15.7.2 **Applications**

ECDs can detect chemicals either by oxidation, in which the working electrode is kept at a positive potential, or by reduction, in which the working electrode is negative. At very high positive or negative potentials the current becomes large owing to the solvent reacting; these are termed the anodic and cathodic limits of solvent.

Most biological applications of ECDs involve the oxidation of the molecule releasing electrons and giving rise to a current (see Fig. 15.12). Aromatic phenols, aromatic amines, heterocyclic nitrogen atoms and sulphur-containing molecules can all be detected by oxidation. Thus, drugs such as aspirin, paracetamol, morphine, nicotine and caffeine can be analysed by oxidation mode. ECD has become the method of choice for the analysis of catecholamines and neurotransmitters, and ions such as sulphide, cyanide and iodide (Table 15.5).

| **Table 15.5** | Common applications of HPLC-ECD |

Anions
e.g. SCN^-, SO_3^{2-}, NO_2^-

Aromatic alcohols
Phenols, e.g. thyroxine
Catechols, e.g. adrenaline, dopamine, L-dopa
Morphine

Aromatic amines
Anilines, e.g. benzidine
Sulphonamides

Indoles
Indole-3-derivatives, e.g. indole 3-acetate acid, melatonin
5-Hydroxyindoles, e.g. serotonin

Phenothiazines
e.g. promethazine

Purines
e.g. uric acid, xanthine, guanine

Thiols
e.g. cysteine, glutathione

Unsaturated alcohols
e.g. ascorbic acid

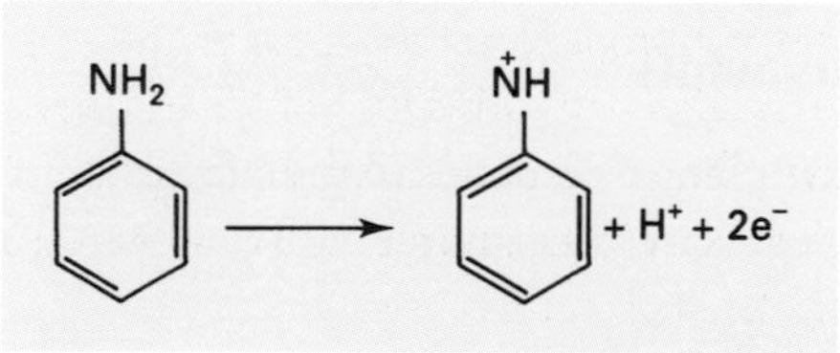

Fig. 15.12. Oxidative of an aromatic amine (aniline).

Oxygenating compounds such as quinones, peroxides and amides can be detected by reduction. This approach is also suitable for aromatic nitro and nitroso groups and halogen compounds. From an electrochemical point of view, however, reductions are more difficult to carry out than oxidations because it is often difficult to obtain ideal experimental conditions. Solvents must therefore be thoroughly degassed, as oxygen will undergo electrochemical reactions, and meticulous care has to be taken to ensure that oxygen cannot re-enter the solution.

Advanced modern ECDs also offer the possibility of operating in a pulse mode, which is well suited to the detection of compounds such as carbohydrates that lack reproducible response in the traditional DC mode of operation.

15.8 **BIOSENSORS**

15.8.1 **Introduction and principles**

A biosensor is an analytical device consisting of a biocatalyst (enzyme, cell or tissue) and a transducer, which can convert a biological or biochemical signal or response into a quantifiable electrical signal. The biocatalyst component of most biosensors is immobilised onto a membrane or within a gel, such that the biocatalyst is held in intimate contact with the transducer, and may be reused.

Biosensors are already of major commercial importance, and their significance is likely to increase as the technology develops. This is because they can be made to respond specifically and with high sensitivity to a wide range of molecules, including those of industrial, clinical and environmental importance. The best-developed systems are undoubtedly within the field of clinical medicine, where glucose responsive biosensors play a vital role in the measurement of blood glucose that is necessary for the management of diabetes.

Biosensors may be categorised as first-, second- or third-generation instruments according to the degree of intimacy between the biocatalyst and transducer. In first-generation instruments the two components (biocatalyst and transducer) may be easily separated and both may remain functional in the absence of the other. In second-generation instruments the two components interact in a more intimate fashion and removal of one of the two components affects the usual functioning of the other. In third-generation instruments the biochemistry and electrochemistry are even more closely linked and where the electrochemistry occurs at a semiconductor the term biochip may be applied to describe such instruments.

15.8.2 **First-generation instruments**

The biocatalyst within a biosensor responds to the substrates in solution by catalysing a reaction. Glucose oxidase, for example, will catalyse the reaction

glucose $+ O_2 \rightarrow$ gluconic acid $+ H_2O_2$

By the use of first-generation technology, the rate of this reaction can be measured as follows:

(i) The rate of consumption of the substrate O_2 can be measured by its reduction at a platinum cathode polarised at -0.6 V versus the standard calomel electrode (i.e. with a Clark oxygen electrode).
(ii) The rate of production of the product H_2O_2 can be measured by its oxidation at a platinum anode polarised at $+0.7$ V versus the standard calomel electrode.
(iii) The rate of production of the product gluconic acid can be measured using a pH electrode to measure the associated decrease in pH.

The actual rate of reaction determined by these transducers will depend on the rate of enzyme reaction, the rate of diffusion of substrate from the bulk phase into the enzyme layer, and the rate of diffusion of substrate within the enzyme layer. Which of these three rates is limiting depends on a number of factors of sensor design. However, although the theoretical kinetics are complex, in practice it is usual to find a rather linear relationship between rate of reaction and substrate concentration over a limited range of concentrations (see Section 15.8.5 for more detail). Within this linear range or useful range it is relatively easy to calibrate the device, requiring just two standard solutions of known glucose concentration. Once the device is calibrated, the measurement of the rate of reaction by the biosensor can be used to quantify the concentration of glucose in solution.

This principle of operation was suggested by L. C. Clark Jr and C. Lyons in 1962, which led to the development of the Yellow Springs Instruments Model 23 in 1974, linking the enzyme glucose oxidase to a probe to measure H_2O_2. Immobilisation of the enzyme on a laminated membrane that covers the probe tip results in rapid response times of 40s, and efficient reuse of the enzyme such that the membrane typically lasts two weeks before renewal becomes necessary. The analyser is able to measure the glucose content of whole blood, plasma or serum, requiring only a 25 mm^3 sample.

The YSI model 23 is now unavailable, having been replaced by the more advanced YSI 2300 STAT Glucose and L-Lacate Analyser. The YSI 2700 SELECT Biochemistry Analyser essentially uses the same technology but allows the glucose oxidase membrane to be replaced with membranes containing other enzymes, enabling the analysis of a wide variety of substances of biological interest (see Table 15.6).

A great variety of other devices may be used as transducers. Many of the devices listed in Table 15.7 have been considered in previous sections. A photomultiplier is a device that can be used to detect the light emitted from enzymes such as luciferase (obtained from *Photinus pyralis*, the firefly) (Section 7.4.2). The photomultiplier is a sensitive photoelectric cell in which electrons emitted from a photocathode are accelerated to a second electrode where several electrons are liberated from each photoelectron. This amplification even may be repeated several times to enable the detection of very low levels of light. A thermistor is a semiconductor device in which the resistance decreases as the temperature increases. It

Table 15.6 **Enzyme membranes available for analysers with H_2O_2 measuring probes as the transducer**

Analyte	Enzyme	Reaction
Alcohol	Alcohol oxidase	Ethanol + O_2 → H_2O_2 + acetaldehyde
D-Glucose	Glucose oxidase	β-D-Glucose + O_2 → H_2O_2 + gluconic acid
Lactose	Galactose oxidase	Lactate + O_2 → H_2O_2 + galactose dialdehyde derivative
L-Lactate	L-Lactate oxidase	L-Lactate + O_2 → H_2O_2 + pyruvate
Starch	{ Amyloglucosidase	Starch + H_2O → β-D-glucose
	{ Glucose oxidase	β-D-Glucose + O_2 → H_2O_2 + gluconic acid

Table 15.7 **Types of transducer used in biosensors**

Type	Principle of operation/cross-reference	Detectable species
Amperometric	Section 15.2.5	O_2, H_2O_2, I_2, NADH
Ion-selective electrode	Section 15.2.4	H^+, Na^+, Cl^-
Field effect transistor	Section 15.5.1	As ion-selective electrodes
Gas-sensing electrode	Section 15.5.1	CO_2, NH_3
Photomultiplier	Light emission	ATP (with luciferase present)
Thermistor	Heat of reaction	Universal

can be used to measure very small temperature changes that take place as reactions proceed. Linking such transducers to appropriate enzymes allows biosensors to be constructed that are responsive to a wide variety of biologically important molecules (Table 15.8).

15.8.3 Second-generation instruments

There are a number of ways in which the degree of intimacy between biocatalyst and transducer can be increased. In sensors utilising oxidoreductases, second-generation instruments can be constructed by designing an electrode surface that is capable of capturing electrons, which are usually transferred in the oxidation or reduction reaction.

A good example of a commercially available second-generation instrument is provided by the ExacTech blood glucose meter (Fig. 15.13). In this device the rate of oxidation of glucose is measured not by the rate of disappearance of substrate or appearance of product, but by the rate of electron flow from glucose to an electrode surface. The reactions that occur in this device may be summarised as follows:

$$\text{glucose} + \text{GO/FAD} \longrightarrow \text{gluconic acid} + \text{GO/FADH}_2$$
$$\quad\ \ \text{(red)} \qquad \text{(ox)} \qquad\qquad \text{(ox)} \qquad\qquad \text{(red)}$$

$$\text{GO/FADH}_2 + 2M^+ \longrightarrow \text{GO/FAD} + 2M + 2H^+$$
$$\text{(red)} \qquad \text{(ox)} \qquad\quad \text{(ox)} \quad \text{(red)}$$

At the electrode,

$$2M \longrightarrow 2M^+ + 2e^-$$
$$\text{(red)} \qquad \text{(ox)}$$

where GO/FAD represents the FAD redox centre of glucose oxidase in its oxidised form, GO/FADH_2 represents the FAD redox centre of glucose oxidase in its reduced form, and M is a mediator, which in the ExacTech blood glucose meter is ferrocene. The electrons donated to the electrode surface then go to form a current that is proportional to the rate of oxidation of glucose, and hence proportional to the glucose concentration in the blood.

Table 15.8 Examples of biosensors

Analyte	Biocatalyst	Transducer	Immobilisation	Stability	Response time
Alcohol	Alcohol oxidase	O_2	Glutaraldehyde	> 2 weeks	1–2 min
Arginine	*Streptococcus faecium*	NH_3	Physically entrapped	20 days	20 min
Cholesterol	*Nocardia erthyropolis*	O_2	Physically entrapped	4 weeks	35–70 s
D-Glucose	Glucose oxidase	O_2	Chemical	3 weeks	1 min
Glutamate	Glutamate decarboxylase	CO_2	Glutaraldehyde	1 week	10 min
NAD^+	NADase and *Escherichia coli*	NH_3	Dialysis membrane	1 week	5–10 min
Nitrate	*Azotobacter vinelandii*	NH_3	Physically entrapped	2 weeks	7–8 min
Penicillin	Penicillinase	H^+	Polyacrylamide	> 2 weeks	15–30 s
Urea	Urease	NH_4^+	Polyacrylamide	> 19 days	20–40 s

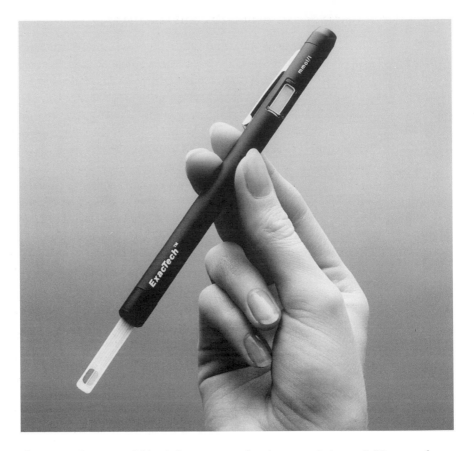

Fig. 15.13. The ExacTech blood glucose meter, showing test strip inserted. (Photograph courtesy of Medisense Britain Ltd.)

Devices of this type are far more suitable for miniaturisation. Whilst the ExacTech meter is itself only the size of a pen, devices using similar technology are now being produced that are so small they can be implanted under the skin to produce a blood glucose-measuring system *in situ*. Work is ongoing to link such sensors to appropriate logic circuits and an insulin reservoir to provide diabetic patients with exactly the insulin they need throughout the day.

15.8.4 Third-generation instruments

Such instruments are essentially at the research level, rather than under commercial development. They involve the most intimate interactions of the biocatalyst and transducer. A glucose biosensor operating on the principle of the ExacTech meter (Section 15.8.3) but in which the enzyme was directly reduced at the electrode surface (obviating the need for a mediator) would be an example of such an instrument.

15.8.5 **Sensor response: linearity and sensitivity**

At first sight, it might be expected that the response of an enzyme-based biosensor to variation in substrate concentration would follow the Michaelis–Menten equation (Section 7.3.2). Under such conditions a first-order response (in which the sensor signal varies linearly with the substrate concentration) would only be approximated at substrate concentrations well below the K_m of the enzyme employed within the sensor. However, in many cases, since the enzyme within the biosensor will be immobilised to a surface, and since the bulk phase substrate solution is generally unstirred, the activity of the enzyme will rapidly deplete the concentration of the substrate around the catalyst itself. With such a localised depletion of substrate, further substrate will diffuse towards the enzyme and the rate of such diffusion will be linearly related to the concentration of substrate in the bulk phase. Thus the sensor is considered to be under diffusion control rather than enzyme kinetic control, and under these conditions a linear sensor signal can be obtained over a wide range of analyte concentrations, up to and beyond the K_m of the enzyme involved. Indeed many biosensors employ a membrane over the enzyme, not only to retain the enzyme and to prevent interfering materials from being detected, but also to increase the degree of substrate diffusional limitation and ensure that the sensor has a linear response over an analyte range that is of relevance to the commercial application. An unfortunate consequence of operating biosensors under diffusional control is that the response time is usually increased.

In many cases, however, sensors are developed to measure very low analyte concentrations. Signal linearity is still an issue, but so is the sensitivity of the device. A variety of electrical signal enhancement techniques may be employed within biosensors, depending on the nature of the transducer component. Also of importance is biochemical signal enhancement, which involves the immobilisation of additional enzymes on the sensor surface. Consider the case of a sucrose biosensor employing two enzymes immobilised close to a hydrogen peroxide sensitive transducer:

$$\text{sucrose} + H_2O \xrightarrow{\text{invertase}} \alpha\text{-D-glucose} + \beta\text{-D-fructose}$$

$$\beta\text{-D-glucose} + O_2 \xrightarrow[\text{oxidase}]{\text{glucose}} \text{gluconic acid} + H_2O_2$$

Since glucose oxidase only accepts the β-anomer of glucose as substrate, the reaction is limited by the rate of spontaneous interconversion of the α- to β-anomer. However by co-immobilising a third enzyme – mutarotase – this interconversion takes place rapidly, and sensor sensitivity may be enhanced 10-fold. The term biochemical amplification is usually reserved for situations where signal enhancement results from cyclic reaction relationships, with one enzyme producing a product which is the substrate or cofactor for a second enzyme, and the second enzyme producing a product which is once again the substrate or cofactor for the first enzyme. Such amplification mechanisms have been used extensively to recycle products in sensors employing thermometric detection (measuring heat generation upon reaction) where signal enhancements of greater than 100-fold have been attained.

15.8.6 Cell-based biosensors

Whilst much of the pioneering work on biosensors has involved purified enzyme preparations as the biocatalyst component, there is a considerable amount of interest in the use of immobilised whole cells and tissues to produce biosensors. Such sensors are usually cheaper to produce than sensors depending on enzymes, as there is no requirement for complex biocatalyst isolation and purification procedures. However, cells contain many enzymes and care has to be taken to ensure selectivity of response (e.g. by adding specific enzyme or electron transport inhibitors to stop undesirable enzyme reactions). Cell-based electrodes may also have longer response times than do enzyme-based sensors, but a more serious problem is the time taken for cell-based sensors to return to baseline potential after use.

When cell-based sensors were first developed, they involved the use of harsh immobilisation procedures such as polyacrylamide gel entrapment, and the immobilised cells were not usually viable. However, the enzymes within them were still active. More recent immobilisation techniques have tended to use gentler physical methods such that cell viability is retained. The advantage of this is that such cells may be involved in converting substrate into product via a complex multienzyme pathway, without having to immobilise each of the enzymes and then provide them with expensive coenzymes.

A good example of a cell-based sensor is that using *Nocardia erythropolis* immobilised in polyacrylamide or agar on an oxygen electrode. The reaction carried out is:

$$\text{cholesterol} + O_2 \xrightarrow[\text{cholesterol oxidase}]{\textit{N. erythropolis}} \text{cholest-4-en-3-one} + H_2O_2$$

The oxygen electrode measures the rate of oxygen uptake and this can be related to the cholesterol content of the biological sample (probably plasma).

More than one cell type can be incorporated into the electrode, thereby increasing the number of potential applications. Thus the biochemical oxygen demand (BOD) of organic matter in waste-water can be detected by a mixed culture of bacteria obtained from soil, since a single microorganism would be unable to use all of the organic compounds likely to be found in the sample.

It is also possible to combine an enzyme preparation with a cell type. For example purified NADase (from *Neurospora crassa*) plus *Escherichia coli* (high in nicotinamide deaminase activity) will produce the following reaction:

$$NAD^+ + H_2O \xrightarrow{\text{NADase}} \text{nicotinamide} + \text{ADP-ribose}$$

$$\text{nicotinamide} + H_2O \xrightarrow{\textit{E. coli}} \text{nicotinic acid} + NH_3$$

The ammonia released can be detected by a gas-sensing electrode (transducer) to produce an NAD$^+$-sensitive biosensor.

Cell types other than microorganisms may also be utilised. A dopamine-sensitive biosensor has been produced by immobilising banana pulp in an oxygen electrode. Banana pulp is rich in the enzyme polyphenol oxidase, which causes the browning of the tissue. The pulp can thus be used as a rich source of the enzyme, and the enzyme found in banana has a high selectivity for the neuroactive agent dopamine.

15.8.7 Enzyme immunosensors

Several kinds of enzyme immunosensors have been developed. They combine the molecular recognition properties of antibodies with the high sensitivity of enzyme-based analytical methods. There are great similarities between such methods and ELISA techniques (Section 2.6).

Probably the commonest method of immunosensing depends on the competition between enzyme-labelled antigen and unlabelled antigen (the analyte) for an antibody immobilised on an appropriate transducer. For example, an immunosensor for IgG may be produced from an amperometric oxygen electrode that contains a membrane onto which has been bound an anti-IgG antibody. Free IgG is then labelled with the enzyme catalase and a known amount of this labelled IgG is mixed with a sample containing an unknown amount of unlabelled IgG. This mixture is then placed into the chamber of the oxygen electrode and the labelled and unlabelled IgG compete for the antibody on the membrane. After exposure to the mixture, the sensor is rinsed to remove any non-specifically associated IgG, and then filled with a hydrogen peroxide solution which acts as a substrate for the catalase. The more unlabelled IgG present, the lower the amount of labelled IgG (and therefore catalase) present, and the lower the rate of oxygen evolution. Finally, the biosensor is regenerated by rinsing with an appropriate acidic buffer such as glycine-HCl to dissociate the antigen from the antibody, though in many cases regeneration is deemed unnecessary and the antibody membrane is simply discarded after a single use.

Similar sensors using amperometric and potentiometric transducers have been developed for the analysis of for human chorionic gonadotrophin (a diagnostic hormone in pregnancy), α-fetoprotein (in the diagnosis of spina bifida), insulin, and a variety of other analytes.

Attempts to construct immunosensors with higher sensitivity have often involved optical transducers measuring fluorescence, bioluminescence or chemiluminescence. Such sensors have been able to measure a variety of analytes down to nmol l^{-1} concentrations.

In many cases the major practical problem in using such devices is the length of time taken for each assay. It may take several hours for the antigen–antibody coupling process to occur, and further time to rinse the unbound antigen. If such processes take place within the sensor itself, the device may be capable of measuring very few samples per day. A practical solution is to carry out the binding and rinsing processes as a separate stage, and only introduce the membrane to the transducer (together with the substrate) for the measurement of the enzyme activity. Such a mode of operation allows one sensor to be used with several antibody-linked membranes and measure numerous samples over a short time.

15.9 KEY TERMS

AC voltammetry	first-generation instruments	chain
activity	flush top sensor	pO_2 probes
anode	galvanic cell	polarographic wave
anodic limit of solvent	gas-sensing electrodes	potential difference
anodic stripping voltammetry	glass electrode	potentiometry
asymmetry potential	half-cells	probe-type
biosensor	half-wave potential	pulse voltammetry
calomel electrode	hanging mercury drop electrode	Q-cycle
Calvin cycle	Hansatech LD2	quantum yield
cathode	Ingold pO_2 electrode	Rank electrode
cathodic limit of solvent	ion-selective electrode	redox couple
cathodic stripping voltammetry	ion-selective field effect transistors	redox electrode
chemiosmotic theory	ionic strength adjustor	redox potential
Clark oxygen electrode	isopotential point	reference electrode
combination electrode	junction potential	respiratory control
cyclic phosphorylation	kinetic control	salt bridge
differential pulse voltammetry	leaf disc electrodes	second-generation instruments
diffusion control	limiting current	silver-silver chloride electrode
double junction reference electrode	liquid junction	spearhead microelectrodes
dropping mercury electrode	Nernst equation	standard hydrogen electrode
electrochemical cell	Nernst factor	stripping voltammetry
electrochemical detection	Nernst slope	third-generation instruments
electrode potential	non-cyclic electron transport	tightly coupled
electrolytic cell	non-cyclic phosphorylation	uncoupled
electrolytic half-cell	oxygen electrode	voltammetry
electron transport chain	pH electrode	wall jet electrochemical detector
endergonic	pH-stat	
field effect transistors	photosynthetic electron transport	

15.10 CALCULATIONS

Question 1   Calculate the pH of a solution containing $0.001\ mol\ H^+\ l^{-1}$.

Answer $pH = \log\left(\dfrac{1}{[H^+]}\right)$

so $pH = \log\left(\dfrac{1}{0.001}\right)$

$= \log(1000)$

$= 3$

Question 2   What is the H^+ concentration at pH 7.8 ?

Answer $pH = \log\left(\dfrac{1}{[H^+]}\right)$

$$7.8 = \log\left(\frac{1}{[H^+]}\right)$$

$$\text{Antilog } 7.8 = \frac{1}{[H^+]}$$

$$6.31 \times 10^7 = \frac{1}{[H^+]}$$

$$[H^+] = \frac{1}{6.3 \times 10^7}$$

$$= 1.58 \times 10^{-8} \text{ mol } 1^{-1}$$

Question 3 Using the data presented in Table 15.1 calculate the standard redox potential change ($\Delta E_o'$) and the standard free energy change ($\Delta G^{0\prime}$) for the following reactions at pH 7.0.

cyt b (Fe^{2+}) + cyt c (Fe^{3+}) → cyt b (Fe^{3+}) + cyt c (Fe^{2+})
(reduced)   (oxidised)   (oxidised)   (reduced)

Answer This may be written as two separate half-reactions:

cyt b (Fe^{2+}) → cyt (Fe^{3+}) b + e$^-$
$E_o' = -0.08$ V (value in Table 15.1 is $+0.08$ V for reaction in opposite direction)

cyt c (Fe^{3+}) + e$^-$ → cyt c (Fe^{2+})
$E_o' = {}^+0.25$ V (from Table 15.1)

Overall $\Delta E_o'$ is sum of two half-reactions
$= -0.08 + 0.25 = +0.17$ V

$$\Delta G^{0\prime} = -nF\Delta E_o'$$
$$= -1 \times 9.648 \times 10^4 \,(\text{J V}^{-1}\text{mol}^{-1}) \times 0.17 \,(\text{V})$$
$$= -16402 \text{ J mol}^{-1}$$
$$= -16.4 \text{ kJ mol}^{-1}$$

Question 4 In carrying out some studies on mitochondrial electron transport we have an oxygen electrode containing 0.1 ml mitochondrial suspension, 0.1 ml succinate solution and 2.7 ml buffer. The oxygen uptake rate (respiration rate) is negligible. We then add 0.1 ml of a 10 mM ADP solution and obtain a rapid rate for a few seconds before the rate again becomes negligible. During this brief time the oxygen concentration within the electrode chamber falls from 200 to 110 μmol 1^{-1}. Calculate the P:O ratio for the mitochondrial suspension and comment on the results.

Answer First we need to calculate the *amount* of ADP added.

10 mM ADP $= 10$ mmol 1^{-1}
$= 10 \,\mu\text{mol ml}^{-1}$
$= 1.0 \,\mu\text{mol in the 0.1 ml we add to the system}$

Next we calculate the *amount* of oxygen consumed.

Change in oxygen concentration $= 200 - 110 \,\mu\text{mol } 1^{-1} = 90 \,\mu\text{mol } 1^{-1}$
90 μmol $1^{-1} = 0.09 \,\mu\text{mol ml}^{-1}$

Since the volume within the electrode chamber is 3 ml, the amount of oxygen consumed is $3 \times 0.09 = 0.27$ μmol.

Since each molecule of oxygen has two atoms, 0.27 μmol O_2 = 0.54 μmol O atoms.

$$\text{Therefore P : O ratio} = \frac{\text{phosphorylation (μmol ADP} \rightarrow \text{ATP)}}{\text{oxidation (μmol O atoms consumed)}}$$

$$= \frac{1.0}{0.54} = 1.85$$

A P : O ratio of 2 is expected for succinate, since it feeds electrons into the electron transport chain as shown in Fig. 15.1. Our result of 1.85 is thus in good agreement with expectations.

15.11 SUGGESTIONS FOR FURTHER READING

ANON. (1976). Classification and nomenclature of electroanalytical techniques (rules approved 1975). *Pure and Applied Chemistry* **45**(2), 81–97. (A fairly well accepted scheme for classifying electrochemical techniques.)

CASS, A. E. G. (ed.). (1990). *Biosensors: A Practical Approach.* IRL Press, Oxford (Useful and detailed description of practical aspects of biosensor design and operation.)

DZWOLAK, W., KONCKI, R. AND GLAB, S. (1996). Immunosensors in analytical chemistry. *Chemia Analityczna* **41**, 715–36. (A very readable text describing the principles and applications of electrochemical, piezoelectrical and optical immunosensors.)

HALL, E. A. H. (1990). *Biosensors.* Open University Press, Milton Keynes. (An excellent introductory text to biosensor technology.)

NICHOLLS, D. G. and FERGUSON, S. J. (1992). *Bioenergetics* **2**. Academic Press, London. (Excellent coverage of membrane bioenergetics and the chemiosmotic theory.)

PARVEZ, H., BASTART-MALSOT, M., PARVEZ, S., NAGATSU, T. and CARPENTIER, G. (eds.) (1987). *Progress in HPLC*, vol. 2. VNU Science Press, Utrecht. (An advanced text detailing the diverse applications of HPLC-ECD; containing a very readable introductory chapter on the subject.)

RILEY, T. and TOMLINSON, C. (1987). *Principles of Electroanalytical Methods.* Wiley, Chichester. (An open learning text covering the basic theory and practical aspects of individual techniques.)

WALKER, D. (1988). *The Use of the Oxygen Electrode and Fluorescence Probes in Simple Measurements of Photosynthesis*, 2nd edn. Hansatech Instruments Ltd, King's Lynn, Norfolk. (Contains much information on the Hansatech leaf disc electrode, together with useful coverage of Rank type electrodes and their applications.)

Index